**Swanton's
Cardiology**

To Lindsay and Robin: with all our thanks for their patience, and for keeping our tummies full when our minds were empty.

Swanton's Cardiology

A concise guide to clinical practice

R.H. Swanton MA, MD, FRCP, FESC, FACC

Consultant Cardiologist
The Heart Hospital
University College London Hospitals
Westmoreland Street
London W1G 8PH

S. Banerjee MBChB, MD, MRCP

Consultant Cardiologist
East Surrey Hospital
Surrey and Sussex NHS Healthcare Trust
Canada Avenue, Redhill
Surrey RH1 5RH

The Heart Hospital
University College London Hospitals
Westmoreland Street
London W1G 8PH

SIXTH EDITION

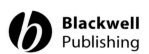

Blackwell
Publishing

First published 1984	Italian edition 1991	Polish edition 1998
Italian edition 1986	German edition 1994	Fifth edition 2003
Spanish edition 1986	Third edition 1994	Italian edition 2006
Second edition 1989	Polish edition 1994	Russian edition 2008
Yugoslav edition 1990	Fourth edition 1998	Sixth edition 2008

1 2008

Library of Congress Cataloging-in-Publication Data

Swanton, R. H.
    Swanton's cardiology : a concise guide to clinical practice/ by R.H. Swanton, S. Banerjee. – 6th ed.
       p. ; cm.
    Rev. ed. of: Cardiology / R.H. Swanton. 5th ed. c2003.
    Includes bibliographical references and index.
    ISBN 978-1-4051-7819-8
1. Cardiology–Handbooks, manuals, etc.   I. Banerjee, S. (Shrilla)   II. Swanton, R.H. Cardiology.   III. Title.
    [DNLM: 1. Heart Diseases–Handbooks.   WG 39 S972c 2008]

    RC682.S837 2008
    616.1′2–dc22
                                        2007037459

ISBN: 978-1-4051-7819-8

A catalogue record for this title is available from the British Library

Set in 9.5/12 pt Palatino by SNP Best-set Typesetter Ltd., Hong Kong
Printed and bound in Singapore by Markono Print Media Pte Ltd

Commissioning Editor: Gina Almond
Development Editor: Victoria Pittman
Editorial Assistant: Jamie Hartmann-Boyce
Production Controller: Debbie Wyer

For further information on Blackwell Publishing, visit our website:
http://www.blackwellpublishing.com

The publisher's policy is to use permanent paper from mills that operate a sustainable forestry policy, and which has been manufactured from pulp processed using acid-free and elementary chlorine-free practices. Furthermore, the publisher ensures that the text paper and cover board used have met acceptable environmental accreditation standards.

Contents

Preface

I am delighted and very grateful that Dr Shrilla Banerjee has agreed to become a co-author of the sixth edition of this cardiology handbook. Her enthusiasm, knowledge and ideas have proved invaluable.

It is hoped that the book will be of practical help to doctors, nurses and cardiac scientific officers confronted by typical management problems in the cardiac patient. As a practical guide it is necessarily dogmatic and much information is given in list format or in tables, especially in the sections dealing with drug therapy.

Some subjects in cardiology are often not well covered in clinical training and it is hoped that some sections will help fill any gaps in doctors' or nurses' clinical course, e.g. sections on congenital heart disease, pacing and cardiac investigations. In addition, scientific officers and technical staff should find that the clinical side of cardiology covered here complements their technical training. And we hope that anaesthetists and intensive care unit physicians will find the book of value.

Since the publication of the fifth edition 4 years ago there have been enormous advances in many aspects of cardiology and we have tried to highlight these. Many sections have been extensively revised, and in particular those on the cardiomyopathies, coronary disease, heart failure, echocardiography and the heart in systemic disease. For ease of access the book now has 17 chapters. The rhythm section has been split into two: bradycardias, pacing, implantable cardioverter defibrillators and pacing for heart failure are dealt with in one chapter, and tachycardias and ablation in another. There is a new, badly needed chapter on pregnancy in patients with heart disease. A summary of the *At a Glance Guide* for driving in the UK for patients with heart disease is now included in appendix 6 by kind agreement of the DVLA. It should be remembered that the full guidance is updated on their website every 6 months.

In response to suggestions we are now able to include many more figures and illustrations and we hope that these will increase the appeal of the book without significantly increasing its bulk or expense. With regret we have still decided not to have a separate section on nuclear cardiology but have included its use in diagnosis where relevant.

Practical procedures such as cardiac catheterization cannot be learnt from a book. However, interpretation of catheter laboratory data is discussed and it is hoped that the book will be helpful to the doctor learning invasive cardiology or the scientific officer monitoring it. Echocardiography is very much a 'hands-on' technique and cannot be covered in depth in a book of this size. However, this section has been considerably expanded with many more illustrations.

Of all the specialities in medicine cardiology is right at the front in evidence-based practice. There are literally hundreds of trials to guide us in our day-to-day management decisions. Most of the trials have acronyms, which have now become part of the language of cardiology. We have referred to the most important trials in the text with the reference section expanded in Appendix 4. To save space we have used abbreviations liberally – but only those that are in common use in everyday cardiology practice. The list of abbreviations in Appendix 7 should cover these.

Drug names are changing. We have switched where appropriate from the British Approved Name (BAN) to the Recommended Non-proprietary Name (rINN) for medicinal substances. Adrenaline and noradrenaline remain unchanged, however.

Finally, we are very grateful to colleagues who have suggested improvements or the inclusion of new material and would encourage the reader to contact us with suggestions of subjects that are not covered at all or dealt with inadequately.

R.H. Swanton

Acknowledgements

The work of a large number of authors has contributed to the body of knowledge in this book and it would be impossible to thank them individually or provide detailed references to their work. In the list of trials, references and further reading we have been able to incorporate their work and our thanks to them all. We are very grateful to many cardiology colleagues, registrars and cardiac technical staff for their enthusiastic help in providing so many ECG pressure tracings and echocardiograms.

Our thanks also to Ms Kalaiarasi Janagarajan, Mr Justin O'Leary, Ms Vivienne Palmer-White and Dr Stavros Kounas and all our colleagues who have made suggestions for new material or alterations.

We are indebted to Dr Richard Sutton and Medtronic Ltd for permission to modify their pacing code diagrams, to Dr Simon Horner for his diagram on VT provocation, to Dr PE Gower for permission to include the nomogram for body surface area, to Dr Diana Holdright for the illustrations on septal ablation pressure measurement, to Dr James Moon and Dr Sanjay Prasad for their MRI pictures and to Dr Denis Pellerin for help with the echocardiography section. Thanks to Fiona England for her patient acquisition of angiograms and CT scans. Our thanks to Medtronic for permission to include the coronary stent diagram and to Boston Scientific Ltd for the picture of the rotablator and the Taxus stent. Our thanks to Cheryl Friedland for her invaluable and patient tuition on ICDs and to Rhian Davies for her tireless help with drug queries. A particular thanks to Dr Ewa Dzielicka from Krakow who has been of great help in bringing several sections up to date.

Finally, and last but not least, we would like to thank Gina Almond and Vicky Pittman from Wiley-Blackwell who have been towers of strength and encouragement. We are grateful to them for their ideas, their patience and their gentle but regular persistence without which we would never have got this far.

R.H. Swanton
S. Banerjee

Special Thanks

A big thank you to Lindsay and Tracy Harvey for their work in preparing the early manuscript and to Jo Goddard for her tireless help sorting out numerous emailed illustrations and references.

RHS

My thanks to my parents, Robin and family, and special thanks to my son, Arun Lalit George – for being as inspiring as his namesakes.

SB

1 Cardiac Symptoms and Physical Signs

1.1 Common Cardiac Symptoms

Angina

Typical angina presents as a chest tightness or heaviness brought on by effort and relieved by rest. The sensation starts in the retrosternal region and radiates across the chest. Frequently it is associated with a leaden feeling in the arms. Occasionally it may present in more unusual sites, e.g. pain in the jaw or teeth on effort, without pain in the chest. It may be confused with oesophageal pain, or may present as epigastric or even hypochondrial pain. The most important feature is its relationship to effort. Unilateral chest pain (submammary) is not usually cardiac pain, which is generally symmetrical in distribution.

Angina is typically exacerbated by heavy meals, cold weather (just breathing in cold air is enough) and emotional disturbances. Arguments with colleagues or family and watching exciting television are typical precipitating factors.

Stable Angina

This is angina induced by effort and relieved by rest. It does not increase in frequency or severity, and is predictable in nature. It is associated with ST-segment depression on ECG.

Decubitus Angina

This is angina induced by lying down at night or during sleep. It may be caused by an increase in LVEDV (and hence wall stress) on lying flat, associated with dreaming or getting between cold sheets. Coronary spasm may occur in REM sleep. It may respond to a diuretic, calcium antagonist or nitrate taken in the evening.

Swanton's Cardiology, sixth edition. By R. H. Swanton and S. Banerjee. Published 2008 Blackwell Publishing. ISBN 978-1-4051-7819-8.

Unstable (Crescendo) Angina

This is angina of increasing frequency and severity. Not only is it induced by effort but it comes on unpredictably at rest. It may progress to myocardial infarction.

Variant Angina (Prinzmetal's Angina)

This is angina occurring unpredictably at rest associated with transient ST-segment elevation on the ECG. It is not common, and is associated with coronary spasm often in the presence of additional arteriosclerotic lesions.

Other Types of Retrosternal Pain

• Pericardial pain: described in Section 10.1. It is usually retrosternal or epigastric, lasts much longer than angina and is often stabbing in quality. It is related to respiration and posture (relieved by sitting forward). Diaphragmatic pericardial pain may be referred to the left shoulder.
• Aortic pain (Section 14.2): acute dissection produces a sudden tearing intense pain, retrosternally radiating to the back. Its radiation depends on the vessels involved. Aortic aneurysms produce chronic pain especially if rib or vertebral column erosion occurs.
• Non-cardiac pain: may be oesophageal or mediastinal with similar distribution to cardiac pain but not provoked by effort. Oesophageal pain may be provoked by ergonovine, making it a useless test for coronary spasm. Oesophageal spasm causes intense central chest pain, which may be relieved by drinking cold water. Chest wall pain is usually unilateral. Stomach and gallbladder pain may be epigastric and lower sternal, and be confused with cardiac pain.

Dyspnoea

This is an abnormal sensation of breathlessness on effort or at rest. With increasing disability, orthopnoea and PND occur. Pulmonary oedema is not the only cause of waking breathless at night: it may occur in non-cardiac asthma. A dry nocturnal cough is often a sign of impending PND. With acute pulmonary oedema, pink frothy sputum and streaky haemoptysis occur. With poor LV function Cheyne–Stokes ventilation makes the patient feel dyspnoeic in the fast cycle phase.

Effort tolerance is graded by New York Heart Association (NYHA) criteria as follows.

Class I

Patients with cardiac disease but no resulting limitations of physical activity. Ordinary physical activity does not cause undue fatigue, palpitation or angina.

Class II

Patients with cardiac disease resulting in slight limitation of physical activity. They are comfortable at rest. Ordinary physical activity results in fatigue, palpitation, dyspnoea or angina (e.g. walking up two flights of stairs, carrying shopping basket, making beds). By limiting physical activity, patients can still lead a normal social life.

Class III

Patients with cardiac disease resulting in marked limitation of physical activity. They are comfortable at rest, but even mild physical activity causes fatigue, palpitation, dyspnoea or angina (e.g. walking slowly on the flat). Patients cannot do any shopping or housework.

Class IV

Patients with cardiac disease who are unable to do any physical activity without symptoms. Angina or heart failure may be present at rest. They are virtually confined to bed or a chair and are totally incapacitated.

Syncope

Syncope may be caused by several conditions:
- *Vasovagal* (vasomotor, simple faint): the most common cause. Sudden dilatation of venous capacitance vessels associated with vagally induced bradycardia. Induced by pain, fear and emotion.
- *Postural hypotension*: this is usually drug-induced (by vasodilators). May occur in true salt depletion (by diuretics) or hypovolaemia.
- *Carotid sinus syncope*: a rare condition with hypersensitive carotid sinus stimulation (e.g. by tight collars) inducing severe bradycardia (see Section 7.6).
- *Cardiac dysrhythmias*: most common causes are sinus arrest, complete AV block and ventricular tachycardia; 24-hour ECG monitoring is necessary.
- *Obstructing lesions*: aortic or pulmonary stenosis, left atrial myxoma or ball-valve thrombus, HCM, massive pulmonary embolism. Effort syncope is commonly secondary to aortic valve or subvalve stenosis in adults and Fallot's tetralogy in children.
- *Cerebral causes*: sudden hypoxia, transient cerebral arterial obstruction, spasm or embolism.
- *Cough syncope*: this may result from temporarily obstructed cerebral venous return. Profound bradycardia can be the cause mediated via the vagus.
- *Micturition syncope*: this often occurs at night, and sometimes in men with prostatic symptoms. It may result partly from vagal overactivity and partly from postural hypotension.

The most common differential diagnosis needed is sudden syncope in an adult with no apparent cause. Stokes–Adams attacks and epilepsy are the main contenders (Table 1.1).

A prolonged Stokes–Adams episode may produce an epileptiform attack from cerebral hypoxia. It is not always possible to distinguish the two clinically.

Table 1.1 Differentiation of Stokes-Adams attacks from epilepsy

Stokes-Adams attacks	Epilepsy
No aura or warning	Aura often present
Transient unconsciousness (often only a few seconds)	More prolonged unconsciousness
Very pale during attack	Tonic–clonic phases
Rapid recovery	Prolonged recovery; very drowsy
Hot flush on recovery	Absent

Cyanosis

Central cyanosis should be detectable when arterial saturation is <85% and when there is >5 g reduced haemoglobin present. It is more difficult to detect if the patient is also anaemic. Cardiac cyanosis may be caused by poor pulmonary blood flow (e.g. pulmonary atresia), right-to-left shunting (e.g. Fallot's tetralogy) or common mixing situations with high pulmonary blood flow (e.g. TAPVD).

Cyanosis from pulmonary causes should be improved by increasing the Fio_2. The child breathes 100% O_2 for 5 min. The arterial Po_2 should increase to >21 kPa (160 mmHg) if the cyanosis is pulmonary in origin. Cyanosis caused by right-to-left shunting should change little in response to 100% O_2 and certainly <21 kPa (160 mmHg).

Peripheral cyanosis in the absence of central cyanosis may be the result of peripheral vasoconstriction, poor cardiac output or peripheral sludging of red cells (e.g. polycythaemia).

Embolism

Both systemic and pulmonary embolisms are common in cardiac disease. Predisposing factors in cardiology are shown in Table 1.2.

Table 1.2 Predisposing factors to pulmonary and systemic emboli

Pulmonary emboli	Systemic emboli	Either or both
Prolonged bed rest	Atrial fibrillation	Myocardial infarction
High venous pressure	Aortic stenosis (calcium)	Dilated cardiomyopathy
Central lines	Mitral stenosis AF > SR	CCF
Femoral vein catheterization	Infective endocarditis	Polycythaemia
Pelvic disease (tumour,	LA myxoma	Diuretics
inflammation)	HCM	Procoagulable state
Tricuspid endocarditis	Prosthetic aortic or mitral	Eosinophilic heart disease
Deep vein thrombosis	valves	
	Floppy mitral valve	
	Closed mitral valvotomy or	
	valvuloplasty	
	Mitral annulus calcification	

Oedema

Factors important in cardiac disease are: elevated venous pressure (CCF peri-cardial constriction), increased extracellular volume (salt and water reten-tion), secondary hyperaldosteronism, hypoalbuminaemia (liver congestion, anorexia and poor diet), venous disease and secondary renal failure.

Acute oedema and ascites may develop in pericardial constriction. Protein-losing enteropathy can occur, with a prolonged high venous pressure exacer-bating the oedema.

Other Symptoms

These are discussed in the relevant chapter:
- Palpitation: principles of paroxysmal tachycardia diagnosis – see Section 8.1
- Haemoptysis: mitral stenosis – see Section 3.2
- Cyanotic attack: catheter complications – see Section 16.3.

1.2 Physical Examination

Hands

It is important to check for the following:
- Dilated hand veins with CO_2 retention
- Temperature (?cool periphery with poor flows, hyperdynamic circulation)
- Peripheral cyanosis
- Clubbing: cyanotic congenital heart disease, infective endocarditis
- Capillary pulsation, aortic regurgitation, PDA
- Osler's nodes, Janeway's lesions, splinter haemorrhages (Figure 1.1), infec-tive endocarditis
- Nail-fold telangiectases: collagen vascular disease
- Arachnodactyly: Marfan syndrome (see Figure 14.12)

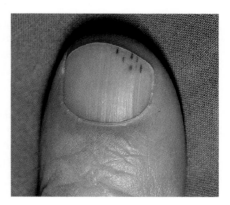

Figure 1.1 Splinter haemorrhages in a man with prosthetic valve endocarditis.

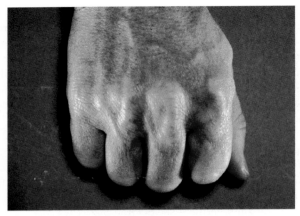

Figure 1.2 Hypercholesterolaemia: knuckle xanthomas.

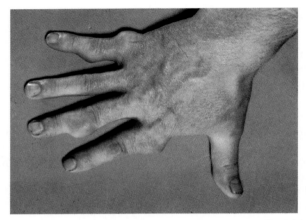

Figure 1.3 Familial hypercholesterolaemia: large xanthomas; serum cholesterol 14.1 mmol/l.

- Polydactyly, syndactyly, triphalangeal thumbs: ASD
- Tendon xanthomas: hypercholesterolaemia (Figures 1.2–1.5)
- Peripheral digital infarcts: hyperviscosity, cryoglobulinaemia (Figure 1.6).

Facial and General Appearance
- Down syndrome (AV canal)
- Elf-like facies (supravalvar aortic stenosis)
- Turner syndrome (coarctation, AS)
- Moon-like plump facies (pulmonary stenosis)
- Noonan syndrome (pulmonary stenosis, peripheral pulmonary artery stenosis)
- Mitral facies with pulmonary hypertension

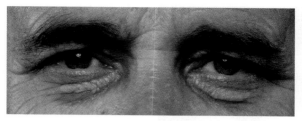

Figure 1.4 Xanthelasma.

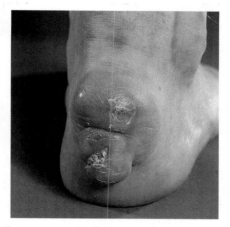

Figure 1.5 Tendon xanthomas: severe familial hypercholesterolaemia with massive cholesterol deposition in Achilles' tendon.

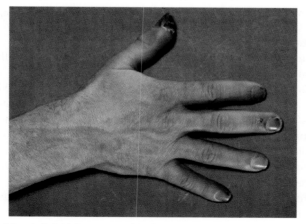

Figure 1.6 Peripheral digital infarcts: cryoglobulinaemia.

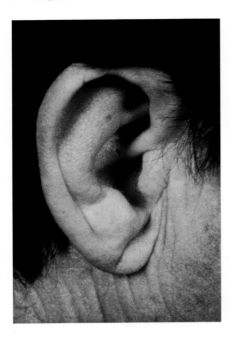

Figure 1.7 Ear-lobe crease: in a young patient may be a sign of coronary disease.

- Central cyanosis
- Differential cyanosis in PDA + pulmonary hypertension or interrupted aortic arch
- Xanthelasma (see Figure 1.4)
- Ear-lobe crease in the young patient (Figure 1.7) association with coronary disease
- Teeth: must be checked as part of general CVS examination
- Dyspnoea at rest. ?Accessory muscles of respiration.

The Jugular Venous Pulse

Waveform examples are shown in Figure 1.8. The JVP should fall on inspiration. Inspiratory filling of the neck veins occurs in pericardial constriction (Kussmaul's sign). The waves produced are as follows:

- 'a' wave: atrial systole. It occurs just before the carotid pulse and is lost in AF. Large 'a' waves indicate a raised RVEDP (e.g. PS, PHT). Cannon 'a' waves occur in: junctional tachycardia, complete AV block, ventricular ectopics (atrial systole against a closed tricuspid valve).
- 'c' wave: not visible with the naked eye. Effect of tricuspid valve closure on atrial pressure.
- 'x' descent: fall in atrial pressure during ventricular systole caused by downward movement of the base of the heart.

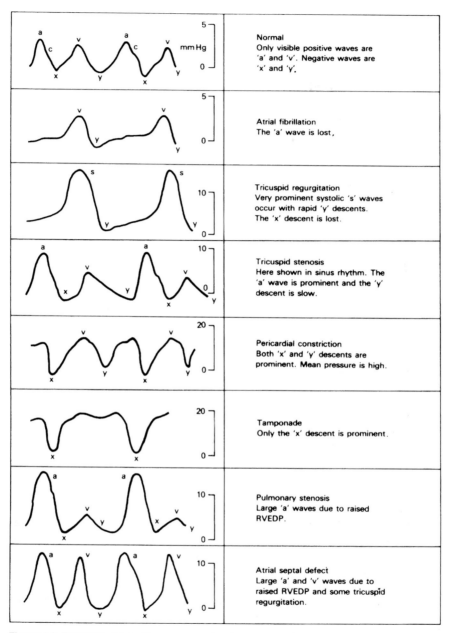

Figure 1.8 Examples of waveforms seen on jugular venous pulse.

- 'v' wave: atrial filling against a closed tricuspid valve.
- 'y' descent: diastolic collapse after opening of the tricuspid valve. Slow 'y' descent in patients with tricuspid stenosis or mechanical tricuspid valve replacements.
- 's' wave occurs in tricuspid regurgitation. Fusion of 'x' descent and 'v' wave into a large systolic pulsation can occur with rapid 'y' descent.

The normal range of JVP is −7 to +3 mmHg. The patient sits at 45° and the sternal angle is used as a reference point.

Distinction between the JVP and the Carotid Pulse

Distinction of the JVP from the carotid pulse involves the following five features:
1 Timing
2 The ability to compress the JVP
3 The ability to obliterate the JVP
4 The demonstration of hepatojugular reflux, the alteration of the JVP with position
5 The site of the pulsation itself.

Although transient pressure on the liver is classically used to augment the JVP, pressure anywhere on the abdomen will have the same effect. The congested liver is often tender and is pulsatile in severe tricuspid regurgitation.

Transient obliteration of the JVP to confirm that a pulse is venous is not easy. The internal jugular vein is wide at the base of the neck and using the point of a finger to obliterate it is often unsuccessful and thereby misleading. Use the whole of the side of the index finger pushed firmly and briefly against the side of the base of the neck. In addition the fact that a pulse is palpable does not necessarily mean that it is arterial. Strong venous pulsations are also palpable.

Using the external jugular vein to decide on the height of the JVP is not always reliable. In some patients there may be a slight positional kink between the junction of the external jugular vein with the subclavian vein. The external jugular vein may thus appear full when the JVP (taken from the internal jugular vein) is in fact normal.

The Carotid Pulse

Waveform examples are shown in Figure 1.9. There are three components to the carotid pulse: percussion wave, tidal wave and dicrotic notch.

Percussion Wave

This is a shock wave transmitted up the elastic walls of the arteries.

Tidal Wave

This is reflection of the percussion wave with a forward-moving column of blood. It follows the percussion wave and is not usually palpable separately.

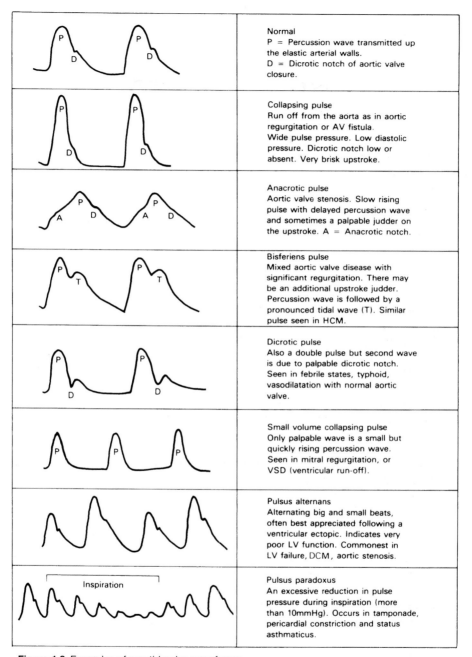

Figure 1.9 Examples of carotid pulse waveforms.

Dicrotic Notch

This is timed with aortic valve closure.

All the pulses are felt, radials and femorals simultaneously (coarctation). Any pulse may disappear with dissection of the aorta. Right arm and carotid pulses are stronger than left in supravalvar aortic stenosis (see Section 3.4).

An absent radial pulse may occur:

- after a peripheral embolus
- after a Blalock shunt on that side
- after brachial artery catheterization with poor technique on that side
- after a radial artery line for pressure monitoring, or after the use of the radial artery for cardiac catheterization
- with subclavian artery stenosis.

Palpation

This checks for: thrills, apex beat, abnormal pulsation and palpable sounds. Systolic thrill in the aortic area suggests aortic stenosis. Feel for thrills in other sites as follows.

- *Left sternal edge*: VSD or HCM
- *Apex*: ruptured mitral chordae
- *Pulmonary area*: pulmonary stenosis
- *Subclavicular area*: subclavian artery stenosis.

Diastolic thrills are less common: feel for apical diastolic thrill in mitral stenosis with patient lying on left side and breath held in expiration. A left sternal edge diastolic thrill is occasionally felt in aortic regurgitation.

Apex beat and cardiac pulsations

Heart is displaced, not enlarged (e.g. scoliosis, pectus excavatum?). Normal apex beat is in the fifth left intercostal space in the midclavicular line. It is palpable but does not lift the finger off the chest. In abnormal states distinguish:

- normal site but thrusting, e.g. HCM, pure aortic stenosis, hypertension, all with good LV
- laterally displaced and hyperdynamic, e.g. mitral and/or aortic regurgitation, VSD
- laterally displaced but diffuse, e.g. DCM, LV failure
- high dyskinetic apex, e.g. LV aneurysm
- double apex (enhanced by 'a' wave), in HCM, hypertension
- left parasternal heave; RV hypertrophy, e.g. pulmonary stenosis, cor pulmonale, ASD
- dextrocardia with apex in fifth right intercostal space.

Abnormal pulsations are very variable, e.g. ascending aortic aneurysm pulsating in aortic area, RVOT aneurysm in pulmonary area, collateral pulsation round the back in coarctation, pulsatile RVOT in ASD, pulsatile liver (felt in the epigastrium and right hypochondrium) in severe tricuspid regurgitation.

Palpable heart sounds represent forceful valve closure, or valve situated close to the chest wall, e.g. palpable S_1 (mitral closure) in mitral stenosis, P_2 in pulmonary hypertension, A_2 in transposition, or both S_1 and S_2 in thin patients with tachycardia.

1.3 Auscultation

Heart Sounds

First and second heart sounds are produced by valve closure. Mitral (M_1) and aortic (A_2) are louder than and precede tricuspid (T_1) and pulmonary (P_2) heart sounds. Inspiration widens the split.

A widely split second sound in mitral regurgitation and VSD is the result of early ventricular emptying and consequent early aortic valve closure. However, the widely split sound is rarely heard because the loud pansystolic murmur usually obscures it. A summary is shown in Table 1.3.

Third Sound (S_3)

This is pathological over the age of 30 years. It is thought to be produced by rapid LV filling, but the exact source is still debated. Loud S_3 occurs in a dilated LV with rapid early filling (mitral regurgitation, VSD) and is followed

Table 1.3 The first and second heart sounds

First sound (S_1) = M_1 + T_1

Loud	Soft	Variable	Widely split
Short PR interval	Long PR interval	Third-degree AV block	RBBB
Tachycardia	Heart block	AF	LBBB
Mitral stenosis	Delayed ventricular contraction (e.g. AS, infarction)	Nodal tachycardia or VT VT	VPBs

Second sound (S_2) = A_2 + P_2

Loud A_2	Widely split	Reversed split	Single
Tachycardia	RBBB	LBBB	Fallot's tetralogy
Hypertension	PS (soft P_2)	Aortic stenosis	Severe PS
Transposition	Deep inspiration	PDA	Pulmonary atresia
	Mitral regurgitation	RV pacing	Eisenmenger syndrome
	VSD		Large VSD
	Hypertension		

Loud P_2	Fixed split		
PHT	ASD		

by a flow murmur. It also occurs in a dilated LV with high LVEDP and poor function (post-infarction, DCM). A higher-pitched early S_3 occurs in restrictive cardiomyopathy and pericardial constriction.

Fourth Sound (S_4)
The atrial sound is not normally audible but is produced at end-diastole (just before S_1) with a high end-diastolic pressure or with a long PR interval. It disappears in AF. It is most common in systemic hypertension, aortic stenosis, HCM (LV S_4), pulmonary stenosis (RV S_4) or after an acute MI.

Triple Rhythm
A triple/gallop rhythm is normal in children and young adults but is usually pathological over the age of 30 years. S_3 and S_4 are summated in SR with a tachycardia.

S_3 and S_4 are low-pitched sounds. Use the bell of the stethoscope and touch the chest lightly.

Added Sounds
• *Ejection sound*: in bicuspid aortic or pulmonary valve (not calcified), i.e. young patients
• *Midsystolic click*: mitral leaflet prolapse
• *Opening snap, mitral*: rarely tricuspid (TS, ASD, Ebstein's anomaly)
• *Pericardial clicks* (related to posture).

Innocent Murmurs
Probably 30% of healthy young children have a heart murmur but <1% will have congenital heart disease. This is usually the result of a pulmonary flow murmur heard best at the left sternal edge radiating into the pulmonary area.

Characteristics of Innocent Murmur
• Ejection systolic: diastolic or pansystolic murmurs are pathological. The only exceptions are a venous hum or mammary soufflé.
• No palpable thrill.
• No added sounds (e.g. ejection click).
• No signs of cardiac enlargement.
• Left sternal edge to pulmonary area. May be heard at the apex.
• Normal femoral pulses.
• Normal ECG: chest radiograph or echocardiogram may be necessary for confirmation.
The venous hum is a continuous murmur, common in children, reduced by neck vein compression, turning the head laterally, bending the elbows back or lying down. It is at its loudest in the neck and around the clavicles. It may reappear in pregnancy.

Pathological Murmurs

These are either organic (valve or subvalve lesion) or functional (increased flow, dilated valve rings, etc.). They are discussed under individual conditions in subsequent chapters.

They should be graded as just audible, soft, moderate or loud. Grading on a 1–6 basis is unnecessary and unhelpful. The murmur should also be classified as to site, radiation, timing (systolic or diastolic, and which part of each), and behaviour with respiration and position. Many murmurs can be accentuated with effort. Alteration of the murmur with position (e.g. squatting) is important in HCM, mitral prolapse and Fallot's tetralogy. The quality of the murmur itself should also be described, e.g. low- or high-pitched, rasping, musical or honking in quality.

Some systolic murmurs can be accentuated by particular manoeuvres. Pansystolic murmurs of VSD and mitral regurgitation are increased by hand grip, and decreased by amyl nitrate inhalation. The systolic murmur of hypertrophic obstructive cardiomyopathy is typically accentuated during the Valsalva manoeuvre and by standing suddenly from a squatting position. The murmur in HCM is reduced by passive leg elevation, hand grip and squatting from a standing position (see Section 4.2).

Accurate documentation of the murmur is important because murmurs may change over time. With a closing VSD the murmur shortens from a pansystolic to an ejection systolic murmur (see Section 2.1). With a floppy mitral valve, a soft late systolic mitral murmur may lengthen to become a pansystolic murmur as the mitral leak becomes worse (see Section 3.3).

Finally, it is important to remember that the loudness of a murmur bears no relationship to the severity of the valve lesion. In summary any of the following features suggest that the murmur is organic/pathological:

- Symptoms
- Cyanosis
- Thrill
- Large heart clinically or on chest radiograph
- A diastolic murmur
- A very loud murmur
- A pansystolic murmur
- Added sounds: ejection clicks, opening snaps, etc. (not S_3 which is normal in young people).

Special Points in Neonates and Infants

- A murmur heard immediately after birth is usually the result of a stenotic lesion. Murmurs from a small VSD or PDA are usually heard a few days later, and from a large VSD still later, as the pulmonary vascular resistance falls. The absence of a murmur does not exclude congenital heart disease. Undersized neonates may have an innocent murmur that arises from relatively hypoplastic pulmonary arteries waiting to grow. This sort of murmur usually disappears by the age of 6 months.

- Does the child have other features? For example:
  - Turner syndrome: coarctation or atretic aortic arch
  - Noonan syndrome: pulmonary stenosis
  - Down syndrome: AV canal
  - Williams syndrome: supravalvar aortic stenosis, pulmonary artery stenoses.
- Clubbing will not be apparent until the child has been cyanosed for ≥6 months. Cyanosis in a neonate always needs investigation.
- Pectus excavatum rarely causes any cardiac embarrassment, but may cause slight displacement of the heart on a chest radiograph. Sometimes associated later with a straight-back syndrome and floppy mitral valve. Pectus carinatum (pigeon chest) is not caused by cardiac enlargement. It may sometimes be the result of a large main pulmonary artery in large left-to-right shunts.
- Tachypnoea, hepatomegaly, sweating forehead and Harrison's sulci all suggest cardiac failure that is most likely to be caused by a left-to-right shunt.
- Midline liver, aspenia, polysplenia, etc. suggest complex congenital heart disease.
- Poor pulses in the legs suggest coarctation or hypoplastic left heart syndrome. Bounding pulses in the legs: PDA, truncus arteriosus or aortic regurgitation.

2 | Congenital Heart Disease

Congenital heart disease occurs in approximately 8 in 1000 live births. Although divided into cyanotic and acyanotic, there are several conditions that start acyanotic and become cyanotic with time, e.g. Fallot's tetralogy, Ebstein's anomaly and left-to-right shunts developing into the Eisenmenger syndrome (1897) (see Section 2.10).

Table 2.1 shows the most common lesions presenting in a neonate and those presenting in the infant and older child. Most congenital heart disease should be detected by a good neonatal examination or at a 6-week check-up.

Cyanotic Congenital Heart Disease

Table 2.2 shows the cyanotic group divided into those conditions with pulmonary plethora or oligaemia, and those with LV or RV hypertrophy. The addition of pulmonary stenosis to a lesion causes oligaemic lung fields and RV hypertrophy.

Grown-up Congenital Heart Disease (GUCH)

Before surgical correction <20% children with congenital heart disease survived to adulthood but now 85% of patients do. GUCH has become a specialty in its own right with approximately 1600 new cases annually in the UK. The GUCH population is increasing at about 5%/year and there are now more GUCH patients than children with congenital heart disease. In addition the population base is changing: there are no adult ASDs or PDAs now with all these defects closed percutaneously in childhood. Typical medical problems that develop in GUCH patients are as follows:

• Arrhythmias: half of the emergency admissions in GUCH patients are for arrhythmias; skilled electrophysiological expertise is needed in every GUCH unit.

Swanton's Cardiology, sixth edition. By R. H. Swanton and S. Banerjee. Published 2008 Blackwell Publishing. ISBN 978-1-4051-7819-8.

Table 2.1 Differentiation of congenital heart disease

	Neonate	Infant and older child
Cyanotic	TGA Tricuspid atresia Obstructed TAPVD Severe PS Pulmonary atresia Severe Ebstein's anomaly with ASD Hypoplastic left heart	TGA Fallot's tetralogy
Acyanotic	Congenital aortic stenosis Coarctation + VSD/PDA	VSD ASD PDA Congenital aortic stenosis Coarctation Pulmonary stenosis Partial APVD + ASD

• Cardiac failure: right heart failure in Fallot's tetralogy, systemic ventricular failure in corrected transposition.
• Pulmonary hypertension (see Section 13.1).
• Thrombosis (see Section 5.7).
• Degenerative change in surgical implants: conduit calcification, xenograft or homograft valve deterioration, baffle obstruction in the Mustard procedure.

Table 2.2 Differentiation of cyanotic congenital heart disease

Pulmonary plethora	Pulmonary oligaemia
TGA Single atrium AV canal Truncus arteriosus TAPVD DORV Primitive ventricle Tricuspid atresia with no PS	Fallot's tetralogy DORV + PS Single ventricle + PS Ebstein's anomaly + PS + ASD Pulmonary atresia with poor collaterals

With RV hypertrophy	With LV hypertrophy
Fallot's tetralogy DORV + PS Single ventricle + PS/subPS TGA + PS (LVOTO) Pulmonary atresia + VSD TAPVD Severe PS	Tricuspid atresia Pulmonary atresia with no VSD Single ventricle

Checking Connections in Congenital Heart Disease

Two-dimensional and Doppler echocardiography have in many cases obviated the need for invasive investigation. Among the factors that need to be assessed are the following:

- Aortomitral continuity: the posterior wall of the aorta should be continuous with the anterior mitral leaflet. Absence of aortomitral continuity is seen in double-outlet right ventricle, some patients with Fallot's tetralogy and truncus arteriosus.
- Aortoseptal continuity: the anterior aortic wall is normally continuous with the interventricular septum. Overriding of the aorta can be seen in Fallot's tetralogy in the long axis view.
- Which AV valve is continuous with which vessel? In transposition of the great vessels (TGA) the posterior AV valve (mitral) is continuous with the posterior pulmonary artery. The anterior tricuspid valve is continuous with the aorta. Distinction of the great vessels depends on size (larger aorta in adults), venous injections of contrast (or agitated 5% dextrose) in children and the recognition of a possible end-diastolic A wave on the pulmonary valve. Unfortunately, both AV valves may look identical and the distinction of the great vessels is important.

2.1 Ventricular Septal Defect

The most common congenital heart lesion is an isolated VSD (2 per 1000 births). It also occurs as part of more complex lesions (Table 2.3).

Table 2.3 VSD in congenital heart disease

Often associated with a VSD	VSD an integral part of the syndrome
Tricuspid atresia	Fallot's tetralogy
Pulmonary atresia	DORV
TGA	Truncus arteriosus
Coarctation	

Pathophysiology and Symptoms

The immediate effects of a VSD in the neonate depend on its size and the pulmonary vascular resistance (PVR). The site of the VSD becomes important later.

As the PVR falls in the first few days of life, and RV pressure falls below systemic LV pressure, the VSD results in a gradually increasing left-to-right shunt. If the defect is large ($>1\,cm^2/m^2$ body surface area) the PVR does not fall with the large left-to-right shunt. The neonatal LV cannot cope with the large volume load and pulmonary oedema develops. These are the typical features of heart failure in infancy:

- tachypnoea
- failure to thrive, feeding difficulties, failure to suck adequately
- sweating on feeding
- intercostal recession (increased respiratory work with stiff lungs)
- hepatomegaly.

Persistent high pulmonary blood flow results in frequent chest infections, retarded growth and chronic ill-health in the untreated case.

Irreversible pulmonary changes start from about the age of 1 year with initial hypertrophy and secondary thrombotic obstruction of pulmonary arterioles.

Physical Signs

These are summarized in Table 2.4. Cases in which the VSD murmur is not pansystolic have either very small or very large defects. With increasing defect size, biventricular hypertrophy is evident both clinically and on the ECG. With shunt reversal and pulmonary hypertension at systemic levels, right-sided signs are prominent and the murmurs are softer or disappear.

Cardiomegaly and enlargement of the PA conus are not as great as in ASD, except in infants with big shunts.

The second sound in very small VSDs is normal. A_2 is obscured by the pansystolic murmur of larger defects, and with equal ventricular pressures S_2 is single.

Spontaneous Closure

This occurs in 30–50% of VSDs. It is common in muscular defects, or defects of the membranous septum. It does not occur in defects adjacent to valves, infundibular (supracristal) defects, AV canal-type defects or malalignment defects.

Sites of VSD

Figure 2.1 shows the four common sites simplified.

Membranous (Infracristal)

This is the most common, just behind the medial papillary muscle of the tricuspid valve, which may oppose it and help to close it spontaneously. On closure, an aneurysm of the membranous septum may occur.

Muscular

This is variable in site and may be multiple. Acquired muscular VSD after septal infarction is usually of the Swiss-cheese type.

Posterior (AV Defect)

This is a paratricuspid defect similar to the site of a VSD in AV canal defect, but this VSD may be present with normal AV valves: 'inlet' VSD.

Table 2.4 Grades of VSD

	Very small	Small	Moderate	Large	Eisenmenger syndrome
Thrill	No	Yes	Yes	Yes	No
Murmur and site	Early ejection systolic LSE only	Loud pansystolic. LSE → apex and PA	As in small, but additional mitral diastolic at apex	Pansystolic decrescendo to S_2 Pulmonary ejection systolic + click Possible pulmonary regurgitation	None at LSE Ejection systolic PA (soft) and pulmonary regurgitation
Apex	Normal	Normal or LV+ slight	LV+ RV+ slight	LV+ RV+	RV++ PA palpable
S_2	Normal A_2 easily heard	A_2 obscured by murmur, but S_2 split on inspiration	Obscured by murmur	A_2 obscured. P_2 may be loud	Loud single palpable S_2
ECG	Normal	Normal	LV+ LA+ LAD	LV+ LA+ RV+	RV+ RA+ RAD
Chest radiograph	Normal	Normal heart size. Mild pulmonary plethora	Slight cardiomegaly PA+ Pulmonary plethora	Cardiomegaly (both ventricles) Large PAs Pulmonary plethora	Large PAs No plethora Peripheral pruning
Differential diagnosis	Mild AS or sub-AS Mild PS or infundibular PS	MR, TR, HCM, PS	MR, TR, PS	Severe MR, mixed AVD	Eisenmenger's ASD, PDA, etc.
Prognosis or treatment	Spontaneous closure	Probable spontaneous closure. Observe	Surgery	Surgery	Medical treatment

Infundibular ('Supracristal')
This is a high VSD just beneath the pulmonary valve and below the right coronary cusp of the aortic valve. It may be inadequately supported and prolapse, causing aortic regurgitation. This VSD does not close spontaneously.

The infundibular VSD may be associated with malalignment of the infundibular septum, e.g.
- VSD + shift of septum to right: Fallot's tetralogy
- VSD + shift of septum to left: double-outlet LV with subaortic stenosis.

Cardiac Catheterization
This confirms a step-up in O_2 saturation in the RV and can quantitate the left-to-right shunt. LV cines in the 45° and 60° LAO views visualize the interventricular septum with head-up tilt. Aortography checks aortic valve competence and excludes PDA or coarctation. RV angiography checks the RVOT. The site of the VSD can be diagnosed at catheter. Muscular VSDs are usually lower in the septum and may be multiple. The infundibular VSD is high, immediately subaortic, and there is no gap between the aortic valve and the VSD jet. The membranous VSD is usually a discrete jet with a slight gap between the jet and the aortic valve (Figure 2.1).

Antibiotic prophylaxis (dental procedures, etc.) is used for all grades.

Complications of VSD

Aortic Regurgitation
This occurs in about 5% of VSDs. It may occur with membranous (infracristal) or infundibular (supracristal) defects. The right coronary cusp is unsupported in the infundibular defect and often prolapses into or through the VSD, obscuring it on angiography. With membranous defects the non-coronary cusp may also be involved.

Infundibular Stenosis
Muscular infundibular obstruction develops in about 5% of VSDs and is progressive – more common in older patients and those who have had pulmonary artery banding. Infundibular stenosis improves flooded lungs but causes shunt reversal and cyanosis.

Infective Endocarditis
This is possible with any VSD with a risk of 0.2% per year. The risk is reduced by VSD closure. All should have antibiotic prophylaxis for dental procedures, etc. Successfully patched VSDs should have antibiotic cover for 3 months after surgery until the patch endothelializes. Infective endocarditis in a VSD with a typical left-to-right shunt presents with pulmonary complications as the infected material is driven into the pulmonary circuit. Patients may present with recurrent atypical pneumonia or pleurisy.

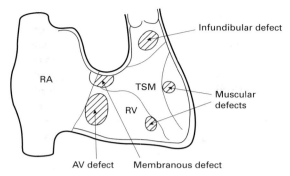

Ventricular septal defects and left ventricular angiography

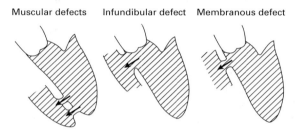

Figure 2.1 Ventricular septal defect. The sites of the four common VSDs are shown, top. TSM = trabecula septomarginalis. The bottom panel shows an LV cineangiogram diagrammatically in the 45° LAO projection with 30° cranial tilt. Muscular VSDs tend to be low in the septum and are often multiple. The infundibular defect is immediately subaortic. The membranous defect tends to be a more discrete jet with a small gap between the jet and the aortic valve.

Pulmonary Hypertension

VSD is the most common cause of hyperkinetic pulmonary hypertension (large PAs on the chest radiograph and pulmonary plethora). Calculation of PVR at catheter is important because this gradually rises as irreversible intimal hypertrophy develops without causing much change on the chest radiograph.

Associated Lesions

• AV canal or simple secundum ASD (see Section 2.2).
• Aortic regurgitation (see above).
• PDA: a common association (10% of VSDs). The early diastolic murmur heard in the left upper chest may be confused with aortic or pulmonary regurgitation. Aortography is mandatory in VSDs.
• Pulmonary stenosis: valvar (congenital), infundibular (congenital or acquired). The effects depend on the size of the VSD, the severity of the pulmonary stenosis and the systemic vascular resistance. With mild PS, a left-to-right shunt persists. If PS is severe and the VSD small, the condition mimics

severe PS alone. If PS is severe and the VSD large, right-to-left shunting occurs (effects similar to Fallot's tetralogy).
- Coarctation.
- TGA, or corrected transposition.
- More complex lesions: DORV, DOLV, truncus arteriosus, tricuspid atresia.
- Gerbode defect: LV-to-RA shunt. Either direct or through the membranous septum first to RV, then to RA via tricuspid regurgitation.

Management

In infancy, digoxin and diuretics are administered in an attempt to hold the situation. With large defects the baby is catheterized early, with a view to surgery at about 3 months should the child fail to thrive on medical treatment. The VSD is closed or, if multiple, PA banding is performed to reduce pulmonary flow.

If medical treatment is successful and there are only moderate size defects, the VSD is closed in pre-school years (e.g. age approximately 3 years).

Closure of small defects may be justified on the grounds of infective endocarditis risk, but minute defects are usually left.

The high incidence of spontaneous closure in the first year of life (approximately 50%) must encourage medical management at this age where possible. Generally surgical closure is indicated for:
- Failure to thrive in infancy
- Large defects (>1 cm^2/m^2); left-to-right shunts ($Q_p:Q_s$) $> 2:1$; increasing heart size on chest radiograph
- RV systolic pressure $> 65\%$ LV systolic pressure if PVR < 8 Wood units (see below)
- Increasing aortic regurgitation
- Doubly committed VSD (e.g. Fallot's tetralogy)
- Previous endocarditis on the VSD.

Management of the child with elevated PVR is more difficult. If the PVR is <8 units the VSD is usually closed. If the PVR is >8 Wood units a lung biopsy may be indicated to assess the severity of intimate proliferation before deciding on surgery (see Table 16.4 for calculation).

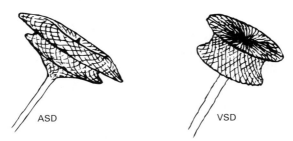

Figure 2.2 Amplatzer devices for closing a secundum ASD (left) and a muscular VSD (right). Both are delivered through a catheter made of nitinol mesh (with a memory) and contain polyester fabric to ensure good closure.

Device Closure

The Amplatzer device can be used for non-surgical closure of some muscular VSDs that have not closed spontaneously. Unfortunately, the device is not suitable for the more common membranous VSDs because it can interfere with the aortic or tricuspid valve or cause LVOTO. The device is made from nitinol mesh filled with polyester fabric to increase its closing ability (Figure 2.2).

2.2 Atrial Septal Defect

From the fifth week of intrauterine life the fetal common atrium starts to be divided by the septum primum. This crescentic ridge grows down from the cranial and dorsal part of the atrium towards the endocardial cushions. The foramen primum develops at the junction of the septum with the endocardial cushions. The foramen secundum develops at the top of the septum primum as the foramen primum closes. The septum secundum develops as a second crescentic ridge to the right of the septum primum, which fuses with the endocardial cushions. The limbic ledge forms the lower part of the septum secundum and the foramen ovale maintains right-to-left atrial flow in fetal life.

Types of ASD (Figure 2.4)
- Patent foramen ovale (PFO)
- Primum
- Secundum (Figure 2.3)

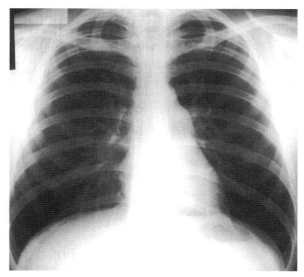

Figure 2.3 Small secundum ASD. Slight enlargement of PA conus.

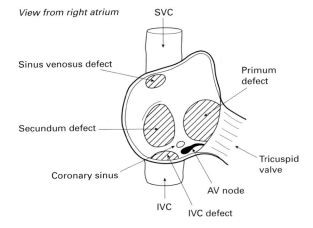

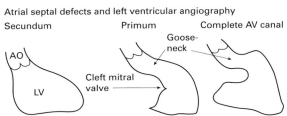

Figure 2.4 Atrial septal defect. The upper diagram shows the sites of the common ASDs. The lower diagram shows the LV cineangiogram in the RAO projection diagrammatically. In the secundum ASD this may be normal or show a prolapsing mitral valve. The typical 'goose-neck' of primum ASDs or AV canal is shown with a horizontal outflow tract, grossly abnormal AV shape and cleft mitral valve.

- Sinus venosus defect
- IVC defect
- Coronary sinus anomalies
- AV canal.

Patent Foramen Ovale
This is not strictly an ASD. It may occur in up to 25% of young children. There is no physiological interatrial shunting unless an additional cardiac lesion is present (e.g. pulmonary stenosis when a high RA pressure may cause right-to-left shunting). A PFO does not require closure unless this situation arises. It is useful in catheterization, allowing left atrial catheterization easily. On withdrawal from the LA to the RA, however, there is a difference in mean pressures. This differentiates a PFO from an ASD, where the mean pressures are the same or virtually the same. A PFO does not need prophylactic antibiotics for dental procedures, etc.

PFO and Paradoxical Emboli

Rarely, a PFO may allow the passage of a paradoxical embolus – particularly if associated with an atrial septal aneurysm. This is increasingly recognized as a cause of stroke, often in young people, after a Valsalva manoeuvre (e.g. straining, heavy lifting). Release of a Valsalva manoeuvre results in a sudden rise in RA pressure with a surge in venous return and possible transient right-to-left shunting through a PFO. This can be checked with transthoracic echocardiography using microbubble injection, with microbubbles seen shunting into the LA. Surgical or device closure in these patients must be considered as a preferable alternative to life-time anticoagulation. It is particularly indicated:

- in younger patients
- if there is a contraindication to anticoagulation
- in procoagulant conditions
- in recurrent cerebral events, or multiple infarcts on MRI
- in additional atrial septal aneurysms.

Device closure should not be considered if there is any other possible embolic source (e.g. AF, carotid disease or any thrombus in the pelvic veins or IVC).

PFO and Migraine

Interest in closing PFOs increased when it was noted that the presence of a PFO was often associated with migraine. With the possibility that right-to-left shunting of microemboli or vasoactive substances might be causing migraine the MIST (Migraine Intervention with Starflex Technology) trial was designed. The Starflex closure device did not reduce the number of patients whose headaches were completely abolished but did seem to reduce the overall headache burden (migraine days). It is possible that these rather disappointing results were the result of incomplete PFO closure and residual shunting. Further trials are under way.

Pathophysiology and Symptoms of an ASD

Left-to-right shunting at the atrial level occurs during the first months of life as the RV becomes more compliant than the LV (which becomes thicker and stiffer in response to systemic pressures). High pulmonary flow results, with flow murmurs audible over pulmonary and tricuspid valves. Pulmonary flow may be five times as great as the systemic flow.

In young adults the development of pulmonary hypertension is not common but it results in RV pressure approaching systemic levels and the start of shunt reversal (Eisenmenger's ASD). It does not occur in infancy.

The sites of the common ASDs are shown in Figure 2.4. The lower panel shows the LV cineangiogram in the RAO projection diagrammatically. In the secundum ASD this may be normal or show a prolapsing mitral valve. The typical 'goose neck' of primum ASDs or AV canal is shown with a horizontal outflow tract, grossly abnormal AV shape and cleft mitral valve (see also Figures 2.5, 2.6, 2.7, 2.8, 2.9).

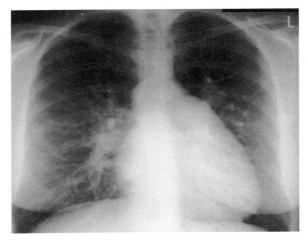

Figure 2.5 CXR. Large secundum ASD. Pulmonary plethora. RV dilatation.

Secundum ASD patients are often asymptomatic in childhood and may not be diagnosed until age 40–50 years. Primum ASDs are picked up earlier. Table 2.5 delineates differences in the types.

Symptoms or reason for diagnosis:

- The chesty child: resulting from high pulmonary flow.
- Dyspnoea on effort and occasionally orthopnoea (stiff lungs, not LVF).

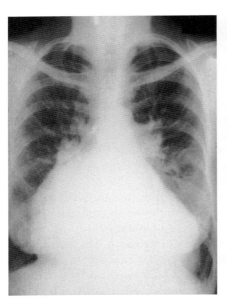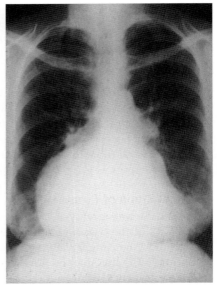

Figure 2.6 Secundum ASD pre- and post-surgical closure. Reduction in pulmonary plethora and right ventricular mass, but no change in atrial size.

Table 2.5 Principal types of ASD

	Secundum ASD	Primum ASD	AV canal
Presentation	Child or adult	Usually childhood	Infancy
Appearance	Normal	Normal	Down syndrome
Colour	Normal	Normal	Cyanosis
Signs	Secundum ASD	As secundum ASD ± MR	As VSD, but S_2 split
Ventricular septum	Intact	Intact	VSD component
Pulmonary hypertension	–	–	+
EGG	RBBB + RAD	RBBB + LAD	RBBB. LAD. Long PR or worse
Mitral valve	Occasionally prolapsing usually normal	Cleft anterior leaflet, varying degrees of MR	Severe MR. Grossly abnormal MV and TV

- Symptomatic: routine school medical or mass radiographs.
- Palpitation: all varieties of atrial dysrhythmias are common, particularly AF or atrial flutter. They may occur postoperatively and are more likely in those in whom the defect is closed after the age of 40 and in those with higher PA pressures preoperatively. Defect closure at any age is no guarantee against the development of subsequent atrial dysrhythmias.
- The development of AF and cardiac failure: this is a serious problem in ASDs. RV compliance is reduced, the tricuspid ring dilates further, and tricuspid regurgitation and hepatomegaly occur. Systemic flow falls, and the left atrium may enlarge as progressive CCF develops. (In SR the left heart is small in secundum ASD.)
- Paradoxical embolism or cerebral abscess may occur in patients with high RV pressures and shunt reversal.

Infective endocarditis is not a problem with an ASD as such, unless there is an associated mitral valve lesion.

Physical Signs of Secundum ASD

This type is more common in females. It may occur as part of the Holt–Oram syndrome (triphalangeal thumbs, ASD or VSD).

Right heart signs are dominant:
- Raised JVP with equal 'a' and 'v' waves.
- RV prominence with precordial bulge in children and large pulmonary conus and flow.
- Pulmonary systolic ejection murmur (flow).

• Fixed split A_2 and P_2 on any phase of respiration is typical, although occasionally very slight movement of P_2 can be detected.
• Tricuspid diastolic flow murmur with large left-to-right shunts.
• Systolic thrill in the pulmonary area may occur from high flow and does not necessarily mean additional pulmonary stenosis.
• With AF, signs of tricuspid regurgitation.
• Pulmonary hypertension results in a softer ejection systolic murmur, often an ejection click, the tricuspid flow murmur disappears and P_2 is loud. Pulmonary regurgitation may occur (Graham Steell early diastolic murmur).

Differential Diagnosis
In the simple secundum, ASD is seen with mild pulmonary stenosis (P_2 delayed, is softer and moves with respiration).

With larger hearts, pulmonary hypertension and the development of cardiac failure, the conditions confused with an ASD include: mixed mitral valve disease (see Figure 3.6); pulmonary hypertension and/or cor pulmonale; and congestive cardiomyopathy.

Patients with ASDs are usually in SR, with right heart signs most obvious. In AF with low output it is more difficult, but on chest radiograph the PA is very large in ASDs and there is pulmonary plethora.

Associated Lesions
• *Floppy mitral valve* (often overdiagnosed on angiography).
• *Pulmonary stenosis*: this will cause right-to-left shunting if severe.
• *Anomalous venous drainage*: the sinus venosus defect is almost always associated with anomalous drainage of the right upper PV to the RA. However, more than one PV may be involved. This is checked at cardiac catheter.
• *Mitral stenosis (Lutembacher syndrome, 1916)*: probably rheumatic mitral stenosis associated with an ASD. Congenital mitral stenosis is a rare possibility.
• As part of more complex congenital heart disease, e.g. TAPVD, TGA, tricuspid atresia, pulmonary atresia with intact ventricular septum.
The sinus venosus defect behaves as a small secundum ASD with its associated right upper lobe anomalous venous drainage.

Chest Radiograph
• Small aortic knuckle; large pulmonary artery conus (Figure 2.3, 2.5)
• Pulmonary plethora, cardiac enlargement is the result of RV dilatation (Figure 2.5)
• Right atrial enlargement common (Figure 2.6)
• Progressive enlargement of both atria once in AF.

ECG
• Incomplete or complete RBBB
• Right axis deviation.

Echocardiography
This is all that may be needed in children when PVR is usually normal.

Cardiac Catheterization
Cardiac catheterization is performed to document the diagnosis, assess the shunt with a saturation run, check pulmonary and coronary sinus drainage, and check RV function and the mitral valve with an LV injection. Thus LV, RV and PA angiograms with follow-through are usually required.

Oximetry is performed early in the catheter before angiography. If the oxygen step-up is high in the RA there may be a sinus venosus defect. In secundum ASD the step-up is in mid-RA. If the oxygen step-up is very low in the RA near the tricuspid valve and the ASD cannot be crossed with the catheter, consider the possibility of anomalous pulmonary veins draining into the coronary sinus.

In secundum ASD the LV is small and normal. The mitral valve may appear to prolapse. Late mitral regurgitation may occur through an associated floppy valve years after secundum ASD closure. In primum ASD there is the so-called 'goose-neck' appearance with a cleft in the mitral valve (see Figures 2.4, 2.7, 2.8) plus some mitral regurgitation, which may fill the RA if severe. In complete AV canal the cleft becomes a large gap and the LV has a characteristic appearance in the RAO view. The LAO views visualize the septum. The aorta is small, shifted to the left (large RA).

Treatment

Surgical Closure
Device or surgical closure is recommended between the ages of 5 and 10 years to avoid late-onset RV failure, tricuspid regurgitation and atrial arrhythmias. Late-onset pulmonary hypertension is uncommon because this is usually established in the first year of life. The calculated left-to-right shunt on saturations should be 2:1 or more at atrial level to recommend closure. Small ASDs can be left alone. As the child grows the size of the ASD will also increase and device closure operators must take this into account. In the older patient, closure of an ASD is still worthwhile, symptomatic improvement being associated with a reduction in RV size (especially if there is low voltage on RV leads preoperatively).

Patients with secundum ASDs may have an associated floppy mitral and/ or tricuspid valve and regurgitation, although this may cause problems years after ASD closure.

Device Closure
Recently small- or moderate-sized ASDs have been closed percutaneously through the right heart using a variety of different devices. The clam-shell device developed in the 1980s was followed by the Sideris, buttoned, double-disc device. Most recently, the Amplatzer device (different design from the

device for closing muscular VSDs, but same material) can be inserted through a 7 F sheath. Transoesophageal echocardiography during the procedure is helpful. The ASD should be <40 mm diameter, clear of the AV valves and pulmonary veins and have a rim of normal atrial septum (>5 mm) to make device closure possible. Approximately 50% of secundum ASDs may be suitable for device closure. About one-third of patients have small residual leaks, and device embolization occurs in a small number necessitating catheter removal or surgery.

ASDs will grow in size with the growing child – so care in sizing the device is important. The devices used for ASD and VSD closure are shown in Figure 2.2. Antibiotic cover is given intravenously before the procedure (see Section 9.7). Aspirin and clopidogrel are given for 6 months after the procedure. If the patient is already on warfarin this is continued for 6 months.

There are several contraindications to device closure:

- Ostium primum ASD
- Sinus venosus ASD
- Anomalous pulmonary venous drainage
- Established severe pulmonary hypertension
- Associated congenital heart lesions requiring surgery.

Primum ASD (see Figure 2.7 and 2.8)
A more complex and serious lesion than the secundum ASD, this forms part of the spectrum of AV canal defects. It is caused by maldevelopment of the septum primum and endocardial cushions. Its most simplified subdivisions are as follows.

Primum ASD
There is no VSD component. Mitral valve (anterior leaflet) is cleft with associated mitral regurgitation of varying degrees, from none to severe. Sometimes called 'partial AV canal'.

Complete AV Canal
Primum type ASD plus VSD component: mitral and tricuspid valves are abnormal with abnormally short chordae and bridging leaflets stretching across the VSD and joining the mitral and tricuspid valves.
It accounts for only 3–5% of congenital heart disease in the first year of life, and less than a tenth of all ASDs.

Associated Lesions
- Down syndrome (very common), Klinefelter syndrome, Noonan syndrome, renal and splenic abnormalities.
- Cardiac abnormalities: common atrium; unroofed coronary sinus (left SVC to LA); pulmonary stenosis; coarctation.

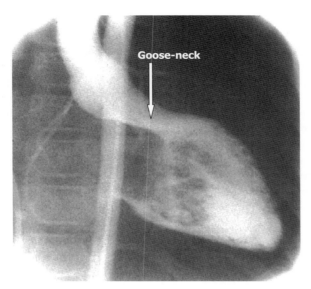

Figure 2.7 Primum ASD. LV angiogram. RAO projection. End-diastolic frame. Goose-neck deformity of LV outflow tract.

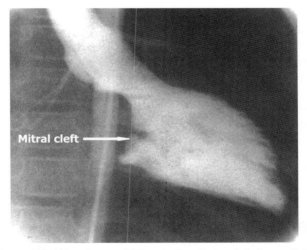

Figure 2.8 Primum ASD. LV angiogram. RAO projection. End-systolic frame. Cleft mitral valve.

Presentation

Primum ASD usually presents in childhood and the complete AV canal in infancy (heart failure and failure to thrive in infancy with signs of VSD, early childhood with dyspnoea and chest infections and central cyanosis if pulmonary vascular disease develops).

Chest Radiograph

Chest radiograph of a simple primum defect resembles a secundum ASD. The AV canal chest radiograph has a large globular heart with pulmonary plethora.

ECG

- RBBB
- Left axis deviation (compare right axis in secundum defect)
- Long PR interval.

Conduction defects are common (the AV node is in the inferior portion of the defect), especially junctional rhythms or complete AV block. If right axis deviation develops, it suggests the development of pulmonary hypertension or additional pulmonary stenosis.

Treatment

Primum ASD

Fifty per cent reach surgery before age 10 years. Early surgery may help prevent RV dysfunction. The cleft mitral valve is repaired if there is significant mitral regurgitation and the defect is closed with a patch.

Complete AV Canal

Fifty per cent die within 1 year if untreated. Options in infancy are banding the pulmonary artery or closure of ASD and VSD components dividing the bridging leaflets. Subsequent mitral valve replacement may be necessary, as well as permanent pacing for AV block. The presence of pulmonary hypertension makes operative mortality high.

Rarer Defects

The IVC defect may be large and allow shunting of IVC blood into the LA, with children becoming slightly cyanosed on effort. It may also occur after surgical closure of a primum ASD.

Unroofed coronary sinus with a left SVC draining to LA usually occurs as part of a more complex lesion (e.g. common atrium).

2.3 The Patent Ductus Arteriosus

In fetal life the duct allows flow from the pulmonary circuit to the aorta. It normally closes spontaneously within the first month after birth. In premature babies it is more likely to remain patent for longer or permanently. Up to 50% of premature babies have a PDA, especially those with respiratory distress syndrome. The duct responds less well to a rise in Po_2 in prematurity and the duct may be silent. The PDA is more common:

- in children born at high altitudes
- in females

• where there has been history of maternal rubella in the first trimester of pregnancy (PDA is the most common congenital heart lesion after maternal rubella).

Pathophysiology and Symptoms

Most children with a PDA are asymptomatic, e.g. the condition having been diagnosed at a school medical. With larger ducts a significant left-to-right shunt occurs, causing an increased LV volume load similar to a VSD. Symptoms of LVF are similar. Irreversible pulmonary hypertension may develop in a few cases, causing Eisenmenger syndrome (approximately 5%).

Differential cyanosis and clubbing may be noticed by the patient who has shunt reversal (blue feet, pink hands), with preferential flow of pulmonary arterial blood down the descending aorta.

In rare instances death is the result of either CCF or infective endocarditis.

Physical Signs to Note

Very small ducts have few signs apart from the continuous machinery murmur in the second left interspace.

The following are signs to note in a moderate PDA:
• Collapsing pulse with wide pulse pressure (feel the foot pulses in babies)
• Thrill, second left interspace, systolic and/or diastolic
• LV+: hyperdynamic ventricle
• Machinery murmur: loud continuous murmur obscuring second sound in second left interspace and just below the left clavicle, louder in systole. It is not present in the neonate (with the high PVR), but appears as the PVR falls in the first few days
• Mitral diastolic flow murmur at apex
• The second sound is usually inaudible.

Pulmonary Hypertensive Ducts

The diastolic component of the murmur may disappear, and the systolic become shorter with an ejection quality. The second sound is single (loud P_2). Occasionally it is reversed audibly (prolonged LV ejection).

Dilatation of the pulmonary trunk causes an ejection sound and sometimes pulmonary regurgitation.

Associated Lesions
• VSD
• Pulmonary stenosis
• Coarctation
• As part of more complex lesions, e.g. pulmonary atresia with intact septum. If collaterals are poor, pulmonary flow is duct-dependent. Drug control in this instance is important. In interrupted aortic arch or hypoplastic left heart syndrome, the PDA maintains flow round the body.

Pharmacological Control of the PDA

Helping to Close the Duct in Neonatal LVF
Important points are: avoiding fluid overload, normal blood glucose and calcium, and diuretics rather than digoxin (AV block in babies). Then use indomethacin 0.2 mg/kg via nasogastric tube given at 6-hourly intervals for a maximum of three doses. An intravenous preparation is not generally available.

There is a risk of renal damage (unlikely with this regimen) and the drug should be avoided if there is an elevated serum creatinine (>150 mmol/l or 1.7 mg/100 ml). Also avoid indomethacin if there is a bleeding disorder.

Helping to Keep the Duct Patent in Pulmonary Atresia
This is more difficult because sudden deaths have been reported following the use of prostaglandin E_1 (PGE_1), and the cause is unknown.

PGE_1 is infused at 0.1 µg/kg per min via an umbilical artery catheter. The PO_2 rises. Vasodilatation may drop the mean aortic pressure and increase the right-to-left shunt if there is one already. After a few minutes the dose is reduced to 0.05 or even 0.025 µg/kg per min.

Other side effects include fever and irritability. Taken orally, the drug produces troublesome diarrhoea. It should not be tried except at experienced neonatal centres.

Differential Diagnosis
This includes the following:
- AP window
- VSD with aortic regurgitation
- Coronary AV fistula
- Pulmonary AV fistula
- Ruptured sinus of Valsalva
- Innocent venous hum
- Mammary soufflé (pregnancy)
- Surgical shunts (Waterston, Blalock, etc.).

Cardiac Catheterization
This is performed if additional lesions are suspected. The right heart catheter follows a characteristic course from the PA down the descending aorta. Associated lesions are excluded by a saturation run (VSD). Aortography indicates duct size and site. LV cine is necessary if a VSD is suspected in addition.

Treatment
Spontaneous closure of the PDA is rare after 6 months of age and a PDA should be closed by the preschool year to avoid the risk of infective endocarditis and the rarer development of LVF or the Eisenmenger reaction. Infective endocarditis on a very small duct is extremely rare and can be left alone.

Infection risk is related to duct size and ducts >4.0 mm should be occluded. Many of the problems encountered by surgical closure (e.g. haemorrhage, 'recanalization' as a result of inadequate ligation, phrenic and left recurrent laryngeal nerve palsy) have been obviated by the use of duct occluders implanted in the catheter laboratory.

The first of these was the ivalon plug implanted retrogradely via the femoral artery. The introducing catheter was too big for children. The Rashkind double umbrella device followed in 1979. Femoral arterial and venous sheaths were needed. A pair of miniature back-to-back umbrellas was positioned across the duct under screening, and angiography at the end confirmed correct positioning and successful duct occlusion. This device has now been superseded by a variety of implantable coils that can be positioned in the duct using only a femoral venous sheath. Smaller guiding catheters can be used than with the Rashkind device. The procedure can now be done as a day case.

Problems with the technique are few in skilled hands. The duct may be too large for the occluder or multiple coils, resulting in a persistent leak. Usually a single coil is enough to occlude the duct. Embolization of the device down a pulmonary artery occurs in about 1% of cases but it can usually be retrieved with a catheter snare. Turbulent flow in the left pulmonary artery may be seen on colour Doppler echocardiography after coil deployment, which can cause a degree of LPA obstruction.

2.4 Coarctation of the Aorta

This is a congenital narrowing or shelf-like obstruction of the aortic arch. The constriction is usually eccentric, distal to the left subclavian artery, opposite the duct and termed 'juxtaductal'. In extreme form the arch may be interrupted. Recognized types are as follows (Figure 2.9).

Infantile Type
Associated with hypoplasia of the aortic isthmus (a diffuse narrowing of the aorta between the left subclavian artery and duct), this was called 'preductal' coarctation. Presentation occurs in the first month of life, with heart failure and associated lesions, which are extremely common.

Adult Type
This coarctation is juxtaductal or slightly postductal (Figure 2.9). The obstruction develops gradually and presentation is commonly between the ages of 15 and 30 years with complications. Associated cardiac lesions are much less common than with the infantile type, apart from a bicuspid aortic valve.

Pseudo-coarctation
This is just a tortuosity of the aorta in the region of the duct. There is no stenosis, just a 'kinked' appearance. It is of no haemodynamic significance. Other severe stenotic lesions may occur in the aorta (e.g. supravalvar aortic

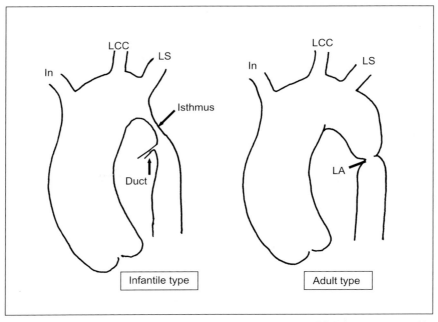

Figure 2.9 Types of coarctation of the aorta. In: Innominate artery. LCC: left common carotid artery, LS: left subclavian artery, LA: ligamentum arteriosum.

stenosis, descending thoracic or abdominal stenoses). The abdominal and descending thoracic aorta stenoses may be the result of an aortitis. Classic coarctation may be caused by abnormal duct flow *in utero* associated with other anomalies, and the two types are not strictly comparable. Children with coarctation are usually male. Coarctation in females suggests Turner syndrome.

Associated Lesions

These are very common:
• Bicuspid aortic valve (which may become stenotic and/or regurgitant); about 50% of cases, but series vary enormously.
• PDA: the most common associated shunt:
    – *postductal coarctation* + PDA: usually left-to-right shunt into the pulmonary artery; if the duct is large, pulmonary hypertension may occur
    – *infantile coarctation* + PDA: high PVR results in right-to-left shunt, with distal aorta, trunk and legs supplied by RV flow through the PDA; differential cyanosis results (blue feet, pink hands) and heart failure
• VSD: in isolation or with:
    – *transposition of the great arteries* + VSD + PDA: complex lesion with differential cyanosis (blue hands, pink feet)

– *mitral valve disease*: congenital mitral valve anomalies, stenosis or regurgitation
– *other complex lesions*: primitive ventricle, primum ASD or AV canal
– *aortic arch anomalies*: hypoplastic left heart with hypoplastic aortic root; aortic atresia; aortic root aneurysms
– *non-cardiac associations*: berry aneurysms, renal anomalies (especially Turner syndrome).

Symptoms
• Infantile heart failure is expected in >50% preductal coarctation. It may also occur with postductal coarctation plus a large PDA (see above).
Postductal coarctation may be missed in childhood presenting in adolescence or early adult life with one or more of the following:
• Noticing a vigorous pulsation in the neck or throat
• Hypertension: may be symptomless, routine medical
• Tired legs or intermittent claudication on running
• Subarachnoid haemorrhage from a berry aneurysm
• Infective endocarditis on coarctation or bicuspid aortic valve
• LV failure
• Rupture or dissection of the proximal aorta: distal aortic rupture has occurred (e.g. into the oesophagus), aortic rupture is more common in pregnancy
• Angina pectoris, premature coronary disease occurs.

Physical Signs to Note
• Blood pressure in both arms (?left subclavian involved or not). Hypertension with wide pulse pressure in right ± left arm.
• Weak, delayed, anacrotic or even absent femoral pulses compared with right radial. Low blood pressure in legs.
• Prominent carotid and subclavian pulsations.
• Collaterals in older children (not before age 6 years) and adults. Bend the patient forward, with arms hanging down at the sides. Feel round the back with the palm, over and around the scapulae and around the shoulders. Collaterals do not develop in preductal coarctation with PDA because distal aorta supply is from the pulmonary artery.
• Tortuous retinal arteries; frank retinopathy is not common.
• JVP is usually normal.
• LV hypertrophy.
• Murmurs:
   – a result of a bicuspid aortic valve (see Section 3.4)
   – from the coarctation itself: a continuous murmur with small, tight coarctation (<2 mm) heard over the thoracic spine or below the left clavicle; with larger coarctation the murmur is ejection systolic only
   – from collaterals: ejection systolic, bilateral, front or back of chest. In interrupted aorta (complete coarctation) the murmurs are the result of collaterals

 – from an associated PDA or VSD
 – from lower thoracic or abdominal coarctation
It may be difficult to decide the source of an ejection systolic murmur in coarctation!
• Second sound: A_2 is usually loud, but not usually delayed beyond P_2.

Chest Radiograph
Rib notching occurs from the age of 6–8 years from dilated posterior intercostal arteries (Figures 2.10 and 2.11). It does not occur in the first and second ribs. (The first two intercostals do not arise from the aorta.) The heart is usually normal in size unless there are associated lesions. The typical aortic knuckle is absent and is replaced by a double knuckle (in postductal coarctations). The upper part is the dilated left subclavian, the lower the poststenotic dilatation of the descending aorta.

ECG
This shows LV hypertrophy; RBBB is common.

Echocardiography
This may obviate the need for cardiac catheter in the infant with no associated lesion. Transoesophageal echocardiography (and MRI) is needed to study narrowing of the aortic arch and isthmus.

Cardiac Catheterization
This is required in children with atypical signs or associated lesions. Babies can be catheterized from the right heart via a PFO or from a right axillary cut-down in older children. Additional lesions are checked (bicuspid aortic valve, PDA, VSD, etc.) and aortography performed in the LAO projection to show the coarctation. A coarctation gradient of >20 mmHg is significant, particularly if the patient is hypertensive. The gradient increases with exercise. The size of the descending aorta is noted, as are site and size of the collaterals.

Balloon Angioplasty and Stenting
Some paediatric centres now advocate this as an alternative to surgery as first-line treatment for both infantile and adult-type coarctation, but this is controversial as first-line treatment. Balloon dilatation results in an intimal and medial tear. It is not a satisfactory procedure in neonates and infants because there is a high re-stenosis rate (up to 80%), and patients with a long narrow segment at the isthmus do badly with little or no reduction in coarctation gradient. There is also a risk of a small saccular aneurysm developing at the site of the dilatation (in which case surgical repair is necessary). Surgery itself carries a re-stenosis risk of 15%.

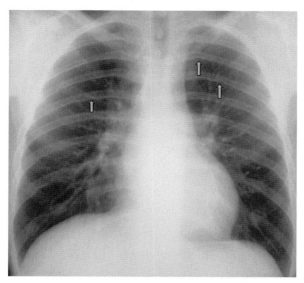

Figure 2.10 CXR coarctation. Note absent aortic knuckle. Rib notching arrowed.

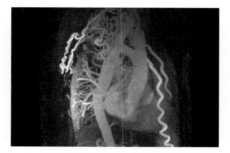

Figure 2.11 Coarctation of the aorta on cardiac MRI (arrow). Note collaterals and large tortuous internal mammary arteries on the right.

The technique is much more suitable for re-stenosis after primary resection than as an initial procedure, and the risk of aneurysm formation is much less for dilatations of re-stenosis (approximately 7%) than as a primary procedure. A close look around the whole of the circumference of the aorta at the coarctation site is needed after dilatation to check for the small aneurysm. The major complication is aortic rupture and death within 36 h of the procedure in about 2.5% cases.

Stenting

Balloon dilatation with stent deployment (Figures 2.12–2.16) reduces elastic recoil, controls any possible dissection flap and reduces re-stenosis. Greater

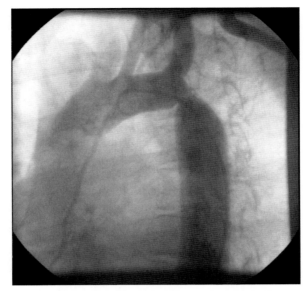

Figure 2.12 Aortogram. Left anterior oblique view. Coarctation pre-stenting.

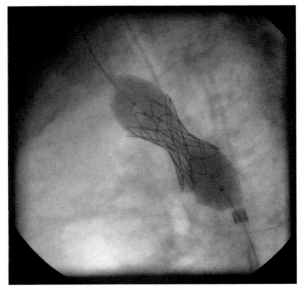

Figure 2.13 Coarctation stenting. Balloon half-inflated.

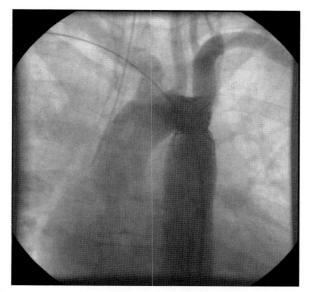

Figure 2.14 Recoarctation stenting. Aortogram following stent deployment. Slight residual waist seen.

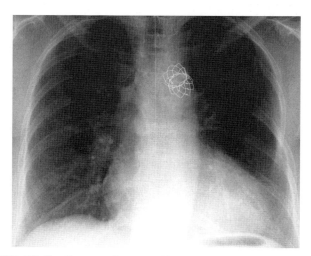

Figure 2.15 CXR. P/A film. Recoarctation treated by stenting.

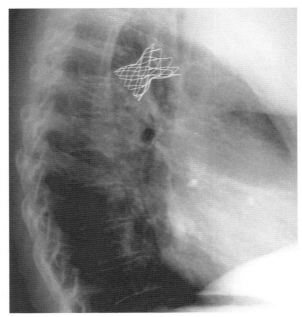

Figure 2.16 CXR. Right lateral. Recoarctation treated by stenting. Slight residual waist in centre of stent.

reduction in gradient is achieved than with balloon dilatation alone. It is likely that there will be a residual gradient after dilatation of a hypoplastic aortic arch. Covered stents are available. Rare complications include: death from aortic rupture, stent migration, aneurysm formation or CVA. Risks are higher in patients >30 years, and those with a bicuspid aortic valve, aneurysmal aortic root or aortic valve replacement.

Surgery

The prognosis without surgery or balloon dilatation is poor: most patients die before age 40 from complications. Severe preductal coarctation in infancy or interrupted aortic arch (usually with PDA + VSD) may require urgent reconstructive surgery.

In postductal coarctation, surgery is performed between 5 and 10 years or at the time of diagnosis, which may be later. Patients with both coarctation and aortic stenosis have the coarctation resected first, and a subsequent aortic valve replacement if necessary.

Recently, extra-anatomical bypass surgery has been developed for coarctation or interrupted aortic arch in older children or adults in which a Dacron graft is anastomosed from the ascending aorta to the descending aorta either above or below the diaphragm. This avoids all the problems of surgery at the coarctation site itself, such as re-stenosis or aneurysm formation at the site of the patch aortoplasty.

Choice of Treatment

This depends on the child's age, and the site and extent of the coarctation, e.g.

- Surgery: hypoplastic isthmus
- Balloon-only angioplasty: discrete coarctation with a normal aortic arch in children aged 6 months–8 years
- Stenting: age >8years, discrete or short segment coarctation. Isthmus normal or mildly hypoplastic.

Follow-up

Postoperative hypertension is expected, usually requiring nitroprusside, labetalol, trimetaphan and/or chlorpromazine in the immediate postoperative phase.

Long-term hypertension is also common. Histological changes with medial hypertrophy in the aorta decrease its compliance in the adult. Patients should be followed up for life after coarctation resection to check:

- continued hypertension
- the possibility of premature coronary artery disease.

Repeat cardiac catheter in infants or early adult life is often performed to check the coarctation site and possible residual gradient, especially if hypertension persists.

Death in untreated coarctation is usually a result of CCF, intracerebral haemorrhage or coronary artery disease.

2.5 Transposition of the Great Arteries (Complete Transposition, D-Transposition)

In its most common form the aorta arises from the right ventricle and the PA from the left ventricle. The aorta lies anterior and to the right of the pulmonary artery (D-loop). There is thus atrioventricular concordance and ventriculoarterial discordance. Unless there is an associated shunt (ASD, VSD, PDA), the two circuits are completely separate and life is impossible once the duct closes.

TGA occurs in approximately 1 per 4500 live births (100–200 cases per year in the UK). It is more common in males. Untreated mortality is high (10% 1-year survival rate).

Presentation

This presents at birth, with cyanosis that increases in the first week as the PDA closes. Birthweight is normal or high. Progress is poor and progressive cardiac enlargement occurs. As PVR declines in the first weeks of life, high pulmonary flow develops and LVF occurs. CCF is the most common cause of death.

When pulmonary vasculature is protected from high flow by pulmonary stenosis, children are often quite active even though very cyanosed. Squatting and cyanotic attacks are uncommon in contrast to the very cyanosed child with Fallot's tetralogy.

Physical Signs to Note

• The most common cyanotic congenital heart disease causing cyanosis at birth.
• Initially hyperdynamic circulation: bounding pulses in a blue baby.
• Loud (palpable) A_2 retrosternally from anterior aorta. P_2 not heard.
• Murmurs often absent: high pulmonary flow may cause a soft midsystolic ejection murmur; ejection sound may arise from either aorta or PA; right-to-left shunt through VSD may cause a soft early systolic murmur; left-to-right shunt through VSD (high PVR or LVOTO) does not usually cause a murmur.

The signs depend on the level of the PVR, the presence or absence of LVOTO and/or a VSD.

ECG

This is very variable. Usually shows RA+, RV+ and RAD. Additional LV+ and LA+ occur with high pulmonary flow and LV volume overload. It is not so prevalent in patients with additional pulmonary stenosis.

Chest Radiograph

This shows pulmonary plethora. Heart has an 'egg on its side' appearance and the pedicle is small (aorta in front of PA). The left heart border is convex.

Echocardiography

This is usually diagnostic. The anterior aorta and posterior PA are seen. Additional defects such as ASD or VSD, LVOTO, PDA or abnormalities of the AV valves should be looked for.

Differential Diagnosis

• All causes of cyanosis and pulmonary plethora (see Table 2.2) but TGA is the most common.
• Also consider Eisenmenger's VSD.
• If there is LVOTO, lung fields are not plethoric, and the condition may then resemble Fallot's tetralogy or DORV with pulmonary stenosis.

Associated Lesions
• PDA may be life saving if there is no VSD; differential cyanosis occurs
• VSD in 70%
• VSD + LVOTO (fibrous shell or fibromuscular tunnel beneath pulmonary valve) = TGA + VSD + LVOTO; these patients have poor pulmonary flow and may have frank cyanotic spells
• ASD: usually without PS, and high pulmonary flow occurs
• Coarctation
• Juxtaposed atrial appendages.
Prognostically the best situations are TGA + ASD, or TGA + VSD + moderate pulmonary stenosis. The child can survive the early months and does not get the irreversible pulmonary vascular changes (these are usually present by 1 year of age) in children with TGA + large VSD but no protective pulmonary stenosis.

Cardiac Catheterization
This confirms normal AV connections, but RV injection fills anterior aorta. The associated shunt is identified. An aortogram shows coronary anatomy plus a possible PDA or coarctation. Injection into the LV shows possible LVOTO. If possible, the PA should be entered to check for PVR (usually easiest via aorta through RV → VSD → LV → PA).

Options for Treatment

Prostaglandin Infusion
This may be needed for the intensely cyanosed neonate with duct-dependent pulmonary flow until a balloon atrial septostomy can be performed (see Section 2.3).

Rashkind Balloon Septostomy
This may be life saving in the neonate, and is performed at diagnostic catheterization. A PFO is enlarged by inflating the balloon catheter carefully in the left atrium, and sudden traction of the balloon into RA increases atrial mixing. About 70% of babies can be helped through the first year with this technique, and atrial septectomy is not generally needed.

Intra-atrial Reconstruction: Senning (1958) or Mustard (1964) Operation
This is usually performed between the age of 6 months and 1 year; these operations separate systemic venous and pulmonary venous return at atrial level.
    In the Mustard operation, systemic venous return is diverted through the mitral valve via an intra-atrial baffle into the LV, and thence to the PA. Pul-

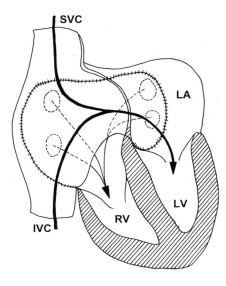

Figure 2.17 Mustard operation for transposition of the great vessels. PA view. Aorta and pulmonary artery not included in the diagram for clarity. After excision of the inter-atrial septum an atrial baffle is constructed to separate the two circulations. Blood from the SVC and IVC is directed into the LV and thence into the pulmonary artery, and pulmonary venous blood is directed into the RV and thence into the anterior aorta.

monary venous return is diverted through the tricuspid valve to the right ventricle, and thence to the aorta (Figure 2.17).

Advantages
- Circuits are separated
- Cyanosis disappears
- Child grows with reasonable exercise tolerance.

Disadvantages
- RV bears load of systemic circulation; both RV muscle and tricuspid valve may not be up to it with RV failure and TR leading to atrial dysrhythmias. ACE inhibitors are used although there is no evidence base to support them in this situation.
- It is not strictly anatomical total correction.
- Postoperative supraventricular dysrhythmias are common (especially with the Mustard procedure).
- Baffle obstruction may occur. This is the Achilles' heel of the operation and baffle dysfunction may occur in up to 50% of asymptomatic patients 6 years after surgery. SVC obstruction is more common than IVC obstruction. Balloon dilatation and stenting may be necessary to relieve this.

Rastelli Procedure for TGA, VSD and LVOTO (i.e. PS)
These patients may be shunted early (Blalock). Then, at ages 3–4 years, the Rastelli procedure is performed. The VSD is enlarged, the pulmonary valve closed and the pulmonary artery ligated just above the pulmonary valve. The

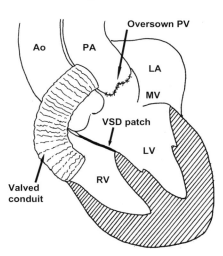

Figure 2.18 Rastelli operation for transposition of the great vessels. Left lateral view. The pulmonary valve is oversown and a valved conduit constructed from the anterior RV to the posterior PA as shown. The VSD patch separates the two circulations and directs LV blood into the anterior aorta.

LV is connected to the aorta by means of an intracardiac patch. Then an extracardiac valve conduit connects the anterior RV to the pulmonary artery. This is total correction, with the LV bearing the systemic load (Figure 2.18).

Problems that can result are a residual VSD, tricuspid regurgitation, conduit compression by the sternum and conduit valve degeneration and stenosis, which are almost inevitable and necessitate further surgery. Atrial and ventricular dysrhythmias are frequent and regular follow-up with echocardiography is necessary.

Anatomical Correction: The Arterial Switch (Jatene 1975)

Switching the great arteries to their correct ventricles is becoming increasingly popular and is anatomical correction. Surgery is performed in the first few weeks of life while the LV is still capable of generating systemic pressures. LV mass will fall as PVR falls and, if the switch is performed too late, the LV will fail. Otherwise a two-stage procedure may be needed, with PA banding to 'tone up' the left ventricle. Problems are primarily surgical on account of the delicate surgery of coronary artery relocation. Distortion of the RVOT, aortic root dilatation and coronary stenoses may occur in time.

An initial Rashkind balloon septostomy, followed later by a Senning or Mustard procedure, was the standard treatment for TGA but has now been replaced by the arterial switch where possible.

2.6 Corrected Transposition (L-Transposition)

In its most common form the aorta lies anterior and to the left of the pulmonary artery (l-loop). It is physiologically corrected in that the circulation proceeds on a normal route although the ventricles are 'switched', i.e.

RA → morphological LV but in RV position → PA → LA → morphological RV but in LV position → Ao

There is thus atrioventricular discordance and ventriculoarterial discordance. There is usually situs solitus with the atria normally placed. Rarely, the condition presents with situs inversus and dextrocardia. A few cases of corrected transposition have no associated lesions and the individual can live a normal adult life with no symptoms, the RV coping well with systemic load. The presence of associated lesions usually results in presentation in childhood, and the condition is not particularly benign.

Associated Lesions: The Four Most Common Ones (Figure 2.19)
• VSD: shunt from systemic (RV) to venous (LV) ventricle. Occurs in 70–90% of cases depending on series. A 'malalignment' defect: as there is malalignment between the atrial and ventricular septum.
• Pulmonary stenosis in 40%: often subvalvar as a result of an aneurysm of the membranous septum bulging out beneath the pulmonary valve.
• AV valve regurgitation: usually a problem with the tricuspid valve (left-sided) not coping with systemic pressures produced by the RV. Also it is often dysplastic with a typical Ebstein malformation. Mitral (right-sided) prolapse also may occur.
• Complete AV block: the AV node is anterior and the bundle runs beneath the pulmonary valve and anterior to the VSD.
Pulmonary valve or VSD surgery runs the risk of inducing AV block (which may also occur spontaneously).

Presentation
• Systemic ventricular failure (RV) resulting from tricuspid (left AV valve) regurgitation.
• Congenital complete AV block: not a benign type of AV block; children may be symptomatic from this alone.
• Cyanotic heart disease mimicking Fallot's tetralogy (subpulmonary stenosis + VSD with venous-to-systemic ventricular shunting).
• Paroxysmal tachycardia as in Ebstein's anomaly. Anomalies of the conducting system may occur (e.g. additional posterior AV node, Wolff–Parkinson–White syndrome).
• Abnormal EGG in adult life: mimicking anteroseptal infarction (Figure 2.20).

Physical Signs
The best clues to corrected transposition are the clinical findings of second- or third-degree AV block in a child, e.g. cannon 'a' waves in the JVP + variable intensity S_1 in third-degree AV block.

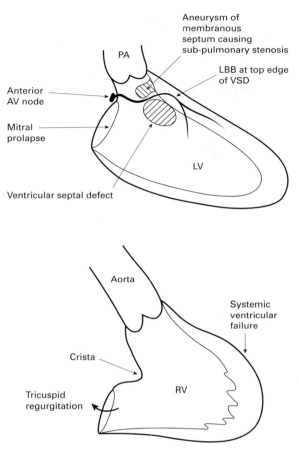

Figure 2.19 Problems in corrected transposition. The upper diagram shows the left (venous) ventricle and the position of the VSD in relation to the bundle. An aneurysm of the membranous septum is shown causing subpulmonary obstruction. The lower diagram shows the right (systemic) ventricle, which is trabeculated. Dysplastic tricuspid valve associated with tricuspid regurgitation. Systemic (RV) ventricular failure is a common cause of death.

As in TGA (complete D-transposition), A_2 is loud and palpable. In corrected transposition it is heard best in the second left intercostal space – mimicking the loud P_2 of pulmonary hypertension.

There may be signs of left AV valve regurgitation (pansystolic murmur from left sternal edge to apex). There may be an ejection click from the anterior position of the aortic valve.

Chest Radiograph
The left-sided aorta produces a 'duck's back' appearance with a straight left heart border, and AV valve regurgitation causes the respective ventricles and

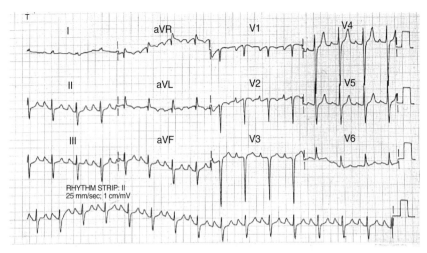

Figure 2.20 12 lead ECG in corrected transposition. Q waves in anterior chest leads resemble old anterior infarction.

atria to enlarge. The left pulmonary artery may be hidden behind the heart and aorta. The pedicle is narrow (Figure 2.21).

ECG (Figure 2.20)
- Long PR interval
- Higher degrees of AV block
- Prominent Q waves in right chest leads (V1–3) but absent Q waves in left precordial leads
- Left axis deviation
- Q wave in standard lead 3, but no Q wave in lead 1.

Treatment
The most common early symptom is from complete AV block (20–30%) requiring pacing. Atrial arrhythmias are common (SVT or AF) from about the age of 40 and digoxin and/or amiodarone therapy will be needed. Beware the negative inotropy of other drugs.

Medical treatment for CCF may be needed if the systemic ventricle (RV) fails to cope with systemic workloads. CCF is the most common cause of death in patients with no associated anomalies. ACE inhibitors should be started early.

Patients may require left AV valve (tricuspid) replacement or repair plus VSD closure. The latter risks the development of complete AV block with the conducting system in the roof of the VSD (see Figure 2.19).

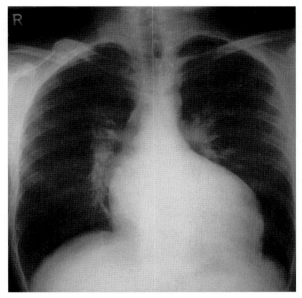

Figure 2.21 PA CXR in corrected transposition. Enlarged ventricular mass. Narrow pedicle.

Intracardiac mapping helps identify and avoid bundle damage. Unusual coronary artery anatomy may make ventriculotomy of the venous (LV) ventricle difficult.

Even with the greatest care, permanent pacing may be needed. The establishment of a permanent system is not without problems either. The transvenous wire must grip the endocardial surface of the non-trabeculated (venous) left ventricle.

Double-switch Surgery
The long-term 10-year survival rate after surgery was only 67% in one series (many deaths resulting from systemic RV failure). As a result of this, combined operations are now being tried: a double-switch using a Senning or Mustard venous switch plus an arterial switch procedure that allows the LV to take the systemic load.

2.7 Fallot's Tetralogy

This is the most common cyanotic congenital heart disease presenting after 1 year of age. It forms part of a spectrum of complex cyanotic congenital heart disease, and is very similar in many respects to double-outlet right ventricle with pulmonary stenosis (DORV + PS), VSD with severe infundibular stenosis, and pulmonary atresia with VSD.

Development of Fallot's Tetralogy

In Fallot's tetralogy there is a failure of the bulbus cordis to rotate properly so that the aorta lies more anterior and to the right (dextroposed) than normal. The aorta moves nearer the tricuspid valve and overrides the septum with a 'malalignment' VSD beneath the aortic valve.

Infundibular stenosis develops, with hypertrophy of the septal and parietal bands of infundibular muscle that form part of the crista (Figure 2.22). Obstruction to RV outflow is usually a result of a combination of infundibular and valve stenosis, but may be either alone. In addition, RV outflow obstruction may be caused by the small size of the pulmonary valve ring or main pulmonary trunk. Peripheral pulmonary stenoses are common. The original tetralogy described by Fallot in 1888 is:

- pulmonary stenosis (Figure 2.22)
- VSD
- overriding of the aorta
- RV hypertrophy.

The following are additional anomalies or problems commonly associated:

- Right-sided aortic arch (in 25%)
- Absent or hypoplastic left PA (more common if arch is right sided)
- Aortic regurgitation caused by large aortic ring plus subaortic VSD
- ASD.

Pathophysiology and Symptoms

With the large VSD, both ventricles are at the same (systemic) pressure. Pulmonary flow and the degree of right-to-left shunt across the VSD depend on the severity of pulmonary stenosis and the level of SVR. Increasing SVR will

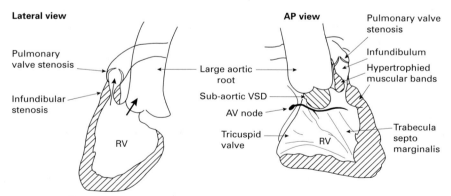

Figure 2.22 Fallot's tetralogy. The left diagram shows a lateral view of the right ventricle with the large aorta overriding the VSD. The severe infundibular stenosis results in the diversion of RV blood straight up into the aorta (heavy arrow). The right panel shows the right ventricle in the AP projection. The VSD is subaortic. Note the hypertrophied bands of the infundibulum. The bundle lies immediately beneath the VSD and is at risk during VSD closure.

reduce the right-to-left shunt and increase pulmonary flow. Mild pulmonary stenosis may be associated with the 'acyanotic' child with Fallot's tetralogy. Pulmonary blood flow may be increased by a PDA, although the association is not that common. Bronchial collaterals develop with increasingly severe pulmonary stenosis.

Infundibular stenosis is a variable obstruction. It increases with time (muscle and fibrous tissue accumulation) and also with hypoxia or acidosis, which may result in cyanotic attacks (infundibular spasm). Infundibular shutdown results in a severe reduction in pulmonary flow and an increased right-to-left shunt of blood from the right ventricle straight into the aorta. Squatting helps cyanosis in two ways: by increasing pulmonary flow and reducing right-to-left shunting:

• increasing SVR
• reduction in venous return – especially of acidotic blood from the legs (acidotic blood promotes infundibular spasm).

Typical Clinical Presentation (also see Section 2.10)
• Patients are not cyanosed at birth (compare TGA). It usually appears at 3–6 months and increases with time.
• Cyanotic attacks develop: often with 'stress', crying or feeding. Increasing cyanosis results in syncope and convulsions (see Section 16.3). The pulmonary stenotic murmur may disappear during attacks. Cerebral blood flow may be so severely compromised that permanent neurological damage results.
• Poor growth; delayed milestones.
• Squatting is common in older children once walking starts. In more severe cases, children may squat at rest (knees up to chest and buttocks on the ground).
• Symptoms of polycythaemia: arterial or venous thromboses, particularly cerebral; children must not be allowed to get dehydrated, which can precipitate this. Later in life: gout, acne, kyphoscoliosis, recurrent gingivitis.
• Infective endocarditis.
• Cerebral abscess (absence of lung filter with right-to-left shunt).
• Paradoxical embolism.

Physical Signs
• Developing cyanosis, clubbing and polycythaemia
• JVP: 'a' wave is usually absent (contrast with pulmonary stenosis with intact septum)
• Parasternal heave of RV hypertrophy
• Palpable A_2 is common (large aorta, too anterior)
• Ejection systolic murmur from left sternal edge, radiating up to pulmonary area, systolic thrill
• Single second sound (A_2 only).
The systolic murmur is a result of the PS, not the VSD. With cyanotic attacks the murmur becomes quieter or may disappear:

• A diastolic murmur in a patient with Fallot's tetralogy may be the result of aortic regurgitation (very large aortic root).

• A continuous murmur is caused by large aortopulmonary collaterals (heard in the back).

Chest Radiograph

The classic heart shape is of a *coeur en sabot* (heart in a boot) appearance with the apex lifted off the left hemidiaphragm by RV hypertrophy. There is a concavity in the usual site of the PA. Lung fields are usually oligaemic and PAs small. A network of collaterals may be seen around the main bronchi at the hilum. The aortic knuckle is a good size and may be right-sided in about 25% of cases.

ECG

This shows sinus rhythm, right axis deviation and RV hypertrophy with incomplete or complete RBBB. Ventricular ectopics are common, and paroxysmal ventricular tachycardia may be found on 24-hour ECG taping.

Cardiac Catheterization (Figure 2.23)

This is needed to assess the anatomy of the RVOT and the main PA branches, RV and LV function, site and size of VSD, and competence of the aortic valve, coronary anatomy to exclude a PDA or coarctation, and to visualize any previous shunt.

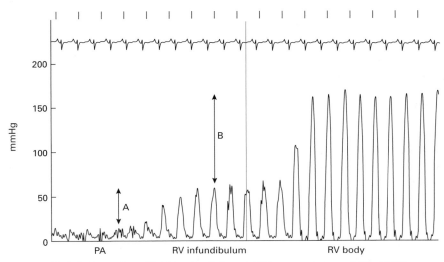

Figure 2.23 Fallot's tetralogy. Right heart withdrawal. PA pressure is normal. The RVOT gradient is both at valve level and subvalve level (infundibular). Valvar gradient (A) = 45 mmHg, and the infundibular gradient (B) = 105 mmHg. Total gradient = 150 mmHg.

This is best managed with biplane RV injection (and craniocaudal tilt on the AP projection helps visualize the main pulmonary trunk and its bifurcation). An LV injection in the LAO projection will show the VSD and LV function. An aortogram is essential in Fallot's tetralogy.

It is important to visualize the size and anatomy of the PAs because this determines the choice of subsequent operation. With severe PS or pulmonary atresia these may not be seen adequately on RV injection. A retrograde pulmonary vein handshot injection (catheter through a PFO or ASD) may show up small true PAs.

The most difficult differential diagnosis is from double-outlet right ventricle with subaortic VSD and PS. In Fallot's tetralogy less than half the aortic valve should straddle the VSD, and in DORV more than half. The final arbiter may be the surgeon. Medical treatment of cyanotic attacks and management of polycythaemia (see Section 16.3 and 2.10).

Surgery

Initial enthusiasm for complete one-stage repair in the first year of life was tempered by high mortality in many patients, especially those needing a transannular patch on the RV outflow tract. However, improved surgical techniques, postoperative care and careful selection have resulted in total correction at 4–6 months of age being the preferred option if possible rather than a two-stage repair. This particularly helps PA growth.

Some patients will have unsuitable anatomy for an initial one-stage repair, and will need a shunt first. Conditions favouring an initial shunt include: hypoplastic PAs, single PA, virtual pulmonary atresia and anomalous coronary anatomy – particularly an anomalous LAD arising from the right coronary artery with its course across the RV outflow tract.

Blalock–Taussig Shunt

The original Blalock shunt was performed (Figure 2.24) if the anatomy was unfavourable (subclavian artery to PA). However, complications of this operation in small children were ischaemia of the arm, or neurological damage to the sympathetic chain or phrenic or recurrent laryngeal nerves. The modified Blalock operation is now used in children with small PAs using a polytetrafluoroethylene (PTFE) end-to-side graft between (usually) the left subclavian and left PA. Problems with the anastomoses include haemorrhage, pseudoaneurysm or kinking of the PA at the graft junction.

Waterston or Potts Shunts

Under the age of about 3 months a Waterston shunt may be preferred, because the subclavian artery may be too small for a good Blalock. A second-stage total correction is then performed when the child is larger (age > 2 years). Problems with the Waterston and Potts procedures are the risk of pulmonary vascular disease from high flow if the shunt is too large. In addition it may

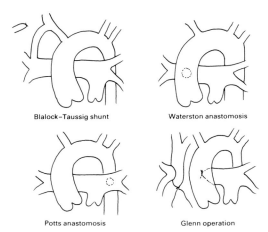

Blalock–Taussig shunt   Waterston anastomosis

Potts anastomosis   Glenn operation

Figure 2.24 Shunt operations for cyanotic congenital heart disease. Blalock–Taussig shunt: either subclavian artery to respective pulmonary artery. Waterston shunt: back of ascending aorta to pulmonary artery. Potts anastomosis: back of pulmonary artery to descending aorta. Glenn operation: SVC to right pulmonary artery only. The Potts operation is rarely used now. The bidirectional Glenn (to both pulmonary arteries) is increasingly popular.

be a difficult shunt to take down at the second stage with an associated increase in mortality risk – not seen with the Blalock.

Pulmonary Valvuloplasty

An alternative to shunting is to try pulmonary valvuloplasty, ballooning the outflow tract and valve, to attempt to improve pulmonary flow and PA size as a palliative method before total correction. Pulmonary valve damage resulting from the balloon will cause late pulmonary regurgitation. Recently resection of infundibular muscle, using a modified atherectomy device, has been attempted and percutaneous infundibular resection may become a useful treatment in time.

Total Correction

First performed by Lillehei in 1954 this operation now carries a mortality risk rate of <5% in expert hands. The VSD can be patched (Dacron or autologous pericardium) using a transatrial route through the tricuspid valve, with a transpulmonary approach to the RVOT obstruction. A transventricular approach gives better access to both with easier infundibular resection, but carries the risk of postoperative ventricular arrhythmias. A transannular patch needed for severe RVOT obstruction may involve an additional monocusp to prevent subsequent severe pulmonary regurgitation. Attempts to preserve pulmonary valve function now involve two patches: above and below the valve.

After total correction there may be further problems:
- RV failure
- Tachyarrhythmias
- Heart block (see position of bundle just beneath VSD)
- Pulmonary regurgitation
- RVOT aneurysm
- Problems from initial shunt
- Reopened VSD
- Aortic regurgitation (dilated root) – substrate for infective endocarditis.

RV failure and rhythm problems are the most important. Repeat cardiac catheterization is sometimes necessary in patients after total correction to assess all these factors.

Late Fallot's Arrhythmias

Virtually any arrhythmia may develop in time. Junctional bradycardia or complete AV block requiring permanent pacing, AF requiring anticoagulation and rate control, or paroxysmal VT requiring antiarrhythmics – usually amiodarone in view of poor RV function or implantation of an implantable cardioverter defibrillator (ICD) (see Section 7.10, 7.11).

RV dilatation, QRS prolongation >180 ms on the ECG and increased QT dispersion are thought to predict malignant ventricular arrhythmias and the risk of sudden death. Patients thought to be at risk should have a ventricular provocation study (see Section 8.5) to check if VT is inducible, it is suppressible with amiodarone or an ICD is required.

Pulmonary Regurgitation

Pulmonary regurgitation is being recognized as increasingly important in the late development of RV failure. Surgical correction involving a transannular patch often involves late pulmonary regurgitation. It is more likely if there is unrelieved PA branch stenosis. Reduction of pulmonary regurgitation using a monocusp valve or a homograft is being attempted to preserve RV function. There is an increasing trend towards transatrial repair for the same reason. Additional peripheral PA stenoses can be dealt with by balloon dilatation and stent implantation.

Recently percutaneous pulmonary valve replacement has become a possibility with the valve inserted via the right femoral vein on the catheter table.

Long-term Results of Surgery

In one recent study the 32-year survival rate was 86% (compared with 96% in age-matched controls). Surgery after the age of 12 reduced survival rates to 76%. Outcome was poorer in those patients who had a previous Potts or Waterston anastomosis (but not in those with a previous Blalock shunt). Redo surgery (in about 10%) may in time be needed for:
- residual pulmonary stenosis (an RV to PA conduit may be needed)
- pulmonary regurgitation

- VSD patch closure if the Qp:Qs ratio >1.5:1
- aortic valve replacement for aortic regurgitation
- ASD closure.

2.8 Total Anomalous Pulmonary Venous Drainage

In TAPVD all four pulmonary veins drain directly or indirectly into the right atrium. There is an associated ASD to allow flow to the left heart. Pulmonary flow is increased and the child is cyanosed. The degree of cyanosis and the severity of symptoms depend on:
- the size of the ASD
- the degree of pulmonary hypertension
- the presence of pulmonary venous obstruction.

   Cyanosis is more severe if pulmonary flow is reduced (e.g. with irreversible pulmonary hypertension) and if mixing in the atria is poor (e.g. with small ASD or PFO). The child with the least cyanosis is the one with high pulmonary flow, low PVR and good atrial mixing (large ASD). Pulmonary venous obstruction reduces pulmonary flow and increases cyanosis, and is most common with infracardiac TAPVD (see below).

Anatomical Possibilities (Figure 2.25)
A variety of venous pathways can conduct pulmonary venous blood to the right atrium. They can be divided into three.

Supracardiac
Venous drainage is to the left SVC, which joins the left innominate vein, and thence to the right SVC. This vein may occasionally be compressed between the left main bronchus (behind) and the pulmonary trunk (in front).

Cardiac
Venous drainage is into a venous confluence (a sort of miniature LA) joining the coronary sinus. Venous drainage is directly into the RA via one or more ostia.

Infracardiac
This is the rarest variety. The venous confluence at the back of the heart joins a vertical vein passing down through the diaphragm to join either the IVC or the portal vein. The vein may be obstructed at the diaphragm, or at the liver if it drains into the portal system. Crying will increase the obstruction and increase cyanosis.

Various combinations of these three are possible (e.g. left lung to vertical vein, right lung direct to RA).

Pathophysiology and Symptoms
In many ways the condition is similar to an ASD (left-to-right shunt into RA, pulmonary plethora, RV hypertrophy) but the patients are cyanosed. As in

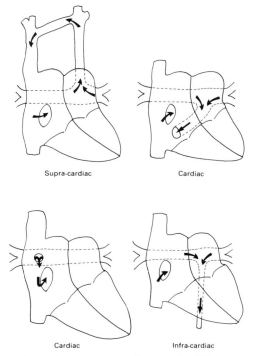

Supra-cardiac   Cardiac

Cardiac   Infra-cardiac

Figure 2.25 Total anomalous pulmonary venous drainage. An ASD is part of the lesion.

ASD, the LV is usually small, the RV doing the extra shunt work. Most infants also have a PDA. High pulmonary flow in a child causes cardiac failure, recurrent chest infections and poor growth development.

Additional pulmonary venous obstruction causes cyanosis at birth, dyspnoea and early death in pulmonary oedema.

Patients with high pulmonary flow plus a large ASD may be only slightly cyanosed, tolerate the lesion well and survive into adult life.

Physical Signs

In patients with no venous obstruction (usually supracardiac TAPVD), the physical signs are similar to those in ASD (Section 2.2), with additional:
- cyanosis (mild to moderate, depending on pulmonary flow)
- a continuous murmur (hum) either high up the LSE or in the aortic area; this is the venous hum of high flow in the SVC with TAPVD to the left innominate vein (supracardiac).

In patients with venous obstruction (usually infracardiac TAPVD), look for:
- prominent 'a' wave in JVP with pulmonary hypertension, but difficult to see in babies
- sick infant, vomiting, deeply cyanosed, tachypnoea, CCF
- no murmurs, loud P2, gallop rhythm.

Chest Radiograph

The supracardiac type shows the 'cottage loaf' heart, or the 'snowman in a snowstorm'. The wide upper mediastinal shadow is caused by the dilated SVC and anomalous vein (left SVC) to the left innominate. The pulmonary plethora and pulmonary venous congestion cause the snowstorm appearance. Pulmonary plethora may not be obvious in the neonate. With additional pulmonary venous obstruction there are additional signs of pulmonary oedema. The left ventricle and left atrium are small, so marked cardiomegaly is uncommon.

ECG

This is similar to a secundum ASD in mild cases. With pulmonary hypertension marked RAD and RV hypertrophy occur with P pulmonale and RV strain pattern (T-wave inversion V1–4).

Echocardiography

May be useful in defining cases with pulmonary venous obstruction.

Septal motion is paradoxical in patients with high pulmonary flow and unobstructed PVs (RV volume overload). In children with pulmonary hypertension and pulmonary venous obstruction, septal motion is usually normal. Two-dimensional echocardiography is useful in defining pulmonary venous anatomy, the venous confluence and the site of drainage.

Differential Diagnosis

The sick neonate: consider other pulmonary causes for cyanosis and tachypnoea (respiratory infection, aspiration of meconium, etc.). Arterial Po_2 should improve by these patients breathing 100% O_2 for 5 min. Echocardiography is helpful.

In cyanosed children with pulmonary plethora on the chest radiograph consider: TGA, primitive ventricle, truncus arteriosus, single atrium.

In patients with gross pulmonary venous obstruction, other causes have to be considered, e.g. cor triatriatum, congenital mitral stenosis.

Cardiac Catheterization

Pulmonary angiography with follow-through is necessary in order to detect the pulmonary venous anatomy. A saturation run is needed with sampling also in the low IVC and left innominate vein. All pulmonary veins must be identified.

If infants are <2 months old, Rashkind balloon septostomy may help by increasing ASD size and allowing better mixing, with reduction in cyanosis and an increased Po_2.

Surgery

Total correction is necessary for all cases of TAPVD, because there is no long-term palliative operation and medical treatment alone carries about a 90%

1-year mortality rate. Most of the infracardiac type have some form of venous obstruction and a low cardiac output. This means surgery on a sick infant with a high operative risk (15–20%). Children with a supracardiac or cardiac type with a large ASD and good mixing initially fare better but develop established pulmonary vascular disease unless totally corrected early. Deep hypothermia and total circulatory arrest may be needed for the operation:

• Supracardiac type: the common pulmonary vein is anastomosed to the back of the LA. ASD is closed and left SVC ligated.

• Cardiac type: the interatrial septum is refashioned, depending on the exact anatomy, to include the drainage site of the pulmonary veins into the LA. The coronary sinus may be included in the LA.

• Infracardiac type: the common pulmonary vein is anastomosed to the back of the LA. The ASD is closed and the descending anomalous vein ligated.

Recurrence of pulmonary venous obstruction postoperatively is uncommon but carries a very poor prognosis.

2.9 Tricuspid Atresia

Anatomy (Figure 2.26)
This is a rare cause of cyanotic heart disease. The tricuspid valve is completely imperforate or more commonly non-existent, being replaced by muscle and/ or fibrous tissue. Systemic venous blood crosses an essential ASD into a large LA and LV. The mitral valve is usually normal. The circuit is usually completed by a VSD. Blood flows from left to right through this VSD into a small RV into the pulmonary arteries. Pulmonary flow may be limited by pulmonary stenosis or too small a VSD. There may in addition be a coarctation or a PDA.

Pathophysiology and Symptoms
There are two main types of tricuspid atresia that dictate the early symptoms:

Common Type
The common type is normal great vessel position (normal ventriculoarterial connections). They usually have pulmonary stenosis, with poor pulmonary flow, small pulmonary arteries or a small VSD.

The poor pulmonary flow in infancy results in intense cyanosis from birth. Cyanosis may deteriorate after the first year, with the additional development of infundibular stenosis resulting in cyanotic attacks.

The chest radiograph shows small heart, straight right heart border and oligaemic lung fields. ECG shows RA strain, left axis deviation and LV hypertrophy. This pattern is uncommon in cyanotic congenital heart disease (see Table 2.2).

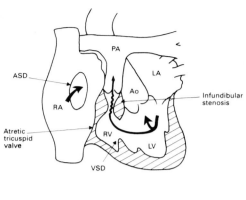

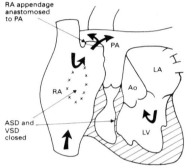

Figure 2.26 Tricuspid atresia. Classic Fontan operation

Less Common Type

This has transposed great vessels (discordant ventriculoarterial connections). PA arises from LV and is of good size with no pulmonary stenosis. As the PVR falls in the first few weeks of life, pulmonary flow increases (unrestricted by pulmonary stenosis), the circulation becomes hyperdynamic with pulmonary congestion and possible additional mitral regurgitation (functional from a dilated LV and mitral annulus). If uncorrected, patients develop CCF (mostly LV) and pulmonary vascular disease.

The chest radiograph shows a large heart with pulmonary plethora and congestion. ECG shows normal or even right axis.

Echocardiography

This is vital. It shows one large AV valve (mitral), and a large RA with bulging septum into the LA. Connections of the great vessels and size of the VSD should be seen. Doppler studies will quantify degree of mitral regurgitation and presence of a possible PDA.

Cardiac Catheterization

The most important pieces of information that cannot be established with the two-dimensional echo are the PA pressure and anatomy (and subpulmonary stenosis). Unfortunately it is commonly impossible to reach the PA with a catheter if the great vessels are not transposed. The surgeon may have to be content with pictures of the pulmonary arteries from the LV injection or MRI. Aortography is needed to check for PDA or coarctation.

Options for Surgical Treatment

Pulmonary Flow too Small

- Rashkind balloon septostomy if ASD too small
- Consider shunt (e.g. bidirectional Glenn, or Blalock) to enlarge PAs; pulmonary flow too great
- PA banding in first year of life: all with a view to one of the following:
  - the classic Fontan operation, 'total correction' from about age 2 years onwards (Figure 2.26)
  - bidirectional Glenn operation
  - total cavopulmonary connection (TCPC).

The Classic Fontan Operation (1968) (Figure 2.26)

The systemic and venous circulations are separated using the LV as the systemic pumping chamber, dispensing with the small RV and connecting the right atrial appendage directly to the right or divided main PA. The ASD and VSD are closed. Blood from the venae cavae thus flows to RA → PA → PV → LA → LV → aorta. There is a variety of modifications of the Fontan procedure depending on the exact great vessel anatomy. Caval valves are unnecessary. PA flow is passive and depends on SVC/IVC pressure. The ASD may be left 'fenestrated', which depressurizes the RA, but will result in some persistent RA-to-LA shunting and persistent mild systemic desaturation postoperatively. The fenestration can later be closed using an Amplatzer device (see Figure 2.2).

The Fontan operation has become a generic term for a group of operations involving a single ventricle with no pumping chamber to the PAs.

The best results with all these procedures occur if:
- child still in sinus rhythm with minimal atrial dysrhythmias
- normal or low PA pressures with low PVR; good-sized PAs
- normal unobstructed pulmonary venous return
- good LV function
- minimal or no mitral regurgitation, or stenosis
- no LVOT obstruction or coarctation.

With the best haemodynamics to start with, operative mortality rate is now <10%, but late complications do occur and atrial arrhythmias can prove a major problem. One-year survival rate is 93% and 5-year survival rate 82%.

Possible Complications
- Atrial dysrhythmias: cardiac output falls sharply if the child develops atrial flutter/fibrillation with signs and symptoms of right heart failure. Long-term antiarrhythmics may be needed to attempt to maintain sinus rhythm. Atrial flutter is a particular problem and there is often more than one circuit. This

may be improved by catheter ablation of the flutter circuit(s) in the RA, or by cryoablation (right atrial maze surgery).
- Hepatomegaly.
- Protein-losing enteropathy from dilated gut lymphatics. Results in oedema, ascites and hypocalcaemia. Manage with a low-salt, high-protein diet and diuretics.
- Coagulation disorders: liver dysfunction results in reduction in levels of protein C, protein S, prothrombin and antithrombin III.

Bidirectional Glenn
This is performed more commonly than the original Fontan operation. The SVC is anastomosed to the right PA as in Figure 2.24 but flow is to both PAs because the main PA is not ligated.

Total Cavopulmonary Connection
This may be performed as the final stage after a bidirectional Glenn rather than as a first operation. The IVC is also connected to the PAs by an extra- or intracardiac conduit. Streamlining flow in this way, excluding the RA, seems to improve cardiac output.

2.10 Cyanotic Congenital Heart Disease in the Adult

Eisenmenger Syndrome
In adults, inoperable cyanotic congenital heart disease is usually a result of the Eisenmenger situation with PA pressure at systemic level and bidirectional shunting through an ASD, VSD or PDA. It may also be caused by incompletely corrected Fallot's tetralogy, or more rarely Ebstein's anomaly, pulmonary atresia or truncus. High pulmonary blood flow in the first year of life results in a reactive medial hypertrophy of the pulmonary arterioles. There is additional intimal hyperplasia and narrowing of the arteriolar lumen results. PA pressure rises and the shunt becomes bidirectional. The PVR rises to $>800\,dyn{\cdot}s/cm^5$ (normal $<200\ dyn{\cdot}s/cm^5$). There is thus a combination of vasoconstriction and vascular remodelling. The rate of progression seems to depend on the shunt site: in infancy and childhood 80% of patients with Eisenmenger syndrome have a VSD; in adults most have an ASD. This diagnosis may be missed in childhood.

The PVR is fixed if it does not fall on breathing 100% oxygen. Patients with a fixed PVR seem to survive better than those with primary pulmonary hypertension (see Chapter 13). Median survival is into the 30s. The heart in these patients is very pre-load dependent. A drop in venous pressure (haemorrhage, dehydration, etc.) is poorly tolerated. Ventricular function is usually maintained.

Bosentan, a dual endothelin antagonist, may improve exercise capacity in these patients. Endothelin levels are known to be raised in Eisenmenger syndrome (see also Section 13.5).

In a few young patients, heart–lung transplantation has offered the only hope of a cure for Eisenmenger syndrome. Early results are good and at least one woman has had a child after heart–lung transplantation.

Careful follow-up of these patients is essential because there is also a great number of non-cardiac problems that must be considered.

Polycythaemia

This is caused by erythropoietin production secondary to chronic hypoxaemia. Oxygen delivery is increased with the rise in haemoglobin. Although theoretically physiological, it is counterproductive because it results in hyperviscosity and hypervolaemia. This causes headaches, blurred vision and a 'muzzy' head with reduced cognition. Patients appear plethoric with suffused conjunctivae. Retinal veins are engorged and tortuous. Scotomata leading to total blindness in one eye may develop with retinal vein thrombosis. Pruritus may be a nuisance, particularly after getting out of a hot bath. More serious complications include venous (and less often arterial) thrombosis, gout and peptic ulceration.

Venesection is necessary if the patient develops these symptoms or if the haematocrit or packed cell volume (PCV) exceeds 0.65. Earlier enthusiasm for venesection at lower PCVs resulted in iron-deficient cells. These are more spherical and less deformable than normal cells and may themselves result in sludging. Aim to keep the PCV between 0.55 and 0.6 (55–60%). Two drip lines are required for simultaneous venesection and the administration of the same volume of a plasma expander/colloid. It is important to avoid any fall in circulating volume. A strict aseptic technique is required because these patients often have acne and are vulnerable to infection. Generally it is sensible just to remove 1 unit of blood (450–500 ml) over 1–2 h and to measure the PCV the following day once equilibration has occurred.

After venesection, the patient should feel improved with a clearer head, better exercise tolerance, less dyspnoea and a better appetite.

It is better to decide on venesection on the basis of the PCV rather than the haemoglobin level. Iron deficiency may develop with repeated venesection and should be treated with low dose oral iron (e.g. ferrous sulphate 200 mg once daily). Bigger doses will result in the patient requiring more frequent venesection. There is a fine balance between excessive venesection causing dyspnoea from anaemia and inadequate venesection causing it from hyperviscosity.

Bleeding Disorders

Paradoxically in a condition where thrombosis is common, bleeding abnormalities also occur. Platelet function may be abnormal and clotting factors may be deficient. There may be occult gastrointestinal bleeding from peptic ulceration and aspirin and non-steroidal anti-inflammatory agents should be avoided. Patients may have troublesome epistaxes or haemoptysis. The latter may be the result of rupture of aortopulmonary collaterals or larger PAs. This may be catastrophic and fatal. Fresh frozen plasma and/or platelet transfusions may be needed, especially pre- and post-cardiac catheterization or surgery. Cardiac catheterization should be avoided in the severely polycythaemic patient and delayed until after venesection, with the risks of contrast media inducing a deterioration in renal function and the risk of venous thrombosis.

Dental Hygiene
Frequent visits to the dentist are often necessary, because adults may contract periodontal disease and gingivitis. A dental brace is a particular hazard for this group, with the risks of infected gums seeding the circulation and causing a cerebral abscess.

Skin
Acne is a common problem and septic foci must be treated early. Long-term tetracycline therapy may be indicated.

Cerebral Abscess
This is a recognized hazard of dental or skin sepsis, the passage of bacteria across a septal defect being the result of the bidirectional shunt. The development of neurological symptoms or signs, drowsiness or a pyrexia of unknown origin (PUO) requires urgent investigation, a cerebral CT scan and a neurological expert.

Gout and Bone Pain
A common complaint that can usually be managed with long-term allopurinol 100–300 mg once daily. Renal function must be checked in these patients. Hypertrophic pulmonary osteoarthropathy may cause bone pain, with the periosteum reacting to an increase in growth factors.

Pregnancy and Contraception (see also Chapter 15)
This is contraindicated because it carries a very high maternal mortality rate (>60% with Eisenmenger VSDs). Spontaneous abortion is very common. It is very important to give early and clear contraceptive advice to all women with cyanotic congenital heart disease. The pill is best avoided (thrombosis risk); the intrauterine contraceptive device is also best avoided (bleeding and endocarditis risk). The best advice is sterilization by tubal ligation, which is probably achieved most safely by a mini-laparotomy rather than by a laparoscopic technique.

In the very unlikely event of a woman refusing all this advice and coming to term the outlook is grim. Caesarean section should be considered electively at 36–38 weeks, with great care paid to volume replacement and oxygenation. Epidural anaesthesia has been recommended rather than a general anaesthetic (see below) but the systemic vascular resistance must not fall.

High Altitudes
Heights of >1000 m should be avoided unless inhaled oxygen is available. Patients should receive inhaled oxygen throughout commercial flights and should avoid flights in light aircraft without oxygen.

Vigorous Exercise
This should be avoided. Right-to-left shunting may increase as SVR falls with muscle bed dilatation. Arrhythmias and sudden death have been provoked by effort.

Antibiotic Prophylaxis
This is routinely given before any dental or surgical procedure.

General Anaesthesia
This is not contraindicated but may be hazardous. Dehydration and hypotension must be avoided, with the risk of increasing the right-to-left shunt. Ketamine 1–2 mg/kg is a good drug for induction, having little effect on systemic or pulmonary vascular resistance. Volume replacement and small doses of phenylephrine (2 µg/kg) may be needed to keep up the arterial pressure. Postoperative heparinization will help prevent venous thrombosis.

Heart–Lung Transplantation (see also Section 6.15)
With a very limited donor supply, it is sensible to refer patients who may be suitable for this early rather than to wait for a crisis. Patients generally should be <50 years old. Results are not as good as for heart transplantation alone. The main indication for this is a rapid deterioration in symptoms, e.g.
• end-stage pulmonary vascular disease
• frequent haemoptysis
• syncope at rest
• refractory arrhythmias
• severe hypoxaemia causing angina
• refractory right heart failure.

Single-lung transplantation with correction of the intracardiac defect may be a possibility in the younger patient who is deteriorating. The results of this operation are not yet quite as good as combined heart and lung transplantation. Problems with the single-lung transplant include postoperative early pulmonary oedema in the transplanted lung, breakdown of the bronchial anastomosis and late obliterative bronchiolitis.

Relative contraindications to transplantation include:
• malignant disease
• moderate or severe renal or hepatic dysfunction (creatinine clearance <50 ml/min)
• severe chest deformity
• previous lung resection or pleurectomy
• positive serology (HIV, hepatitis B or C)

- pulmonary aspergillosis
- active infection
- on high-dose steroids
- multisystem disease, e.g. diabetes, collagen vascular disease
- active peptic ulceration
- peripheral vascular disease
- psychiatric condition, drug or alcohol abuser.

The final decision is team-based and also involves assessment of the patient's social circumstances, family support, etc. Both the patient and his or her family need to know both the risks of the operation and the subsequent management, which places considerable demands on them.

3 Valve Disease

3.1 Acute Rheumatic Fever

Although there has been a sharp reduction in the incidence of rheumatic fever in the last century in the western world, it is still the cause of almost half of the cardiac disease in the developing world, especially in the younger age groups. The decline of the disease in the UK has been ascribed partly to a reduction in virulence of *Streptococcus* species, partly to the reduction in over-crowding and improved living conditions, and partly to the early use of antibiotics for tonsillitis by general practitioners. However, we should not get complacent about rheumatic fever and think of it as a disease of the past; new cases still occur in the UK and recently there have been several outbreaks in the USA, not necessarily confined to the poorer areas. Peak age is 5–15 years. The disease is rare under the age of 5 years. It tends to be a recurrent illness unless prevented, with patients often having three or more attacks by the age of 20 years.

Aetiology

Pharyngeal infection with Lancefield group A streptococci triggers a subsequent attack of rheumatic fever about 2–3 weeks later in >3% of children.

Antigenic mimicry is thought to be the most likely explanation. A carbohydrate in the cell wall of the group A streptococci is similar to a glycoprotein in the human cardiac valve. It is thought that an autoimmune reaction occurs. Antibodies to the streptococcal cell wall cross-react with valve tissue: hence the latent period after the initial pharyngeal infection while the antibody response is mounted. Other cross-reacting antibodies have been found; one cross-reacting with the myocardial sarcolemma could account for the myocarditis, and another to the caudate nucleus for Sydenham's chorea. Anti-heart antibodies found during an acute attack may be the cause or the effect.

Swanton's Cardiology, sixth edition. By R. H. Swanton and S. Banerjee. Published 2008 Blackwell Publishing. ISBN 978-1-4051-7819-8.

Diagnosis

This is purely clinical. The Jones criteria (1944) have been revised several times and are shown below. For diagnosis there must be:
- evidence of a preceding β-haemolytic streptococcal infection
- two major criteria or
- one major and two minor criteria.

Revised Jones criteria for rheumatic fever diagnosis are listed in Table 3.1.

The differential diagnosis includes acute juvenile arthritis (Still's disease), a connective tissue disease, infective endocarditis, serum sickness, drug hypersensitivity and many viral illnesses causing pericarditis. Children frequently present with a fever and joint pains and have a soft, innocent mid-systolic flow murmur and a third heart sound. These alone are very non-specific.

Rheumatic fever can affect any of the cardiac tissues. It causes a pancarditis of the pericardium, myocardium (including the conduction tissue) and endocardium (including the valves). The histological marker is the Aschoff node (1904), which may persist in the myocardium long after the disease is over. Aschoff nodes may be found in the atrial appendage of patients who have had a closed mitral valvotomy.

Clinical Features

Carditis and arthritis are the only common features.

Carditis

This usually causes no symptoms in a first attack. The most common evidence is a soft pericardial rub or a soft apical pansystolic murmur of mitral regurgitation. An early diastolic murmur is very unusual in a first attack. Valve stenosis does not occur at this stage. There may be a soft mid-diastolic murmur (Carey Coombs' murmur) but this does not necessarily indicate subsequent mitral stenosis. There may be a small pericardial effusion, but tamponade or constriction does not occur. A prolonged PR interval on the ECG is non-specific.

Arthritis

This is a migrating polyarthritis, usually of larger joints, flitting from one joint to another. It does not cause chronic arthritis. If arthritis is used as a major criterion for the diagnosis, arthralgia cannot be used as a minor one.

Table 3.1 Revised Jones criteria for rheumatic fever diagnosis

Major	Minor	In addition
Carditis	Fever	Recent streptococcal infection
Arthritis	Previous rheumatic fever	History of scarlet fever
Sydenham's chorea	Raised ESR or CRP	Positive throat swab
Erythema marginatum	Arthralgia	Raised ASO titre
Subcutaneous nodules	Long PR interval	Raised anti-DNase B titre

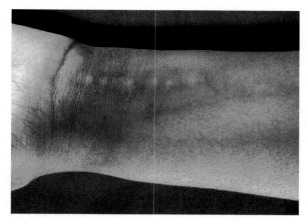

Figure 3.1 Acute rheumatic nodules.

Nodules
These are small (often smaller than a pea), mobile and painless on extensor surfaces of the elbows, wrists, ankles and spine. They are rare: probably <5% of cases (Figure 3.1).

Erythema Marginatum
This is also unusual. It occurs mainly on the trunk but not on the face. It is an evanescent geographical-type rash with slightly raised red edges and/or clear centre. The patches change shape with time. It does not itch and is not indurated.

Sydenham's Chorea (St Vitus' Dance)
This does not occur until several months after rheumatic fever. Unilateral or bilateral, involuntary, quasi-purposeful movements are sometimes associated with facial grimacing. As the initial illness is easily missed this may be the first manifestation of the disease.

Investigations
There are no specific tests. ESR and CRP, anti-streptolysin O and anti-DNase B titres are measured and should be raised, or be rising, on the second estimate. Anti-hyaluronidase antibody also serves as a measure of previous streptococcal infection. Echocardiography is used to detect the very early changes of stretching of the anterior mitral chordae.

Treatment
Treatment with salicylates or steroids does not prevent the development of subsequent rheumatic heart disease. It is important to establish the diagnosis, which may mean waiting until arthritis or carditis is definite. Treatment includes the following:

• Salicylates rapidly reduce fever and arthritis. Dose is 100 mg/kg per day in children. Serum salicylate levels should be 15–20 mg/100 ml. Toxicity produces tinnitus and hyperventilation.
• Steroids are used rather than salicylates for patients with definite carditis. Prednisolone about 3 mg/kg per day in divided doses for 2 weeks, tapering off quickly. If symptoms recur the course is restarted.
• Diazepam is used for Sydenham's chorea. Neither salicylates nor steroids have any effect on this.
• Penicillin: immediate treatment with benzathine penicillin 1.2 MU i.m. eliminates any remaining streptococci. Prevention of further attacks by using phenoxymethylpenicillin 250 mg twice daily on a regular basis until the patient is considered beyond risk (e.g. up to the age of 30 years). For penicillin hypersensitivity use sulfadiazine 500 mg twice daily.

Most cases settle within 4–6 weeks. Occasional cases need longer courses of therapy plus treatment for CCF. Long-term myocardial damage is often forgotten in the concentration on valve lesions.

3.2 Mitral Stenosis

This is almost always secondary to rheumatic fever, although only half the patients have a positive history. The incidence is declining although many cases from developing countries are severe. Two-thirds of patients are female.

Aetiology

Valvar
• Rheumatic: almost all cases; all the rest are rare
• Congenital: isolated lesion or associated with ASD (Lutembacher syndrome); some of these cases may be rheumatic mitral stenosis plus a patent foramen ovale
• Mucopolysaccharidoses: Hurler syndrome; glycoprotein deposition on the mitral leaflets
• Endocardial fibroelastosis spreading on to the valve
• Prosthetic valve: rare and usually only in earlier design mechanical valves (e.g. Starr–Edwards, Björk–Shiley)
• Malignant carcinoid.

Inflow Obstruction
Conditions that mimic mitral stenosis, e.g.
• Left atrial myxoma (see Section 11.6)
• Left atrial ball valve thrombus
• Hypertrophic obstructive cardiomyopathy (see Section 4.2)
• Cor triatriatum (stenosis of a common pulmonary vein).

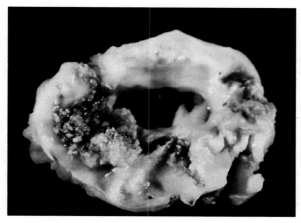

Figure 3.2 Rheumatic calcific mitral stenosis: excised valve.

Pathogenesis

Group A (usually type 12) streptococci have cell wall antigens that cross-react with structural glycoproteins of the heart valves. Very small nodules (macrophages and fibroblasts) develop on the valve edge and the cusp gradually thickens. Stenosis occurs at three levels:

1 Commissures: these fuse with the valve cusps still mobile.
2 Cusps: the valve leaflets become thick and eventually calcified.
3 Chordae: these fuse, shorten and thicken.

A combination of all three results in a 'fish-mouth' buttonhole orifice (Figure 3.2).

Pathophysiology and Symptoms

Dyspnoea on Effort

This is orthopnoea and PND. A rising left atrial pressure is transmitted to pulmonary veins. Secondary pulmonary arterial hypertension results. Pulmonary oedema may be precipitated by:

- development of uncontrolled AF
- pregnancy
- exercise
- chest infection
- emotional stress
- anaesthesia.

Fatigue

This is caused by low cardiac output in moderate-to-severe stenosis. A doubling of cardiac output quadruples the mitral valve gradient. The loss of atrial transport when AF develops results in a fall in cardiac output. Exercise tolerance on the basis of four classes is based on the New York Heart Association (NYHA) criteria (see Section 1.1).

Haemoptysis

This may be a result of the following:
- Bronchial vein rupture: 'pulmonary apoplexy', large haemorrhage but not usually life-threatening
- Alveolar capillary rupture: pink frothy sputum in pulmonary oedema
- Pulmonary infarction: in low-output states and immobile patients
- Blood-stained sputum: in chronic bronchitis associated with attacks of dyspnoea.

Systemic Emboli

These occur in 20–30%.

Thrombus develops in large 'stagnant' left atrium and atrial appendage, mainly in patients with AF, low output and large atria. It may be the presenting symptom. Mesenteric, saddle and iliofemoral emboli are common. Ball valve thrombus may occur in LA.

Chronic Bronchitis

This is common in MS, and is caused by oedematous bronchial mucosa.

Chest Pain

This is similar to angina. In patients with RV hypertrophy secondary to pulmonary hypertension – even with normal coronaries. Coronary embolism may occur.

Palpitations

These cause paroxysmal AF with fast ventricular response.

Symptoms of Right Heart Failure

These are pulmonary hypertension and possible functional tricuspid regurgitation: hepatic pain on effort (hepatic angina), ascites, ankle and leg oedema.

Symptoms of Left Atrial Enlargement Compressing Other Structures
- Left recurrent laryngeal nerve, hoarseness (Ortner syndrome)
- Oesophagus, dysphagia (beware potassium replacement tablets causing oesophageal ulceration)
- Left main bronchus, very rarely causing left lung collapse.

Infective Endocarditis

This is rare in pure MS (see Section 9.1).

Physical Signs (Figure 3.3)

- Mitral facies (Figure 3.4)
- Dilated telangiectases on cheeks and bridge of nose.

The cause is unknown but occurs with the development of pulmonary hypertension.

The differential diagnosis includes: weather-beaten appearance, butterfly rash of SLE, acne rosacea and carcinoid syndrome. Mitral facies disappear if the mitral stenosis is corrected and PA pressure falls.

Other Points to Note

- S_1 is loud, because the mitral valve is open throughout diastole and is suddenly slammed shut by ventricular systole. It indicates mobile leaflets.
- A_2–OS interval shortens with increasing severity of stenosis (OS is the opening sound). LA pressure 'climbs' up LV pressure curve, approaching in time aortic valve closure (Figure 3.5) (see Cardiac Catheterization below).

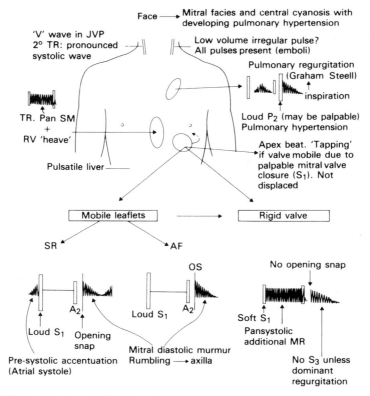

Figure 3.3 Physical signs of mitral stenosis.

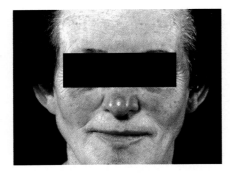

Figure 3.4 Mitral facies.

- The length of the diastolic murmur is an indication of the severity of the stenosis.
- As the mitral valve calcifies, S1 and the opening snap disappear, and additional mitral regurgitation appears.

Differential Diagnosis
- Causes of inflow obstruction (HCM, LA myxoma, ball-valve thrombus)
- Causes of rumbling mitral or tricuspid diastolic murmur:
  - aortic regurgitation (see Section 3.5; Austin–Flint)
  - flow murmur in ASD; this may be confusing (Figure 3.6)

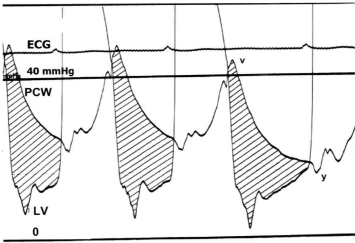

MITRAL STENOSIS and REGURGITATION

Figure 3.5 Mixed mitral valve disease: measurement of LV pressure and pulmonary capillary wedge pressure (PCW) with the mitral valve gradient shaded. Prominent 'v' wave resulting from additional mitral regurgitation. The wedge pressure traces are always slightly delayed compared with direct LA pressure measurement.

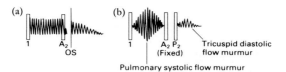

Figure 3.6 Similarity on auscultation between (a) mixed mitral valve disease and (b) ASD.

   – tricuspid stenosis, diastolic murmur accentuated by inspiration; best sign is slow 'y' descent on JVP
* Causes of early diastolic sound resembling opening snap:
   – constrictive pericarditis
   – restrictive myopathy
   – sudden cessation of early rapid ventricular filling
* Causes of loud S1: tachycardia and hyperdynamic states (valve still open at end diastole, and forceful closure by hypercontractile LV).

ECG
* AF (in sinus rhythm P mitrale)
* RV hypertrophy
* Small voltage in lead V1
* Progressive right axis deviation.

Echocardiography (see Section 17.3)
In pure MS with mobile leaflets this obviates the need for cardiac catheterization. It may show the following:
* Thickened mitral leaflets with the posterior leaflet moving anteriorly in diastole. Mitral opening coincides with snap on phonocardiogram.
* Reduced diastolic closure rate (E–F) slope of mitral anterior leaflet.
* Small LV (unless additional MR present). Slow diastolic filling.
* Pulmonary valve may be flat with absent 'a' wave opening (in pulmonary hypertension).
* Calcification of mitral leaflets or mitral annulus.

   Echocardiography is also very useful in distinguishing the 'mimics' of MS. It will diagnose a left atrial myxoma, HCM and aortic regurgitation. It is very useful as a guide to the severity of mitral stenosis and to document the results of mitral valvotomy. The mobility of the mitral leaflets is easily seen with this technique.

Cardiac Catheterization
This should be unnecessary in a young patient with a mobile valve and no signs of mitral regurgitation. It is contraindicated in pregnancy when echocardiography is essential. A patient with an atrial myxoma diagnosed by echocardiography should not be catheterized unless there is a particular suspicion of

coronary disease, in which case coronary angiography alone may be necessary. (The LV catheter may knock fragments off a prolapsing myxoma.) A myxoma requires urgent surgery (see Section 11.6).

Cardiac catheterization is advisable in patients who have had a previous valvotomy in order to assess the mitral valve and the degree of regurgitation. It is necessary in patients with signs of mitral regurgitation. Doppler echocardiography can be diagnostic (see Section 17.3).

Catheterization is also required in patients with signs of other valve disease, symptoms of angina (coronary angiography), signs of severe pulmonary hypertension and when the mitral valve is calcified on chest radiograph (Figures 3.7, 3.8 and 3.9). If mitral valve replacement is envisaged, coronary angiography is usually performed (especially in elderly people).

The mean mitral gradient is calculated at rest and, if this is low, also on exercise (straight-leg raising). The mitral valve area can be calculated if the cardiac output is measured (see Section 16.3). Grades of severity in MS are shown in Table 3.2.

Table 3.2 Assessment of severity of mitral stenosis from echocardiography or catheter data

	Mild	Moderate	Severe
Mean mitral gradient (mmHg)	<5	5–10	>10
PA systolic pressure (mmHg)	<30	30–50	>50
Mitral valve area (cm^2)	>1.5	1.0–1.5	<1.0

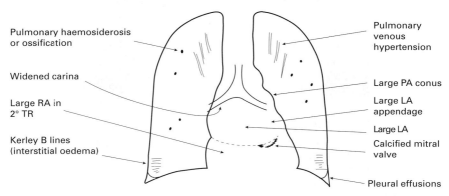

Figure 3.7 Chest radiograph in mitral stenosis.

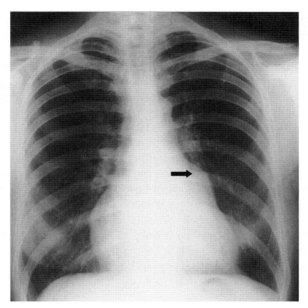

Figure 3.8 PA Chest radiograph: moderate mitral stenosis – enlarged left atrial appendage (arrowed), LV size normal, small aortic knuckle.

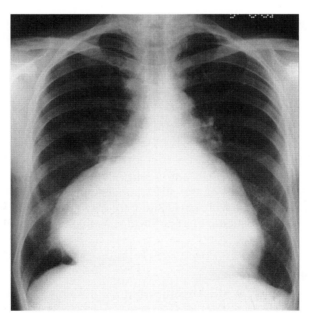

Figure 3.9 Severe long-standing mitral stenosis, pulmonary hypertension, giant atria.

Medical Treatment
• Digoxin: in AF only. If fast AF is not slowed by standard doses, either a small dose of verapamil or β-blocking agent should be added. There is no evidence that digoxin prevents the development of AF in patients who are still in sinus rhythm.
• Diuretics are necessary to reduce preload and pulmonary venous congestion. They may help delay the need for surgery.
• Anticoagulants are still controversial. They should be used in patients who:
  – have had a previous systemic/pulmonary embolism
  – have a mitral prosthesis (tissue or mechanical)
  – have low-output states with right heart failure
  – are in AF with moderate mitral stenosis and who have not had an atrial appendicectomy.
Anticoagulants are not of proven benefit in sinus rhythm. They should be avoided in pregnancy if possible (see Section 3.8 and 15.7). Patients who have had a mitral valvotomy and atrial appendicectomy can probably be managed without anticoagulants provided that they do not fall into the above categories.

Cardioversion (see Section 8.3)
This may be attempted if the development of AF is recent and the patient is anticoagulated. If not, there is a risk of systemic emboli.

Heparinization for 24 hours before cardioversion is not adequate. There is nothing to be gained by repeated cardioversions. AF should be accepted and the ventricular rate slowed. Amiodarone β blockade or flecainide may help prevent the development of AF in patients who have been successfully cardioverted.

Infective Endocarditis (see Section 9.1)
This is rare in pure MS.

Acute Rheumatic Fever
This should be thought of in any young patient presenting for the first time with MS. Histology of the atrial appendage will help in diagnosis. Prevent further attacks with penicillin 250 mg twice daily or sulfadiazine 500 mg twice daily. It should be continued in young women to the age of 40 years.

Intervention
Symptomatic decline in MS is gradual but the development of AF usually causes a sharp deterioration in symptoms. Some form of intervention is needed in those patients with class 3 or 4 NYHA effort tolerance and some

patients with class 2 who find it difficult to work or to manage the housework. Mitral valve area <1 cm^2 is an indication for intervention. This now consists of mitral valvuloplasty, open mitral valvotomy or mitral valve replacement. There is still no perfect mitral prosthesis, and intervention aims to preserve, where possible, the native mitral valve, especially in the younger patient.

Mitral Valvuloplasty

The development of the Inoue balloon is a great advance from the original double-balloon and two-wire technique, and mitral valvuloplasty has now replaced the operation of closed mitral valvotomy. It is the technique of choice for patients with pure MS but no regurgitation or mitral valve calcification. It can be performed in any age group; however, the results are best in the younger age group where the subvalve mitral chordae have not become thickened and fused. It can be performed in the mid-trimester of pregnancy.

Before mitral valvuloplasty it is important to establish, using transoesophageal echocardiography, that there is no thrombus in the left atrial appendage. Transthoracic echocardiography cannot be relied on for this information. Valvuloplasty is avoided with:
- left atrial or left ventricular thrombus
- a history of systemic emboli
- >grade 1 mitral regurgitation
- thickened rigid mitral leaflets
- thickened fused mitral chordae
- moderate or severe mitral calcification.

Figures 3.10, 3.11 and 3.12 show the technique. The procedure requires only light sedation, as with a routine cardiac catheter. The choice of balloon size (26, 28 or 30 mm) is dictated by the patient's height (Table 3.3).

After trans-septal puncture via the right femoral vein, the Inoue balloon is advanced into the left atrium over a curly guidewire (Figure 3.10a). The distal portion of the balloon is inflated slightly and the balloon advanced to the apex of the left ventricle (Figures 3.10b and 3.11). The balloon is then gradually withdrawn until it is positioned across the mitral valve and free of the sub-valve apparatus (Figure 3.10c). On balloon inflation the distal portion inflates first, then the proximal portion, to form an hourglass shape with the waist across the mitral valve (Figures 3.10d and 3.12). Finally, with continuing

Table 3.3 Calculation of Inoue balloon size

Patient height (cm)	Maximum balloon diameter (mm)
≤147	24
>147	26
>160	28
>180	30

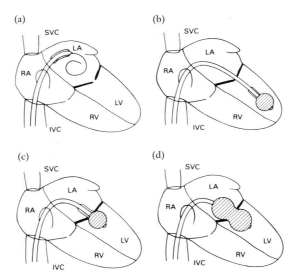

Figure 3.10 Stages in mitral valvuloplasty: (a) the balloon is advanced to the left atrium via a trans-septal puncture and curly guidewire through the fossa ovalis. (b) The guidewire is withdrawn, the distal portion of the balloon is inflated and advanced to the left ventricle. (c) The balloon is drawn back to the mitral valve. (d) The balloon is fully inflated. The proximal portion of the balloon now inflates forming an hourglass shape, and this waist finally disappears with maximum inflation.

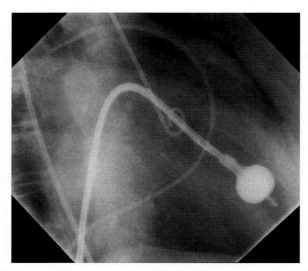

Figure 3.11 Mitral valvuloplasty. Inoue balloon: initial inflation of distal part of balloon in left ventricle.

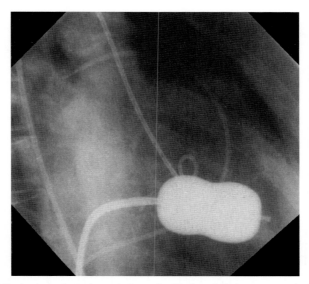

Figure 3.12 Mitral valvuloplasty. Inoue balloon: final balloon inflation across mitral valve.

inflation the waist disappears and the commissures are split. The residual mitral valve gradient is measured directly (Figure 3.13) and the degree of mitral regurgitation, if any, assessed by left ventriculography or Doppler echocardiography. In correctly selected patients the results are startlingly good with at least a doubling of the valve area. A tiny ASD is left but this is of no significance and the shunt if any is trivial. Long-term results are as good as a closed valvotomy with benefit expected for 10–15 years.

An echocardiographic score has been devised (Wilkins) that is useful prognostically, but does not include information on commissural fusion. Valve leaflet mobility, thickening, calcification and subvalve chordal thickening are graded 0–4 and added together (worst possible score 16). High scores (>10) fare badly. A low LVEDP is also important as a good prognostic indicator.

Surgery
Closed Mitral Valvotomy (Closed Commissurotomy)
This is performed through a left thoracotomy without bypass. It is rarely performed now as a result of the development of mitral valvuloplasty. The contraindications to a closed valvotomy are the same as for valvuloplasty (see above), but also include patients with severe lung disease or chest deformity, and elderly frail patients in whom a valvuloplasty may still be possible.

Open Mitral Valvotomy (Open Commissurotomy)
This is performed on cardiopulmonary bypass (CBP) through a median sternotomy. It is used in patients who have already had a mitral procedure (previous closed valvotomy or valvuloplasty) or in whom there are other features,

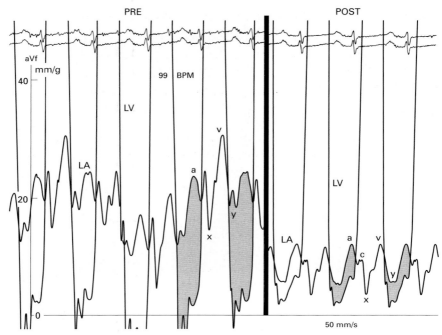

Figure 3.13 Mitral valvuloplasty: recordings of left atrial pressure (LA) and left ventricular pressure (LV) in a woman with mitral stenosis pre- and post-valvuloplasty. Sinus rhythm throughout. The mitral gradient is shaded for comparison in two representative beats. There is a fall in LA pressure after successful valvuloplasty and a reduction in the mitral valve gradient.

e.g. mild mitral regurgitation or calcification, a history of emboli or demonstrable thrombus in the left atrium, or in whom there is concern about the subvalve chordae.

Mitral Valve Replacement

This is needed for heavily calcified and rigid mitral valves (see Figure 3.2), or for those with unacceptable mitral regurgitation, severe chordal thickening and fusion or two previous valvotomies or valvuloplasties.

Mitral re-stenosis occurs over a period of years after valvuloplasty or valvotomy. It is caused by turbulent flow across thickened valve leaflets resulting in platelet and fibrin deposition. It is least likely to occur where a good valvuloplasty or valvotomy with pliable leaflets results in good mitral flow. Early re-stenosis (within 5 years) usually means an inadequate valvuloplasty or valvotomy. Patients may do well with an open valvotomy. Late re-stenosis may need valve replacement as a result of degenerative change and calcification in the valve.

3.3 Mitral Regurgitation

This may be caused by abnormalities of the mitral annulus, mitral leaflets, chordae or papillary muscles. Chordal or papillary muscle dysfunction gives rise to subvalvar mitral regurgitation. Many disease processes affect the valve at more than one level.

Aetiology (Table 3.4)

Functional Mitral Regurgitation
This is probably a combination of mitral annulus dilatation and papillary muscle malalignment. It occurs in LV dilatation from any cause, commonly in dilated cardiomyopathy (DCM) and ischaemic heart disease.

Annulus Calcification
This occurs in elderly people and is more common in women, and people with diabetes or Paget's disease. It commonly affects the posterior part of the mitral annulus and is often visible as a calcified band at the back of the heart on the lateral chest radiograph with calcium in the posterior AV groove. The calcium may involve the mitral leaflets, causing mitral regurgitation, and eventually the conducting system. Very severe ring calcification may make mitral valve replacement (MVR) impossible. In its milder form it causes no mitral valve problem and may be a chance finding on chest radiograph or echocardiography.

Mitral annular calcification is an independent risk factor for stroke with a relative risk twice that of controls. This is independent of other risk factors such as AF or CCF.

Valvar Regurgitation
This is commonly caused by rheumatic fever, infective endocarditis or a floppy valve. In rheumatic causes the cusps are thickened, with fused commissures and often a 'fish-mouth' orifice (Figure 3.2). Patients commonly have combined MS and MR.

Chordal Rupture
This is often idiopathic. Myxomatous degeneration in the floppy valve syndrome may also involve the chordae, which stretch and eventually rupture. Ischaemia may cause chordal rupture.

Papillary Muscle Dysfunction
Inferior infarction commonly causes posterior papillary muscle dysfunction with characteristic signs (see below). Anterior papillary muscle dysfunction is much rarer and signifies a large anterior infarct with probable additional right coronary artery disease.

Table 3.4 Aetiology of mitral regurgitation

Mitral annulus	Mitral leaflets	Connective tissues disorders	Chordae	Papillary muscles
Senile calcification	*Infective*	*Connective tissues disorders*	*Elongation/rupture*	*Dysfunction/rupture*
Degeneration	Endocarditis	Marfan syndrome	Marfan syndrome	Ischaemia
Functional dilatation	Rheumatic	PXE	Ischaemia	Infarction
Ring abscesses		Osteogenesis imperfecta	Endocarditis	Abscess
Marfan syndrome		Ehlers–Danlos syndrome	Trauma	Infiltrations
			Rheumatic	Sarcoid
			Idiopathic	Amyloid
			Ehlers–Danlos syndrome	Myocarditis
			Parachute MV	Hurler syndrome
		Floppy valve		*Malalignment*
				LV dilatation
				LV aneurysm
				HCM
				Endocardial fibroelastosis
				Corrected TGA

The Floppy Valve

This forms a spectrum of conditions from an asymptomatic patient with a midsystolic click, to one with severe MR from chordal rupture. It has also been called mitral leaflet prolapse, mitral click systolic murmur syndrome, Barlow syndrome, myxomatous degeneration of the mitral valve and billowing mitral valve syndrome. The condition occurs as the following:
• An isolated lesion often in asymptomatic patients
• Associated with other conditions, e.g. secundum ASD, Turner syndrome, PDA, Marfan syndrome, osteogenesis imperfecta, PXE, cardiomyopathy, Wolff–Parkinson–White (WPW) syndrome.

It occurs in approximately 4% of the normal asymptomatic population. It has been grossly overdiagnosed echocardiographically and may become a cause of cardiac neurosis. It is caused by progressive stretching of the mitral leaflets, with weakening as a result of acid mucopolysaccharide deposition in the zona spongiosa. The chordae are also involved. Tricuspid prolapse may coexist.
• Some patients have non-specific atypical chest pain (non-anginal) and palpitations.
• Infective endocarditis prophylaxis is necessary for those patients with a murmur. An isolated mid-systolic click does not merit it.
• Rarely, complications develop, e.g.: progressive MR requiring MVR; cerebral emboli; dysrhythmias may be ventricular with associated re-entry and pre-excitation pathways; sudden death.
• In an extreme form aneurysmal dilatation of a leaflet may occur (Figure 3.14).

Pathophysiology and Symptoms

Mild cases of MR may be asymptomatic for many years. Most patients fall into one of two groups depending on the time course of events and the size/compliance of the left atrium (Table 3.5).

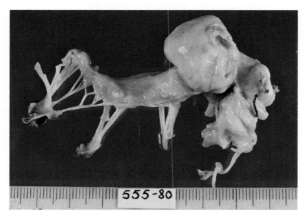

Figure 3.14 Mitral valve aneurysm (not infected).

Table 3.5 Acute versus chronic mitral regurgitation

Acute	Chronic
Sudden-onset dyspnoea and pulmonary oedema	Chronic dyspnoea and fatigue
Small left atrium	Large left atrium
'Non-compliant'	'Compliant'
Usually still in SR	Usually in AF
? Apical thrill if chordal rupture	? Associated mitral stenosis
Often honking ejection systolic murmur	Pansystolic murmur
Pulmonary hypertension	Pulmonary hypertension less severe
Large 'v' wave in wedge trace (Figure 3.17)	Lower 'v' wave on wedge trace except on effort
Common causes	
Chordal rupture	Rheumatic valve
Acute inferior infarction with posterior papillary muscle dysfunction (rupture is rarer)	Floppy valve
Infective endocarditis	Functional MR

In acute MR the small LA cannot absorb the regurgitant fraction and the systolic wave is transmitted to the pulmonary veins, with resulting acute pulmonary oedema. In long-standing MR the LA is large; it can absorb the regurgitant fraction and the 'v' wave transmitted to the pulmonary veins is smaller (Table 3.5).

Symptoms are similar to MS in the chronic state. Haemoptysis and systemic emboli are less frequent.

Generally, pulmonary hypertension and right heart symptoms are not as frequent in MR as in pure MS. Infective endocarditis is more common in MR, however.

Physical Signs in the Floppy Valve Syndrome
These vary with the degree of MR. With mild or moderate degrees of MR, the following signs peculiar to the floppy valve syndrome occur. With severe regurgitation physical signs are less specific.

Apex Beat
A double apex may be noted in some patients with a floppy valve. Tensing of the chordae in midsystole may cause this midsystolic dip. It is felt best when the patient is lying on his or her left side.

Murmurs
As LV volume diminishes in midsystole the floppy valve starts to prolapse and a midsystolic click (tensing of chordae) often precedes the murmur of MR (there may be more than one click). In very mild cases a midsystolic click with no murmur is common.

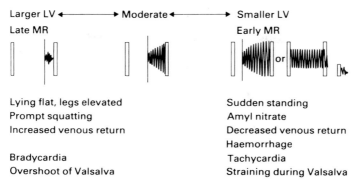

Larger LV ◀──────▶ Moderate ◀──────▶ Smaller LV

Late MR   Early MR

Lying flat, legs elevated	Sudden standing
Prompt squatting	Amyl nitrate
Increased venous return	Decreased venous return
	Haemorrhage
Bradycardia	Tachycardia
Overshoot of Valsalva	Straining during Valsalva

Figure 3.15 Mitral regurgitation in the floppy valve syndrome.

The smaller the ventricle the earlier the systolic click and the longer the murmur, which gets louder up to S2 (crescendo in quality). The signs may be altered by various manoeuvres in a similar way to HCM (see Section 4.2) (Figure 3.15).

Differential Diagnosis
• *Aortic valve stenosis*: the floppy valve has a normal or slightly collapsing pulse. The midsystolic click occurs after the carotid upstroke.
• *HCM*: this is more difficult because both may have similar pulses, double apex beats and murmurs getting louder on amyl nitrate inhalation. HCM does not have a midsystolic click and has more LV+.
• *VSD*: here the murmur is usually pansystolic with a thrill, both maximum at the left sternal edge. Differentiation from subvalvar regurgitation with posterior chordal rupture may be impossible clinically, especially if associated with MI.
• *Papillary muscle dysfunction*: classically post-inferior infarct. The murmur may be late systolic but without a click. In the more severe cases the murmur is pansystolic.
• *Tricuspid regurgitation*: an 'inspiratory' murmur loudest at the left sternal edge. Best sign is prominent systolic waves in the JVP.

Physical Signs in Chronic Valvar MR (Figure 3.16)
• Sudden premature ventricular emptying as a result of MR causes early aortic valve closure. The murmur may continue through A_2. S_2 is thus more than normally split and P_2 may be loud if additional pulmonary hypertension is present.
• Features to suggest chordal rupture as opposed to valvar regurgitation:
  – sinus rhythm
  – apical thrill in systole
  – murmur, which is more ejection in quality and sometimes mid- to late systolic.

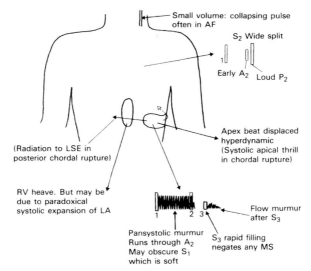

Figure 3.16 Physical signs in chronic valvar mitral regurgitation.

• In posterior chordal rupture the jet is directed to the anterior wall of the left atrium. The murmur is often loudest at the left sternal edge. In anterior chordal rupture the jet is directed posteriorly and the murmur may be loudest in the back.

Important Points in MR Clinically
• The intensity of the systolic murmur is absolutely no guide to the severity of the regurgitation. Prosthetic valve regurgitation may be inaudible
• A murmur maximal at the left sternal edge may be MR
• Mitral regurgitant murmurs may be pansystolic, late-crescendo systolic or ejection systolic in quality
• Check that P_2 moves on inspiration to exclude an ASD.

ECG
• AF in chronic disease; if in SR: LA+
• LVH
• A few cases show RVH in addition.

Echocardiography (see Section 17.3)
• To show left atrial size with systolic expansion
• May show a flail mitral leaflet with chaotic movement
• May show posterior mitral leaflet prolapse – late or pansystolic: vegetations on mitral valve, mitral annulus calcification
• Dilated LV with rapid filling; dimensions relate to prognosis

Table 3.6 Assessment of severity of mitral regurgitation using Doppler signal or echo measurements

	Mild	Moderate	Severe
Doppler vena contracta width (cm)	<0.3	0.3–0.69	>0.7
Regurgitant volume (ml/beat)	<30	30–59	>60
Regurgitant fraction	<30	30–49	>50
Regurgitant orifice area (ROA) (cm^2)	<0.2	0.2–0.39	>0.4
Angiographic grade	1	2	3–4

• Rapid diastolic mitral closure rate (steep E–F slope) caused by rapid filling
• Mean VCF (circumferential fibre shortening) often increased with good LV function
• Possibly additional floppy tricuspid or aortic valves
• Doppler will establish size and site of regurgitation jet (Table 3.6 and Section 17.3)
• Transoesophageal echocardiography will give the clearest view of the mitral leaflets or of a malfunctioning prosthetic valve.

Chest Radiograph
• LV dilatation enlarging the ventricular mass and left heart border.
• LA dilatation in chronic cases. Rarely, giant left atrium may occur with calcified wall.
• Mitral valve calcification, signs of pulmonary venous congestion, Kerley B lines as in MS.

Cardiac Catheterization
It is necessary to confirm the diagnosis and exclude other valve and coronary disease. LV function is assessed. Coronary angiography is also performed.

The size of the 'v' wave in the pulmonary wedge or left atrial pressure trace depends on the severity of MR and the size of the left atrium. In severe cases of acute MR the 'v' wave may reach 50 mmHg or more (Figure 3.17). The height of the 'v' wave increases sharply with effort.

LV angiography in the 30° RAO projection will show the severity of the regurgitation. In severe cases the regurgitant jet fills the pulmonary veins in one systole. The angiogram will also help identify the cause. In rheumatic MR there are usually one or more discrete jets through an immobile valve with associated stenosis.

In the floppy valve or chordal rupture the regurgitant jet is over a broad front, and the prolapsing leaflet can usually be seen. Posterior papillary muscle dysfunction is usually associated with inferior hypokinesia. Spurious MR may be produced by ectopic beats or by a catheter too near the mitral valve or subvalve apparatus.

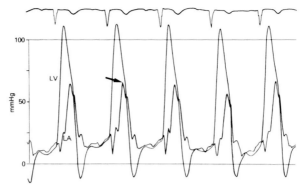

Figure 3.17 Mitral regurgitation: simultaneous recordings of LV and LA pressures (recorded from PA wedge position) in a patient with acute mural regurgitation from ruptured chordae. The 'v' wave reaches 60 mmHg as a result of the severe regurgitation and the small left atrium. The patient is still in sinus rhythm. The peak of the 'v' wave is arrowed.

Medical Treatment (see Section 6.4; heart failure)
- As in mitral stenosis fast AF is treated with digoxin.
- Anticoagulants are not indicated unless there is: a history of systemic embolism; a prosthetic mitral valve, either xenograft or mechanical; additional mitral stenosis with a low output or AF.
- Diuretics are needed to reduce pulmonary venous congestion and LV preload.
- Afterload reduction with intravenous nitrates or nitroprusside is indicated in acute MR by helping to reduce the regurgitant fraction and increase forward stroke volume. Afterload reduction in acute MR is less successful than in aortic regurgitation. ACE inhibitors are used routinely but with little evidence of their long-term benefit.
- In acute MR with chordal rupture and pulmonary oedema, a continuous positive airway pressure (CPAP) mask or artificial ventilation and full monitoring as in cardiogenic shock may be necessary (see Section 6.14).
- Infective endocarditis should be considered (see Section 9.1).

Prognosis
As in chronic aortic regurgitation, chronic MR is a relatively well-tolerated lesion if LV function is preserved. About 60% of patients with chronic MR are alive 10 years later. The problem is that LV deterioration is masked by the unloading effect of the leaking mitral valve. Patients may remain virtually asymptomatic while LV function deteriorates, and this determines prognosis. The following are poorer prognostic features:
- Symptomatic history >1 year
- AF
- Patients aged >60 years
- Angiographic ejection fraction <50%

- Angiographic LVEDV >100 ml/m^2 and LVESV >60 ml/m^2
- Echocardiographic dimensions of left ventricle: end-systolic dimension >5 cm; end-diastolic dimension >7 cm.

Surgery

All patients with pure MR should have transoesophageal echocardiography (TOE) before the operation to help determine which are suitable for mitral valve repair. In severe acute MR with pulmonary oedema, this will need to be done on a ventilated patient. The TOE is repeated intraoperatively immediately after the repair to check for residual valve regurgitation. Up to 40% of cases thought to be suitable for valve repair need a valve replacement. MVR for pure MR has been less successful than for pure MS, possibly because MVR has been delayed until LV function is irreversibly impaired. The overall operative mortality rate is 6% for elective surgery. Chordal preservation at surgery helps preserve LV function. Some recovery of LV function after surgery is possible but this may take many months.

Acute MR with Chordal Rupture

Surgery is necessary in most cases because medical treatment alone carries a poor prognosis. Mitral valve repair may be possible in some cases (e.g. plication of mitral cleft or commissure, advancement of posterior cusp in floppy valve). Generally repair is reserved for a single prolapsing leaflet, with valve replacement preferred if both leaflets are involved.

Chronic MR

MVR should be performed before LV function deteriorates irreversibly. Surgery is indicated for symptoms of increasing fatigue and dyspnoea (NYHA classes 3 and 4), and in patients with class 2 symptoms who have enlarging heart on chest radiograph and increasing dyspnoea. Annuloplasty is generally not a very satisfactory procedure although is sometimes useful in patients with a grossly dilated mitral annulus (as in a dilated cardiomyopathy).

Post-infarct MR

Papillary muscle infarction or rupture usually requires urgent MVR without delay. Intensive vasodilator therapy or IABP may hold the situation for a few hours but is no substitute for surgery.

3.4 Aortic Stenosis

Levels of Aortic Stenosis

Aortic stenosis may occur at three levels and the three are not mutually exclusive:

1 Valvar aortic stenosis
2 Supravalvar aortic stenosis
3 Subvalvar aortic stenosis. This may be result from:

– discrete fibromuscular ring
– HCM
– tunnel subaortic stenosis
– anomalous attachment of anterior mitral leaflet, e.g. in AV canal, or parachute deformity of mitral valve with fused papillary muscles.

Various anatomical combinations may occur: a discrete fibromuscular ring with supravalvar stenosis and/or a grossly hypertrophic upper septum. In severe cases in childhood the term 'higgledy-piggledy' left heart has been used by Somerville to describe pathology in the subvalve region, the valve and aorta occurring together.

The term 'fixed subaortic' stenosis has been used to describe a group of conditions: discrete fibromuscular ring and tunnel subaortic stenosis as opposed to variable obstruction caused by muscular hypertrophy in HCM. The division is artificial because the conditions may coexist, and 'fixed' obstruction may be gradually acquired.

Valvar Aortic Stenosis

This is the most common cause of aortic stenosis. It does not have a single aetiology (Figure 3.18).

Congenital Valvar Abnormality

The most common cause of isolated aortic stenosis, 72% in one series. More frequent in males (4:1):

• Bicuspid valve (about 1% of the population): the most common form of congenital heart disease. Both types become increasingly fibrotic and calcified with age, the bicuspid valve being the most common cause of aortic valve stenosis in the age group 40 to ≥60 years.

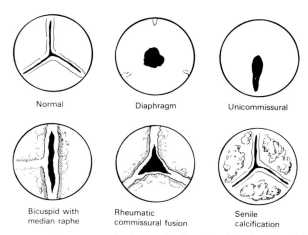

Normal Diaphragm Unicommissural

Bicuspid with median raphe Rheumatic commissural fusion Senile calcification

Figure 3.18 Diagrammatic summary of valvar aortic stenosis with valve viewed from above.

• Other degrees of commissural fusion: unicommissural with eccentric hole, or even diaphragm (three fused cusps) with central orifice. Unicuspid aortic valve is the most common cause of aortic stenosis presenting under the age of 1 year. It often presents as part of the hypoplastic left heart syndrome.

Senile Calcification of a Normal Valve
Occurs in those aged >60 years. The valve is tricuspid. The commissures are not fused, but the cusps are immobilized by heavy calcification. This often causes an ejection systolic murmur, although frank aortic valve stenosis is not so common.

Inflammatory Valvulitis
Rheumatic fever results in commissural fusion of a tricuspid valve. The valve is usually also regurgitant also (Figure 3.18). Rheumatoid arthritis may cause nodular thickening of aortic valve leaflets and, rarely, a degree of aortic stenosis usually with regurgitation.

Atherosclerosis
Severe hypercholesterolaemia in homozygous type II hyperlipoproteinaemia. Gross atheroma involves aortic wall, major arteries, aortic valve and coronary arteries.

Disease Progression
Valvar obstruction gradually increases even in children who may be asymptomatic. Progressive valve calcification occurs and may be visible on the chest radiograph from about the age of 40 years onwards. The severity of the calcification correlates roughly with the degree of stenosis.

Pathophysiology and Symptoms
• *Compensated*: good LV function with valve area >$1\,cm^2$. May be asymptomatic. Children may be asymptomatic even with severe disease. Adults may not present until age > 60 years.
• *Angina*: occurs with normal coronary arteries. Caused by imbalance of myocardial oxygen supply/demand (Table 3.7).
• *Dyspnoea*: occurs as a result of high diastolic pressures in the left ventricle increasing with exercise. As LV function deteriorates (or AF occurs) orthopnoea or PND supervenes.
• *Giddiness or syncope on effort*: possible reasons are:
  – high intramural pressure on exercise, firing baroreceptors to produce reflex bradycardia and vasodilatation
  – skeletal muscle vasodilatation on exercise with no increase in cardiac output or additional rhythm disturbance
  – development of complete AV block with aortic ring calcium extending into the upper ventricular septum.
• *Systemic emboli*: often retinal or cerebral. Amaurosis fugax may be the presenting symptom, especially when the valve is calcified. Small flecks of

Table 3.7 Mechanisms of angina in aortic stenosis

Increased demand	Decreased supply

↑Cardiac work
↑Muscle mass from hypertrophy
↑Wall stress from high intracavity
  pressure: in both systole and diastole
	Prolonged systole with shorter diastole
	Reversed coronary flow in systole from the
	  Venturi effect of narrow valve orifice
	High intramural pressure in systole preventing
	  systolic coronary flow
	Low aortic perfusion pressure in diastole with
	  high LVEDP
	Rarely calcification extending to coronary
	  ostia

calcium and/or platelet emboli may be seen wedged in retinal arterioles on ophthalmoscopy.

• *Sudden death*: may occur in 7.5% of cases, even before severe ECG changes develop, e.g. in children.

• *Infective endocarditis* (see Section 9.1).

• *Congestive cardiac failure*: severe aortic stenosis may present for the first time as CCF with a large heart, very low pulse volume and soft murmurs, or no audible murmurs at all.

• *Gastrointestinal bleeding*: the calcified stenotic aortic valve can cause acquired von Willebrand syndrome; von Willebrand's factor (which sticks platelets to damaged endothelium) circulates as large multimers (250 kDa), which can be damaged by the high shear stress passing through the aortic valve. The presence of a coincidental angiodysplasia in the colon, combined with this haemostatic abnormality, can cause chronic iron deficiency anaemia that is cured by an aortic valve replacement.

• *Aortic dissection:* Increased risk with bicuspid aortic valve, especially in preguancy (see Section 15.6)

Physical Signs
See Figure 3.19.

Coexisting Lesions
In addition to the fact that an aortic valve abnormality may coexist with subvalvar stenosis, both lesions may occur with certain other congenital cardiovascular defects, e.g.

• Aortic valve stenosis (bicuspid valve) + coarctation of the aorta (e.g. Turner syndrome)

• Aortic valve stenosis + coarctation + PDA

• VSD ± pulmonary stenosis

• As part of the hypoplastic left heart syndrome

• Corrected TGA

• Supravalvar stenosis with pulmonary artery branch stenosis.

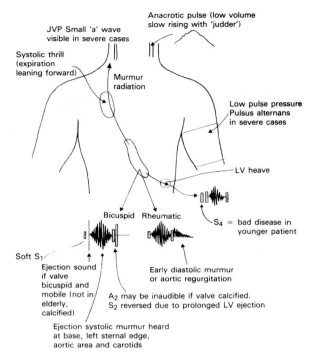

Figure 3.19 Typical signs in valvar aortic stenosis.

ECG in Aortic Valve Stenosis
- Should be in sinus rhythm. If in AF, suspect additional mitral valve disease or ischaemic heart disease.
- P mitrale with prominent negative P-wave component in V (caused by high LVEDP).
- LV hypertrophy.
- 'Strain pattern' in lateral chest leads. In children T-wave inversion in inferior leads often occurs first. Severe aortic stenosis may occur with a normal ECG in children.
- Left axis deviation (caused by left anterior hemiblock).
- Poor R-wave progression in anterior chest leads.
- LBBB or complete heart block with calcified ring (in about 5% of cases).

After aortic valve replacement there is often a reversion of the P- and T-wave changes gradually over the years, and a reduction in LV voltage as the LV mass is reduced.

Chest Radiograph (Figure 3.20)
This may show the following:
- LV hypertrophy
- Calcified aortic valve (in age ≥40 years): calcium on lateral view will be above and anterior to oblique fissure

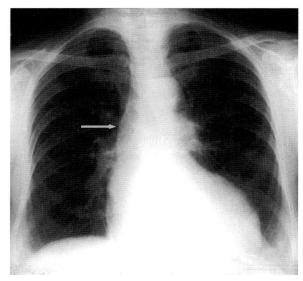

Figure 3.20 Chest radiograph P/A: mixed aortic valve disease. LV hypertrophy. Mild post-stenotic dilatation of ascending aorta (arrowed).

- Post-stenotic dilatation of ascending aorta (not specific for valvar stenosis, e.g. may occur with fibromuscular ring in subvalvar stenosis)
- Pulmonary venous congestion and signs of LVF.
Note: check for rib notching and small or 'double' aortic knuckle in coarctation (Figure 2.10).

Echocardiography (see also Section 17.3)
This may show the following:
- Bicuspid valve (eccentric 'closure' line on M mode) with reduced valve opening
- Calcified valve (multiple echo-bands)
- LV hypertrophy: assess LV function
- Diastolic fluttering of anterior mitral leaflet if additional aortic regurgitation is present
- Assessment of aortic valve gradient from Doppler echocardiography (Table 3.8). This may be a substitute for cardiac catheterization in the younger patient. Peak systolic gradient is $= 4V^2$ where V is the peak velocity of the continuous wave Doppler signal across the aortic valve recorded from the apex (see Section 17.3). Valve gradient is dependent on both aortic valve area and LV function.
- Two-dimensional echocardiography gives more information about the valve and LV function, but cannot provide coronary artery anatomy
- Estimate of aortic valve area from the Bernouille equation (see Section 17.3).

Table 3.8 Assessment of severity of aortic stenosis from echocardiography

	Mild	Moderate	Severe
Peak velocity (m/s)	<3.0	3.0–4.0	>4.0
Aortic valve area (cm²)	>1.5	1.0–1.5	<1.0
Aortic valve gradient (mmHg)	<25	25–50	>50

Transthoracic Dobutamine Stress Echocardiography (DSE)

This can be used to determine contractile reserve in the LV in cases where the LV function is known to be poor, but where the aortic valve gradient is relatively low (e.g. 30 mmHg). This situation may result from genuinely severe aortic valve stenosis, or 'pseudo-severe' aortic stenosis where LV dysfunction is the primary problem – perhaps from additional coronary disease.

In experienced hands this is a safe procedure. The test can be performed with a minimum increase in heart rate and should be stopped if the heart rate exceeds 10% above baseline. An increase in ejection fraction and stroke volume (by >20%) indicates a contractile reserve, and this is an important guide to surgical risk.

Surgery is best avoided in cases of no contractile reserve or in pseudo-severe AS, which is suggested if the final aortic valve gradient is <30 mmHg, and the aortic valve area is >1.2 cm².

Cardiac Catheterization

This may be performed to:
• document the aortic valve gradient (Figures 3.21 and 3.22) or calculate the valve area (see Chapter 16, Figure 16.21); peak systolic gradient of >100 mmHg and valve area <0.5 cm² = severe aortic stenosis; peak instantaneous gradient > peak-to-peak gradient (Figure 3.21)
• assess LV function
• perform coronary angiography to document possible CAD and check the coronary ostial anatomy; bicuspid aortic valve is associated with a dominant left coronary artery and short main stem
• check the aortic root.

Rate of Progression of Aortic Stenosis

This is very variable and symptoms may occur at any stage of the disease and any valve area. Generally an average annual change to be expected would be:
• gradient increase by 5–10 mmHg/year
• peak velocity on continuous wave Doppler: increase of 0.2–0.3 m/s per year (see Section 17.3)
• aortic valve area: reduction of 0.1 cm²/year.

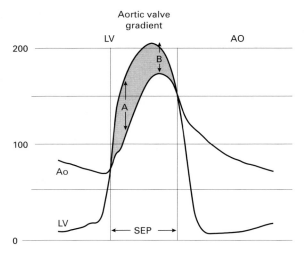

Figure 3.21 Simultaneous pressure recordings in left ventricle (LV) and aorta (AO) in a man with mild aortic stenosis. A: the peak instantaneous gradient of 54 mmHg is greater than B – the peak-to-peak gradient of 32 mmHg. SEP, systolic ejection period. The peak-to-peak gradient is conventionally used as it is easier to measure.

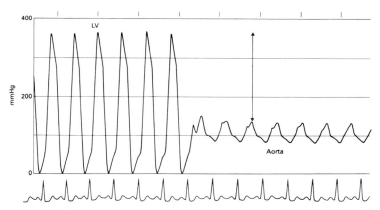

Figure 3.22 Severe aortic stenosis: withdrawal of catheter from left ventricle to aorta in a man with severe aortic stenosis resulting from a calcified bicuspid aortic valve. LV pressure is 360/0–40 and aortic pressure is 130/80. Peak-to-peak gradient is 230 mmHg (arrowed).

Indications for Surgery

• *Aortic valvotomy or valvuloplasty* may be performed in children who are symptomatic or asymptomatic with severe stenosis. This may buy time until they are large enough for a conventional valve replacement.

• *Ross operation (1967)*: this is the alternative for children and young adults The pulmonary valve is used as an autograft in the aortic position and a homograft is used for the removed pulmonary valve. The pulmonary autograft grows with the patient and anticoagulation is not needed. Both autograft and homograft dysfunction can occur and are the Achilles' heel of this operation with potential dilatation and failure of either or both ventricles. Redo surgery for a failed Ross operation is very demanding surgery.

• *Aortic valve replacement* is recommended once symptoms develop in adults. The natural history of medically treated patients who are symptomatic is poor. (Average survival is 2–3 years with angina or syncope, 1–2 years with cardiac failure.)

Adults who are absolutely asymptomatic can be managed medically but must be kept under close observation in the outpatient clinic every 6 months. Surgery is necessary as soon as symptoms develop. Only 21% of patients are still asymptomatic at 2 years if their peak aortic jet velocity exceeds 4 m/s. This is the best predictor of trouble ahead and is a superior guide in the asymptomatic patient to aortic valve area, valve gradient or LV ejection fraction. The severity of aortic valve calcification is also a useful prognostic guide.

The decision to operate on the elderly patient must depend on:
• adequate hepatic and renal function
• adequate lung function (forced expiratory volume in 1 second, FEV1 preferably >0.8–1.0 l)
•   reasonable adult weight (>40 kg)
• the severity of additional coronary disease or LV dysfunction.

Average operative mortality for isolated aortic valve replacement is now <2%. The need for additional coronary revascularization, the presence of poor LV function and very heavy valve calcification increase the risk (10–20%). Long-term survival post-AVR depends on presence of:
• additional CAD and history of infarction
• heart size increasing preoperatively
• low cardiac output
• pulmonary hypertension.

Aortic Valvuloplasty

This technique has proved of some value in a very small group of elderly patients with severe AS who are considered inoperable (very poor lung function, renal failure, etc.). It is of more value to the paediatric cardiologist in a child with AS who is too small for an aortic valve replacement. It is performed percutaneously in the catheter laboratory. The technique involves insertion of one or two balloons across the aortic valve via guidewire(s). The balloon can usually be advanced across the valve retrogradely but the distal end of the balloon may damage the left ventricular septum and cause arrhythmias. The balloon is usually inflated to 4–9 atm for up to 1 min. The procedure usually causes an abrupt reduction in cardiac output during inflation and the patient should be well atropinized and not hypovolaemic.

After valvuloplasty there is a gradient reduction, and usually an increase in aortic valve area. Long-term results vary, and some workers have found only a temporary improvement in aortic valve area. Complications include profound bradycardia, hypotension, tamponade, systemic emboli and death in a few cases. In addition there is a significant problem with entry site complications, some patients needing femoral artery repair. This problem is receding with use of a long arterial sheath.

Aortic valvuloplasty cannot be considered an alternative to aortic valve replacement. It is of some value to a very small group of infirm patients, or a group of children with congenital aortic stenosis. Its benefits may only be temporary but in children it may gain time until they have grown enough for an aortic valve replacement. It has even been performed on the fetus *in utero* with success.

Percutaneous Aortic Valve Replacement
This is now possible in a few centres using a stent valve mounted at the tip of a catheter, which can be advanced into position retrogradely via the femoral artery using a long sheath. Balloon inflation in the centre of the native valve deploys the stent valve. This avoids the need for cardiac surgery. A steerable retroflex catheter aids passage round the aortic arch. Sizes 23–26 mm are currently available and the original Cribier–Edwards valve is being replaced by the Sapien valve. Careful positioning is needed to avoid the left coronary ostium. A mild degree of paravalve aortic regurgitation is to be expected.

The procedure is reserved for patients who are too frail to undergo conventional aortic valve replacement, or where there are co-morbidities such as chronic renal failure. A porcelain aorta is not a contraindication.

The principal risks are:
- Femoral artery damage
- Aortic root or arch dissection
- Thromboembolism from atheroma in the ascending aorta
- Malposition deployment.

In skilled hands this technique can rescue patients who are moribund from end-stage aortic stenosis. The technique will increase in use as the technology improves. An alternative transapical approach has been performed in theatre successfully with the stent valve advanced anterogradely.

Supravalvar Aortic Stenosis (Figure 3.23)
This is caused by a constricting ridge of fibrous tissue at the upper margin of the sinuses of Valsalva. The coronary ostia are below the stenosis. Rarely, the obstruction is a more generalized hypoplasia of the ascending aorta.

Associated Conditions
Williams syndrome (autosomal dominant with variable penetration): children with:
- elfin facies (large mouth with protruding upper lip, high forehead, epicanthic folds, recessed nasal bridge, learning disability, strabismus, low-set ears)

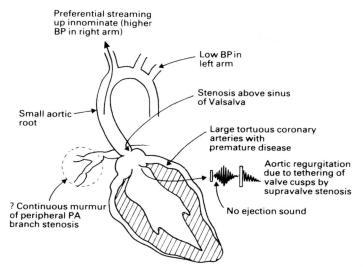

Figure 3.23 Diagrammatic summary of supravalvar aortic stenosis.

- hypervitaminosis D and hypercalcaemia
- other cardiac lesions: peripheral pulmonary artery stenoses, valvar pulmonary stenosis, aortic valve regurgitation
- mesenteric artery stenoses, thoracic aortic aneurysms
- rubella syndrome.

Cardiac Lesion and Signs

Supravalvar aortic stenosis should also be considered in a child who has
additional aortic regurgitation, no ejection sound and blood pressure in the
left arm lower than the right. The chest radiograph does not show post-stenotic dilatation of the ascending aorta.

Symptoms are those of valvar stenosis. Coronary arteries are characteristi-
cally large but tend to have premature arterial disease as a result of the high
pressure below the supravalvar stenosis.

The supravalvar shelf and the adherent aortic cusps may rarely isolate the
coronary artery orifice ('house-martin's nest' appearance on angiogram) and
acute MI or sudden death occurs.

The pulmonary arterial stenoses may improve with time and the RV pressure then falls. The left-sided lesions often gradually get worse. In patients
initially managed medically, repeat catheterization is often needed to check
for possible deterioration of the supravalvar aortic lesion. An example of a
catheter withdrawal tracing from LV to aorta in this condition is shown in
Figure 4.6.

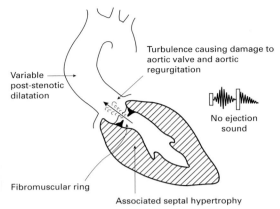

Figure 3.24 Diagrammatic summary of discrete fibromuscular subaortic stenosis.

Surgery
This is less satisfactory than for aortic valve stenosis. It may be possible only if the ascending aorta is of reasonable size. A gradient from LV to ascending aorta of >70 mmHg would be an indication for operation. The narrowed segment may be enlarged by inserting an ellipse- or diamond-shaped patch of woven Dacron or pericardium. The aortic wall is often thickened, increasing the difficulties of surgery.

Discrete Fibromuscular Subaortic Stenosis
Occurs in about 10% of congenital aortic stenosis. The fibromuscular ring obstructs the LV outflow tract immediately beneath the aortic valve. It never presents under the age of 1 year and is probably an acquired lesion associated with congenital abnormality of the ventricular muscle. About half the affected patients have additional cardiovascular lesions.

Distinction from valvar aortic stenosis may be very difficult. Discrete fibromuscular subaortic stenosis is a possibility if:
• there is aortic regurgitation (thickening of valve as a result of high-velocity jet through obstruction or even attachment to the right coronary cusp)
• absent ejection sound (Figure 3.24)
• no valve calcification.

Post-stenotic dilatation of ascending aorta may or may not occur and is not reliable diagnostically.

Echocardiography
This is invaluable in establishing the diagnosis. On M-mode it may show the following:
• Very early systolic closure of aortic valve (right coronary cusp especially) and systolic fluttering of aortic leaflets (Figure 17.6)
• Cluster of subaortic echoes above anterior mitral leaflet.

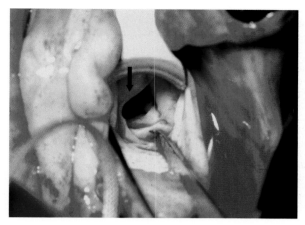

Figure 3.25 Subaortic stenosis at surgery: fibromuscular ring (arrowed) viewed through aortic valve.

Two-dimensional echocardiography may show the subaortic shelf clearly in the long-axis view in older children. The differentiation of the echoes from the aortic valve itself may be difficult in younger children.

Cardiac Catheterization
This confirms subaortic obstruction. The ring is visualized on LV angiography. The degree of the obstruction can be measured and additional aortic regurgitation assessed.

Surgery
Excision of the fibromuscular ring is possible, but often residual abnormal LV muscle remains (very similar to HCM). The ring is excised through the aortic valve (Figure 3.25). There is usually a small residual gradient and sometimes mild aortic regurgitation. Follow-up with repeat cardiac catheterization is necessary to exclude recurrent obstruction. Occasionally, aortic valve replacement is required later for aortic regurgitation.

3.5 Aortic Regurgitation

This may be caused by primary disease of the aortic valve or by aortic root disease with dilatation and stretching of the valve ring (Table 3.9). The regurgitation may be through the valve or, rarely, down a channel adjacent to the valve ring (e.g. ruptured sinus of Valsalva aneurysm, aorto-LV tunnel).

Pathophysiology
Often moderate aortic regurgitation is tolerated with no symptoms:
• Aortic regurgitation results in an increase in LV end-diastolic volume (LVEDV) and end-systolic volume (LVESV)

Table 3.9 Aetiology of aortic regurgitation

Congenital	Acquired
Valve disease	
Bicuspid valve	Rheumatic fever
Supravalvar stenosis	Infective endocarditis
Discrete subvalvar fibromuscular	Rheumatoid arthritis (valve nodules)
ring	SLE
Supracristal VSD with prolapse	PXE
of right coronary cusp	Hurler syndrome and other mucopolysaccharidoses
Aortic root disease	
Ruptured sinus of Valsalva aneurysm	Dissection (type A)
	Hypertension
	Cystic medial necrosis, e.g. Marfan syndrome
	Osteogenesis imperfecta
	Giant cell aortitis
	Arthritides with aortitis, e.g. ankylosing spondylitis, Reiter syndrome, psoriasis
	Syphilis
	Trauma

- The stroke volume (SV) is high in compensated cases
- LV mass is raised with LV hypertrophy
- Compensatory tachycardia reduces the regurgitant flow per beat by shortening diastole, and allows an increase in cardiac output.

As the regurgitation increases and LV function deteriorates:

- LVEDP rises and may eventually equal aortic diastolic pressure
- Premature mitral valve closure occurs, preventing diastolic forward flow through the mitral valve
- LVEDV rises further, but stroke volume falls.

Symptoms

As in aortic stenosis, but angina and syncope are much less common.

Unlike aortic stenosis, aortic regurgitation is a well-tolerated lesion if gradual compensatory mechanisms can occur. Even moderate aortic regurgitation may be tolerated for years. However, acute valvar aortic regurgitation or ruptured sinus of Valsalva is poorly tolerated and quickly produces LVF or CCF. Intensive medical therapy followed by investigation and surgery is often necessary.

Eponyms Associated with Aortic Regurgitation (Figure 3.26)

- Austin–Flint murmur: a low-pitched low-frequency mitral diastolic murmur. Caused by vibrations in diastole of both mitral leaflets, particularly the anterior leaflet, which oscillate between the aortic regurgitant jet and the anterograde blood flow from the left atrium. Very similar to mitral stenosis,

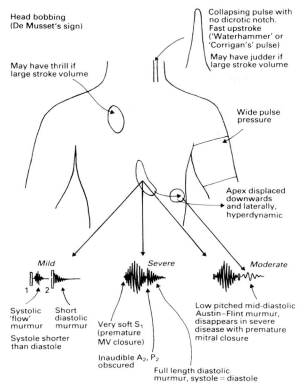

Figure 3.26 Typical signs of aortic regurgitation: left sternal edge – use stethoscope diaphragm with patient sitting forward and breath held in expiration. Apex (to hear S_3 and Austin-Flint murmurs): use bell with patient lying on left side.

but S1 is quiet and there is no opening snap. Figure 3.27 shows an apical phonocardiographic recording of an Austin–Flint murmur recorded with an M-mode echo of the mitral valve. The fluttering frequency is identical in both recordings.

- Duroziez's sign: to-and-fro murmur audible over femoral arteries.
- Quincke's pulse: capillary pulsation in fingertips or mucous membranes.
- Traube's sign: 'pistol-shot' sound audible over femoral arteries. Presence of additional aortic stenosis is detected by the bisferiens carotid pulse.
- De Musset's sign: head bobbing as a result of collapsing pulses.

Differential Diagnosis
- Pulmonary valve regurgitation, e.g. in patients who have had total correction of Fallot's tetralogy or post-pulmonary valvotomy. Patients with pulmonary hypertension secondary to mitral valve disease (Graham Steell murmur).

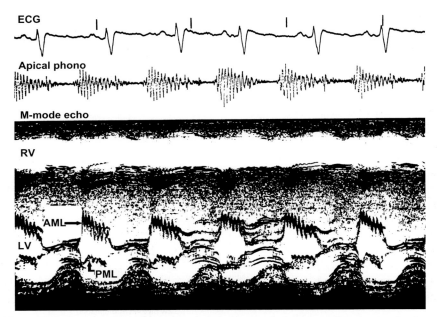

ECG

Apical phono

M-mode echo

RV

AML→

LV

PML

Figure 3.27 M-mode echocardiogram recorded with an apical phonocardiogram showing the Austin–Flint murmur in a man with moderately severe aortic regurgitation. There is diastolic fluttering of both anterior and posterior mitral leaflets (AML and PML) generating the low frequency diastolic murmur.

- PDA: machinery murmur usually loudest in second left interspace.
- VSD with aortic regurgitation: usually right coronary cusp prolapses into or through a supracristal VSD. The prolapsing cusp may cause RV outflow tract obstruction (retrosternal thrill, harsh pansystolic murmur, early diastolic murmur).
- Ruptured sinus of Valsalva aneurysm: usually right coronary sinus ruptures into RV outflow tract or RA. Sudden-onset chest pain and CCF with high JVP. Consider this in patients with aortic regurgitation and signs of right heart failure because it is unusual in aortic regurgitation.

More rarely:
- Coronary AV fistula: this presents during adult life with LVF as a result of a left-to-right shunt (into RA, RV or coronary sinus).
- Pulmonary AV fistula, e.g. in patients with Osler–Rendu–Weber syndrome + bronchiectasis, cyanosis and second-degree polycythaemia.
- Aortopulmonary window: usually large communication with resultant pulmonary hypertension. Rarely survive to adult life.
- Aorto-LV tunnel.
- Persistent truncus arteriosus: again patients rarely survive to adult life (early pulmonary hypertension, cyanosis, VSD + truncal valve regurgitation).

ECG
LVH with diastolic overload pattern (prominent Q waves in anterolateral leads). ST depression and T-wave inversion occur as the condition deteriorates.

Echocardiography
This may show the following:
• LV function and dimensions: exercise may help detect early LV dysfunction.
• Aortic valve thickening: possible 'vegetations' on aortic valve.
• Diastolic fluttering of anterior mitral leaflet which may be audible as the Austin–Flint murmur (see Figure 3.27).
• Premature mitral valve closure: occasionally only the 'a' wave opens the mitral valve at all in severe cases.
• Aortic root dimensions and possible 'double' wall in aortic dissection.
• Flail aortic leaflet prolapsing into LV outflow tract.
• Colour Doppler will help document size and direction of regurgitant jet (Table 3.10 and Section 17.3).
• Confirms that the aortic regurgitant jet is into the LV, and the diagnosis is not one of many other possibilities (see Differential Diagnosis, p. 109).

Chest Radiograph
This may show the following:
• Aortic valve calcification uncommon in pure AR
• Large LV
• Ascending aorta may be very prominent (e.g. dissection) or aneurysmal (e.g. Marfan syndrome, syphilis)
• Calcification of ascending aorta (syphilitic AR)
• Signs of pulmonary venous congestion or pulmonary oedema.

Cardiac Catheterization
It is necessary to document the following:
• The severity of the aortic regurgitation:

Table 3.10 Assessment of severity of aortic regurgitation using Doppler signal or echocardiographic measurements

	Mild	Moderate	Severe
Vena contracta width (cm)	<0.3	0.3–0.6	>0.6
Colour Doppler jet width (% LVOT)	<25	25–65	>65
Regurgitant volume (ml/beat)	<30	30–59	>60
Regurgitant fraction (%)	<30	30–49	>50
ROA (cm²)	<0.1	0.1–0.29	>0.3
Mitral pressure half-time (PHT) (ms)	>500	200–500	<200
Angiographic grade (see below)	1	2	3–4

ROA: regurgitant orifice area.

  – grade I: dye just regurgitant, not filling the ventricle
  – grade II: dye gradually accumulating to fill the whole ventricle
  – grade III: dye filling the whole ventricle, but cleared each systole
  – grade IV: dye filling the ventricle in one diastole, never cleared.
- The anatomy of the aortic root, and to check that the regurgitation is valvar and not ruptured sinus of Valsalva, to exclude dissection, to check for rarer congenital defects mimicking aortic regurgitation.
- To assess LV function; with severe aortic regurgitation the LVEDP equals the aortic end-diastolic pressure.
- To check coronary arteries and coronary ostia.
- Additional valve disease.

Outpatient Follow-up
All patients need antibiotic cover for dental or surgical procedures (see Section 9.7). The activity of patients with mild regurgitation need not be restricted. Patients with moderate or severe regurgitation should avoid isometric exercise and competitive sports and need 6-monthly follow-up. Long-acting nifedipine has been shown to delay the development of LV dysfunction in chronic aortic regurgitation. Digoxin is not of benefit unless the patient is in AF.

Indications for Surgery
The aortic valve must be replaced before irreversible LV dysfunction develops and this may occur in the asymptomatic patient. Consider AVR if:
- Symptoms of increasing dyspnoea and LVF.
- In the patient with no heart failure symptoms: exercise test. If abnormally symptomatic during exercise refer for AVR.
- In the asymptomatic patient with a satisfactory exercise test refer for AVR if:
  – enlarging heart on chest radiograph (>17 cm on PA film), or increasing LV dimensions on echocardiography: LVEDD >70 mm (35 mm/m^2), LVESV >50 mm (25 mm/m^2) or LVEF < 50%
  – pulse pressure >100 mmHg (especially if diastolic <40 mmHg)
  – ECG deterioration with T-wave inversion in lateral chest leads.
  Of patients with all three of these criteria 65% will either die or develop CCF within 3 years if untreated.
- Ruptured sinus of Valsalva aneurysm.
- Infective endocarditis not responding to medical treatment.

3.6 Pulmonary Stenosis

Obstruction to RV outflow may be at several levels, as in aortic stenosis.

Peripheral PA Stenosis
This includes stenoses of main trunk of PA or more distal stenoses. These stenoses may be localized or diffuse. Commonly associated with supravalvar

aortic stenosis and infantile hypercalcaemia. Also part of the rubella syndrome associated with PDA.

Pulmonary Valve Stenosis
This is a common isolated lesion (7% of congenital heart lesions). Also occurs as part of Noonan syndrome, Fallot's tetralogy or rubella syndrome. It is rarely acquired, e.g. carcinoid syndrome.

Pulmonary Infundibular Stenosis
This is rare as an isolated lesion. Usually associated with a VSD, or as part of Fallot's tetralogy, or just in association with pulmonary valve stenosis.

Subinfundibular Stenosis
This rarest form has been described. It may occur as part of right-sided HCM.

Pathophysiology and Symptoms
The effects of pulmonary stenosis depend on its severity and the structure and function of the rest of the right heart, i.e. RV function (systolic and diastolic), competence of the tricuspid valve, presence or absence of a VSD, presence or absence of an ASD/PFO, maintenance of sinus rhythm.

With good RV function and a competent tricuspid valve plus sinus rhythm, moderate pulmonary stenosis can be tolerated with no symptoms.

Very severe 'pinhole' pulmonary stenosis is virtual pulmonary atresia and may lead to early infant death, especially if the duct closes.

The additional presence of an ASD or PFO may lead to right-to-left shunting (e.g. on effort), with cyanosis.

RV failure is the most common cause of death, with gross cardiac enlargement. Common symptoms are thus:
- dyspnoea and fatigue (low cardiac output), not orthopnoea or PND
- cyanosis (if ASD or PFO)
- RV failure with ascites, leg oedema, jaundice, etc.
- retarded growth in children.

Symptoms that are uncommon (unlike aortic stenosis) are angina, syncope on effort and symptoms from infective endocarditis. Patients may be aware of pulsation in the neck from the giant 'a' wave in the JVP.

Physical Signs to Note
Characteristic facies may be:
- rounded plump face with isolated pulmonary valve stenosis
- Noonan syndrome ('male Turner')
- Williams syndrome (hypercalcaemia + supravalvar aortic stenosis + pulmonary artery stenoses), elf-like facies, JVP: prominent or giant 'a' wave, RV hypertrophy, palpable RVOT thrill.

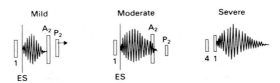

Figure 3.28 Grades of pulmonary stenosis.

Valve Stenosis (Figure 3.28)

With mild valve stenosis there is an ejection sound, ejection systolic murmur, and A_2 and P_2 clearly heard and widely split. As the stenosis becomes more severe, the murmur is longer and obscures A_2. P_2 is delayed still further and is softer. With severe stenosis P_2 becomes inaudible and the ejection sound disappears as the valve calcifies. The murmur radiates towards the left shoulder and over the left lung posteriorly.

With infundibular stenosis there is no ejection sound and the murmur may be more prominent at the left sternal edge.

Differential Diagnosis

Differential diagnosis is from aortic valve or subvalvar stenosis, VSD, Ebstein's anomaly, ASD and innocent RVOT murmurs in children.

ECG

This shows right axis deviation, right atrial hypertrophy, 'P pulmonale', RV hypertrophy, incomplete or complete RBBB.

Chest Radiograph

There is post-stenotic dilatation of the pulmonary artery (Figure 3.29) but lung fields are oligaemic, in contrast to ASD. RV hypertrophy causes some cardiac enlargement with the apex lifted off the left hemidiaphragm.

With severe long-standing pulmonary stenosis the heart may be very large with an enormous right atrium (the wall-to-wall heart). This appearance is seen in:
- severe pulmonary stenosis in the adult
- Ebstein's anomaly
- large pericardial effusion (chronic)
- mitral stenosis with giant atria
- dilated cardiomyopathy
- Uhl's anomaly (RV hypoplasia).

Cardiac Catheterization

This is necessary to document the gradient and site of the stenosis.

The size of the PAs and possible additional stenoses. Additional lesions must be excluded, especially PDA, VSD, ASD and left-sided obstructive lesions. RV functions are important. The position and comparative size of the

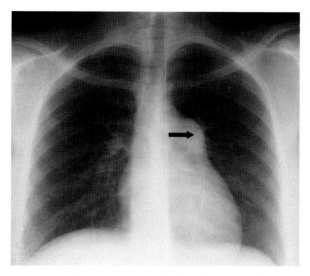

Figure 3.29 Mild pulmonary stenosis: post-stenotic dilatation of main PA conus (arrowed).

great vessels are important in more complex lesions (e.g. Fallot's tetralogy, DORV with PS, TGA with VSD and PS).

Pulmonary Valvuloplasty
Pulmonary valvuloplasty is now an acceptable alternative to surgery. Good reduction of pulmonary valve gradient is obtained, long-term results are good and RV hypertrophy on the ECG regresses.

Percutaneous Pulmonary Valve Replacement
Pioneered in the UK by Bonhoeffer, a stent valve manufactured from bovine jugular vein mounted on a catheter tip can now be used as an alternative to redo surgery in selected patients. The best cases are patients who have had pulmonary homograft that has now calcified and degenerated. The calcium acts as a useful anchor for the stent, which is advanced into position via a femoral vein. Only sizes 22 and 24 mm are currently available so that large main pulmonary arteries, or outflow tracts that have had a transannular patch, are not suitable.

Surgery
Pulmonary valvotomy and/or infundibular resection should be considered if there is RV failure, or if peak systolic gradient at valve/subvalve level is >70 mmHg. Emergency surgery may be needed in infants. An additional PFO/ASD or VSD is usually closed. With severe valve stenosis a transannular patch may be needed.

3.7 Tricuspid Valve Disease

The most common tricuspid valve disease is functional regurgitation second-ary to pulmonary hypertension. Tricuspid valve destruction from infective endocarditis is increasingly seen in drug addicts. Other forms of tricuspid valve disease are uncommon (Table 3.11).

Tricuspid Regurgitation
Dilatation of the tricuspid valve ring with deteriorating RV function is common in patients with pulmonary hypertension from any cause. It often occurs in patients with rheumatic mitral valve disease and pulmonary hypertension. The development of AF in ASDs is associated with TR. AF is expected with any significant degree of TR, both RA and RV dilate with the change to AF and the regurgitation worsens.

Symptoms
If any, there may be fatigue, hepatic pain on effort, pulsation in the throat and fullness in the face on effort, ascites and ankle oedema.

Signs
- Systolic 's' wave in the JVP with rapid 'y' descent
- If still in sinus rhythm (rare) prominent 'a' wave also
- RV heave
- Soft inspiratory pansystolic murmur at LSE
- Pulsatile liver
- Ankle oedema and possible ascites
- Jaundice
- Peripheral cyanosis.

Treatment
Some degree of TR can be tolerated in the ambulant patient by conventional diuretic therapy and digoxin. Spironolactone, amiloride or an ACE inhibitor

Table 3.11 Aetiology of tricuspid valve disease

Congenital lesions	Acquired lesions
Tricuspid atresia	Functional regurgitation
Tricuspid hypoplasia	Destruction from infective endocarditis (see
Ebstein's anomaly (see below)	Chapter 9)
Cleft tricuspid valve (AV canal)	Rheumatic involvement
	Floppy valve
	Endocarditis caused by hepatic carcinoid
	Fenfluramine, dexfenfluramine, phentermine,
	dopamine agonists (pergolide, capergoline),
	ergot derivatives (methysergide, ergotamine)

should be part of the regimen. Support stockings may help prevent trouble-some ankle oedema and venous ulceration.

In more severe and symptomatic patients a period of bed rest and intrave-nous diuretic therapy is needed. The symptoms quickly recur, usually once the patient has been mobilized. In these cases tricuspid valve replacement must be considered. Tricuspid annuloplasty does not often result in any lasting benefit.

Tricuspid Stenosis

This is rare, almost always rheumatic, and associated with additional mitral or aortic valve disease. Symptoms are as in TR.

Signs

- Slow 'y' descent in JVP
- Prominent 'a' wave if in SR
- RV heave absent
- Tricuspid diastolic murmur at LSE best heard on inspiration and after effort.

At cardiac catheterization even a gradient of 3–4 mmHg across the tricuspid valve is highly significant. RV angiography usually shows additional TR. The only treatment is valvuloplasty or valve replacement.

Drug-induced Valve Disease

Increasing evidence points to drugs that are 5-HT_{2B} agonists causing valve regurgitation on both sides of the heart. Carcinoid heart disease results from high levels of 5-HT (serotonin) released from the tumour reaching the tricus-pid valve and causing fibrotic change on the leaflets and chordae. There are many 5-HT_{2B} receptors on heart valves. Fenfluramine and dexfenfluramine are 5-HT agonists, and were withdrawn when they were found to have similar effects. As well as these two drugs being used for migraine prevention, ergot-amine and methysergide can induce valve fibrosis (in addition to pulmonary, pericardial and retroperitoneal fibrosis). Recently the dopamine agonists per-golide and capergoline have also been shown to cause this fibrotic reaction. These agents are also ergot derivatives.

Ebstein's Anomaly

This is a tricuspid valve dysplasia with downward displacement of the valve into the body of the right ventricle. The tricuspid leaflets are abnormal; they may be fused, perforated or even absent and their chordae are abnormal. The clinical picture depends on the following:

- Severity of TR.
- RV function: the atrialized portion of the RV is thin-walled and functions poorly.
- Rhythm disturbances. These are frequent. Both SVT and VT. There is often an abnormal conducting system with type B (right-sided) WPW syndrome.

• Associated lesions, commonly ASD or PFO; PS; corrected transposition. Less commonly MS, Fallot's tetralogy.

Presentation

Infancy
It presents as heart failure from severe TR with chronic low output, and cyanosis from right-to-left shunting at the atrial level (PFO or ASD). This may increase when a PDA closes because pulmonary flow is reduced still further. Prognosis at this age is poor.

Older Child or Young Adult
This may be with a murmur noticed at a school medical, or paroxysmal SVT. Mild forms may be asymptomatic.

Physical Signs

These depend on the above lesions. Usually the child is cyanosed, with elevated JVP and hepatomegaly.

At LSE listen for pansystolic murmur (TR), S_3 (RV), tricuspid diastolic murmur.

Chest Radiograph

Shows very large right atrium in symptomatic cases often with oligaemic lung fields. With large globular hearts consider: pericardial effusion PS and dilated cardiomyopathy as alternatives.

ECG

This shows RBBB, RAD, RA+ (P pulmonale). Sometimes type B WPW syndrome. Echocardiography is diagnostic.

Treatment

This is medical initially to control symptoms of right heart failure and arrhythmias if present.

RV angiography is diagnostic, but frequently produces rhythm disturbances that may be difficult to control. Simultaneous measurement of intracardiac pressure and electrogram shows, at one point, an RA pressure but an RV cavity electrogram.

Tricuspid valve replacement plus closure of an ASD is possible but results are generally not good.

Alternatively a tricuspid annuloplasty can be performed with plication of the atrialized portion of the right ventricle.

3.8 Prosthetic Cardiac Valves

Types

There is no perfect valve prosthesis. Knowledge of possible valve problems and complications is necessary for long-term management of these patients,

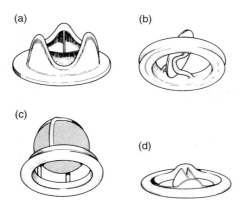

Figure 3.30 Examples of prosthetic valves: (a) Carpentier–Edwards porcine xenograft. Only the three wire stents (cloth-covered) are radio-opaque. (b) Björk–Shiley disc valve: the single disc is pyrolite carbon and is not radio-opaque. (c) Starr–Edwards ball valve: the mitral valve shown has four struts, and the aortic prosthesis has three. The Silastic ball is not seen on the chest radiograph. (d) St Jude medical bileaflet valve shown in this picture in the open position. This is a low-profile valve with two pyrolite carbon discs. The CarboMedics and MIRA valves are similar.

and regular follow-up by experienced physicians is essential. Currently there are three main types of prosthesis.

1 Mechanical Valves (Figure 3.30)
These may be of the ball-in-the-cage type (Starr–Edwards, introduced in 1960), single-tilting disc (Björk–Shiley, introduced in 1969, Medtronic Hall) or double-tilting disc (St Jude, CarboMedics, MIRA). All patients with mechanical valves require anticoagulation for life. The valves are very durable, but have a higher thromboembolism rate than xenografts. Very occasionally a patient or his or her partner may be disturbed by the audible valve clicks. The double tilting disc valves have much better flow profiles than the Starr–Edwards ball valve and have largely superseded it.

Biological Valves

2 Xenografts
These are manufactured from porcine valves (Carpentier–Edwards, Hancock, Wessex) or from pericardium (Ionescu–Shiley, Hancock, Edwards Perimount) mounted on a frame. Aortic xenografts can be managed without anticoagulants, but most patients with mitral xenografts are in AF and should also be anticoagulated. Biological valves do not have as good long-term durability as mechanical valves and may need replacing at about 8–10 years (mitral) or 10–15 years (aortic). Unfortunately they have poorer durability in young patients and are better in elderly patients.

Nevertheless there is a gradual shift towards the use of tissue valves, particularly in the USA. The operative mortality of redo surgery is falling, but the long-term morbidity of redo surgery must be considered.

3 Homografts

These are cadaveric aortic or pulmonary valves. They are either transferred into a nutrient antibiotic medium and stored for up to 4 weeks, or frozen in liquid nitrogen for long-term storage. Availability is limited. A homograft should be considered the valve of first choice in a young patient requiring an aortic valve replacement. The use of an inverted homograft in the mitral position is not successful. Anticoagulation is not needed. Durability is better than xenografts, but deterioration in valve function is possible with time. They are also useful in replacing infected aortic valves, being more resistant to reinfection than other valves.

Outpatient Follow-up Problems

Systemic Embolism

This may occur with any valve prosthesis, but is most common with mechanical valves: about 1% per year even with the best anticoagulant control. Absolutely rigorous anticoagulant control is necessary: aim to keep the INR between 3.0 and 4.0 for all mechanical valves. If a patient with good warfarin control has a small (e.g. retinal) systemic embolism and the valve prosthesis sounds normal, then do the following:

- Check for infective endocarditis, blood cultures, FBC, ESR, CRP
- Echocardiography for possible visible vegetations or intracardiac thrombi; transoesophageal echocardiography is superior to transthoracic echocardiography for both aortic and mitral prosthetic vegetations or LA thrombus
- Consider transient rhythm changes (e.g. paroxysmal AF); check 24-hour tape
- Consider non-cardiac source, e.g. innominate or carotid bruit.

If all tests are negative and valve function is normal then dipyridamole 100 mg three times daily or clopidogrel 75 mg once daily is added to the warfarin. If a further event occurs add soluble aspirin 75 mg once daily after the biggest meal of the day. Aspirin is a more effective anti-platelet agent than dipyridamole in this situation, but carries a greater risk of bleeding from the gut. Dipyridamole and clopidogrel can cause dyspepsia.

If further emboli occur on this triple regimen, a redo valve replacement must be considered. The risks of redo valve surgery are higher with a mitral (10%) than an aortic (5%) prosthesis. In the absence of infection and a functionally otherwise normal valve it may be preferable to 'ride out' the episodes, especially in elderly people.

Dental Care

Meticulous dental care is absolutely vital for patients with prosthetic cardiac valves, and physicians should check that 6-monthly dental visits are made. Much dental work may need to be done before valve surgery, such as extraction of infected roots, but more complex restorative work usually has to wait until several months after valve replacement. Close liaison with the dentist is essential. Extractions are usually easier to manage with a short hospital admission. There are two big problems: the need both to stop the warfarin and for parenteral antibiotic cover.

• Warfarin can be stopped for about 4–5 days before dental work, provided that it is restarted immediately afterwards. Attempts to reverse the INR with vitamin K should be avoided because it makes subsequent anticoagulation difficult. If bleeding is a problem, FFP is needed but its effects are only temporary and repeated doses are usually necessary. If vitamin K has to be given, use small incremental doses, e.g. 1–3 mg only.

• Antibiotic cover is given orally but must be intravenous if there is a previous history of endocarditis. This is detailed in Chapter 9. For previous endocarditis patients: ampicillin 1 g plus gentamicin 120 mg i.v. before the procedure with amoxicillin 0.5 g orally at 6 h. For patients who are sensitive to penicillin: vancomycin 1 g slowly intravenously over at least an hour plus gentamicin 120 mg i.v., or teicoplanin 400 mg i.v.

Infection (see also Chapter 9)

Prosthetic valve endocarditis (PVE) carries a mortality rate of up to 40% and is a condition requiring urgent referral to a cardiothoracic centre. Patients should be reminded, in the clinic, to report any unexplained malaise, fever, weight loss, dyspnoea, etc. and should avoid antibiotics until seen by a cardiologist.

Endocarditis developing within the first 4–6 months of valve replacement is usually caused by *Staphylococcus epidermidis*, which colonizes the valve at the time of operation. Patients with a history of a perioperative wound infection need particularly careful follow-up. PVE occurring 6 months or more after surgery may result from a wide variety of organisms, as in native valve endocarditis. A high index of suspicion is needed, particularly if patients have:

• had dental treatment in the last 6 months, not covered by parenteral antibiotics

• noticed a change in their valve sounds

• a new symptom, however vague: dyspnoea, night sweats, myalgia, anorexia, etc.

• had a recent course of antibiotics.

Clinically the search for signs of PVE is as for native valve infection. Additional points to note are as follows:

• In mechanical valves the opening and closing sounds of either ball or disc should be clear and sharp, not muffled. Vegetations may restrict ball or disc movement and muffle the relevant prosthetic sounds.

• A mitral xenograft should have no murmurs. An aortic xenograft may have a soft ejection systolic murmur only.

• Very significant PVE may have developed without the presence of an audible regurgitant murmur. A new murmur is a vital clue, but unchanged sounds cannot be relied on. New murmurs in PVE occur late.

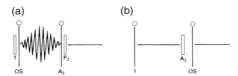

Figure 3.31 Normal Starr–Edwards prosthetic valve sounds. (a) *Aortic valve*: a normal first sound is followed by a prosthetic opening sound. There should be a soft aortic systolic ejection murmur. The ball closing sound is equivalent to A$_2$. The pulmonary component (P$_2$) is only heard in patients with wide RBBB. Diastole should be silent. (b) *Mitral valve*: the first heart sound is the mitral ball valve closing. There should be no systolic murmur. A$_2$ is soft but should be heard distinct from the ball opening sound (OS) that follows. The A$_2$–OS Interval gives an indication of left atrial pressure as in mitral stenosis, a short interval indicating high LA pressure. Diastole should be silent.

- Splinter haemorrhages are common.
- Check for mild haemolysis even in the absence of a new murmur. ?Urinary urobilinogen.
- Check ECG for PR interval prolongation (septal abscess).
- Echocardiography is vital, to look for vegetations and abscess formation. Doppler echocardiography is needed to establish valve regurgitation or a paraprosthetic leak. Transoesophageal echocardiography is particularly valuable if available.
- Radiological screening may show rocking of the prosthetic valve ring as a result of dehiscence. This usually occurs in the presence of obvious valve regurgitation and is a late and ominous sign.

If there is any doubt, the patient should be admitted and fully investigated preferably in a cardiothoracic centre (see Chapter 9). Most cases of PVE need a redo valve replacement, and this should be performed early.

A knowledge of normal prosthetic valve sounds is important. Figure 3.31 shows normal Starr–Edwards aortic and mitral prosthetic sounds.

Pregnancy (see also Chapter 15)
In a woman of childbearing age the choice of valve prosthesis is difficult. A xenograft involves a further valve operation at 8–10 years but avoids the problems of anticoagulation. A mechanical valve may avoid the need for a further operation but anticoagulation is mandatory. In young women who want to have children a homograft is the valve of choice in the aortic position, accepting the need for a redo valve replacement at about 10 years or more. In the mitral position a mitral valve repair may be possible in patients with a floppy valve. If a valve replacement is unavoidable it is better to opt for a mechanical valve and its long-term durability. A redo mitral valve replacement carries twice the risk of an aortic redo and a mitral xenograft deteriorates faster in younger patients. Xenografts may deteriorate particularly rapidly during pregnancy.

Problems with Warfarin in Pregnancy
• *Fetal haemorrhage*: warfarin crosses the placenta but vitamin K-dependent clotting factors do not – the immature fetal liver cannot manufacture them. Good maternal anticoagulant control unfortunately does not prevent fetal haemorrhage.
• *Teratogenicity*: fetal malformation occurs in 5–30% of reported cases. Chondrodysplasia punctata and stippled epiphyses may occur with abnormal development of the brain (learning disability, corpus callosum agenesis, ventral midline dysplasia with optic atrophy) and face (nasal hypoplasia). The typical embryopathy occurs with exposure to warfarin at 6–12 weeks' gestation. CNS abnormalities may occur as a result of exposure in the second trimester.
• *Spontaneous abortion*: the risks of this are increased partly as a result of fetal and placental haemorrhage.
• *Delivery*: the patient must be switched from warfarin to heparin at about 36 weeks. This is a good time to admit the patient; administer the heparin intravenously (1000 units/h initially).
• *Breast-feeding*: not a problem with warfarin. Mothers can be restarted on warfarin and continue to breast-feed.

Problems with Heparin in Pregnancy
Heparin does not cross the placenta and hence does not cause fetal malformation or fetal haemorrhage. Retroplacental bleeds and spontaneous abortion can still occur. There are, however, additional major problems with heparin:
• *Administration and compliance:* this has to be by subcutaneous self-injection throughout pregnancy from 6 to 36 weeks. Low-dose heparin (5000 U twice daily) is ineffective. The recommended dose is 7000 U s.c. three times daily or 10 000–12 500 units s.c. twice daily. This is a major undertaking for any patient and often unacceptable. It has to be started very early to avoid the teratogenic effect of warfarin in the first trimester. The switch from warfarin to heparin has to be immediately on obtaining a positive pregnancy test. However, a patient may not realise that she is pregnant for several weeks, by which time warfarin may have had its effect.
• *Osteoporosis:* this may occur after >5 months of heparin therapy, with demonstrable reduction in bone density. The cause is unknown. There is a little evidence that it may be reversible on stopping the heparin.
• *Alopecia:* may occur in some patients.
• *Thrombocytopenia:* this is common but usually asymptomatic. It is more common with heparin derived from bovine lung than from porcine gut (an IgG–heparin immune complex is formed). It usually occurs 3–15 days after starting the heparin and returns to normal if the drug is stopped within 4 days.
• *Lipodystrophy and bruising:* may occur at injection sites.

Recommendations for Anticoagulant Regimen during Pregnancy
There is no ideal regimen. Earlier enthusiasm for subcutaneous heparin has waned because of the major logistical problems and the dangers of ineffective anticoagulation.

It is safer from the mother's point of view to continue with effective warfarin control throughout the pregnancy and then to switch to intravenous heparin with a hospital admission at 36 weeks. These patients often require a short labour with a low threshold for caesarean section, and heparin is stopped about 6 h before delivery. It is restarted as soon as possible after delivery with the warfarin being restarted 2 days post partum.

With this regimen the mother must appreciate the fetal malformation risk, which is realistically <10%.

Haemolysis

This may occur with either mechanical or tissue valves. Although unusual it is more common in patients who have mechanical valves. It may develop severely acutely, usually associated with acute valve regurgitation (e.g. a flail mitral leaflet Figure 3.33), or on a milder, more chronic basis. Mild haemolysis may easily be missed. Additional intercurrent infections will exacerbate the anaemia. Prosthetic valve endocarditis must be considered in any patient with haemolysis.

Starr–Edwards valves with cloth-covered struts were introduced in 1967 in an attempt to reduce systemic emboli. Unfortunately, cloth disruption and haemolysis tended to develop and these valves were replaced by metal-tracked valves.

Patients are anaemic and possibly mildly jaundiced. There is urobilinogen and haemosiderin in the urine. Serum LDH levels are raised and haptoglobins lowered. The blood film shows fragmented cells (schistocytes), microcytosis and polychromasia. The Coombs' test is negative.

Mild haemolysis in the absence of infection may be managed with iron and folic acid supplements and occasional transfusion. Usually redo valve surgery is required.

Structural Valve Failure

Mechanical Valves
Failure is fortunately rare with mechanical valves. Ball variance with early Starr–Edwards valves was a result of absorption of lipid by the Silastic ball: the ball altered shape or even split.

The Björk–Shiley 60° convexo-concave single-disc valve (C–C valve) had problems, with minor strut fracture allowing the disc to escape. All Björk–Shiley valves manufactured after 1975 have a radio-opaque ring marker in the edge of the tilting disc. In a patient presenting in acute LVF, where valve sounds are inaudible, screening the valve will show that this ring is missing if the strut is fractured. The disc may be spotted in the peripheral circulation

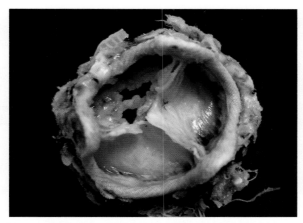

Figure 3.32 A 22-year-old aortic Carpentier–Edwards xenograft excised because of severe aortic regurgitation. One of the valve cusps has disintegrated. Not infected.

wedged in an artery. About 4000 patients are alive in the UK with C–C valves and the risk of strut fracture is about 7 per 10 000/year of whom two-thirds die acutely. The risk of a mitral redo valve replacement far exceeds this. Some patients may request a redo operation but most will just require close follow-up. The greatest risk seems to be in patients with a large-size mitral prosthesis (31 and 33 mm) and a weld date between 1/1/1981 and 30/7/1982.

Duramedics bileaflet valves (withdrawn in 1988) also rarely had a problem with fracture of the valve housing mechanism. Most will have been explanted now.

Tissue Valves (Xenografts or Homografts)
Gradual deterioration in all tissue valve function is to be expected, particularly in the young patient. Usually there is a gradual increase in valve regurgitation, often as a result of degeneration in a single cusp (Figure 3.32) but the valve may calcify and stenose. Most tissue valves will require a redo replacement at 10–15 years. Tissue valves in the aortic position last longer than in the mitral one. Tissue valves degenerate quickly in the young patient and particularly in pregnancy.

Acute tissue valve deterioration is due to a cusp tear (Figure 3.33). It is a difficulty with any tissue valve, and has been a problem with pericardial valves. The patient presents in acute pulmonary oedema. In patients with a mitral xenograft there is often a characteristic apical whooping systolic murmur and apical systolic thrill. The diagnosis is confirmed by Doppler echocardiography. Urgent redo valve replacement is needed. The torn cusp is not suitable for repair.

There is a gradual increase in the use of tissue valves with improving durability of modern valves. The risks of redo surgery now (particularly

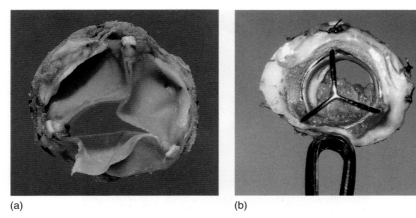

(a)   (b)

Figure 3.33 Prosthetic heart valve problems: (a): a 9-year-old xenograft (pericardial valve) removed from the mitral position in a woman presenting with acute pulmonary oedema and haemolysis. One of the three leaflets has torn and is flail. (b) A Starr–Edwards aortic valve removed from a 78-year-old woman with a history of recurrent transient ischaemic attacks. The Silastic ball has been removed to show a mass of thrombotic pannus occluding two-thirds of the valve orifice. Anticoagulant control had been inadequate.

in the aortic position) may well be less than a life sentence with warfarin and its complications. The patient's views must be included in the decision.

Valve Dehiscence

This occurs when sutures cut out, causing paraprosthetic valve regurgitation. It may occur in patients requiring valve replacement for uncontrolled infective endocarditis because the surrounding tissue is so oedematous and friable (Figures 3.34 and 3.35). It is common in patients with aortic valve endocarditis who have a mycotic aortic root aneurysm and need an aortic valve replacement. Patients with Marfan syndrome are at risk, with the surrounding tissue friable from cystic medial necrosis. It may also occur after a mitral valve replacement where the annulus is heavily calcified. As a sign of prosthetic valve endocarditis it usually occurs at a late stage.

A mild paraprosthetic leak may be tolerated well and treated medically, provided that it is not infected. Haemolysis is common. Echocardiography with colour flow mapping is diagnostic. Transoesophageal echocardiography is superior for mitral leaks. A moderate amount of haemolysis can be tolerated remarkably well by the patient, provided that the valve is not infected, the situation is stable and the patient is receiving folate and iron supplements.

Valve Thrombosis

This is usually the result of inadequate anticoagulant control and is fortunately rare. Patients present with symptoms from valve obstruction and valve

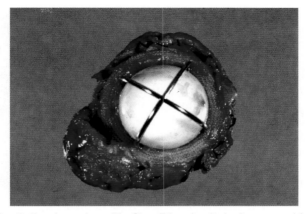

Figure 3.34 Prosthetic valve endocarditis: Starr–Edwards mitral valve removed for severe valve dehiscence with annular vegetations.

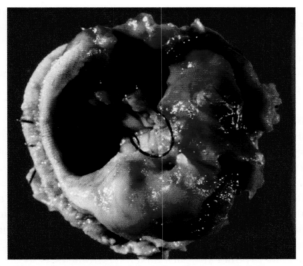

Figure 3.35 Prosthetic valve endocarditis: infected aortic xenograft. A large vegetation is obstructing half of the valve orifice.

sounds are muffled or absent. Large infected vegetations (especially fungal) may also cause valve obstruction. Echocardiography is again diagnostic. Abnormal central regurgitation may be seen. Acute valve thrombosis in the critically ill or pregnant patient may be rescued temporarily by thrombolysis, with the risks being much less than for redo surgery. The stroke risk is 7%. Urgent redo valve replacement is needed for fitter patients.

A chronic non-infected pannus of tissue may rarely encroach on the valve from the annulus and gradually cause valve obstruction (see Figure 3.33). Redo surgery is essential.

Myocardial Failure
This will cause deterioration in a patient's condition in spite of a perfectly functioning prosthetic valve. It may be a result of:
- muscle disease caused by previous rheumatic fever
- ventricular hypertrophy and fibrosis resulting from previous valve disease (e.g. aortic stenosis)
- coronary artery disease
- sepsis from infective endocarditis directly affecting ventricular muscle (see Chapter 9)
- long CPB, especially in patients with ventricular hypertrophy
- systemic or pulmonary hypertension
- coronary emboli
- preoperative poor ventricular function with severe MR; MVR once involved removal of the papillary muscles and it also increases afterload: this may provoke LV failure
- additional uncorrected valve disease
- rarely unrelated myocarditis or muscle infiltration.

Treatment will depend on the cause. Most patients will improve with the addition of diuretics and an ACE inhibitor (see Section 6.1).

Rhythm Problems
The three most common are the development of complete heart block after an aortic valve replacement, AF after a mitral valve replacement and ventricular arrhythmias in patients with myocardial disease.

Complete Heart Block
This is common after aortic valve replacement for severely calcified aortic valves and usually occurs during or very soon after surgery. Dual-chamber pacing is needed with the presence of LV hypertrophy. VVI pacing alone in this situation may produce the pacemaker syndrome (see Section 7.6).

CHB may also result from a septal abscess in infective endocarditis. In patients with native endocarditis it is an indication for urgent temporary pacing, followed by valve surgery with epicardial pacing for a day or two, followed by the implantation of a permanent pacemaker before the warfarin is started.

AF and Atrial Flutter
These are common after CPB, and particularly so in patients in sinus rhythm undergoing an MVR. Preoperative treatment with amiodarone (see Section 8.9) may help prevent this. Treatment when it occurs is along standard lines (see Section 8.3). If sinus rhythm was present preoperatively, DC cardioversion should be considered before the patient goes home.

Malignant Ventricular Arrhythmias (see Section 8.4)

These may occur in patients with severe ventricular hypertrophy, or in patients who have very poor ventricular function. They may cause sudden death in patients who have apparently made a good recovery from surgery. Diuretic-induced hypokalaemia and hypomagnesaemia must be avoided, as must digoxin toxicity. The proarrhythmic effects of antiarrhythmic drugs must be remembered.

4 | The Cardiomyopathies

Classification

These heart muscle diseases are a heterogeneous group of conditions associated with inappropriate hypertrophy or dilatation. The disease may be confined to the heart or be part of a systemic disorder. Mechanical and/or electrical dysfunction may lead to cardiac failure or cardiovascular death.

The diseases were originally divided by Goodwin into four functional categories:

1 Dilated cardiomyopathy (DCM), formerly congestive cardiomyopathy
2 Hypertrophic cardiomyopathy (HCM)
3 Restrictive cardiomyopathy
4 Obliterative cardiomyopathy.

The obliterative group included endomyocardial fibrosis and/or eosinophilic heart disease in which the apex of either or both ventricles was obliterated by fibrous tissue. The functional result was a small stiff ventricle and they subsequently became classified with the restrictive group.

However, with the passage of time this classification has proved too narrow and a broader classification was needed to include so many other heart muscle diseases (Table 4.1). This classification is based more on aetiology where this is known rather than function.

4.1 Dilated Cardiomyopathy

This is a common and usually irreversible form of heart muscle disease. One or both ventricles are dilated with poor systolic function. Coronary arteries are normal. The definite diagnosis can only be made following coronary angiography, because ischaemic heart disease may sometimes present as heart failure in patients who have never had angina. Prevalence is approximately 1 : 2500.

Swanton's Cardiology, sixth edition. By R. H. Swanton and S. Banerjee. Published 2008 Blackwell Publishing. ISBN 978-1-4051-7819-8.

Table 4.1 Classification of cardiomyopathies

Primary cardiomyopathies	Secondary cardiomyopathies (with systemic disease)[a]
Genetic	**Infiltrative and storage diseases**
Hypertrophic cardiomyopathy (HCM)	Amyloid heart disease
Arrhythmogenic RV cardiomyopathy (ARVC)	Gaucher's disease
Isolated ventricular non-compaction (IVNC)	Hurler's disease
Mitochondrial myopathies	Hunter's disease
	Haemochromatosis
	Anderson-Fabry disease
	Niemann-Pick disease
	Glycogen storage diseases
	Sarcoidosis
Mixed	**Autoimmune/collagen vascular disease**
Dilated cardiomyopathy (DCM)	Systemic lupus erythematosus
Restrictive cardiomyopathy	Scleroderma
	Rheumatoid arthritis
	Polyarteritis nodosa
Acquired	**Endocrine**
Myocarditis	Diabetes mellitus
Takotsubo cardiomyopathy (TTC)	Hyperthyroidism
Puerperal cardiomyopathy	Hypothyroidism
Tachycardia-induced myopathy	Acromegaly
Endomyocardial fibrosis (EMF)	**Toxicity**
Loeffler's eosinophilic endocarditis	Drugs: anthracyclines, trastuzumab, cyclophosphamide, chloroquine
	Radiation
	Heavy metals: lithium, lead, antimony
	Alcohol
	Neuromuscular disorders
	Friedreich's ataxia
	Emery-Dreifuss muscular dystrophy
	Duchenne-Becker muscular dystrophy
	Dystrophia myotonica
	Neurofibromatosis
	Nutritional deficiencies
	Beri-beri (vitamin B_1), kwashiorkor, scurvy, selenium

[a]See Chapter 11.

The left ventricle becomes more globular and spherical. The endocardium becomes diffusely thickened and the atria also dilate with possible thrombus in the atrial appendages. Myocyte attenuation and cell death are associated with increased interstitial fibrosis and possible T-cell and macrophage infiltration.

Aetiology (see Table 4.1)
In most cases no cause is identified. Factors that may cause a dilated cardio-myopathy are:
• Alcohol
• Infective myocarditis: viral infection, Coxsackie virus, adenovirus, parvo-virus, HIV; bacteria; rickettsiae; parasitic: Trypanosoma cruzi (Chagas' disease)
• Thyrotoxicosis (see Section 11.16)
• Drugs: anthracyclines, trastuzumab (see Section 11.7)
• Heavy metal toxicity: lead, cobalt or mercury poisoning
• Nutritional deficiency: beri-beri (vitamin B1), selenium, carnitine
• Catecholamines: phaeochromocytoma (see Section 12.6)
• Autoimmune disease
• Puerperium
• Neuromuscular disease: Duchenne, Emery–Dreifuss muscular dystrophy
• Genetic factors
• Haemochromatosis (see Section 11.9).

Autosomal Forms of DCM
The most common is the mutation of the lamin A/C gene (*LMNA*) coding for the nuclear envelope and associated with autosomal dominant DCM, conduction system disease, mild skeletal myopathy and autosomal dominant Emery–Dreifuss muscular dystrophy. Sinus and AV node disease tend to occur first followed by the DCM.

X-linked Forms of DCM
DCM is associated with a number of X-linked genetic mutations with genes encoding the cytoskeletal proteins dystrophin, α-actin, desmin, sarcoglycans, the nuclear envelope proteins lamin A/C and emerin, the Z disc protein titin, metavinculin and ZASP (the Z line-associated protein), and the mitochondrial respiratory chain gene. In contrast, gene mutations causing HCM code for contractile sarcomeric proteins (see below).

X-linked forms occur early in male adolescents or young adults who develop DCM associated with a muscular dystrophy (Table 4.2).

Table 4.2 Genetic mutations associated with dilated cardio-myopathy and skeletal muscular dystrophy

Gene coding	Type of muscular dystrophy
Dystrophin	Duchenne, Becker's
Tafazzin (gene 4.5)	Barth syndrome (male infants)
Emerin	Emily-Dreifuss
δ-Sarcoglycan	Limb-girdle
Mitochondria	Mitochondrial myopathy

Detailed studies of first-degree relatives of patients with DCM have shown that up to 20% have a degree of ventricular enlargement and 3% have definite DCM. Overall, up to 35% of patients have familial disease. In particular search for a family history of conduction system disease and/or a skeletal myopathy.

Pathophysiology and Symptoms

There is progressive dilatation of both ventricles (usually LV > RV) with a low cardiac output, and tachycardia produces fatigue, dyspnoea, and later oedema and ascites typical of CCF.

Additional problems result from the following:

• Functional valvar regurgitation: dilated mitral and tricuspid valve rings plus poor papillary muscle function.

• Systemic or pulmonary emboli: mural thrombus is common in either ventricle.

• AF: especially in DCM secondary to alcohol. A further reduction in cardiac output occurs with the development of AF.

• Conduction system disease: LBBB is common.

• Paroxysmal ventricular tachycardia or ventricular fibrillation and sudden death.

• Secondary renal failure or hepatic failure: further salt and water retention, secondary hyperaldosteronism and hypoalbuminaemia, all contributing to the oedema.

Typical Signs

A cool, peripherally cyanosed patient with very poor exercise tolerance or a bedridden patient.

• Blood pressure: low. Small pulse pressure (e.g. 90/75).

• Pulse: small volume; thready; may be in AF. If in SR may have pulsus alternans. Usually rapid (>100/min).

• JVP: raised to the angle of the jaw. May have prominent 'v' wave of tricuspid regurgitation.

• Apex: displaced to anterior or midaxillary line; diffuse.

• Auscultation: gallop rhythm (summation if in SR) with functional mitral regurgitation and/or tricuspid regurgitation.

• Pleural effusions and possible crepitations.

• Hepatomegaly; mild jaundice; ascites; oedema of legs and sacrum.

Check also for signs of hypercholesterolaemia, excessive alcohol intake, previous hypertension (fundi) or collagen disease. Check thyroid for bruit.

Investigations

Chest radiograph shows moderate-to-gross cardiac enlargement with signs of LV failure, pleural effusions or pulmonary oedema.

ECG shows sinus tachycardia usually with non-specific T-wave changes. Poor R-wave progression in anterior chest leads may be mistaken for old anterior infarction.

Echocardiography shows large left and right ventricles with very poor septal and posterior wall movement. Two-dimensional echocardiography may show mural thrombus. There is often a small pericardial effusion. Ejection fraction is very low. Doppler studies may quantitate the degree of mitral regurgitation.

Cardiac catheterization can be dangerous in patients with very poor LV function and precipitate acute pulmonary oedema, systemic emboli or arterial occlusion. It may be necessary once a patient has been 'dried out' to:

- confirm the diagnosis and document normal coronaries
- exclude LV aneurysm
- check on the severity of associated mitral regurgitation.

Ventricular biopsy is no longer indicated for the diagnosis but will still be needed for research. Histological confirmation of acute myocarditis with infiltration of the interstitial tissue by T lymphocytes (confirmed on immunohistochemistry) is found in only 10% of patients. There are many non-specific and non-diagnostic changes. Early excitement, with the use of DNA probes and in situ hybridization to find viral RNA within the biopsy fragments, has proved unfounded because this has now been found as frequently in control specimens. The viral genome may persist within the myocardium long after the acute phase of the disease.

Blood Tests

- Viral titres (especially for the Coxsackie virus and enterovirus group) and an autoimmune screen as a routine
- Blood grouping and HLA typing if transplantation is considered
- Measure thyroid function if in AF
- Routine serum iron and iron-binding capacity (see Section 11.9).

Autoantibodies to α- and β-myosin heavy chains are found in $\leq$25% of patients with DCM at the time of diagnosis. The titre may gradually fall after an initial episode of acute myocarditis. They are thought to be a marker of disease rather than pathogenetic: in fact the presence of antibody is associated with a milder disease course and better functional capacity at 1 year.

Management

Complete prolonged bed rest with careful fluid balance monitoring, daily weight measurement and some fluid restriction is required. Intravenous diuretics are usually needed. Digoxin is indicated in AF or if a loud S3 persists in spite of diuretics and bed rest. β Blockers are not used in the acute phase even with an inappropriate tachycardia. An ACE inhibitor is usually necessary but starting with very low doses (see Section 6.6). Anticoagulation is very important in all patients with DCM even if in sinus rhythm. Only small doses of warfarin may be needed (hepatic congestion); 24-hour ECG monitoring is performed to check for AF or VT.

There is no indication to use steroids and immunosuppression, because these have no influence on prognosis even in confirmed myocarditis.

Prognosis

About 50% of patients with DCM will die within 2 years of initial diagnosis and the mortality rate is about 4%/year thereafter. Poorer prognostic features include:

- AF
- LVEDD >7.6 cm
- Increasing mitral regurgitation
- PCW pressure >16 mmHg on treatment
- Myocardial O_2 consumption (Vo_2) <50% predicted value
- Restrictive pattern of filling
- T-wave alternans during stress testing
- Chagas' disease.

Transplantation offers the only hope of long-term survival for patients not responding to medical therapy.

Puerperal Cardiomyopathy (also see Chapter 15)

About 60% of patients with puerperal cardiomyopathy improve. However, there is a significant risk of deterioration in LV function with subsequent pregnancies, whether or not cardiac function has returned to normal after the first episode (about a 20% chance of deterioration if cardiac function has returned to normal and a 44% chance if it has not). Mothers should be warned of this before considering a further pregnancy.

Cardiac Transplantation (see Section 6.15)

Conventional cardiac surgery has little to contribute. Mitral valve replacement is considered when mitral regurgitation is severe but carries an increased risk if the ejection fraction is very low, and even if the patient survives there may be little improvement in ventricular function. LV volume reduction (wedge resection of a segment of the ventricle avoiding the papillary muscles) is an operation of interest but as yet is of unproven long-term benefit. Cardiac transplantation in the younger patient carries the only hope of long-term survival and a good lifestyle. Transplantation centres vary in the top age limit for accepting cases, which is usually between 50 and 60. It is important that the patient be referred early before the development of renal failure, recurrent chest infections and cardiac cachexia, which greatly influence operative risks and postoperative survival.

Patients with systemic disease may not necessarily be refused. Patients with type 1 diabetes have been transplanted successfully. Specific conditions must be discussed in advance with the transplant centre.

Future Trends

Growth Hormone

A small number of patients with DCM have been treated with recombinant human growth hormone 14 IU/week. Over 3 months there was a reduction in LV dimensions, an increase in LV wall thickness and myocardial mass, and an improvement in exercise capacity. The study was uncontrolled but this is an exciting possible alternative to transplantation that needs further study.

Cell Therapy

Randomized controlled trials are under way in attempts to improve the LV ejection fraction using injections of autologous bone marrow stem cells or autologous skeletal myoblasts. It is known that these implanted cell nests survive and develop contractile potential. There are concerns about the possibility of the cells acting as arrhythmogenic foci. Early results are conflicting and may relate to the difficulty of measuring the ejection fraction with the small improvements seen within the reproducibility of the measurement itself.

Exclusions

In patients with suspected DCM it is important to exclude conditions that resemble it and may respond to surgery:
• pericardial constriction
• severe aortic stenosis with LVF
• severe mitral regurgitation
• LV aneurysm
• severe pulmonary stenosis
• severe Ebstein's anomaly.

In low-output states these conditions may produce few or no murmurs. Echocardiography is important in these exclusions.

4.2 Hypertrophic Cardiomyopathy

This was first described in 1958 by Teare, who noted asymmetrical septal hypertrophy in nine adults, eight of whom died suddenly. It is known by other terms, such as IHSS (idiopathic hypertrophic subaortic stenosis), familial hypertrophic subaortic stenosis, ASH (asymmetrical septal hypertrophy) and DUST (disproportionate upper septal thickening), although the last two are really just echocardiographic terms. The prevalence is 0.2% (1 in 500 of the population).

Although the pathology, haemodynamics and natural history of the condition are well described, we are ignorant of the causes of sudden death and have made little difference to the progression of the disease with medical treatment.

Table 4.3 Hypertrophic cardiomyopathy: common genetic mutations

Chromosome	Mutation on gene coding for	Cases (%)	Associations
1q3	Troponin T	15	Worst prognosis
7q3			Wolff-Parkinson-White syndrome
11p13	Myosin-binding protein C	10–15	
14q11	β-Myosin heavy chain	30	
15q2	α-Tropomyosin	3	

Inheritance

The first genetic defect was identified in north Canada in 1989. About 70% of cases are inherited as an autosomal dominant with a high degree of penetrance and equal sex distribution. In the rest genetic defects cannot as yet be identified. Spontaneous mutations occur accounting for sporadic cases. These mutations are in genes coding for sarcomeric contractile proteins (Table 4.3). More than 30 missense mutations (a single amino acid mutation) have been found in the B-myosin heavy chain gene on chromosome 14 alone. This genetic heterogeneity may account for the different clinical spectrum in HCM. The mutation type may be important prognostically and allows preclinical diagnosis. At least 10 different genes have now been identified with recognised mutations.

Pathogenesis

This is unknown. It has been suggested that the abnormal arrangement of myocardial cells in the septum may be the result of excessive catecholamine stimulation caused by a genetic abnormality of neural crest tissue (compare the association of HCM with hypertension, lentiginosis and phaeochromocytoma). A very similar lesion occurs in Friedreich's ataxia.

Pathology

This is hypertrophy of the ventricular septum compared with the LV free wall (Figure 4.1). The abnormal muscle fibres are short, thick and fragmented, with myocardial disarray. There is fibrosis (Figure 4.2). The nuclei are large and the fibres arranged in whorls. These findings may be patchy but are concentrated in the septum. The pathological changes have been found in the RV outflow tract in patients with a VSD and in the RV of infants with pulmonary atresia. The subvalve obstruction occurs between the thickened interventricular septum and the anterior leaflet of the mitral valve and its apparatus (Figure 4.3). The mitral apparatus is either sucked forward in systole (Venturi effect of high-velocity jet) or pulled by malaligned papillary muscles. The mitral valve becomes thickened and may be regurgitant. It is possible to have ASH without obstruction. Hypercontractile ventricles may look like HCM on LV

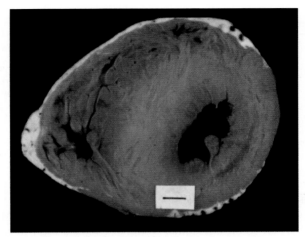

Figure 4.1 Postmortem specimen of hypertrophic cardiomyopathy with marked asymmetrical septal hypertrophy. The interventricular septum was 4.2 cms thick. (Reproduced with permission of the publisher from Crawford MH, DiMarco JP, Paulus WJ in Cardiology, 2nd edn, 2003, Oxford, Elsevier.)

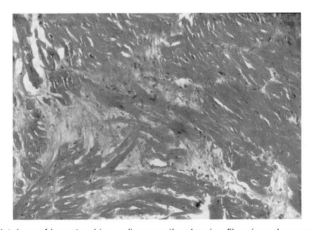

Figure 4.2 Histology of hypertrophic cardiomyopathy showing fibrosis and myocardial disarray.

angiography but have no gradient at rest or on provocation (may be seen in first-degree relatives of patients with HCM). Occasionally the obstruction seems more apical in site. The condition is similar to true HCM. About a third of cases have concentric LV hypertrophy (Figure 4.4).

Myocardial bridging of the left anterior descending may be a risk factor for sudden death in children.

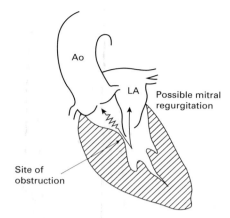

Figure 4.3 Site of obstruction in HCM.

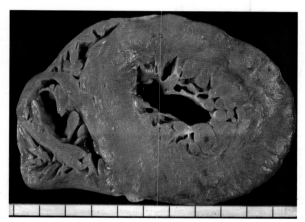

Figure 4.4 Postmortem specimen from a 16-year-old Jamaican girl who died from HCM: massive concentric LV hypertrophy.

Pathophysiology and Symptoms (Figure 4.5)

The symptoms may be identical to aortic valve stenosis. It may present at any age.

Angina, Even with Normal Coronaries

• Possibly as a result of: excessive muscle mass exceeding coronary supply; high diastolic pressures producing high wall tension preventing diastolic coronary flow; high systolic stress increasing myocardial oxygen demand; excessive internal work for any level of external work resulting from increased frictional and viscous drag. The disarrayed hypertrophy results in inefficient transfer of rising muscle tension to muscle shortening. Extravascular compression of coronary vessels and reduced capillary density contribute.

• Abnormal narrowing of small coronary vessels; reduces coronary flow reserve.

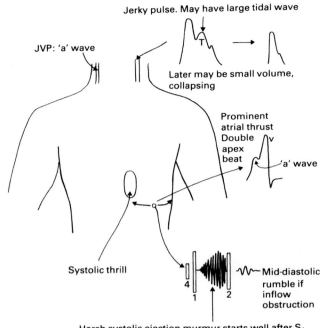

Figure 4.5 Clinical signs of HCM.

Dyspnoea
• Caused by poor LV compliance, resulting in a stiff ventricle in diastole. LVEDP is high. Atrial transport is vital. Symptoms become rapidly worse if AF supervenes. Thick papillary muscles may result in 'inflow obstruction'.
• Caused by associated mitral regurgitation.

Syncope and Sudden Death
This is as in aortic valve stenosis, but also:
• Extreme outflow obstruction caused by catecholamine stimulation (effort or excitement).
• Known association with Wolff–Parkinson–White (WPW) syndrome; rapid AV conduction down accessory pathway leading to VF in patients who develop AF or sinus tachycardia.
• Massive MI.

Risk Stratification
Sudden death occurs annually in about 1% of patients and determining which patients are at risk of sudden death and who should be considered for an ICD remains a great problem. The search for a marker with high predictive accuracy continues. Poor prognostic features are as follows.

History
- Young age at diagnosis (<14 years)
- Syncope as a presenting symptom
- Family history of HCM with sudden premature death (age < 40)
- Previous cardiac arrest: approximately 40% chance of recurrence.

Holter Monitoring for Non-sustained VT in Adults
This occurs in about 25% of adults with HCM, and is defined as three or more consecutive ventricular extrasystoles at a rate of >120/min lasting <30 s. The attacks are usually asymptomatic and often occur at night when vagal tone is high. However, non-sustained VT remains the best non-invasive marker for sudden death, with a sensitivity of 69% and specificity of 80%. However, predictive accuracy is low at 22%, because the incidence is low in children. Sustained monomorphic VT is relatively rare.

Peripheral Vascular Responses
There is a fall in systolic pressure on exercise, or failing to increase systolic pressure by >20 mmHg. About a third of patients with HCM fail to increase their blood pressure normally on effort. The reason for this vasodepressor response is unknown (possibly mediated by LV baroreceptors firing off under very high pressure causing peripheral vasodilatation). It tends to occur in younger patients, those with the smaller LV cavity and those with a family history of sudden death.

Prognostic Genotyping
For details, see Inheritance above. Identification of the mutation type appears to carry prognostic significance, e.g. the troponin-T mutation is the worst, patients often dying in the age range 18–24 years after the puberty growth spurt.

Extreme LV Hypertrophy
Risk of sudden death increases with increasing wall thickness and patients with LV wall thickness >30 mm are at particular risk.

Invasive Electrophysiology

Increased ECG Fractionation
This is still experimental. Preliminary studies involving paced RV electrograms at various RV sites have shown increased fractionation in survivors of VF.

Ventricular Provocation (see Section 8.5)
This is a procedure not without risk in HCM. VT can rapidly degenerate into VF and the prognostic value of inducing VF is uncertain and hence little used.

Other Features

Features that have not proved of prognostic benefit in HCM include the following:

• *Non-invasive electrophysiology*: unfortunately theoretically useful markers such as QT dispersion, heart rate variability and late potentials on the signal-averaged ECG have not proved of prognostic value.

• *Invasive haemodynamics*: the severity of the resting subvalve gradient is of little prognostic value as an isolated risk factor. LVOTO is associated with an increased risk of sudden cardiac death but with low positive predictive accuracy. The asymptomatic patient with LVOTO and no other risk factor is at low risk of sudden cardiac death (0.4%/year).

• *Identification of myocardial ischaemia*: the presence of ST-segment depression is common in baseline ECGs with such marked LV hypertrophy. Neither thallium-201 scanning nor positron emission tomography has proved of value yet in documenting ischaemia. Thallium-201 perfusion defects are common in HCM. Coronary sinus metabolic studies with atrial pacing may prove helpful.

Principal Risk Markers for Sudden Death in HCM

• Previous cardiac arrest
• Non-sustained VT on Holter monitoring
• Abnormal BP response on exercise
• Family history of premature sudden death
• Unexplained syncope
• Severe LV hypertrophy

Natural History

Annual mortality rate in children (<14 years) is 5.9%. Generally children are less symptomatic (apart from syncope). Annual mortality rate in those aged 15–45 years is 2.5%.

Symptom severity is not closely related to haemodynamic estimates of LVOTO. Some patients may develop endstage congestive cardiac failure with rapidly enlarging heart and reduction in LVOT gradient (postmyotomy patients are said to do this more frequently).

Differentiation from Aortic Valve Stenosis (Table 4.4)

The three conditions most likely to be confused with HCM are:

1 Aortic valve stenosis
2 'Subvalve' mitral regurgitation (e.g. chordal rupture)
3 VSD.

'Subvalve' mitral regurgitation, VSD and HCM may have small volume 'jerky' pulses, a harsh ejection systolic murmur and a systolic thrill. The thrill

Table 4.4 Differentiation of aortic valve stenosis from hypertrophic cardiomyopathy

	Valve stenosis	HCM
Carotid pulse	Anacrotic	Jerky
Thrill	Second right interspace	Lower sternum to left
Ejection sound	May be present	Absent
Aortic EDM	Often present	Rare (after surgery)
Manoeuvres to vary obstruction	Fixed	Variable

Table 4.5 Variation in LV outflow obstruction

Increased LVOT obstruction (murmur louder and longer)	Decreased LVOT obstruction (murmur softer and shorter)
Reducing ventricular volume	**Increasing ventricular volume**
Sudden standing	Squatting
Valsalva's manoeuvre (during)	Valsalva's manoeuvre (after release)
Amyl nitrate inhalation	Mueller's manoeuvre (deep inspiration against a closed glottis)
Nitroglycerin	
Hypovolaemia	Handgrip
Excessive diuresis	Passive leg elevation
Increasing contractility	**Decreasing contractility**
β Agonists, e.g. isoprenaline	β Blockade (acute intravenous)
Post-extrasystolic potentiation	
	? Calcium antagonists
Decreased afterload	**Increased afterload**
α Blockade	α Agonists
	Phenylephrine
	Handgrip

in mitral regurgitation is usually apical in chordal rupture (but may be more anterior in posterior chordal rupture).

Therefore the demonstration of variable obstruction is very important (Table 4.5). Some of these manoeuvres can be performed at the bedside and are therefore useful in differentiating from aortic valve stenosis.

Differentiation from the Athlete's Heart (Table 4.6)

Regular intensive athletic training induces concentric LV hypertrophy and LV chamber dilatation. In addition increased vagal tone results in a sinus bradycardia and even an occasional Wenckebach-type AV block at night. Difficulties may arise with a patient thought to have HCM who indulges in a fair amount of exercise. It is important to realize that really intensive athletic training is required to induce LV hypertrophy, which might be confused with HCM, and a weekly game of football is definitely not enough! In addition mild hypertension does not cause the degree of LV hypertrophy seen in HCM.

Table 4.6 Differentiation of hypertrophic cardiomyopathy from the athlete's heart

Pattern	Hypertrophic cardiomyopathy	Athlete's heart
Unusual pattern LVH	Yes	No
LVEDD <45 mm	Yes	No
LVEDD >55 mm	No	Yes
LA enlargement	Yes	No
Bizarre ECG	Yes	No
Abnormal LV filling	Yes	No
Family history	Yes	No
LV reduces on deconditioning	No	Yes
Max Vo$_2$ >45 ml/kg per min	No	Yes

Reproduced from Maron *et al.*, Circulation 1995; 1596–601 with permission of Lippincott Williams & Wilkins.

In spite of these differences it can occasionally be difficult to decide, and the initial diagnosis of HCM may be one of exclusion of other possible causes of LV hypertrophy.

Echocardiography (see Section 17.4 and Figure 17.6, 17.41–17.43)
Several features in association are diagnostic of HCM:
• Midsystolic aortic valve closure (occurring later than discrete fibromuscular ring obstruction): midsystolic fluttering of aortic valve.
• ASH: grossly thickened septum compared with posterior LV wall, with reduced motion of the septum. Angulation of the echo beam may produce false positives on M-mode.
• Small LV cavity with hypercontractile posterior wall.
• Systolic anterior movement (SAM) of the mitral apparatus: this may demonstrate contact between the anterior mitral leaflet and septal wall in systole. This contact has been used to quantitate the severity of the obstruction.
• Reduced diastolic closure rate of anterior mitral leaflet. This is a result of slow LV filling in diastole with low LV compliance. Echocardiography is useful in assessment of the results of drug treatment.
• Continuous-wave Doppler studies using the apical four-chamber view with the sample volume in the LV outflow tract show a characteristic dynamic envelope with a concave leading edge.

Electrocardiography (see Chapter 16, Figure 16.2)
Usually abnormal even in asymptomatic patients (only about 25% have no symptoms plus a normal ECG). The following are the most common abnormalities:
• LV hypertrophy plus ST- and T-wave changes, progressive and steeper T-wave inversion with time
• Deep Q waves in inferior and lateral leads (septal hypertrophy and fibrosis)

- Pre-excitation and WPW syndrome
- Ventricular ectopics
- Ventricular tachycardia on ambulatory monitoring.

Cardiac Catheterization

M-mode and two-dimensional echocardiography have reduced the need for diagnostic catheterization. The LV is very irritable, and entering the LV with a catheter often provokes VT. The procedure should document the following:

- The severity of the resting gradient, or provocation of a gradient if none at rest; a typical withdrawal gradient is seen in Figure 4.6
- The presence of mitral regurgitation
- The possibility of an additional fibromuscular ring

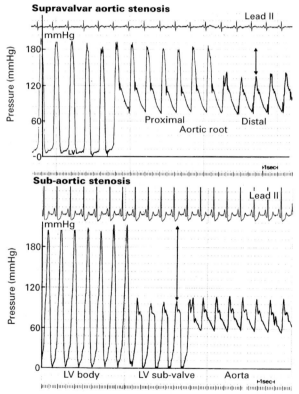

Figure 4.6 Withdrawal of a catheter from left ventricle to aorta in supravalvar aortic stenosis (top panel) and subaortic stenosis (lower panel), in this case hypertrophic obstructive cardiomyopathy. Both were recorded on slow sweep speed. The gradients are represented by vertical arrowed bars. In supravalvar AS the gradient is within the aortic root itself (see Section 3.4). In HCM the gradient is between the LV body and the subaortic chamber (see also Figure 4.3).

- The state of the coronary arteries
- Electrophysiological investigation may be needed in patients with the WPW syndrome
- Postoperative assessment.

Magnetic Resonance Imaging

Although this is not a routine investigation in HCM, cardiac MRI can be of value in determining the severity and possible asymmetry of LV hypertrophy, possible additional mitral regurgitation and LV systolic obliteration (Figures 4.7 and 4.8).

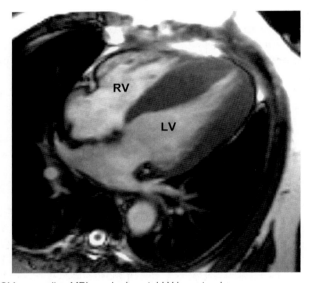

Figure 4.7 HCM on cardiac MRI: marked septal LV hypertrophy.

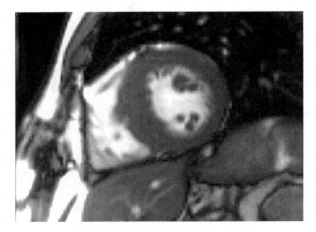

Figure 4.8 HCM on cardiac MRI: septal hypertrophy > posterior wall.

Medical Therapy

- *Patients with angina* caused by HCM should not receive nitrates.
- *Digoxin* should be prescribed only when AF is established and irreversible, or if considerable cardiac enlargement occurs when LV outflow tract obstruction has already fallen.
- *Diuretics* must be used carefully.
- *The role of β blockade:*
  - acute intravenous β blockade is well documented to reduce the subvalve gradient and lower LVEDP; it may increase LVEDV; β blockade is thus the mainstay of therapy for symptoms of angina, dyspnoea, giddiness and syncope

  Long-term studies of its efficacy are awaited. There is still no evidence to suggest that it alters long-term prognosis or reduces the incidence of sudden death. Very large doses of propranolol have been shown to prevent the gradual increase in LV hypertrophy over time.
  - large doses of β-blocking agents are sometimes used (e.g. propranolol >160 mg three times daily).
- *The role of calcium antagonists:*
  - this is still debatable and depends on the balance between the negative inotropic effect and the vasodilating action of the various drugs
  - nifedipine has a more pronounced vasodilating action than a negative inotropic action and should be avoided
  - verapamil has a less vigorous vasodilating effect and more pronounced negative inotropic effect. The claims that it reduces septal thickness have not been substantiated. It should be avoided in patients on β blockade. It not as effective an anti-arrhythmic drug as amiodarone in HCM, but can be used as an alternative to β blockade. As with β blockers, large doses are needed (240–480 mg/day) but the dose should be increased gradually. Verapamil should be avoided in patients if there is a substantial outflow tract gradient because it may precipitate hypotension and pulmonary oedema.
- *Disopyramide:* a small trial of intravenous disopyramide has shown that it can substantially reduce the LVOT gradient. Oral disopyramide is an alternative to β blockade and patients may find a better exercise capacity on this.
- *Dysrhythmias:* AF should be cardioverted as soon as possible even in large hearts. Patients who will not revert should be digitalized. Amiodarone taken orally may induce version to sinus rhythm. Non-sustained VT is common, occurring in 25% of patients on Holter monitoring and is the most likely cause of sudden death (see Risk Stratification above). Propranolol and verapamil are not effective at abolishing this and have no effect on prognosis. Low-dose amiodarone should be tried (plasma levels 0.5–1.5 mg/l), which helps avoid long-term side effects (see Section 8.9) and has been shown to be effective, but there is still no long-term randomised trial using amiodarone. Alternatives

are flecainide, mexiletine and disopyramide. Patients with refractory VT on drug therapy should be considered for an implantable cardioverter defibrillator (ICD).

• *Pregnancy* with HCM is generally well tolerated (see Section 5.5). β-Blocking agents should be withdrawn if possible (small-for-dates babies and fetal bradycardia may occur as side effects of β blockade). Vaginal delivery is possible but excessive maternal effort should be avoided. Haemorrhage may increase the resting gradient and volume replacement should be available. Ergometrine may be used. Epidural anaesthesia is probably best avoided because it may cause vasodilatation and hence an increased gradient. Antibiotic prophylaxis for delivery is advised. There is a strong chance that the child will be affected.

• *Infective endocarditis* may occur in HCM. Routine antibiotic prophylaxis should be given for dental and surgical procedures (see Section 9.7).

• *Systemic emboli* may occur and require anticoagulation.

Dual Chamber Pacing

This was an encouraging alternative to surgery, performed in the absence of the usual conduction indications. Depolarization from the RV apex alters septal motion and reduces the subaortic gradient. Initial results showed that the gradient may be halved with considerable improvement in symptoms. Long-term results and the effects on mitral regurgitation are, however, disappointing with the technique not fulfilling its early promise.

Dual chamber pacing is cheaper and safer than surgery and could still be considered as the initial procedure in older and frailer patients with symptoms resistant to drug therapy and those with mitral regurgitation. The pacemaker should be programmed with a short AV delay to ensure that every ventricular complex is paced. Some patients will, in addition, have chronotropic incompetence (failure of heart rate to increase on effort) and benefit from DDDR pacing rather than just DDD pacing (see Section 7.6).

Implantable Cardioverter Defibrillator (see Section 7.11)

An ICD should be considered in patients with HCM who have multiple risk factors for sudden death, e.g. non-sustained VT, syncope, extreme LVH (>30 mm), abnormal exercise BP responses and family history of sudden death. See risk markers in HCM above.

Percutaneous Septal Ablation

This is the injection of 2 ml 96% alcohol down the first septal artery at cardiac catheterization (Sigwart 1995) has been shown to reduce the outflow tract gradient. The alcohol is injected through the central lumen of an angioplasty balloon. This remains inflated for 5 min after injection to prevent alcohol reflux into the LAD. This reduction in LVOT gradient is maintained in the long term, and LV mass and wall thickness remote from the outflow tract are also reduced. This suggests that the LV hypertrophy results partly from the LVOT obstruction itself.

Case selection is very important and critically depends on septal artery anatomy. Transthoracic echocardiography is used to assess the area of muscle supplied by the first septal artery or one of its branches, with injection of Sonovue down the balloon catheter lumen. If any other part of the LV or RV than the upper septum is highlighted by this injection, the patient is unsuitable for the procedure. After successful septal ablation there is a reduction or abolition of the outflow tract gradient, which does not even appear after an interpolated ventricular ectopic beat (Figures 4.9 and 4.10).

Temporary RV pacing is required before alcohol injection and there is a small risk of permanent complete heart block necessitating permanent dual chamber pacing.

Finally, it is important to remember that septal ablation or surgical myomectomy is a procedure for refractory symptoms. Neither protects the patient from sudden death and an ICD may be necessary in addition.

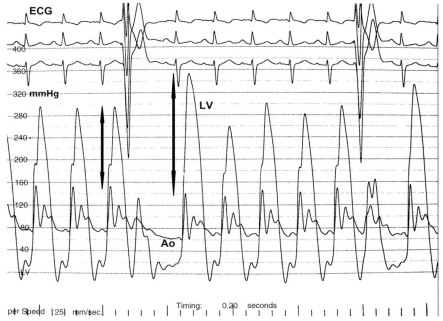

Figure 4.9 HCM with outflow obstruction: baseline recordings from aorta (Ao) and left ventricular (LV) before septal ablation; post-ectopic potentiation. There is a resting LVOT gradient of 140 mmHg. Following an interpolated ventricular ectopic the post-ectopic beat shows an increased gradient of 210 mmHg (vertical arrows), but the pressure in the aorta is typically lower than the pre-ectopic beat.

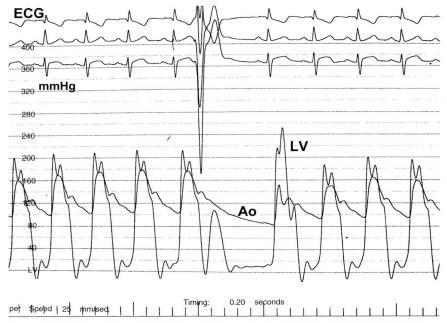

Figure 4.10 HCM: post-septal ablation – simultaneous recordings of aortic and LV pressures. The LVOT gradient is virtually abolished. The post-ectopic beat still shows a small residual gradient.

Surgery

This is reserved for the 5% of severely symptomatic patients who continue to have disabling angina, dyspnoea or syncope in spite of vigorous medical treatment, or those unsuitable for alcohol septal ablation (see above).

A myotomy/myomectomy is performed through the aortic valve (Morrow operation). This reduces the LVOT gradient more substantially than DDD pacing. About 5% of patients will need an additional mitral valve replacement with a low profile valve. Unroofing of the left anterior descending coronary artery may be beneficial in patients with a demonstrable myocardial bridge. The development of LBBB postoperatively may help reduce the obstruction. There is no evidence yet that surgery reduces the incidence of sudden death.

Surgery in early series carried some risk (10–27%), usually as a result of malignant postoperative ventricular dysrhythmias. Large series now have the perioperative mortality rates down to 3.6% with good long-term survival (80% at 10 years). Amiodarone is used for documented VT perioperatively and an ICD may be needed for recurrent VT (see Section 7.11). Surgery can dramatically improve a patient's symptoms. Complete AV block may occur as a result of myomectomy and, if it does, dual chamber pacing is essential with a programmed short AV delay because the LV muscle is stiff and atrial transport vital to maintaining the cardiac output. There is a small risk (<5%) of a VSD with surgery, and an additional small risk of postoperative aortic regurgitation.

Poor prognostic features postoperatively are:

- NYHA class III or IV
- additional procedure at surgery (e.g. MVR or CABG)
- CCF
- AF.

4.3 Restrictive Cardiomyopathy

Clinically this may be identical to constrictive pericarditis. Whereas surgery is necessary for pericardial constriction, it is of no benefit to and possibly harmful to patients with restriction (see Sections 10.3 and 11.3).

Causes
- Iron-storage diseases (see Section 11.9)
- Scleroderma (see Section 11.14)
- Amyloidosis (see Section 11.3)
- Loeffler's eosinophilic endocarditis and endomyocardial fibrosis (EMF), both known as 'eosinophilic heart disease' (see Section 4.7)
- Sarcoidosis (see Section 11.13).

Patients with amyloid heart disease or sarcoidosis may have additional mitral or tricuspid regurgitation. Q waves on chest leads of the ECG are common and may be confused with old infarction. Atrial systolic failure (caused by amyloid infiltration) increases the symptoms of congestion. Stagnation of blood in an inert atrium or AF increases the risk of systemic emboli and anti-coagulation may be needed. Digoxin has an evil reputation in amyloid heart disease.

Differentiation of Constrictive Pericarditis from
Amyloid Heart Disease (see also Section 10.3)

This is difficult. Both restrictive myopathy and constrictive pericarditis may have:

- raised JVP with prominent 'x' and 'y' descents (see Chapter 10, Figure 10.5)
- normal systolic function
- LVEDV <110 ml/m^2
- absence of LV hypertrophy
- rapid early diastolic filling with diastolic dip and plateau waveform (see Chapter 10, Figure 10.6).

The best techniques to differentiate the two conditions are echocardiography, at cardiac catheter, and with cardiac MRI (see Section 10.3)

Echocardiography in Restrictive Cardiomyopathy
(see Section 10.3 Table 10.2)
- Normal pericardium
- Normal septal motion
- No respiratory variation of mitral inflow E velocity
- Reduced E/A ratio
- Slow LV flow propagation velocity.

At Cardiac Catheter
- LVEDP and RVEDP are different, especially at end-expiration in restriction, usually by >7 mmHg (identical in constriction).
- Cardiac biopsy is usually diagnostic.
- The search for amyloid elsewhere, e.g. urinary light chains; gum or rectal biopsy may help but cannot prove cardiac amyloid.
- Technetium pertechnetate scanning is positive in amyloid heart disease, with uptake in the infiltrated muscle.
- SAP scan: I^{123}-labelled serum amyloid protein (SAP) is an alternative to technetium. It is valuable for identifying amyloid in other organs, but unfortunately not particularly good for cardiac amyloid.

4.4 Arrhythmogenic Right Ventricular Cardiomyopathy (ARVC)

Genetics
This is a rare autosomal dominant condition, with variable penetrance, primarily affecting the RV free wall and RV outflow tract. Prevalence is unknown in a condition that is difficult to diagnose but may be as high as 1 in 5000. Linkage analysis has identified several culprit loci on different chromosomes involving specific genes for adhesion molecules (see below) and the ryan-odine receptor gene. There is genetic heterogeneity as with other cardiomyopathies.

Pathophysiology
Fibro-fatty infiltration in the right ventricle may cause supraventricular arrhythmias, VT and a risk of sudden cardiac death. There is relative sparing of the endocardium in the early stages. This is a disorder of cell adhesion molecules: desmoplakin and plakoglobin. Cell separation is followed by cell death and replacement by fibro-fatty tissue, which becomes the substrate for ventricular arrhythmias. In its later stages the left ventricle may be involved, but marked cardiac dilatation is uncommon. The interventricular septum is rarely involved.

Diagnosis
This is difficult. There is no single test and multiple investigations are needed. Young adults are typically affected. Patients may present with palpitation,

presyncope, syncope, fatigue, effort dyspnoea or even sudden death. Arrhythmias are often exercise induced. There may be a relevant family history of premature sudden death. The diagnosis should be suspected in patients presenting with VT with an LBBB and inferior axis morphology (resembling an RVOT tachycardia see Figure 8.10). The diagnosis may be suspected if the ECG shows ε waves (notches at the ST/T junction – see below), or if there are late potentials on the signal-averaged ECG (SAECG). Electrophysiological studies may be unreliable in the young because VT may not be inducible but the patient is still at risk, and the study cannot be used as a prognostic indicator. However, mapping of the tachycardia if induced can be helpful because, unlike RVOT tachycardia, the VT may not start in the RF outflow tract.

Echocardiography, CT and MRI have been used to try to detect the fatty infiltration in the RV wall. This is a difficult area of the heart to image with any modality. ARVC gene mutations have been identified and genetic testing is now possible. Several loci have been identified (14q 23–24).

Diagnostic criteria have now been established (Table 4.7). Two major criteria, one major plus two minor or four minor criteria are regarded as necessary to establish a diagnosis.

Problems with Diagnostic Investigations

Endomyocardial Biopsy

Diagnostic endomyocardial biopsy of the RV is not often successful because the biopsy usually gets samples from the interventricular septum and this

Table 4.7 Diagnostic criteria for diagnosis of arrhythmogenic RV cardiomyopathy

Major criteria	Minor criteria
RV dysfunction	
Severe RV dilatation with low RVEF	Mild RV dilatation and reduced RV function and normal LV function with normal LV
Localized RV aneurysms or severe segmental dilatation and hypokinesia	Regional RV hypokinesia
RV biopsy showing fibro-fatty infiltration	
ECG changes	
ECG showing ε waves	Inverted T waves in V2 and V3 (age >12 and no RBBB)
Localized QRS prolongation (>110 ms) in leads V1–3	Late potentials on signal-averaged ECG
	LBBB tachycardia
	Frequent ventricular ectopics (>1000/24 h)
Family history	
Familial disease at postmortem examination or surgery	Family history of sudden cardiac death (<35 years) or family history of ARVC based on these criteria

condition primarily initially affects the RV free wall, infundibulum and RVOT. Attempts to biopsy the RV free wall percutaneously may lead to perforation.

ECG
There are several non-diagnostic ECG changes including incomplete or complete RBBB, and low voltages in V1–3. The ε wave (a major criterion) is a very small amplitude-positive deflection right at the end of the QRS complex, representing delayed RV depolarisation. Such waves occur in about 30% cases of ARVC and are easily missed.

The differential diagnosis of the VT is with a simple RVOT tachycardia which is a more benign condition and usually easily amenable to VT ablation.

Imaging
Echocardiography in the early stages may be normal. Later a dilated hypokinetic right ventricle with secondary tricuspid regurgitation may be seen, possibly with localized aneurysm formation. Cardiac MRI is probably the best imaging modality. Fatty infiltration in the RV free wall is detected with high signal intensity on T_1-weighted images. Experience is needed in differentiating this from normal fatty deposits (e.g. in the AV groove).

Treatment
Patients at risk of sudden cardiac death need to be identified and prevented from playing competitive sports or taking vigorous exercise. The following are those at particular risk:
- Young age
- Family history of sudden cardiac death
- Extensive RV disease with poor RV function
- History of syncope or cardiac arrest
- Documented VT
- Additional LV involvement.

Drug Treatment
Anti-arrhythmic drug therapy usually involves sotalol initially, which may be more effective than amiodarone. Use additional anti-failure treatment on usual lines (see Chapter 6).

VT Ablation
This may be possible for focal RVOT disease, but multifocal recurrence is possible.

ICD Implantation
Patients with ARVC and VT should be considered for an ICD. Under-sensing of difficulties and problems with high defibrillation thresholds can be expected

with fatty infiltration of the RV, together with an increased risk of lead perforation.

Cardiac Transplantation
This may be the only hope for patients with severe end-stage cardiac failure (as in dilated cardiomyopathy) with recurrent VT.

4.5 Isolated Ventricular Non-Compaction (IVNC)

First described in 1986 this poorly understood condition results from a failure of the myocardium to condense in intrauterine life. The endocardium thus has a spongy appearance with deep trabecular recesses and a more normal compacted outer epicardium. These deep clefts in the endocardium do not connect with the coronary circulation. The non-compacted myocardium is chiefly found at the LV apex and lateral wall.

Genetics
There is an X-linked infantile type caused by a mutation in the G4.5 gene on the X chromosome, associated with the Barth syndrome and possibly showing facial dysmorphism. The adult type is a non-sex-linked autosomal dominant condition with the possible mutant gene on chromosome 11p15. There may be associated neuromuscular disorders.

Diagnosis
This is usually made with echocardiography with possible additional contrast (e.g. Sonovue) injection to enhance the endocardial border. The diagnosis is then based on the following:
• A non-compacted layer of myocardium more than twice as thick as the normal epicardial compacted zone
• The deep inter-trabecular clefts or recesses in communication with the LV cavity (on Doppler screening) and visible on cardiac MRI (Figure 4.11)
• No other cardiac abnormality.

Presentation and Treatment
This is a very heterogeneous condition. Patients may be asymptomatic with good LV function, a normal size left atrium and the diagnosis made incidentally on echocardiography. At the other end of the scale patients present with heart failure with a condition resembling DCM. Arrhythmias and systemic emboli are also possible.

Management is on the usual lines for heart failure with anticoagulation necessary for the dilated left ventricle.

Prognosis
This depends on LV function at presentation. Most patients will have LV systolic dysfunction with a poor long-term prognosis. The minority of patients

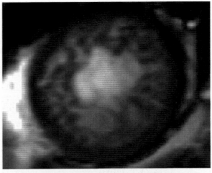

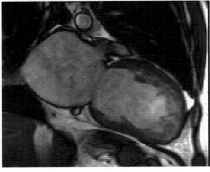

Figure 4.11 Cardiac MRI showing isolated ventricular non-compaction (IVNC). The upper panel (short axis view) shows a thickened myocardium with darker intertrabecular clefts. The apex has a thickened hazy appearance.

who are asymptomatic, with diagnosis picked up incidentally, are thought to have a good prognosis.

4.6 Takotsubo Cardiomyopathy/Apical Ballooning Syndrome

This bizarre condition chiefly affects women and is a form of reversible catecholamine-induced myocardial stunning. It is poorly understood. Initially described in Japan in 1990 the term 'Takotsubo' refers to an octopus bottle used by Japanese fisherman, the shape of which resembles the stunned heart in this condition.

Diagnosis
Patients (usually female) present with chest pain often after a severe emotional upset. This has resulted in the condition being nicknamed the 'broken heart syndrome'.
- The coronaries are normal, or <50% stenoses
- Dynamic ST/T-wave changes on ECG
- Mild elevation of cardiac enzymes only (<twice normal CK)
- There is apical reversible akinesia with a hypercontractile base (Figure 4.12).

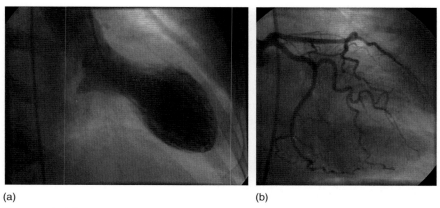

(a)   (b)

Figure 4.12 a) Takotsubo apical ballooning syndrome in a 62 year old woman with acute cardiac pain. End-systolic frame of a left ventriculogram in the right anterior oblique projection. There is apical akinesia with a hypercontractile base. Coronary angiography was normal. b) Normal left coronary angiogram in the right anterior oblique projection.

Studies so far in this condition have failed to identify a definite cause. There is no evidence of myocarditis or MI on MRI or cardiac biopsy. The stunned myocardium may be a result of episodes of transient coronary occlusion followed by reperfusion. Stress echocardiography using dobutamine does not improve the apical akinetic segment. RV involvement occurs in about 25% cases with occasional pleural effusions.

The condition although alarming initially is benign, and a full recovery can be expected in about 3 weeks from symptom onset, with LV function returning to normal.

4.7 Endomyocardial Fibrosis/Loeffler's Eosinophilic Endocarditis

These are now thought to be the same condition, causing a restrictive cardiomyopathy. EMF is a tropical disease common in equatorial African rainforests. Its aetiology is unknown, but a recurrent febrile illness suggests an infective origin, with new cases more apparent in the rainy season. Only a mild eosinophilia is present and common anyway in these regions, with worm infestation.

The cardiac effects of Loeffler's eosinophilic syndrome and eosinophilic leukaemia are similar. Eosinophils in the myocardium degranulate and cause fibrosis, particularly of the endocardium. The ventricular cavity becomes smaller, with encroaching fibrosis and eventually there is complete obliteration of the apex of either or both ventricles. Secondary thrombosis occurs over this endocardial fibrosis, with systemic emboli. There is marked AV valve regurgitation with involvement of the papillary muscles. There may be a pericardial effusion and conduction problems with advanced disease.

The clinical picture depends on which ventricle is involved. The symptoms may be predominantly right sided with ascites and peripheral oedema, left-sided with pulmonary oedema and systemic emboli, or both.

Cardiac catheterization and endomyocardial biopsy will confirm the diagnosis. Degranulated eosinophils may be found between the myocardial cells. Pressure measurements in the right heart in advanced disease show a 'tube-like' heart with identical pressures in PA, RV and RA. Angiography shows typical apical obliteration by fibrous tissue.

Management
Patients with severe eosinophilia should receive steroids and/or hydroxy-urea. Heart failure is managed along conventional lines. Severe AV valve regurgitation warrants valve replacement and some cases have been improved by endocardial resection.

5 Coronary Artery Disease

The Burden of Cardiovascular Disease

Angina accounts for 1% of visits to primary care physicians. An estimated 2.7 million in the UK have symptoms from coronary disease. The annual mortality rate for patients with mild angina and stable symptoms is 0.9–1.7%, but it is much higher for those with unstable symptoms. About 10% patients/year with stable angina will develop worsening symptoms requiring revascularization. There are approximately 105000 deaths per year in the UK from coronary heart disease and an additional 32000 deaths from other forms of heart disease. The overall annual toll of deaths resulting from cardiovascular disease (including stroke) is 216000.

Coronary artery disease in the UK is a major cause of health-care expenditure and the annual cost of coronary disease to the NHS is £7.9 billion.

5.1 Pathophysiology of Angina

Relevance to Medical Therapy

Ischaemia develops if myocardial oxygen (O_2) demand exceeds supply. Cellular acidosis and lactate release occur before ST-segment depression on the ECG, which in turn precedes angina. ST depression occurring in the absence of pain is called silent ischaemia (see below). Oxygen supply is increased by increasing coronary flow (autoregulation) rather than by increasing oxygen extraction from coronary artery blood. Coronary AV O_2 difference remains constant at approximately 11 ml/100 ml blood. Coronary dilatation in response to ischaemia is probably mediated via adenosine, which is the ideal messenger because it has a very short half-life. Adenosine may be the cause of anginal pain when released from the ischaemic cell, acting as a self-protecting mechanism. Determinants of the O_2 supply/demand ratio are shown in Table 5.1. Angina therapy works by improving this ratio.

Swanton's Cardiology, sixth edition. By R. H. Swanton and S. Banerjee. Published 2008 Blackwell Publishing. ISBN 978-1-4051-7819-8.

Table 5.1 Mechanisms of angina therapy

$\uparrow O_2$ supply	$\downarrow O_2$ demand
Length of diastole $\uparrow$: β blockade, I_f blockade	Heart rate $\downarrow$: β blockade, I_f blockade
Coronary tone $\downarrow$: nitrates, calcium antagonists	Contractility $\downarrow$: β blockade
LV diastolic pressure $\downarrow$: nitrates	Wall tension $\downarrow$:
O_2 capacity of blood $\uparrow$: transfusion if anaemic	LV pressure nitrates $\Big\}$ $\downarrow$ nitrates
Aortic perfusion pressure: improve if hypotensive or hypovolaemic	LV cavity radius^2
Coronary atheromatous stenoses: angioplasty or surgery	

Coronary Tone

Coronary tone is under neurogenic and humoral control. Coronary arterial smooth muscle contains α-, $β_1$-, dopamine and parasympathetic receptors. β blockade is avoided in patients with proven coronary spasm (unopposed α-receptor activity). Cardioselective agents are used with care in patients with angina plus possible vasospasm (Raynaud's phenomenon or migraine).

The coronary endothelium is now known to be very important in the release of vasoactive substances, some causing constriction and others dilatation (Table 5.2). Many vasodilators act by releasing endothelial-derived relaxant factor (EDRF) from the endothelial cell, which in turn increases intracellular cyclic guanosine monophosphate (cGMP), which results in muscle relaxation. EDRF is nitric oxide. Some vasodilators work only in the presence of an intact endothelium (e.g. acetylcholine) but others are independent of an intact endothelium (e.g. nitrates and isoprenaline). If the endothelium is denuded, acetylcholine may even cause coronary constriction.

The role of prostaglandins in coronary tone is still poorly understood. Prostacyclin (PGI2) is derived from intact endothelium and acts locally to cause dilatation, by increasing intracellular cAMP (adenosine cyclic 3':5'-monophosphate) (Figure 5.1). It acts in opposition to platelet-derived thromboxane A_2 (TxA_2), a potent vasoconstrictor.

Nitrates probably work by forming NO, which stimulates guanylyl cyclase, increasing intracellular cGMP. The action of some vasodilators on the vascular smooth muscle cell is shown in Figure 5.1. The physiological effects of β-blocking agents are shown in Figure 5.4 and of nitrates in Figure 5.5.

In spite of our increasing knowledge of vasoactive substances released by the coronary endothelium, a few patients still present with absolutely typical angina but angiographically normal coronary arteries (Table 5.3).

Chest Pain with Normal Coronary Arteries

There are many causes of chest pain that may mimic angina in patients with angiographically normal coronary arteries (Table 5.3). There are also a large number of cardiac causes, some of which are ischaemic.

Table 5.2 Regulators of coronary tone

Vasoconstrictors	Examples
Mechanical	Systolic compression (intramural arteries), muscle bridge (epicardial artery)
α-Adrenoceptor agonists	Noradrenaline, adrenaline, high-dose dopamine (>15 μg/kg per min) via noradrenaline, ergotamine, ergonovine (partial α and 5-HT$_2$ agonist)
Endothelium produced	Thromboxane A$_2$ (and from platelets), endothelin, prostaglandin F series
Adventitial nerve plexus	Neuropeptide Y
Other hormones	Vasopressin, angiotensin II

Vasodilators	Examples
Mechanical	Diastolic relaxation
Metabolites from ischaemic myocardium	Adenosine, bradykinin, CO_2, H^+
α-Receptor antagonists	Prazosin, phenoxybenzamine
Angiotensin II antagonists	Captopril, enalapril
β-Receptor agonists	(β$_1$ > β$_2$), e.g. dobutamine, isoprenaline
Dopamine receptor agonist	Low-dose dopamine (<5 μg/kg per min)
Phosphodiesterase inhibitors	Papaverine, methylxanthines (aminophylline)
Voltage-dependent calcium channel blockers	Nifedipine, diltiazem, verapamil
Potassium channel openers	Minoxidil, nicorandil, diazoxide
Purine receptor agonist	Adenosine (A$_2$ receptor), peripheral > coronary vessels
Direct stimulator of intracellular cGMP	Nitrates, atrial natriuretic peptide
Endothelium produced	EDRF: nitric oxide; PGI$_2$, CGRP; substance P; VIP; prostaglandin E series

CGRP, calcitonin gene-related peptide; EDRF, endothelial-derived relaxant factor; PGI$_2$, prostacyclin; VIP, vasoactive intestinal peptide.

Coronary Spasm

This is thought to be the cause of variant angina described by Prinzmetal in 1958. Angina is typical in site but comes on unpredictably at rest, sometimes provoked by cold or hyperventilation, and associated with ST elevation on the ECG. The spasm is usually localized to a segment of an epicardial coronary artery, and in about half the cases there is an associated atheromatous lesion at the site of the spasm, although in the rest the vessels look normal once the spasm has relaxed. Myocardial infarction may occur if the spasm cannot be reversed. Earlier studies provoked spasm at angiography with intracoronary ergonovine, but this has not always proved to be reversible with intracoronary nitrates. Patients are treated with nitrates and calcium antagonists but not β blockade (unopposed α effects). Coronary angioplasty in patients with coexisting atheroma may provoke spasm post-dilatation.

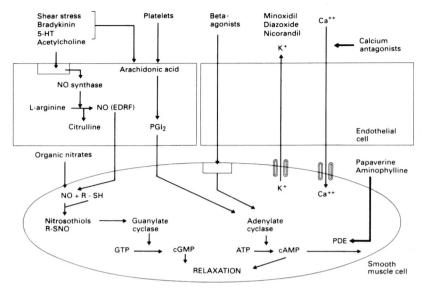

Figure 5.1 Action of vasodilators on smooth muscle cells. Reproduced from Weatherall et al. (1994) *Oxford Textbook of Medicine 3rd edition* Oxford University Press, Oxford with permission.

Cardiac Syndrome X

This term has been applied since 1981 to a group of patients who have:

- typical angina pectoris
- a positive treadmill stress test
- angiographically normal coronary arteries.

Table 5.3 Chest pain with normal coronary arteries

Non-cardiac	Cardiac-ischaemic	Cardiac-non-ischaemic
Poor history	Angiogram misinterpretation, e.g. ostial	Pericarditis
Musculoskeletal pain	stenosis, coronary arteritis, wrong	Mitral valve prolapse
Cervical root pain	projection	Aortic dissection
Thoracic root pain	Coronary spasm	
Anaemia	Microvascular angina	
Thyrotoxicosis	Syndrome X	
Hyperventilation	Linked angina	
Pneumothorax	Coronary emboli, e.g. atrial myxoma,	
Asthma	mural thrombus, vegetation	
Oesophagitis	Aortic valve stenosis	
Oesophageal spasm	Severe LV hypertrophy, e.g. HCM,	
Gastritis	hypertension	
Peptic ulcer		

These patients probably represent a heterogeneous group including some with normal hearts. They are often middle-aged women and in some their chest pain is not always typical, e.g. prolonged or sharp in quality or in the left chest. There is evidence that their angina is ischaemic. Several studies have shown that these patients have abnormal coronary flow reserve: they do not increase coronary flow normally on response to adenosine, dipyridamole or papaverine. This is thought to be a result of inappropriate vasomotor tone of the small resistance vessels (<100 μm diameter – invisible on angiography). There is documented failure of endothelial-dependent dilatation. Slow coronary flow is often seen in the larger epicardial vessels on coronary angiography in patients with syndrome X. Other cardiac abnormalities found in some patients with syndrome X include:

• perfusion abnormalities on stress thallium scanning
• abnormal intramural arteries (<100 μm) on cardiac biopsy
• abnormal systolic and diastolic function (high LVEDP, abnormal filling rates)
• ischaemia proven on coronary sinus lactate studies with atrial pacing
• myocardial damage: conduction abnormalities, e.g. LBBB, mitochondrial swelling.

In such a heterogeneous group, these findings are not always consistent in every patient. Other studies suggest a more generalized smooth muscle abnormality with oesophageal dysmotility and abnormal forearm hyperaemic responses. Oestrogen deficiency in female patients has been suggested as an aetiological factor because oestrogen causes both endothelial-dependent and -independent vasodilatation.

Whatever the cause of syndrome X, patient's angina responds well to nitrates and calcium antagonists. β Blockade should be avoided unless there is a resting tachycardia or systemic hypertension. H_2-receptor antagonists are tried for patients with poor symptom relief or any suggestion of acid reflux (see Linked Angina, below). Low-dose imipramine (25–50 mg at night) may help.

A recent multicentre study – the Women's Ischaemia Syndrome Evaluation (WISE) study – found that on a 5-year follow-up of patients with persistent symptoms the number of adverse events (MI, CVA, CCF) was almost twice that of the group without persistent angina. Their angina should not be dismissed as of little consequence and is clearly more of a risk marker than was originally thought. Follow-up and aggressive risk factor reduction are needed in those with recurrent symptoms.

Linked Angina

This is the generation of angina in patients with syndrome X by oesophageal reflux. Instillation of acid into the oesophagus of patients with syndrome X has been shown to reduce coronary flow reserve, but does not occur in the denervated heart of transplanted patients. A neurogenic cardio-oesophageal reflex has been incriminated, affecting the coronary microvasculature. This compounds an already confusing diagnostic problem. Oesophageal pain may mimic cardiac pain in many respects. Exertion can cause oesophageal reflux anyway, and patients with syndrome X often have gastro-oesophageal problems (e.g. small hiatus hernia in the middle-aged woman).

Silent Myocardial Ischaemia

Episodes of ST depression occurring without chest pain are termed 'silent ischaemia'. This may be documented on an exercise test or during 24-hour Holter monitoring using FM recording equipment (Figure 5.2). Silent asymptomatic ST depression has been found to occur in 2.5% of the male population.

It is now appreciated that silent ischaemia represents impaired myocardial perfusion. It occurs in patients with chronic stable angina and ≤75% of episodes of ST depression on 24-hour Holter monitoring may be silent. Generally the more severe the ST depression, the more likely it is to be felt by the patient as angina. The frequency of silent ischaemia on the 24-hour tape parallels the exercise test result: the more positive the exercise test and the worse the exercise tolerance, the greater the incidence of silent ischaemia.

Silent ischaemia on Holter monitoring occurs more commonly in the morning. This circadian rhythm is mirrored by the increased incidence of MI in the morning. It occurs in about 10% of patients after an MI.

Patients with frequent episodes of silent ischaemia should be investigated along conventional lines, with exercise testing and subsequent coronary angiography if indicated. Conventional medical treatment for stable angina reduces episodes of silent ischaemia. β Blockade will reduce the episodes of silent ischaemia and abolish the early morning peak of silent ST depression.

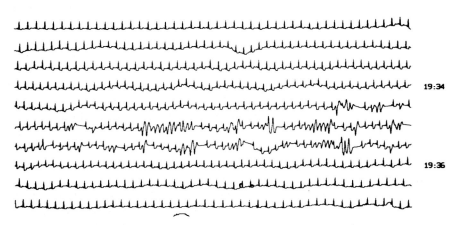

Figure 5.2 Sample from a continuous 24-hour ECG recording, showing the development of silent ST-segment depression followed by a burst of non-sustained ventricular tachycardia. The silent ischaemia gradually resolves.

Prognostic Importance
Silent ischaemia is perhaps surprisingly of no prognostic importance in patients with chronic stable angina, as shown in the TIBET study. Exercise testing is more sensitive at detecting ischaemia and there is no need to perform continuous ambulatory ST-segment monitoring in this group. However, it is of considerable prognostic value in patients with unstable angina, probably representing a ruptured unstable plaque. Patients with unstable angina who have silent ischaemia on ECG monitoring need urgent coronary angiography.

Ischaemic Preconditioning
Brief periods of ischaemia (2–15 min) can protect the myocardium from possible subsequent lethal ischaemia. This protection is probably mediated via the adenosine A_1-receptor activating intracellular protein kinase C. The subsequent target is uncertain. This self-protecting mechanism may explain why patients who have a history of angina before infarction have a better prognosis than those who have a sudden infarct with no preceding angina. It is a phenomenon also noticed during PCI, with second and subsequent inflations being less painful and with less ST segment shift than the initial inflation.

Hibernating Myocardium
This is chronic reversible LV dysfunction caused by prolonged reduction in coronary flow. Oxygen supply is enough to keep myocytes alive and metabolizing, but insufficient to allow them to contract. This is important because inert myocardium on angiography may be assumed to be dead, infarcted tissue, but will recover function after bypass grafting. Hibernating myocardium can be diagnosed by the following:
• Infusion of low-dose dobutamine during echocardiography: hibernating muscle will be induced to contract.
• Positron emission tomography (PET): perfusion is studied using [13]Nammonia, and metabolism with [18]Ffluorodeoxyglucose (FDG). Hibernating myocardium will be highlighted as areas still metabolizing but with no registerable flow. Cyclotron is needed.
• Thallium[201] scanning with rest/redistribution study and late reinjection: this is an alternative to PET and is much more widely available. In one study, >50% patients with coronary disease and poor LV function were found to have hibernating myocardium on PET.

Myocardial Stunning (see also Section 4.6)
This is prolonged but reversible LV dysfunction in the absence of ischaemia. After total occlusion of a vessel with subsequent reopening, LV function gradually returns towards normal. This delayed recovery of regional wall motion occurs after prolonged inflations at PCI, in unstable angina and possibly during non-transmural infarction.

5.2 Management of Angina

This involves alteration of lifestyle, exclusion or treatment of precipitating factors, drug treatment, and possibly surgery or angioplasty if medical treatment fails.

Alteration of Lifestyle

This involves a reduction of physical activity at work and home. It may require a change in job (HGV drivers, airline pilots, divers) or a change within employment (miners, furniture removers, etc.). Smoking must be stopped. Weight reduction may be needed. Many activities (e.g. gardening, sex) can be continued with medical treatment and nitrates taken prophylactically.

Driving may be continued provided that traffic does not induce angina, angina is stable and it is a private car only. Vocational driving licence holders (Group 2 drivers) should not drive their vehicles and should inform the DVLA (see Appendix 6).

Rarely, attention to climate or altitude may help – patients may be helped by moving to warmer climates during winter months.

Flight as an airline passenger is not contraindicated provided that the angina is stable. The airline medical personnel should be informed before the flight, and the patient should not carry heavy luggage and should be well insured for hospital care abroad.

Vigorous competitive sports should be stopped (e.g. squash, rugby). Regular daily exercise within the anginal threshold is important. Swimming is allowed if angina is stable. Patients should not swim alone, should not dive into cold water and should get into water that is only within their depth. Heated pools are obviously preferable.

Skiing is not recommended (high altitude, physical effort, cold air and emotional factors).

Exclusion and Treatment of Precipitating Factors

These include anaemia, high-output states, thyrotoxicosis, diabetes mellitus and hypercholesterolaemia.

The most important cardiac precipitating factors are hypertension, obstruction to LV outflow, aortic valve stenosis, HCM and paroxysmal arrhythmias.

Angina in aortic valve stenosis may be cured by aortic valve replacement. Patients with angina and aortic regurgitation should have a test for VDRL/TPHA especially if there are coronary ostial stenoses. Twenty-four hour ECG monitoring should be performed if the history suggests arrhythmias precipitating angina.

Investigation and Medical Treatment

Exercise testing is performed on patients with stable angina provided that there are no contraindications (see Section 16.2). This helps confirm the diag-

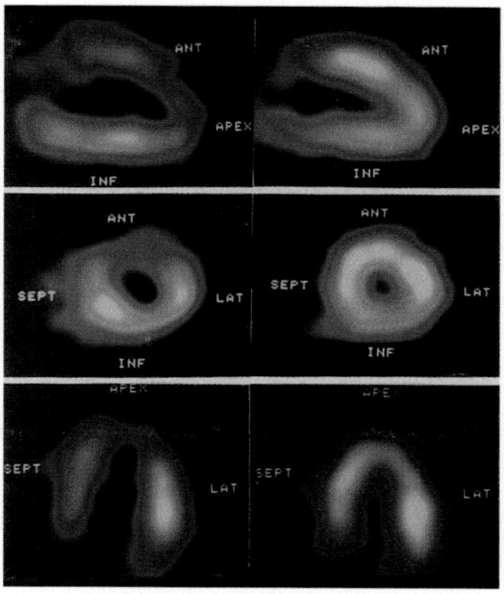

Figure 5.3 Thallium[201] myocardial perfusion scan at peak bicycle exercise (left three panels) and at rest 4 hours later (three right panels). Top two panels: vertical long axis view, middle two panels: short axis view, bottom two panels: horizontal long axis view. There is a reversible perfusion defect in the septal and apical walls as a result of a stenosis in the left anterior descending coronary artery.

nosis and assess the severity of symptoms, and is a guide to the need for coronary angiography. Patients who cannot complete stage 2 of the standard Bruce protocol because of symptoms, or who develop positive ST changes, hypotension or arrhythmias, need angiography.

Some patients with atypical symptoms who are unable to perform a treadmill test or have uninterpretable ECGs (e.g. LBBB or pre-excitation – see Chapter 16) should have stress myocardial perfusion scanning. An example of a positive scan is shown in Figure 5.3 in a man with left anterior descending stenosis.

Drug therapy involves several groups of drugs: nitrates, β-blocking agents and calcium antagonists. Additional diuretic or antihypertensive therapy may be needed. Stable angina is treated initially with a β-blocking agent and glyceryl trinitrate (GTN). Calcium antagonists or long-acting nitrates should be considered when β blockers are contraindicated, i.e.

- low-output state, borderline LVF – i.e. uncontrolled heart failure
- Prinzmetal's variant angina
- high-degree AV block
- sinoatrial disease without a pacemaker implant
- severe peripheral vascular disease, claudication, gangrene
- asthma, moderate or severe bronchospasm
- depressive psychosis in the history
- Raynaud's phenomenon
- bradycardia < 60/min
- hypotension: systolic pressure <100 mmHg
- metabolic acidosis.

Unstable angina is controlled initially medically and then investigated with a view to PCI or surgery. Nocturnal or decubitus angina may respond to a diuretic taken in the evening or a calcium antagonist taken at night.

Table 5.4 β-Blocking agents

Drug (trade name/s)	Fat soluble	Cardioselective	ISA	Plasma half-life (h)	Plasma protein binding (%)	Elimination route	Starting oral dose for angina (mg)	? Single schedule for hypertension (mg)	Intravenous dose (slowly over 5 min) (mg)
Acebutolol (Sectral)	+	Yes	Yes	3	15	Hepatic 60% first-pass renal	200 three times daily	200–400 once daily	10–50
Atenolol (Tenormin)	–	Yes	No	6–9	10	Renal only	100 once daily	100 once daily	5–10
Betaxolol (Kerlone)	–	Yes	No	15–22	50	Renal	10 once daily	Yes	–
Bisoprolol (Emcor, Monocor)	++	Yes	No	10–12	30	Renal 50% Hepatic 50%	10 once daily	Yes	–
Bucindolol*	++	No but α_1 blocker	No	3–4	90	Hepatic	50 once daily	100–200 once daily	–
Carteolol (Cartrol)	–	No	Yes	6–9	15	Mainly renal	10 once daily	Yes	–
Carvedilol (Eucardic)	++	No but α_1 blocker	No	6–7	95	Hepatic	12.5 twice daily	25–50 once daily	–
Esmolol (Brevibloc)	+	Yes	No	9 min	55	Red cell Hepatic	No	No	50–200 µg/kg per min
Celiprolol (Celectolol)	+	Yes + β_2	Yes	5–6	25	Hepatic and renal	200 once daily	Yes	–

Drug								
Labetalol (Trandate)	++	No	No	3–4	85	Hepatic, 90% metabolized	100 three times daily	No	50, repeated if necessary
Metoprolol (Lopresor, Betaloc)	+	Yes	No	3	15	Hepatic and renal	50–100 three times daily	Durules 200 once daily	5–10
Nadolol (Corgard)	–	No	No	16–24	20	Renal only	40 once daily	40–80 once daily	–
Nebivolol (Nebilet)	–	Yes	No	10	98	Renal Hepatic	5 once daily	Yes	No
Oxprenolol (Trasicor)	+	No	Yes	2	75	Hepatic	40 three times daily	Slow oxprenolol 160 once daily	1–10
Penbutolol (Lasipressin)	+++	No	Yes	4–5	80	Hepatic	20 once daily	Yes	–
Pindolol (Visken)	–	No	Yes	3–4	60	Hepatic and renal	5 three times daily	No	–
Propranolol (Inderal)	+++	No	No	3–6	90	Hepatic 95% first-pass metabolism	40 three times daily	Propranolol LA 160 once daily	1–10
Sotalol (Betacardone Sotacor)	–	No	No	12–15	5	Renal only	80 twice daily	No	10–20
Timolol (Betim, Blockadren)	±	No	No	4–6	65	Hepatic and renal	10 twice daily	No	0.5–1

*Bucindolol is not yet available in the UK.

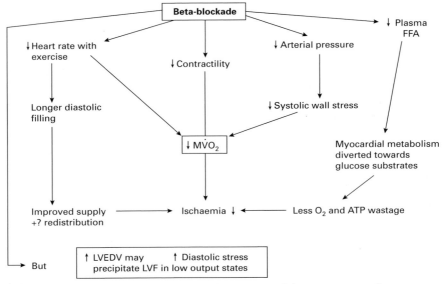

Figure 5.4 Mode of action of β blockade in reducing myocardial oxygen consumption.

5.3 β-Blocking agents (Figure 5.4)

Choice of β Blocker (Table 5.4)

Table 5.4 shows the currently available agents in the UK. Personal preference and experience mainly dictate the choice. Most of the ancillary properties of β blockers, e.g. membrane-stabilizing effect or intrinsic sympathomimetic activity (ISA), matter little clinically. Drugs with an ISA prevent a resting bradycardia. The membrane-stabilizing effect (quinidine-like) may play a role in the antiarrhythmic action, as may the reduction in platelet stickiness that occurs with β blockade. Additional non-cardiac conditions are considered in the choice.

- Patients with cool peripheries, peripheral vascular disease, diabetes mellitus or mild bronchospasm should start with a cardioselective drug such as bisoprolol or celiprolol (which contains in addition β$_2$-agonist properties). In patients with airway obstruction, start on a small dose and monitor peak flows at least twice daily.
- Patients complaining of bad dreams (e.g. on propranolol) should receive a non-fat-soluble drug (atenolol, nadolol or sotalol).
- Hypertensive patients may be best managed with a single-dose schedule taken in the morning (atenolol, sustained-action metoprolol, propranolol). Alternatively they should start labetalol, a combined α- and β-receptor antagonist. Many β blockers can be used as single-dose schedules for hypertension. More frequent dose schedules are usually required for angina.
- Renal failure: choose a β blocker with hepatic excretion (e.g. propranolol, labetalol, carvedilol) but at a lower dose than in patients with normal renal

function. Reduction in cardiac output lowers renal plasma flow and may cause a deterioration in renal function.

- Elderly patients: start with a very low dose (e.g. propranolol 10 mg twice daily, or metoprolol 25 mg twice daily).
- Liver disease: first-pass metabolism occurs with fat-soluble drugs (e.g. propranolol, labetolol, acebutolol). Patients with liver disease should have the dose of fat-soluble drugs reduced or switched to a non-fat-soluble drug (e.g. pindolol, nadolol), which is excreted only by the kidneys.
- Heart failure (see Section 6.10): interest is growing in the use of β blockade in patients with mild-to-moderate heart failure. Three β-blocking agents have been shown to be of benefit in heart failure trials: carvedilol, metoprolol and bisoprolol. However, bucindolol was not shown to be of benefit and a class effect cannot be assumed. Introduced slowly at very low dose, improvement in LV function has been demonstrated over time. Some patients have deteriorated and have been withdrawn from the trials. Patients with heart failure and NYHA (New York Heart Association) class III or IV symptoms should be admitted to hospital for the introduction of β-blockade therapy.
- Diabetes mellitus is not a contraindication to β blockade, even if the patient is on insulin. β Blockade prevents the sympathetic reaction to hypoglycaemia. Muscle glycogenolysis is mediated via β_2-receptors. Hence cardioselective drugs are preferable in patients with diabetes.
- Pregnancy: the evidence that β blockade during pregnancy results in small-for-dates babies is largely retrospective. Prospective trials have shown that β blockade as treatment for hypertension in pregnancy confers a benefit to the fetus compared with methyldopa or hydralazine (see Section 15.2).
- Overdose of β-blocking agents is treated by intravenous β agonists in competitive doses, e.g. dobutamine (10–15 µg/kg per min or more as required) or atropine 1.2 mg i.v. (Complete AV block may occur and not be reversed by atropine.) Temporary pacing is often necessary.

5.4 Nitrates (Figure 5.5)

Sublingual and Buccal Nitrates (Table 5.5)

Isosorbide dinitrate preparations dissolve particularly quickly in the mouth and are often preferred by patients to standard GTN. Nitrates may relieve the pain of oesophageal spasm and renal or biliary colic.

Some patients prefer the long-acting buccal nitrate preparation (e.g. Suscard). The tablet is placed between the upper lip and the gum. The advantage is that the tablet can be removed if side effects such as headache become intolerable.

They are contraindicated in angina caused by HCM because they increase the outflow tract gradient. Patients should be informed of the following:

- To renew the tablets every 6 months – the shelf-life is limited.
- A GTN spray may be preferred.
- To take them prophylactically and concurrently.

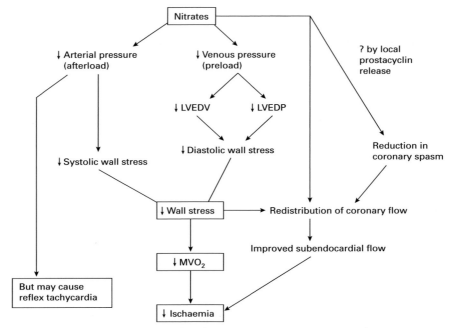

Figure 5.5 Mode of action of nitrates in reducing myocardial oxygen consumption.

- Tablets taken in hot atmospheres may induce postural hypotension or even syncope.
- To expect a headache and/or facial flushing. If these symptoms are intolerable, GTN may be swallowed and absorption is reduced. The tablet may of course be spat out. Isosorbide is absorbed from the mouth and gut.
- The tablets are not addictive. Tolerance is not a problem. Patients should not limit their intake to a fixed number daily. (Methaemoglobinaemia is possible with very high tablet consumption but is rare in clinical practice.)
- Chewing the tablets will speed absorption in severe angina. Patients on additional β-blocking therapy will not develop a reflex tachycardia.
- Sildenafil and longer acting PDE 5 inhibitors are contraindicated in patients on intrates (hypotension).

Care must be taken on prescribing nitrates to patients with cerebral arteriosclerosis. Hypotension may provoke cerebral ischaemia.

Table 5.5 Sublingual preparations

Preparations	Effective time
Glyceryl trinitrate 0.5 mg	10 s–30 min
Isosorbide dinitrate 5 mg	10 s–1 h
Pentaerythritol tetranitrate 10 mg	10 s–45 min

Amyl Nitrite

Ampoules of amyl nitrite are used in echocardiography or in the catheter laboratory to provoke outflow tract gradients in patients with labile LVOTO. They cause headaches to both patients and operators and are used only diagnostically.

Nitrate Sprays

Many patients find these quicker and more convenient than GTN tablets. Coronitro and Nitrolingual Spray both dispense 0.4 mg GTN with each squirt. Approximately 200 puffs are available per dispenser.

Oral Nitrates (Table 5.6)

The drugs considered in this section are longer acting than sublingual nitroglycerin (Table 5.6). Isosorbide mononitrate preparations have the theoretical

Table 5.6 Oral nitrates (longer acting than GTN sublingually)

Drug	Preparation marketed	Tablet strengths (mg)	Dose used (mg)
Glyceryl trinitrate	Suscard	2, 3, 5	2–5 twice daily or three times daily
	Sustac	2.6, 6.4	
Isosorbide dinitrate	Isosorbide dinitrate	10	10–40 twice daily to three times daily
	Cedocard Retard	20, 40	20 twice daily to 40 twice daily
	Isoket Retard	20, 40	20 twice daily to 40 twice daily
Isosorbide mononitrate	Elantan Elantan LA	10, 20, 40 25, 50	10 twice daily to 40 three times daily 25–100 once daily
	Isosorbide mononitrate	10, 20, 40	10 twice daily to 40 three times daily
	Chemydur 60XL	60	30–120 once daily
	Imdur	60	30–120 once daily
	Ismo 10, 20 or 40	10, 20, 40	10 twice daily to 40 three times daily
	Ismo Retard	40	40 once daily
	Isib 60XL	60	60–120 once daily
	Isodur 25 or 50XL	25, 50	25–100 once daily
	Isotard	25, 40, 50 60	25–120 once daily
	Modisal LA	25, 50	25–100 once daily
	Modisal XL	60	60–120 once daily
	Monomax SR	40, 60	40–120 once daily
	Monomax XL	60	60–120 once daily
	Monomil XL	60	60–120 once daily
	Monsorb XL 60	60	60–120 once daily
	Zemon 40 or 60XL	40, 60	40–120 once daily

advantage over the dinitrate preparations in that the mononitrate does not require first-pass metabolism in the liver and bioavailability is thus greater. Both preparations are valuable and the few trials done suggest that GTN requirements were less with the mononitrate.

Transdermal Nitrates

Nitropaste 2% (Percutol)
This ointment is absorbed through the skin and has a prolonged action (3–4 h). Ointment is usually contained in 30 or 60 g tubes and 2.5 cm is squeezed on to the chest and covered by an occlusive plaster. Absorption occurs and, if the patient becomes hypotensive or develops severe headache, it can be wiped off. It is rather messy and dosage control is uncertain. Approximately 800 µg/h is released from 2.5 cm (1 inch) of ointment.

Nitrate Patches
These are preparations of GTN contained beneath a small plaster with a rate-limiting membrane that controls its release. Five different brands and three sizes are available:
1 Transiderm-Nitro 5 and 10: GTN content 25 and 50 mg, respectively.
2 Deponit 5 and 10: GTN content 16 and 32 mg, respectively.
3 Minitran 5, 10 and 15: 5–15 mg GTN release over 24 h.
4 Nitro-Dur: 0.2 mg/h, 0.4 mg/h and 0.6 mg/h (approximately 5–15 mg/24 h).
5 Trintek 5, 10 and 15: 5–15 mg GTN release over 24 h.

In 24 hours 5–15 mg GTN is absorbed, depending on brand and patch size. Only one plaster is needed daily. The plaster is waterproof. It should be removed at night unless the patient suffers from nocturnal angina.

With both transdermal preparations it is important to make sure that the area of skin used each day is different. Inflamed, cracked or icthyotic skin should be avoided (too rapid absorption). Skin sensitivity is not common.

Steady-state plasma levels can be achieved with the once-daily preparation (0.1–0.2 ng/ml) which, although much lower than oral therapy, has been shown to reduce the number of anginal attacks per day.

Nitrate Tolerance
In many patients, tolerance to nitrate therapy develops quite rapidly. The following are mechanisms that have been suggested to cause this:
• Activation of renin–angiotensin system: if this is the cause it should be blocked by captopril, but there is evidence that captopril does not prevent nitrate tolerance in patients with CCF. Activation of the renin–angiotensin system has also been said to account for the rebound phenomenon (vasoconstriction occurring on nitrate withdrawal).
• Plasma volume expansion: this may develop during nitrate therapy. It may also be partly responsible for nitrate tolerance.

• Depletion of sulphydryl (–SH) groups in vascular smooth muscle (see Figure 5.1): administration of N-acetylcysteine has been shown to reduce nitrate tolerance and may well prove to be useful in the future if a palatable way of administering it orally is found.

Tolerance can be avoided by arranging therapy to provide a nitrate-free period during the 24-hour cycle. Oral nitrates should not be given after 6pm in the evening and nitrate patches should be removed also. A nitrate-free period at night can be achieved in this way. A few patients get angina chiefly at night (lying flat increases LV wall stress) and in this group the long-acting nitrate is taken once only on going to bed.

Intravenous Nitrates

Both preparations below are very similar in action and are comparable in price:
• GTN: 5 mg/ml in 5 ml ampoules (Nitrocine, Nitronal are 1 mg/ml in 10 ml ampoules)
• isosorbide dinitrate (Isoket): 1 mg/ml in 10 ml ampoules.

Indications

Intravenous nitrates are used in the following situations:
• Crescendo or unstable angina not responding to medical treatment orally
• LV failure and pulmonary oedema: this may be secondary to acute mitral regurgitation, ruptured ventricular septum, etc.
• Accelerated hypertension (malignant hypertension), although nitroprusside is a better drug in this condition, having more arterial vasodilator properties
• During and after CAB surgery: hypertensive episodes after heart surgery
• During cardiac catheterization: intracoronary injection of nitroglycerin or isosorbide may be necessary if chest pain is associated with ST-segment elevation (i.e. coronary spasm or impending MI)
• Occasionally a prophylactic measure during PCI (see Section 5.9).

Problems and Difficulties with Intravenous Nitrates

Direct measurement of arterial pressure may be necessary. PA wedge (PAW) pressure or PA pressure can also be monitored by a Swan–Ganz catheter but this is rarely necessary.

Hypotension may occur with excessive dosage. The infusion should be stopped, the legs elevated and if necessary plasma expansion/volume replacement given.

Side Effects
Palpitations, giddiness, nausea, retching, sweating, headache, restlessness and muscle twitching have all been seen.

Table 5.7 Nitrate compatibility and giving sets

Incompatible PVC	Compatible polyethylene
Viaflex (Travenol)	Polyfusor (Boots)
Steriflex (Boots)	Bottlepak/Flatpak (Dylade)

Drug Incompatibility

Both nitroglycerin and isosorbide used intravenously are incompatible with PVC infusion bags or giving sets. Up to 30% potency may be lost within 1 h. Polyethylene or glass is not a problem (Table 5.7 gives examples).

The drugs can be given either by drip infusion or by infusion pump using a glass syringe or rigid plastic syringe and polyethylene tubing. They may be mixed in either 5% dextrose or 0.9% (physiological) saline.

Patient Incompatibility

Intravenous nitrates are best avoided in:
- pregnancy
- uncorrected hypovolaemia
- patients with closed-angle glaucoma
- anaemic or hypotensive patients
- patients with severe cerebrovascular disease.
- patients taking PDE 5 inhibitors (eg Sildenafil)

GTN (Nitroglycerin) Dose Calculation

GTN (Nitrocine, Nitronal)

The 10 ml ampoules contain either 1.0 mg/ml (10 mg ampoule) or 5 mg/ml (50 mg ampoule).

Preparation: add 1×50 mg ampoule to 40 ml 5% dextrose in an infusion pump (concentration = 1 mg/ml) or 1×50 mg ampoule to 490 ml 5% dextrose (concentration = 100 µg/ml).

Start at 10 µg/min. Increase every 20–30 min by 20 µg/min until effect has been achieved, to maximum 400 µg/min. Usual range needed 10–30 µg/min. (This range equates to 0.5 mg/h increasing to 2 mg/h.)

Isosorbide Dinitrate Dose Calculation

Isosorbide Dinitrate (Isoket)

This comes as 0.5 mg/ml or 1 mg/ml in 10 ml ampoules (0.05% or 0.1%). In addition it comes as 50 mg in 50 ml ampoules for use in an infusion pump.

Add 5×10 ml ampoules (50 mg) to 450 ml 5% dextrose. Mixture concentration = 1 mg in 10 ml. Start at 10 ml (1 mg)/h, i.e. 10 paediatric microdrops/min. Usual range needed is 1–7 mg/h. In severe cases 10 mg/h may be needed.

5.5 Calcium Antagonists

These are a group of drugs that share the property of inhibition of calcium influx during phase 2 of the cardiac action potential (plateau phase). Calcium enters the cell via two types of voltage-dependent calcium channel (L and T) in myocardial and vascular smooth muscle. These channels are voltage dependent as calcium influx occurs only during depolarization. The inward movement of calcium ions triggers further calcium release from the sarcoplasmic reticulum, which in turn triggers the contractile proteins (excitation–contraction coupling). Hence some calcium antagonists may have a negative inotropic effect. Inhibition of the calcium channel in vascular smooth muscle cells causes muscle cell relaxation and vessel dilatation. Conventional calcium antagonists block the L-type channel. The T-type channel is important in the sinus and AV node: T channel blockade should slow the heart rate without a negative inotropic effect and hopefully this might prove of value in both angina and cardiac failure. β Agonists increase calcium influx via a receptor-operated channel and this is not inhibited by calcium antagonists.

The increasing number of calcium antagonists have varying properties and some seem to have a predilection for certain vascular beds (Table 5.8). The drugs have a wide variety of chemical structures and the nature of the voltage-dependent channel and how the drugs block it are imperfectly understood. There is an overlap in drug effects but Table 5.8 outlines the more specific uses of the drugs.

Although the degree of negative inotropism varies, all calcium antagonists should be used with great care in patients with a history of LV failure or large hearts on the chest radiograph and verapamil definitely avoided.

Table 5.8 Physiological effects of calcium antagonists

Effect	Drug	Condition treated
Negative inotropic effect	Verapamil	HCM
		Hypertension
Effect on AV node conduction	Verapamil	SVT
		Fast AF or flutter
		Fascicular tachycardia
Systemic vasodilatation	Dihydropyridines	Hypertension
		Raynaud's phenomenon
		Aortic regurgitation
Pulmonary vasodilatation	High-dose nifedipine or diltiazem	Primary pulmonary hypertension
Coronary vasodilatation	All	Stable angina
		Microvascular angina
		Coronary spasm
		? Diastolic dysfunction
Cerebral vasodilatation	Nimodipine	Subarachnoid haemorrhage

There is considerable interest in the fact that calcium antagonists can help suppress the development of atheroma in cholesterol-fed rabbits. Preliminary work in humans suggests that calcium antagonists may help delay the development of coronary disease (nifedipine 20 mg four times daily in the INTACT study over a 3-year period and diltiazem 30–90 mg three times daily in heart transplant recipients). The three most commonly used calcium antagonists in the UK are verapamil, nifedipine and diltiazem.

Nifedipine (Dihydropyridine Group)

This is useful in all types of angina, especially when β blockade is contraindicated. It can be used synergistically with β blockade. It dilates both coronary and systemic vessels and is useful in systemic hypertension. It is of great value in Raynaud's phenomenon but of very limited value in intermittent claudication. It should not be used in pregnancy and should be avoided in women who may wish to become pregnant. Its vasodilating properties result in a warm generalized flush from 30 min to 1 h after taking the drug, and a reflex tachycardia. It is of no value in supraventricular or junctional tachycardia.

Side Effects

These include flushing and tachycardia, and ankle and leg oedema gradually developing during the day. This oedema does not respond well to diuretics and is better managed with advice about posture and support stockings, if necessary. Other side effects are pruritus (avoid in inflammatory skin disease) and gum hyperplasia. Some patients notice a diuretic effect.

Dose

Use slow-release preparation only for maintenance. Start with 10–20 mg twice daily after meals up to a maximum of 40 mg daily. The short-acting capsules (5 mg or 10 mg) may be chewed in acute angina and the drug is absorbed through the buccal mucosa. The capsule contents can be squeezed into the mouth of a patient with acute hypertension or coronary spasm during or after cardiac catheterization. An intracoronary preparation is available: 0.2 mg into the heart will help prevent coronary spasm during PCI.

Contraindications to Dihydropyridine Drugs (Nifedipine Group)

- Severe aortic stenosis
- HCM
- Women of childbearing age unless using reliable contraception
- Poor LV function
- Unstable angina as a sole agent: must be used with a β blocker.

Diltiazem (Benzothiazepine Group)

This drug is a potent coronary vasodilator but has less effect on dilating peripheral vascular beds. It causes less flushing and reflex tachycardia than nifedipine. Like nifedipine it can be used synergistically with β blockade but the combination may induce bradycardia especially in the elderly. It increases AV nodal refractoriness and can be used for SVT. It also appears to have an antiplatelet effect, which may be shared by other calcium antagonists. It is useful in the first-line treatment of angina where β blockade is unsuitable. The three most common calcium antagonists (diltiazem, nifedipine and verapamil) all increase coronary blood flow.

Side Effects
These are few and the drug is well tolerated. A small number of patients develop an irritating skin rash, which resolves when the drug is stopped. Rarely, a more serious exfoliative dermatitis and epidermal necrolysis have been reported.

Dose
This is given orally 60–120 mg three times daily. An intravenous preparation is not generally available yet. Slow-release preparations are given – 90 mg twice daily or 120–240 mg once daily.

Verapamil (Phenylalkylamine Group)
Although introduced initially as a drug for angina, it has become very valuable in the treatment of supraventricular and junctional tachycardia because of its effect on AV nodal conduction. It can be used as an alternative to β blockade but should be avoided in patients on β blockers unless they are under close supervision, and have good LV function and no conduction defect. It is useful in decubitus angina. It has a negative inotropic effect and should be used with great care in patients with a history of LVF in the past, or a large heart on the chest radiograph. Reduce the dose in liver disease.

It is of value in the acute management of supraventricular (narrow complex) tachycardia but has been superseded by adenosine, which is safer and better (see Section 8.3). It will increase the degree of AV block in AF and atrial flutter with fast ventricular rates, and can be used with digoxin in the chronic management of these arrhythmias. Given intravenously in atrial flutter with a fast ventricular rate, it will slow the ventricular rate, allowing the flutter waves to appear more clearly. Carotid sinus massage may abort an attack of SVT after or during verapamil administration even if it did not do so before it. It is the drug of choice in fascicular tachycardia (see Figure 8.9).

Side Effects
Constipation is the main drawback with verapamil. Haemorrhoids may be the result. Ankle oedema may also occur at the end of the day.

Dose
Orally: initially 80 mg three times daily increasing to 120 mg three times daily. A slow-release preparation is available (e.g. for hypertensive patients) 240 mg once daily as a single dose.

Intravenously: verapamil 5–10 mg: repeat in 30 min if necessary. ECG monitoring is essential during intravenous administration.

Verapamil should be avoided in the following:
- Patients on β-blocking agents unless under close supervision and LV function is good
- Sinoatrial disease
- Patients with AV block
- Possible digoxin toxicity
- Hypotensive patients
- AF and Wolff–Parkinson–White syndrome (see Section 8.7)
- Wide complex tachycardias: these may be VT rather than SVT with aberrant conduction. Verapamil given to patients with VT may produce hypotension and asystole. The only exception is fascicular tachycardia (RBBB + left axis deviation), which responds to verapamil (see Figure 8.9).

Other Calcium Antagonists

There are a large number of second-generation calcium antagonists of the dihydropyridine group (nifedipine analogues) on the market, with an increasing emphasis on long-acting drugs such as amlodipine or nisoldipine or slow-release preparations of nifedipine, verapamil or diltiazem, which need to be taken once or at most twice daily. There is very little to choose between the increasing number of calcium antagonists with properties that differ only slightly.

Nimodipine

This is more selective for cerebral vessels and of value after subarachnoid haemorrhage, increasing flow to poorly perfused areas. Dose is 1 mg/h i.v. for 2 h then 2 mg/h (or 60 mg 4-hourly for 21 days). Infusion must be protected from the light.

Amlodipine

Longest-acting calcium antagonist with a half-life of 35–50 h. Once-a-day preparation starts with 5 mg once daily for angina or hypertension. The maximum dose is 10 mg once daily. There is slow absorption and 90% is metabolized. There is no need to reduce the dose in renal disease but care must be taken in liver disease. The PRAISE study showed that it was safe in patients with severe heart failure, and was useful in treating coexisting angina or hypertension in this group. It appeared to be of particular benefit in improving the prognosis in patients with dilated cardiomyopathy. The ASCOT-BPLA trial showed it was superior to a beta-blockade regimen in hypertension.

Nicardipine

This is a short-acting water-soluble drug, which is highly protein bound and has weaker negative inotropic action than nifedipine. It is not light sensitive. The dose is 20 mg three times daily, up to 40 mg three times daily.

There is approximately 30% first-pass metabolism. Dose is reduced in both liver and renal diseases. It increases digoxin levels.

Felodipine
This has a high vascular selectivity, and a half-life of 8 h. it is very similar to nifedipine. Dose: start 5 mg twice daily, up to 10 mg three times daily, for hypertension and/or angina. In the VHeFT III trial it was shown to be no better than enalapril and did not improve survival in patients with heart failure, although it was shown to produce a fall in BP and a rise in LV ejection fraction.

Isradipine
This is another dihydropyridine more specific for vascular smooth muscle than the myocardium. There is extensive first-pass metabolism with about 20% bioavailability. It is 95% protein-bound and has a pronounced diuretic effect. Dose: 2.5 mg twice daily up to 10 mg twice daily. It has a half-life of 8 h.

Nisoldipine
This is a drug with high vascular selectivity available as a slow-release coat-core preparation. It has been shown to be safe in patients with moderate LV dysfunction with no negative inotropic effect. Dose is 10–30 mg once daily on an empty stomach. Its predilection for the coronary vascular bed results in few peripheral side effects compared with nifedipine.

Long-term Safety of Calcium Antagonists
Since 1995 there has been a great deal of unrest in both the medical and popular press about the long-term safety of calcium antagonists based on meta-analysis of 16 pooled trials by Furberg and Psaty. This suggested that high-dose, short-acting nifedipine (80 mg daily) carried a threefold, long-term mortality risk compared with placebo. It was suggested that this might have been the result of arrhythmias induced by activation of the sympathetic nervous system secondary to acute vasodilatation. Other concerns have been expressed relating to gastrointestinal bleeding and malignancy. The following came out of all the furore:
- There was considerable dispute about the analysis methods.
- The 80 mg dose of nifedipine exceeded the manufacturer's recommendations.
- There were virtually no long-term prospective data.
   In practical terms:
- Nifedipine is not a recommended drug for acute MI.
- Short-acting calcium antagonists of any type should be avoided, particularly short-acting dihydropyridines, except in the management of acute hypertension or coronary spasm.

• The third generation of calcium antagonists now have long half-lives or are slow-release preparations. Nifedipine is also available in slow-release format and considered perfectly safe, as shown in the prospective STONE study of treating elderly people with long-term hypertension.

Newer Drug Therapy for Angina

Nicorandil

This is a new drug that consists of two components: a nitrate and a potassium channel opener. It dilates both arteries and veins. The activation of the K^+ ATP channel may help with ischaemic preconditioning. It is of use in stable angina, and side effects and precautions are as for nitrates. Headache is the most common side effect. The dose is 10–20 mg twice daily and the half-life is 1 h. It should be avoided in hypotensive patients, children, pregnant women and lactating women. It is less likely to have an effect in patients who are already on a long-acting nitrate, but worth a try in patients with refractory angina. In a large trial (IONA) of 5126 patients with stable angina it reduced cardiac events by 17%. (Primary endpoint: cardiac death, non-fatal MI and admission with angina.)

Ivabradine

This is a new drug that works by blocking the I_f current in the sinus node, resulting in a slowing of the sinus rate both at rest and on exercise. Exercise time and symptoms improve. It is of no value in patients with AF. It is particularly useful in patients who are intolerant of β-blocking drugs (e.g. those with peripheral vascular disease or provoked bronchospasm). The dose is 5 mg twice daily. There is no rebound effect on withdrawal (as with β blockers). In one double-blind trial it was as effective as atenolol.

Metabolic Switching Agents

Although β-blocking agents may reduce plasma free fatty acids and thereby improve metabolic efficiency (see Figure 5.4), three drugs not yet available in the UK inhibit fatty acid oxidation (β oxidation) and switch the heart to more glucose oxidation. This improves metabolic efficiency and wastes less ATP (uses less O_2 for the same ATP). These agents are: trimetazidine, ranolazine and perhexiline.

Trimetazidine

When administered with metoprolol in a randomized trial, trimetazidine improved exercise time to 1 mm ST depression, time to angina onset and total number of weekly episodes of angina. Several small trials comparing trimetazidine with placebo have confirmed its value. The dose is 20 mg three times daily.

Ranolazine

At doses of 500–1000 mg twice daily, this drug has been shown to be of value in several trials in chronic angina. It was approved for use by the FDA in 2006 but is not approved in Europe yet. In a small trial it also appears to reduce the HbA1c in people with diabetes.

Unfortunately it increases the QT interval (see Section 8.6) and should be avoided in patients with a long QT interval, in co-administration with any other drug with the potential to prolong the QT interval or drugs that inhibit CYP3A4 (e.g. diltiazem), and in hepatic disease. In spite of its effect on the QT interval, torsades de pointes resulting from the drug has not yet been documented. Its use in ACS was tested in the MERLIN TIMI 36 trial, but the drug was of no benefit in reducing cardiovascular death or recurrent MI, although it did reduce recurrent myocardial ischaemia and clinically significant arrhythmias on Holter monitoring. There was certainly no proarrhythmic effect.

Perhexiline

This drug, originally used for peripheral vascular disease as well as angina, was withdrawn from use in the UK with reports of hepatotoxicity and peripheral neuropathy. These toxic effects occurred in slow acetylators. The drug is still of value and in use in some countries (e.g. Australia). Plasma concentrations should be maintained between 150 and 600 ng/ml to reduce side effects.

5.6 Unstable Angina/Non-Q-wave MI/Non-ST-segment Elevation MI (NSTEMI)

These conditions are now grouped together as part of the spectrum of acute coronary syndromes (ACS) because their management is identical. Until the results of blood tests are known they are often grouped under the title unstable angina.

Unstable Angina
* Angina occurring with increasing frequency or severity
* Angina occurring at rest, or more frequently at night
* Angina not relieved quickly with nitroglycerin
* Usually associated with ST depression on the ECG.

Subendocardial/Non-Q-wave MI/NSTEMI
Subendocardial/non-Q-wave infarcts account for about 20–30% of all infarcts. A total coronary occlusion usually produces a transmural Q-wave infarct. Incomplete thrombosis or early lysis in a coronary artery produces a non-Q-wave infarct. The diagnosis of a subendocardial/NSTEMI infarct is based on a typical history of chest pain, ECG changes (ST depression or T-wave inversion) plus enzyme or troponin elevation, which is often mild compared with transmural Q-wave infarction (Figure 5.6 and Table 5.9).

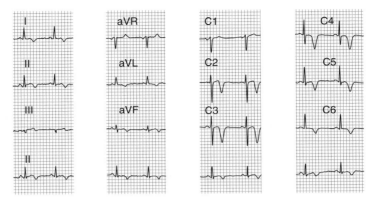

Figure 5.6 Non-ST-segment elevation MI: steep symmetrical T-wave inversion across anterior leads V1–5 without Q waves. This patient had a severe LAD stenosis involving the origin of the first diagonal.

Generally it is an incomplete and small infarct. It may be the result of diffuse three-vessel disease or a single severe stenosis in a large artery. In either case it may occur early in the course of a Q-wave infarct, before the vessel is totally occluded. Frequently it progresses to a Q-wave infarct.

Table 5.9 Acute coronary syndromes

Clinical syndrome/term	ECG changes	Enzyme changes	Thrombolysis
Acute MI	ST elevation New LBBB Posterior MI on ECG Developing Q waves	CK-MB, CK > 2 × normal Troponin T > 0.2 ng/dl Troponin I > 1.0–1.5 ng/dl	Yes
Minimal myocyte necrosis Subendocardial infarction Non-Q-wave MI/non-STEMI	Transient ST elevation ST depression T-wave inversion Non-specific ECG changes	CK-MB, CK < 2 × normal Troponin T 0.01–0.2 ng/dl Troponin I 0.1 or 0.4 ng/dl to 1.0–1.5 ng/dl[a]	No
Unstable angina	Transient ST elevation ST depression T-wave inversion Non-specific ECG changes Normal ECG	CK-MB, CK in normal range Troponin T < 0.01 ng/dl Troponin I < 0.1 or <0.4 ng/dl[a]	No

[a]Depending on assay used.
Non-STEMI: non-ST-segment elevation myocardial infarction.

Outcome of Unstable Angina/Non-Q-wave MI

From the PRAIS-UK data at 6 months of medical management (aspirin and antianginal drugs) there is a 12.2% incidence of death or MI and a 30% risk of death, MI, refractory angina or readmission with unstable angina. This is a high incidence of future events and this figure will be lowered only by intervention in high-risk patients.

• Hospital mortality rate: approximately 2% but up to 12% in one long-term study (12–18% hospital mortality rate in Q-wave infarcts).
• High incidence of late events: 10% mortality rate at 1 month; 30% rate of death/MI/refractory angina at 6 months (PRAIS – UK study).
• ST-segment depression at diagnosis more dangerous than ST elevation.
• High incidence of arrhythmias; 24-hour ECG monitoring needed.
• More incidence of post-infarct angina than after Q-wave infarction.
• LV function may improve transiently after a non-Q-wave infarct. If segmental wall motion can be shown to improve, then that area is at high risk for a full-thickness infarct subsequently.

The Benefit of an Early Invasive Strategy

With limited evidence available from randomized trials there was some contention about early intervention in patients with unstable angina. The problems were under-powered trials with additional high crossover rates to intervention, e.g. TIMI IIIb trial – no difference with early intervention; VAN-QWISH trial – hazard greater with early intervention. However, more recent trials have come down firmly on the side of early intervention (FRISC II and TACTICS-TIMI 18). A meta-analysis of seven randomized trials of 8375 patients comparing an early invasive strategy against a conservative strategy has shown a lower mortality, a lower incidence of recurrent unstable angina requiring readmission and a lower rate of non-fatal MI at 2 years.

Patients with unstable angina should be managed medically initially and risk stratified as soon as possible to determine future management. ECG and blood tests for troponin and CK-MB should be taken on admission and at 8 hours after admission. Patients who are at high risk should be pre-treated with a platelet glycoprotein IIb/IIIa antagonist and proceed to urgent coronary angiography, with a view to possible angioplasty or surgery. Investigation, angioplasty or surgery in the unstable phase carries only a very slightly higher risk than when undertaken in stable angina.

Risk Stratification in Acute Unstable Angina/Non-Q-wave MI

Patients who are not in this high-risk group should have a treadmill exercise test or stress thallium scanning and coronary angiography performed on those with positive tests (Table 5.10).

Stage 1: Initial Medical Management on Admission

• Complete bed rest
• Light sedation

Table 5.10 High-risk features in patients indicating need for urgent coronary angiography

Clinical features	ECG changes	Enzyme changes
Older patient > 65 years	Transient ST elevation or depression during pain	Any elevation of CK-MB, CPK or troponin T or I
Previous MI		
LV dysfunction	Failure of ST depression to resolve on treatment	
Cardiogenic shock		
Continuing chest pain	Deep T-wave inversion	
Hypertension	Ventricular arrhythmias	
Diabetes	LBBB	

- Restricted visitors
- Analgesia as required (diamorphine 2.5–5.0 mg i.v./i.m. p.r.n. 4-hourly)
- Drug therapy started immediately.

β Blockade
For example, propranolol 40 mg three times daily. β Blockade is avoided if there is any evidence of coronary spasm (labile ST segments during pain with some ST elevation) because this avoids unopposed α effects on coronary arteries in patients with spasm.

Diltiazem Slow Release, 90–180 mg Twice Daily
One trial suggested that nifedipine should not be used without a β blocker in unstable angina. Calcium antagonists have not been shown to reduce mortality in unstable angina when used alone but are considered safe and useful as synergistic agents with a β blocker. Diltiazem and a β blocker may produce a marked sinus bradycardia (start with low doses, especially in elderly people). Avoid verapamil/β-blocker combination (combined negative inotropic effect of both drugs).

Nitrates
Start with oral isosorbide mononitrate slow-release 60 mg once daily. Additional GTN spray or tablets should be available as required. If the angina does not settle rapidly switch to intravenous nitrates, e.g. isosorbide dinitrate, starting at 2 mg/h up to 10 mg/h if necessary.

Soluble Aspirin, 75–150 mg Daily
Aspirin has been shown to reduce the incidence of MI and death in unstable angina. It inhibits platelet cyclo-oxygenase, reducing synthesis of thromboxane A_2 and platelet adhesiveness see Figure 5.7. This may help to reduce microthrombi formation on an atherosclerotic plaque, which is known from angioscopy studies to be part of the syndrome of unstable angina.

Clopidogrel
This platelet ADP-receptor antagonist causes less neutropenia than ticlopidine and is started in patients who are proceeding to angiography and possible stenting. Loading dose is 600 mg, followed by 75 mg daily. The CURE trial showed additional benefit in ACSs when combined with aspirin.

Heparin
Low-molecular-weight heparins (Dalteparin and Enoxaparin) have several advantages over intravenous, standard, unfractionated heparin. The drugs have longer half-lives than unfractionated heparin and are given subcutaneously twice daily. No monitoring of coagulation is required because standard clotting tests are unaffected (e.g. APTT), anti-factor Xa activity is higher, administration is easier and can be continued at home for patients waiting for revascularization, and the incidence of thrombocytopenia and osteoporosis seems to be less than with intravenous heparin.

Dalteparin (Fragmin)
This has been shown in the FRISC study to reduce the incidence of new MI and death in patients already taking aspirin in unstable angina. The dose is 120 IU/kg body weight twice daily s.c. for 1 week followed by once daily.

Enoxaparin (Clexane)
This has been shown to be superior to unfractionated heparin when given with aspirin in unstable angina (the ESSENCE and TIMI IIb trials). Dose is 1 mg/kg s.c. twice daily.

Glycoprotein IIb/IIIa receptor antagonists
The value of aspirin and the finding of microthrombi on culprit lesions in unstable angina have led to studies using more specific platelet antagonists. Antibodies to the platelet glycoprotein IIb/IIIa receptor help prevent platelet adhesion and subsequent degranulation. There are three drugs in this group at present in the UK. These drugs block the final common pathway of platelet activation, blocking the receptors linking to other platelets by fibrinogen cross-bridges (Figure 5.7). All three are given by intravenous infusion. Oral agents have proved valueless, just causing increased bleeding. None of the three agents is cheap. The following gives the cost of an average course for a patient:
- Synthetic small molecule IIb/IIIa inhibitors:
  - tirofiban (Aggrastat) £440
  - eptifibatide (Integrilin) £400
- Chimaeric (mouse/man) monoclonal antibody:
  Abciximab (ReoPro) £850.

There is evidence that these drugs reduce events in patients with unstable angina, with the strongest evidence being with abciximab (10 trials) in patients undergoing coronary intervention. There is evidence that abciximab reduces mortality in high-risk cases particularly those with diabetes. High-risk patients

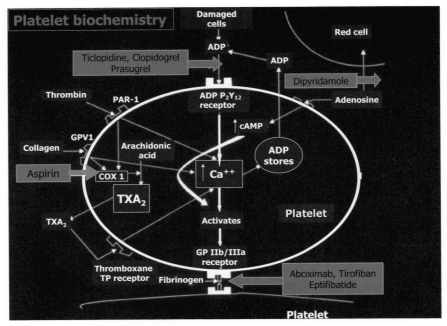

Figure 5.7 Platelet biochemistry: a diagram of a platelet illustrating the sites of drug action. Platelet activation results in an increase in intracellular ionized calcium, which causes a conformational change (pseudopodia) and activation of the final common pathway – the glycoprotein IIb/IIIa receptor. There are approximately 80 000 of these receptors per platelet. Activation of these receptors results in fibrinogen cross-bridging to adjacent platelets. Light arrows: activation pathways. Heavy green arrows: sites of drug inhibition.

should be started on abciximab within 24 hours of the start of the coronary intervention procedure or just before it. Abciximab has been shown to reduce the risk of adverse events further in high-risk patients undergoing PCI for non-ST-elevation ACSs after pre-treatment with clopidogrel. The additional benefit of abciximab on top of clopidogrel was seen only in troponin-positive cases (ISAR-REACT 2 trial).

Abciximab dose: bolus dose: 0.25 mg/kg i.v. stat, followed by 12-hour infusion at 10 μg/min in total of 50 ml 0.9% saline.

Prolonged infusions of abciximab (up to 48 h) did not reduce events in ACSs (GUSTO V). A head-to-head trial of abciximab and tirofiban showed that abciximab was a superior drug at preventing future events after PCI (TARGET). The evidence points to these drugs being more useful in preventing events during and after coronary angioplasty rather than just as adjunctive medical treatment in patients not needing intervention.

Problems with glycoprotein IIb/IIIa blockers. Abciximab may be given to patients if they have received it previously and hypersensitivity reactions are rare. It may also be used in the catheter laboratory even if patients have received a small molecule inhibitor only days before. Severe thrombocytopenia is uncommon but more likely in patients who are also on clopidogrel. Eptifibatide should not be given to patients with chronic renal failure (creatinine clearance <30 ml/min).

The main problem is post-procedural bleeding from the groin entry site. This can be largely prevented by the following:
- Use only intravenous heparin 70 U/kg at the start of coronary intervention.
- Remove the sheath at the end of the procedure using a vascular sealing device (e.g. Angioseal, Starclose).
- Check the platelet count at the end of the PCI and the next morning. Platelet administration may be needed for bleeding. Platelets are not given for asymptomatic thrombocytopenia unless the platelet count drops <10000/mm^3.
- Use a groin compression device if there are any doubts about the oozing groin (e.g. Femostop).

Thrombolysis is not on this list and has not yet been shown to carry any benefit in patients with unstable angina or non-Q-wave infarction.

Stage 2: Coronary Angiography, Angioplasty or Surgery
About 7–10% of patients will have left main stem stenosis, about 70% will have left anterior descending stenosis, <3% will have coronary spasm and a few will have normal coronary arteries (<10%).

Further intervention depends on the coronary arteriographic findings, the facilities available and the expertise of the investigator. The options are:
- PCI
- CABG
- IABP
- continuing medical treatment.

PCI is very valuable in unstable angina. The history is often short and the lesion, if a single one, is often soft: ideal for angioplasty and stenting. In unstable angina stand-by facilities for CAB surgery are necessary.

IABP is rarely used in unstable angina except as a holding mechanism before surgery or to move the patient to a surgical centre. The balloon can be inserted percutaneously without the need for radiological screening. IABP is very useful in the short term for controlling pain. Difficult or high-risk angioplasty can be performed with the balloon pump working (see Section 6.14).

Medical treatment is reserved for patients with normal coronary arteries or dominant coronary spasm. Patients with normal coronaries or spasm will continue calcium antagonists and nitrates with soluble aspirin, but their β-blocking agent is stopped. A very few patients with unstable angina will have severe diffuse coronary disease that is considered inoperable. These patients must also be managed medically.

In the UK, facilities for immediate investigation of high-risk cases are not always immediated available. Patients will need to be managed medically with the above regimen before being transferred to a centre for possible coronary intervention.

Future Trends

Risk Markers

There is increasing evidence that inflammatory markers are raised in unstable angina and have prognostic value. CRP, serum amyloid A protein (both acute phase proteins) and interleukin-6 levels from macrophages and T cells are raised in unstable angina, and the higher the level the worse the prognosis. In the FRISC trial troponin T, CRP and fibrinogen were related to long-term prognosis and risk of cardiac death.

These raised markers must reflect inflammatory cell infiltrate into the atheromatous plaque, and probably a systemic inflammatory process. Aspirin's greatest effect is in patients with higher CRP levels. Cardiac troponins and CK-MB are also risk markers in unstable angina (see above). The inflamed atheromatous plaque generates heat, and measurement of this and identifying the hot (unstable) plaque is now a possibility.

New platelet inhibitors

Inhibitors of the P2y12 platelet receptor (see Figure 5.7) include not only ticlopidine and clopidogrel, but also prasugrel, which may prove to be more effective as a platelet inhibitor. One study has suggested that there is a lower rate of non-responders in coronary disease patients with stable angina treated with prasugrel.

Coated and Drug-eluting Stents

See Section 5.9.

5.7 ST Elevation Myocardial Infarction (STEMI)

Primary Prevention

With over 105000 deaths annually from coronary disease in the UK, primary prevention is of vital importance. The largest case control study ever performed in the identification of modifiable risk factors is the INTERHEART study (2004). Fifty-two countries worldwide contributed to this study, enrolling 15152 cases with 14820 controls.

Nine risk factors were identified that accounted for 90% of the population-attributable risk in men and 94% in women. These risk factors were:

1 current smokers (any tobacco in the last 12 months)
2 diabetes
3 hypertension
4 abdominal obesity (waist:hip ratio: top tertile in men >0.95, and in women 0.90)
5 Apo-B:Apo-A1 ratio (normal ratio 0.8–1.0)
6 in adequate daily consumption of fruit and vegetables

7 psychosocial factors: combination of depression, work or home stress, financial stress or one or more life events.

8 exercise <4 h/week

9 alcohol intake (<three times/week).

The two strongest risk factors after multivariate analysis were smoking and the Apo-B:Apo-A1 ratio, which together accounted for 66.8% of the population-attributable risk. Five of the risk factors together accounted for 80% of the risk (lipids, diabetes, hypertension, smoking, obesity). Consumption of alcohol more than three times a week was protective.

The rate of obesity (BMI >30) is rising in the UK, with 22.5% of men and 23% of women now considered obese. In addition there are 2 million known individuals with diabetes and probably an additional 2 million unknown individuals with diabetes/metabolic syndrome. This represents a major potential health burden both now and in the years ahead.

Acute MI and the Ambulance Service

Fifty per cent of patients who die from an acute MI do so within the first 2 h of symptoms. The great delay in getting patients to hospital is generally a result of the delay in the patient recognizing the importance of his or her symptoms. A large national advertising campaign has encouraged patients to ring for an ambulance if they have symptoms suggestive of an MI, rather than ringing their GP or trying to get to hospital themselves.

Mobile CCUs developed in Brighton and Belfast in the UK have been very successful in the immediate management of MI by:

• reduction of transport deaths
• resuscitation of on-site VF
• possible reduction of infarct size by early treatment of arrhythmias, although this will be impossible to prove
• reduction of the time taken to reach a CCU
• early administration of thrombolysis (see Section 5.8).

Education of laypeople in cardiac resuscitation has proved very valuable (e.g. in Seattle) and static CCUs (e.g. in sports stadia) are being developed. Many cities now have automatic external defibrillators (AEDs) positioned in mainline stations, airports, stadia and concert halls, which can be safely used by the public. Many lives have been saved by the use of these devices.

Hospital mortality has dramatically halved in the last few years with the advent of thrombolysis, aspirin, etc. and now runs <10%. Thrombolytic trials (inevitably including more low-risk patients) show single-figure mortality rates. PPCI centres now run at <5% mortality.

Immediate Pre-hospital Thrombolysis or Primary Percutaneous Coronary Angioplasty (PPCI)?

Both these interventions reduce MI mortality. Some countries (e.g. Poland, Czech Republic) rely exclusively on a highly developed PPCI service. Others (such as the UK) have both interventions running in parallel.

The development of a pre-hospital thrombolysis service in England started in 2003. The thrombolytic drug (either reteplase or tenecteplase) is delivered by paramedics. They diagnose the STEMI independently and the ECG can be telemetered to medical staff if necessary for confirmation. The paramedics have a stringent checklist of indications and contraindications for thrombolysis. The introduction of this service has sharply reduced MI mortality (see below).

Pathology
Approximately 90% of patients with a transmural infarct have total occlusion of the relevant coronary artery (as visualized by angiography) within 4 h of pain onset. Incidence decreases with time (possibly as a result of relaxation of additional spasm or recanalization). Most occlusive thrombi are associated with intimal plaque rupture and haemorrhage into the plaque.

A small proportion of patients will have normal coronary arteries. Emboli and spasm must be the prime mechanisms in these cases.

Home care?
After the original work of Mather and his colleagues in 1971, numerous publications appeared extolling the virtues of both home and hospital care for MI. Can home care still be a possibility in the age of primary angioplasty and pre-hospital thrombolysis?

Fifty per cent of those patients who die do so within 2 h of the onset of their symptoms. Neither thrombolysis nor primary PCI carries any mortality benefits after 12h. Home care with arrangements for subsequent referral may therefore be considered where:
- time from onset of symptoms is >12 h
- the patient is warm, well perfused, out of pain and normotensive
- there are no signs of LVF
- there is no history of diabetes
- the cardiac rhythm is stable.

The wishes of the patient and his or her relatives are considered, together with social circumstances, availability and proximity of a CCU, and available transport facilities.

Immediate Treatment in the Home

Analgesia
Diamorphine is the drug of choice. It should be given intravenously (2.5–5.0 mg) in case subsequent thrombolysis is given. Metoclopramide 10 mg i.v. or i.m. or cyclizine 50 mg i.m. or orally should be administered as an antiemetic. Both opiates and MI cause vomiting. Cyclizine is more sedative than metoclopramide. Numerous other antiemetics are available. Metclopramide has the additional advantage of speeding gastric emptying and increasing the tone of the cardia (oesophagogastric junction).

Oxygen
This is given at 5l/min.

Bradycardia (Sinus or Junctional)
This is treated with atropine 0.6 mg i.v., repeated to a maximum of 3.0 mg.

Amiodarone
In the absence of bradycardia, hypotension or shock, amiodarone 300 mg i.v. may be given for frequent multifocal ventricular extrasystoles, salvos of VT, etc. or before transfer to hospital.

Lidocaine 300 mg i.m. is the alternative if amiodarone is unavailable, but amiodarone appeared to have better outcomes than lidocaine in the ALIVE trial.

Intravenous Furosemide
This is given to the patient in acute pulmonary oedema (also has a venodilator effect). The dose is 40–80 mg initially intravenously. It should not be given for a raised JVP in the presence of an inferior infarct unless the patient also has pulmonary oedema.

Immediate Thrombolysis
This service is now available in most parts of England and parts of Wales delivered by paramedics in the local ambulance service without a physician being present. A stringent checklist is used by the paramedics. The age limit is 80 and the BP must be <180/110.

Diagnosis of MI
This may pose a great problem, and there are no absolutely accepted criteria. A recent consensus from the European Society of Cardiology and the American Heart Association has redefined the diagnosis of MI, which involves including patients who are troponin-positive but CK-negative (less than twice normal) as having minimal myocardial necrosis. See Acute Coronary Syndromes in Section 5.6 and Table 5.9.

The diagnosis is based on the following:
• History: severe typical cardiac pain lasting > 20 min unrelieved by nitrates
• ECG changes
• Cardiac enzyme or troponin elevation
• Postmortem evidence.
    Other criteria that may help but are less reliable include the following:
• Physical signs, e.g. new high dyskinetic apex, pericardial rub
• Fever developing 48 h after the pain
• Elevated WBC and ESR
• Myocardial scintigraphy: not positive until 48 h post-infarction, e.g. hot-spot scanning using isotopes taken up into dead/dying cells (e.g.

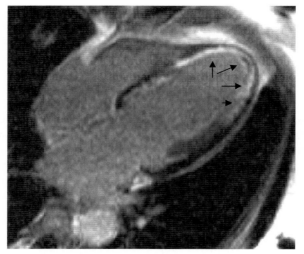

Figure 5.8 Cardiac MR scan in a man with an old anteroapical myocardial infarct. There is late gadolinium enhancement seen as a white rim (arrowed) indicating myocyte loss and replacement by fibrous tissue.

imidodiphosphate) or cold-spot scanning using potassium analogues taken up by living cardiac cells (e.g. thallium)
• Cardiac MRI with gadolinium injection: gadolinium does not diffuse away from infarcted/scar tissue. This late gadolinium enhancement shows up as a white rim in the relevant infarcted territory (Figure 5.8).

Summary of ECG Changes (for examples see Figures 5.9–5.14 and 16.11–16.14)

Pathological Q Waves
New Q waves are the hallmark of so-called transmural infarction. In standard leads pathological Q wave should be not less than 25% of the R wave and 0.04 s in duration with negative T waves. In precordial leads pathological Q waves should be associated with QRS duration <0.1 s (i.e. not LBBB), and with negative or biphasic T waves. Q waves in V4 or V5 should be >0.4 mV and in V6 > 0.2 mV.

Large Q waves occur also with hypertrophy and fibrosis (e.g. HCM) and infiltration (e.g. amyloidosis). It is most valuable to be able to establish that the Q waves are new. Q waves also occur in the chest leads in corrected transposition (see Section 2.6 and Figure 2.20).

Injury Current/ST-segment Elevation
ST-segment elevation should persist preferably for 24 h. (Transient ST-segment elevation occurs with Prinzmetal's angina.) It usually appears within 24 h of

a transmural infarct, and returns to isoelectric baseline in <2 weeks. Persisting ST-segment elevation at >1 month suggests LV aneurysm. (Figure 14.2 and Section 5.10)

For diagnosis there should be >2 mm ST elevation in two adjacent chest leads or >1 mm ST elevation in two adjacent limb leads. In inferior infarction with marked RV involvement, there should be >1 mm ST elevation in V4R.

Reciprocal ST-segment Depression

This is thought to reflect a 'mirror image' of electrical activity on the opposite non-infarcted wall. It is not thought that reciprocal ST-segment depression indicates additional ischaemia and coronary disease in the relevant territory.

T-wave Inversion

By itself this is not diagnostic of infarction. (Occurs in the normal heart in some patients with catecholamine stimulation, reversed by β blockade.)

Steep symmetrical T-wave inversion may occur without new Q-wave development in either ventricular hypertrophy or 'subendocardial' infarction (see Figure 5.6). Enzyme elevation is necessary to confirm infarction in the absence of new Q waves.

Localization of Infarcts from ECG (Table 5.11)

• Anterolateral: Q waves in I, aVL and V3–6. ST elevation with T inversion in I and aVL.
• Anteroseptal: Q waves in V2 and V3 (but often none in lateral precordial or standard leads) with ST elevation and T inversion.
• Anteroapical: Q wave in I with ST elevation. Apparent right-axis deviation (see Figure 5.6). May be Qs in V3–4.
• Inferior (diaphragmatic): Q waves in II, III aVF with ST elevation and T inversion. Additional ST elevation in V4R suggests RV infarction.

Table 5.11 Summary of infarct localization on ECG

Site of infarct	ECG leads showing change	ST elevation/depression
Anterior	V1–4	Elevation
Lateral	I, aVL, V5, V6	Elevation
Inferior	II, III, aVF	Elevation
Right ventricular	V4R	Elevation
Posterior	V1–4	Depression
Posterior	V7–9 (back of left chest)	Elevation

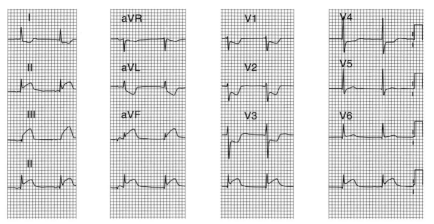

Figure 5.9 Acute inferoposterior MI: ST elevation in leads II, III and aVF, with positive R wave in V1, and ST depression in V1–3. Sinus rhythm initially and then junctional rhythm.

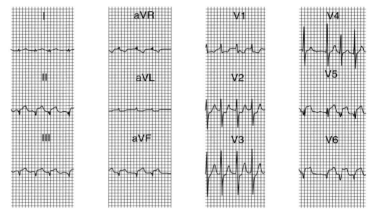

Figure 5.10 Acute inferolateral MI and AF: ST elevation in leads II, III, aVF, V4–6.

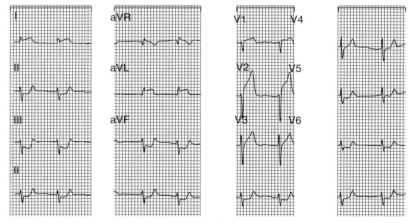

Figure 5.11 Hyperacute anterolateral MI and AF: ST elevation in leads V2–3, I and aVL. Reciprocal changes (ST depression) in inferior leads (II, III and avF). No Q waves yet.

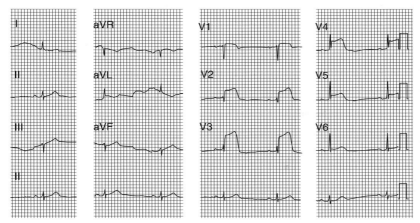

Figure 5.12 Acute anterior MI with sinus bradycardia: ST elevation in V1–5. No Q waves yet.

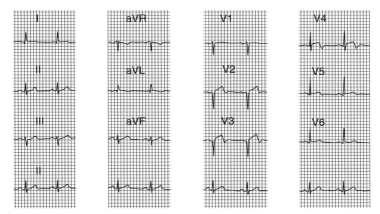

Figure 5.13 Evolving anterior MI: biphasic T waves V2–4. Q waves V2 and V3.

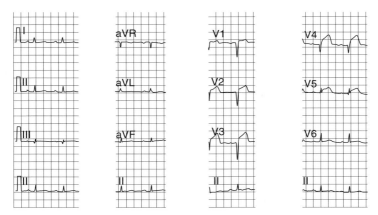

Figure 5.14 Old anterior MI with persistent ST elevation in V1–5 (? LV aneurysm).

- True posterior: tall R waves in V1 and V2 (exclude RV hypertrophy, type A WPW syndrome and RBBB) with negative ST depression in V1–3. This can be confirmed by the oesophageal lead.

Changes on ECG not diagnostic of infarction, but that may be ischaemic, include:

- ST-segment depression
- transient ST-segment elevation (e.g. spasm)
- axis shift – left or right
- transient T-wave inversion
- increase in R-wave voltage (e.g. on exercise testing; see Chapter 16, Figure 16.17, bottom panel)
- LBBB or RBBB
- first-, second- or third-degree AV block
- tachyarrhythmias
- transient, tall, peaked T waves.

Cardiac Enzymes and Cardiac Markers

CPK
MB isoenzyme – the most specific cardiac enzyme – rises and falls within the first 72 h. Cumulative CPK concentrations have been used to estimate infarct size. It has a peak concentration 24 h post-infarction. Other isoenzymes of CPK are CPK-MM (skeletal muscle) and CPK-BB (brain and kidney). Very small amounts of CPK-MB also occur in the small intestine, tongue and diaphragm.

Recent analysis of CPK-MB isoforms has helped discriminate true MI at the very early stage of 4–6 h when thrombolysis may be needed. CPK-MB has two isoforms: MB_1 from serum and MB_2 from myocardial tissue. The normal ratio is 1.0. A ratio of $MB_2:MB_1 > 1.5$ is diagnostic of myocardial damage. This raised ratio occurs before total CPK-MB is elevated by conventional testing.

SGOT
Serum aspartate aminotransferase (AST; formerly known as glutamic–oxaloacetic transaminase SGOT) is less specific than CPK-MB. It rises and falls within 4–6 days, with peak concentration at 24 h. SGOT is also elevated in liver disease, hepatic congestion, pulmonary embolism, skeletal muscle injury, shock or intramuscular injections.

Lactic Dehydrogenase
Again lactic dehydrogenase (LDH) is not cardiospecific; it peaks about 4–5 days post-infarction and may take 2 weeks to return to baseline. LDH is also elevated in haemolysis, leukaemia, megaloblastic anaemia, renal disease, plus all the false-positive causes of elevated SGOT.

The LDH false positives can be separated by isoenzyme electrophoretic studies: LDH_1, cardiac, red cells; LDH_4 and LDH_5, liver and skeletal muscle.

Hydroxybutyrate Dehydrogenase
Hydroxybutyrate dehydrogenase (HBD) measures the activity of LDH_1 isoenzyme and is often used instead of LDH analysis and isoenzyme differentiation.

Myoglobin
Although not strictly an enzyme, peak levels of serum myoglobin occur before peak CPK-MB activity. It is also excreted in the urine. It is not clinically useful, with its origin also from skeletal muscle. It is released after vigorous physical effort.

Troponin T or I
An immunodiagnostic test detects these myofibrillar proteins, which are specific markers for MI. Levels of troponins remain raised for up to 2 weeks after infarction, much longer than CPK (2–3 days). They have prognostic value in patients admitted with unstable angina, raised levels indicating a high likelihood of subsequent infarction (see Section 5.6). Time is the problem with troponins: a second blood sample should be taken 8 h after admission if the first is negative. Raised levels of troponin I may occur in renal failure. The source is still cardiac and indicates coronary disease needing investigation. These tests can be done at the bedside. Elevated troponins can also occur in acute myocarditis, cardiac contusion, as a result of cardiotoxic drugs and in acute pulmonary embolism.

Heart Fatty Acid-binding Protein (HFABP)
This protein carries free fatty acids into the mitochondria. Concentration in heart muscle is 10 times that in skeletal muscle. It is a newer marker that may well supersede troponins as raised levels occur within 15 min of myocardial cell necrosis. It is a low-molecular-weight protein which leaks out of necrotic cells faster than troponin. It is rapidly cleared by the kidneys. A raised HFABP level is independently associated with a worse outcome, whether or not the troponin is raised. As a predictor of risk in ACSs, a combination of troponin and HFABP is better than either alone.

Immediate Treatment in the Hospital
It is important that patients with suspected MI receive immediate treatment in accident and emergency departments with a fast-track system to get them quickly to the catheter laboratory or the CCU. Immediate measures in A&E should include the following:
• Rapid assessment of the patient, e.g. ? shock, hypotension, signs of LVF or RVF, heart murmurs

- Establishing intravenous access
- 12-lead ECG
- Give:
  - oral aspirin 300 mg and 75 mg daily, thereafter if no contraindications
  - oral clopidogrel 300 mg then 75 mg daily
  - O_2 40% if no history of chronic obstructive airway disease
  - diamorphine 2.5–5.0 mg i.v. and repeat as necessary to control pain
  - metoclopramide 10 mg i.v.
  - GTN spray × 2 if not hypotensive
- Portable chest radiograph (or in CCU) if there is any suggestion of an aortic dissection
- Take blood for urgent U&Es, glucose, CPK, HBD and FBC; repeat bloods at 24 and 48 h
- Transfer to catheter laboratory for primary coronary angioplasty or to local cardiothoracic centre.
- If not possible then immediate thrombolytic therapy. This is considered in detail in Section 5.8. It should be administered within 30 min of arrival in A&E. It is important that this is not delayed because of the logistical problems of getting the patient transferred from A&E to CCU. The use of triage nurses in A&E has increased the percentage of patients receiving thrombolytic agents and reduced the door-to-needle time.

In CCUs, consider additional therapy:
- *β Blockade*: β-blocking agents without intrinsic sympathomimetic activity have been shown to reduce mortality and subsequent cardiac events. They probably reduce early mortality by preventing cardiac rupture (analysis of ISIS 1 data). Use atenolol 5 mg i.v., or metoprolol or propranolol 5 mg i.v. Then continue orally thereafter. Contraindicated in patients with pulmonary oedema, third sound gallop, peripheral ischaemia and asthma.
- *Heparin*: low subcutaneous dose (5000 U twice daily) helps prevent deep vein thrombosis. High subcutaneous dose (12 500 U twice daily) helps prevent mural thrombus, but does slightly increase the risk of cerebral haemorrhage. Intravenous heparin is used after fibrin specific thrombolytics for 24 h in an attempt to improve coronary patency and prevent reinfarction. Generally intravenous heparin should be given to patients with large infarcts, who are slow to mobilize, with heart failure, etc.

   Dose: 5000 U as an initial bolus then 1000 U/h. Check APTT at 2–4 × control (see also Section 5.6 for alternative use of low-molecular-weight heparin).
- *Intravenous nitrates*: these are used for selected patients only – those with LVF or continuing pain, e.g. isosorbide dinitrate, starting at 2.0 mg i.v./h (see Section 5.4).
- *ACE inhibitors*: the SAVE trial has shown that captopril started 3–16 days after an MI in patients with abnormal LV function helps reduce long-term

mortality (17%), recurrent heart failure and reinfarction (24%). This is independent of the other agents above and thrombolysis. Captopril appears to reduce LV dilatation with beneficial effects on LV remodelling. The CONSENSUS II trial was unable to show similar beneficial effects with enalapril, possibly because the drug was started too early and was not confined to patients with poor LV function. Therefore on present evidence, use captopril starting at 6.25 mg three times daily on the fourth post-infarct day aiming to reach 12.5–25 mg three times daily by hospital discharge. Alternatively ramipril 1.25 mg bd increasing to 2.5–5 mg bd. Select patients particularly with:

- large infarcts
- heart failure
- large heart on chest radiograph
- anterior Q waves on ECG
- LVEF < 40% on echocardiography or MUGA (multiple gated acquisition) scanning.

• *Magnesium*: evidence from the LIMIT 2 study from Leicester suggested that intravenous magnesium given within 24 h of an acute infarction reduced mortality by 24%. Data from the much larger ISIS 4 trial completely refuted this and there is no indication for routine use of magnesium now. It should be considered in cases of resistant or recurrent VT.

Dose: 8 mmol in 20 ml 5% dextrose over 20 min, followed by 65 mmol in 100 ml 5% dextrose over 24 h.

Contraindications to magnesium: AV block, renal failure (creatinine >300 mmol/l), severe bradycardia.

• *Calcium antagonists*: the evidence that these are beneficial early after infarction is skimpy. The Danish verapamil trial (DAVITT II) with verapamil started 4–5 days post-infarct, suggested a benefit if LV function was normal.

Immediate Primary Angioplasty without
Thrombolysis (Figures 5.15–5.17)

Until 1993 it was accepted that PCI in acute infarction could be delayed until 2–3 weeks after thrombolysis and performed only in those with evidence of continuing ischaemia or a positive stress test (see Section 5.8). The PRAMI trial was an early trial to suggest that immediate PCI without thrombolysis can successfully reduce recurrent angina, reinfarction, death and intracranial bleeding as well as length of hospital stay, compared with conventional thrombolysis.

There seems little doubt now that immediate PCI (mechanical reperfusion) in acute MI is superior to thrombolysis. Although mortality reduction and myocardial salvage appear similar with either technique if the patient is treated within 3 h of symptom onset, angioplasty is superior in patients presenting later and also carries all the other advantages described above.

Stenting is superior to balloon angioplasty alone and the adjuvant use of abciximab appears to be of additional benefit (ADMIRAL study). Figures 5.15–5.17 show immediate angioplasty in a totally occluded right coronary artery treated with multiple stenting and abciximab.

PCI-related Delay

Delay in reopening an artery with an angioplasty balloon is just as important as delay in giving thrombolytic therapy. The quicker TIMI 3 flow (normal coronary flow) can be established the lower the mortality. The decision to send the patient for a PCI will increase the delay to reperfusion with the logistical problems of transfer, calling in the emergency on-call angioplasty team if out of hours, etc. A meta-analysis of 23 trials by Keeley and Grines comparing primary PCI with in-hospital thrombolysis suggests that, if the PCI-related delay is >1 h, then the advantage of primary PCI over thrombolysis is lost.

In patients who did not receive immediate reperfusion therapy there is no point in considering late reopening of an occluded infarct-related artery. In the OAT (Occluded Artery Trial) study, reopening of an occluded vessel 3–28 days after an infarct was of no benefit over a 4-year period. In fact there was a trend to a higher rate of reinfarction in the PCI group.

UK Logistics and Reperfusion Therapy

The logistical difficulties in providing an immediate PCI service in the UK for acute MI are considerable and, in spite of the results of the PRAMI study, most hospitals are still using conventional thrombolysis in acute infarction. About 80% of reperfusion therapy in the UK is thrombolysis but the figure is slowly falling as the primary PCI services get into gear.

In units where primary PCI has become established with a 24-hours-a-day service, the fastest door-to-balloon time is reached by direct transfer of the patient from the ambulance to the catheter laboratory. This requires organization of an on-call team, and good communication with the local ambulance service. The ambulance paramedics or the local hospital can telemeter or fax an ECG through to the PCI hospital if there is any doubt about the diagnosis.

Facilitated PCI (Pre-hospital Thrombolysis Followed by PCI)

Theoretically the combination of pre-hospital thrombolysis followed by PCI should provide the optimal reperfusion strategy: dealing with the thrombus, microcirculation and stenotic plaque. Unfortunately the biggest trial to compare facilitated PCI using full-dose tenecteplase in the pre-hospital setting followed by PCI, with primary PCI alone (no pre-hospital thrombolysis), resulted in a larger number of strokes in the facilitated group (ASSENT IV trial).

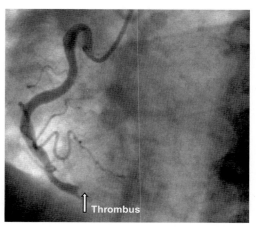

Figure 5.15 Primary coronary angioplasty: 1 –acute occlusion of proximal right coronary artery.

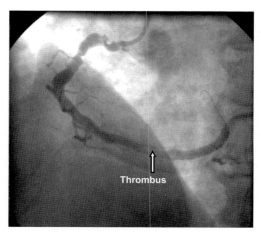

Figure 5.16 Primary coronary angioplasty 2 – vessel reopened with balloon-only dilatation. Dissection flap and/or thrombus visible (arrowed).

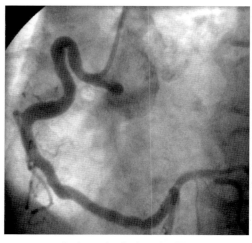

Figure 5.17 Primary coronary angioplasty. 3 – final result with coronary stenting.

Table 5.12 Strategies of PCI and thrombolysis in acute MI

• Primary PCI with no thrombolysis	Preferred strategy
• Facilitated PCI (thrombolysis followed by immediate PCI)	No proven benefit yet
	Potential harm
	Reasonable if very early presentation (<1 h) followed by delayed PCI
• Rescue PCI for failed thrombolysis	Clinical benefit with PCI and stenting
• PCI after successful thrombolysis	Delayed PCI safer than immediate PCI after successful lysis. Best timing still uncertain
• Intracoronary thrombolysis after successful PCI	No proven benefit yet

Strategies of PCI and Thrombolysis in Acute MI (Table 5.12)

Further trials are under way to identify the best immediate antiplatelet and antithrombotic strategy for patients going to the catheter laboratory for a primary PCI.

Post-infarct Management after Thrombolysis

Early investigation is necessary, with exercise testing and coronary angiography. PCI is useful for suitable lesions, or coronary surgery for patients with diffuse three-vessel disease.

Medical management alone is unsatisfactory, but if no other facilities are available, treatment with soluble aspirin and β blockade is recommended for patients with good LV function, and aspirin and captopril for poor LV function.

Early Hospital Discharge

Selection of a low-risk group of patients has allowed early discharge from hospital at about 1 week after infarction, with shorter stays for patients treated with primary PCI. If there have been no complications at the end of the fourth day, there are unlikely to be any. Using an early discharge policy will very rarely result in the release of a patient who later develops problems. Early follow-up is necessary.

Patients who should not be discharged early are those with:
• pulmonary oedema or evidence of LVF
• further chest pain after admission
• diabetes
• arrhythmias
• conduction defects: second- or third-degree AV block, bifascicular block
• persistent fever.

Common sense and the patient's social circumstances are all important.

Early Investigation Post-infarction

Treadmill exercise testing has been performed as little as 1 week after uncomplicated infarcts and is useful in assessing the severity of coronary artery disease and the 1-year prognosis.

Most centres now exercise patients before returning them to work and perform coronary angiography on young patients or those with strongly positive tests and poor exercise tolerance. There is no need to discontinue β blockade before the tests.

Advice to the Coronary Patient before Hospital Discharge

This should also be reinforced at the first outpatient visit 4 weeks later.

Work. The patient should consider returning to work if possible 2 months after an MI. In a few cases this time may be shortened. A return to full-time work is the single most important item in a patient's recovery. A few occupations, however, cannot be restarted after an infarction: Group 2 drivers, airline pilots or air traffic control personnel, divers. (see Appendix 6)

Several occupations should be considered hazardous for the post-infarct patient, e.g. furniture removers, scaffolders, bricklayers, dockers, miners, steelworkers, and if possible the patient should be advised to seek a lighter job.

Exercise. Regular daily exercise is encouraged. The patient should be recommended initially to take two short walks (15–20 min) daily, with prophylactic GTN if necessary. This distance should be increased weekly. Instructions for swimming, etc. are as with angina (see Section 5.2).

Weight. Weight control is important and is often difficult when giving up smoking.

Smoking. This should be stopped. Nicotine replacement therapy is safe.

Diet. A diet that does not produce weight gain is the most important factor. A high-fibre diet with vegetables and cereals should be encouraged. Vitamins C and E are antioxidants and help prevent oxidation of LDL-cholesterol in the blood vessel wall. The CHAOS trial from Cambridge used 400–800 mg vitamin E/day and reduced cardiac events by 77%, but surprisingly had no effect on cardiac mortality. Although theoretically oral antioxidant supplementation should be beneficial, this cannot be recommended, with no evidence that it lowers mortality.

Reduction in saturated fats is important in secondary prevention. Three studies (4S, CARE and WOSCOPS) have provided strong evidence for both primary and secondary prevention in coronary disease and emphasized the importance of lowering even only slightly elevated serum cholesterol (see Section 5.11).

Sex. This should be discussed. Intercourse is probably best avoided for 1 month only after an MI. GTN prophylaxis and β blockade will help patients who suffer with angina on intercourse, but β blockade may cause impotence. A relatively passive role in intercourse should be encouraged initially.

Contraception. The pill should be discouraged and alternative methods suggested for women.

Alcohol. Regular evening alcohol intake in moderation is perfectly satisfactory (e.g. two glasses of wine or a double whisky). Several pints of beer, however, should be discouraged because of its water-load effect.

Travel. Travel abroad should be discouraged for the first 2 months, but may be unavoidable (see Angina Section 5.2).

Secondary Prevention
There is enough evidence now to recommend soluble aspirin 75–150 mg daily, a routine β blocker, a statin and an ACE inhibitor.

Aspirin: meta-analysis of seven randomized prospective trials has shown an overall reduction in mortality of 21% and a reduction in reinfarction of 31% in patients taking aspirin. It should be taken till age 75. There is concern that aspirin intake in those aged over-75 years may increase the risk of cerebral haemorrhage and prophylactic aspirin is best avoided in the long term in this group, particularly if they are hypertensive.

β Blockade: β blockers are continued indefinitely because late withdrawal of the β blocker has been shown to cause a late rise in mortality in both metoprolol and timolol trials. β Blockade reduces reinfarction by about 25%. $β_1$-Receptor blockade is important and a cardioselective drug can be used. Avoid β blockers with intrinsic sympathomimetic activity (e.g. oxprenolol). There have been positive trials with timolol, propranolol, atenolol and metoprolol.

ACE inhibitors, e.g. ramipril, should be used indefinitely in all patients – particularly in those with large hearts or poor LV function (reduction in both future heart failure and further MI). The HOPE trial showed a reduction in ischaemic events over 4.5 years in patients with known vascular disease receiving ramipril (no known LV dysfunction in this group). The largest tolerable dose is recommended: 5 mg twice daily.

Long-term calcium antagonists are of doubtful value. There has been a positive trial for both diltiazem and verapamil, but only if LV function was normal. Generally they should be used only if the patient has angina.

Magnesium: long-term oral magnesium is of no benefit.

Warfarin should be used only for patients in AF, those with LV thrombus visualized on echocardiography, or those with an LV aneurysm or grossly dilated hypokinetic ventricles. Warfarin is less effective than aspirin at preventing recurrent ischaemic events after successful thrombolysis.

HRT: there is not enough evidence for hormone replacement therapy in post-menopausal women as secondary prevention. It should be used only for non-cardiac indications. One large American study suggested an increased risk with HRT. If a patient was on HRT before an MI it should be either discontinued or switched to a selective oestrogen receptor modulator (SERM) such as tamoxifen or raloxifene. We still await data to confirm whether or not SERMs provide benefit in coronary heart disease patients.

Folic acid: supplementation necessary for patients with hyperhomocysteinaemia (>14 μmol/l) is usually prescribed, although there is no data on long term benefit.

Outpatient Follow-up after MI
The first outpatient visit 4 weeks after an infarct is very important. Symptoms must be assessed. Risk stratification, secondary prevention and the possible need for rehabilitation must be considered with a view to getting the patient back to work and to a normal life.

Symptoms
Angina is treated medically initially (see Section 5.2) and the patient is put on the waiting list for coronary arteriography. Priority is given to those at greater risk (see Risk Stratification, below).

Dyspnoea is most commonly the result of poor LV function, which is assessed clinically and on echocardiography. Mitral regurgitation, a possible VSD or developing LV aneurysm must be picked up, as must possible additional anaemia, airway obstruction, etc. Occasionally a patient's symptoms are misinterpreted by the physician as dyspnoea when the patient is in fact complaining of angina. Dyspnoea caused by poor LV function is treated with ACE inhibitors and diuretics (see Section 6.6).

Palpitations (see Section 8.1): 24-hour monitoring is necessary. Isolated ventricular ectopics and non-sustained VT do not necessarily need treatment unless associated with poor LV function. Avoid class 1 antiarrhythmic agents (higher mortality than placebo in the CAST study). Ensure that the serum potassium is >4.0 mmol/l.

Occasional ventricular ectopics should be ignored and the patient reassured. Frequent ectopics (>10/h) with good LV function are managed with β blockade if the patient is symptomatic. If LV function is poor, start with an ACE inhibitor, which also helps keep the potassium up.

Non-sustained VT (bursts of <30s): refer for coronary angiography and treat those with poor LV function with an ACE inhibitor and amiodarone. Sustained VT merits urgent admission and coronary arteriography. Patients are revascularized where possible (either PCI or CABG) and subsequently restudied with Holter monitoring and treadmill testing. Patients who are not suitable for revascularization are considered for an implantable cardioverter defibrillator (ICD) and/or amiodarone (see Section 7.11).

Risk Stratification
It is important to determine which patients are at high risk of sudden death or reinfarction because they need coronary angiography during the first admission or as soon after as is practical.

Those particularly at risk are those with:
- a history of previous MI
- age > 75 years
- diabetes
- resting tachycardia >100/min
- poor LV function as evidenced by:
  - clinical signs; systolic blood pressure < 100 mmHg
  - echocardiography LVEF < 40%
  - MUGA scanning
  - large heart on chest radiograph (CTR > 50%)
- unstable angina; rest or nocturnal angina unrelieved by GTN
- documented VT (sustained > 30s)
- positive treadmill testing; unable to complete stage 2 of the Bruce protocol, 7 METS (add 6 min for the modified Bruce protocol, a gentler test for the post-infarct patient)
- frequent episodes of silent ischaemia on 24-hour monitoring
- depression of heart rate variability.

Unfortunately studies of after-potentials (which are theoretically linked with ventricular arrhythmias) on the signal-averaged ECG after infarction have not yielded as valuable prognostic information as was initially hoped.

Of all of these the single most useful variable is the LV function.

MI with Normal Coronary Arteries
Definite Q-wave infarcts occasionally occur in patients who have normal coronary angiograms at subsequent investigation. It is not always possible to provide an explanation but probable considerations are:
- coronary spasm
- coronary emboli
- recanalization after coronary thrombosis
- thyrotoxicosis
- coronary arteritis
- prothrombotic state.

Cocaine abuse can cause coronary spasm and MI with subsequent normal coronary arteries at angiography. Chemotherapy with vincristine or 5-fluorouracil can also cause an ACS from coronary spasm (see Section 11.7).

Spontaneous thrombus developing in a normal artery is rare but may indicate a hypercoagulable or prothrombotic state. It may occur in heavy smokers, women on the pill and polycythaemic patients. Haematological help is needed but investigations that should be considered include:

- FBC
- platelet count
- prothrombin time, partial thromboplastin time and thrombin time
- platelet aggregation to ADP; ?spontaneous aggregation of platelets in platelet-rich plasma
- lupus anticoagulant: check dilute Russell viper time
- anticardiolipin antibody
- antithrombin III deficiency
- protein C deficiency
- protein S deficiency
- activated protein C resistance (factor V Leiden)
- homocystinuria/hyperhomocystinaemia.

The haematologist will want the patient off aspirin for at least 2 weeks before all these tests can be done, and they are best organized in outpatients about a month after the infarct.

5.8 Coronary Thrombolysis

It is now well established that thrombolysis has an important part to play in acute MI. Several studies have shown a significant reduction in early (1 month) and late (1 year) mortality in those patients receiving thrombolytic agents even up to 12 h of onset of pain.

The pre-existing high-grade stenosis in the coronary artery suddenly becomes occluded by thrombus, usually secondary to plaque rupture. The cause of plaque rupture remains unknown. Acute occlusion of the coronary artery results in MI in the dependent territory. Coronary angiography at the time of acute infarction shows total occlusion of the relevant vessel in 90–100% of cases. Progressive myocardial damage develops and becomes irreversible at 6 h. The aim of thrombolysis is to produce reperfusion of the distal artery and to improve the microcirculation. The high-grade stenosis can be dealt with by coronary angioplasty on a subsequent occasion.

Thrombolytic Agents (Table 5.13)
- *Non-specific thrombolytic*: streptokinase (Streptase)
- *Fibrin-specific agents*:
  - rtPA (recombinant tissue plasminogen activator): alteplase (Actilyse) – single chain (double-chain duteplase no longer marketed)

Table 5.13 Summary of commonly used thrombolytic agents (see Section 5.8 for choice)

	Streptokinase (SK)	Alteplase (tPA)	Reteplase (rPA)	Tenecteplase (TNK)
Approximate cost per patient (£)	89	600	666	612
Intravenous dose	1.5 MU	80–100 mg	10 MU stat plus 10 MU at 30 min	0.5 mg/kg
Infusion time	1 h	90 min–3 h	Double bolus 30 min apart	Single bolus 5–10 s
Half-life (min)	30	4	13–16	20
Storage	Room temperature	Room temperature	Room temperature	Room temperature
Source	Bacterial	Recombinant human protein	Recombinant deletion mutant of tPA	Recombinant multiple mutant of tPA
Anaphylaxis	0.1%	Nil	Rare	Rare
Allergic reaction	2–3%	Nil	Rare	Rare
Fibrin-specific, adjuvant heparin needed	No	Yes	Yes	Yes

– tenecteplase (TNK, Metalyse); compared with tPA in ASSENT-2 trial
– reteplase (rPA, Rapilysin); compared with tPA in GUSTO III trial
– lanoteplase (nPA); compared with tPA in the InTIME II trial
– urokinase and its inactive precursor pro-urokinase.

Streptokinase and tPA were the two agents most commonly used in the UK, but the simplicity of TNK (single bolus) and rPA (double-bolus) administration make these agents increasingly popular. Streptokinase can be given either intravenously or via the coronary artery catheter. Disadvantages are that it causes a systemic lytic state and depletes fibrinogen and α_2-antiplasmin levels. It is antigenic and often causes a fever and allergic reaction (see Complications below).

Fibrin-specific agents work only at the site of the thrombus and deplete fibrinogen and α_2-antiplasmin levels less (Figure 5.18).

Although the newer fibrin-specific agents have been shown to achieve better vessel patency than tPA they have not improved survival.

Indications for Thrombolysis

• Patients with a typical history of cardiac pain within the previous 24 h and ST-segment elevation on the ECG. There should be 1 mm ST elevation in standard leads or at least ≥2 mm ST elevation in adjacent chest leads.
• Chest pain plus LBBB on ECG.

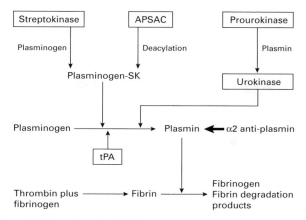

Figure 5.18 Thrombolytic agents: site of action.

If the ECG is doubtful on arrival, thrombolysis should be withheld and the ECG repeated at 15 and 30 min. Thrombolysis should not be given if the ECG remains normal. There is as yet no evidence that patients with isolated ST depression benefit from thrombolysis, even though they may represent true posterior infarction.

Patients whose pain started 12–24 hours previously should receive thrombolysis only if they are in continuing pain or if their general condition is deteriorating.

Patients with unstable angina (NSTEMI) should not receive thrombolysis unless thrombus is seen in a coronary artery at angiography.

Special Benefit
Trials have so far shown that the following groups particularly benefit from thrombolysis:
- anterior infarction
- pronounced ST elevation
- people >75 years
- poor LV function or LBBB, systolic pressure <100 mmHg
- very early administration (within the first hour of symptoms): 'the golden hour'.

Contraindications to Thrombolysis
- Recent CVA (in last 6 months)
- Recent gastrointestinal bleed
- Haemorrhagic diathesis or warfarin therapy
- Recent abdominal surgery, neurosurgery, eye surgery, liver biopsy, dental extraction, lumbar puncture within 1 month
- Pregnancy or post partum
- Trauma

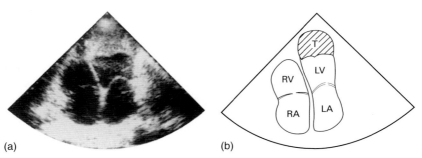

(a)   (b)

Figure 5.19 Transthoracic echocardiogram in a man with an anterior infarct, showing, in the apical four-chamber view, extensive apical thrombus (T). This patient should not receive thrombolysis.

- Aortic dissection; beware wide mediastinum on chest radiograph or absent pulse
- Aortic aneurysm
- LV aneurysm containing thrombus (Figure 5.19) (see Complications below).
- Prolonged cardiopulmonary resuscitation (>5 min)
- Systemic hypertension: >180/100 not responding to immediate therapy.

Although not contraindications care should be taken with:
- liver or renal disease
- menstrual bleeding: avoid thrombolysis only in women with menorrhagia
- intramuscular injections in A&E: a large intramuscular haematoma may develop with thrombolysis
- ulcerative colitis
- heart block requiring pacing
- diabetic retinopathy: background retinopathy is not a contraindication but recent photocoagulation for proliferative retinopathy is.

It is important to note that cardiogenic shock and advanced age are not contraindications to thrombolysis. Unfortunately only about 30% of patients suitable for thrombolysis actually receive it. The GRACE study has found that patients who had diabetes, presented without typical chest pain, or had a history of previous MI or CABG were less likely to receive thrombolytic treatment.

Administration

Streptokinase
Before streptokinase administration, the patient should receive hydrocortisone 100 mg i.v. and chlorpheniramine 10 mg i.v. The need for this prophylactic antiallergic regimen is debated. It is sensible to consider it in any patient with a history of a recent sore throat. Streptokinase is given intravenously 1.5 MU in 100–200 ml 0.9% saline over 60 min.

Intracoronary streptokinase is rarely given now as the advantages over the intravenous route are minimal and the logistics much more difficult. The intracoronary dose is 10 000 U stat followed by an infusion of 4000 U/min for 60–120 min.

Accelerated ('Front-loaded') tPA
This regimen was used in one arm of the GUSTO trial. The full dose of tPA is given over 90 min with two-thirds of the dose given in the first 30 min. Dose regimen: 15 mg bolus; 0.75 mg/kg over 30 min (not to exceed 50 mg); then 0.5 mg/kg over 60 min (not to exceed 35 mg). Heparin dose: 5000 U bolus followed by 1000 U/h. Most benefit: anterior infarcts within 4 h. Use this regimen within 6 h of symptoms; beyond this time the dose is 40 mg i.v. over the first hour and 40 mg over the next 2 hours.

Role of Adjuvant Heparin
The ISIS 3 trial showed no advantage in mortality reduction in using heparin with any of the three agents in addition to aspirin. Heparin has not been shown to reduce mortality or, fortunately, to increase strokes. The GUSTO trial showed a benefit of heparin only with the accelerated tPA regimen. The three fibrin-specific agents need to be followed by additional heparin for 24 h. Heparin is not used routinely after streptokinase.

Choice of Thrombolytic Agent
Although results from the GUSTO trial show a slight benefit in mortality reduction in patients receiving accelerated tPA, streptokinase is the thrombolytic agent of choice in first infarcts because of its considerable cost saving. The ISIS 3 trial showed no clear benefit for tPA (3 h infusion regimen not accelerated) over streptokinase. Fibrin-specific agents are more expensive and any additional benefit in mortality reduction is small (1%). The ease of bolus administration (reteplase and tenecteplase) means that they have become the agents of choice for pre-hospital thrombolysis and are increasingly used in the hospital setting also.

Accelerated tPA, TNK or reteplase should be considered the agents of choice in the following circumstances:
• Previous streptokinase therapy, because neutralizing antibodies are still present in about 30% of patients even after 1 year and persist for at least 4 years. Streptokinase should not be repeated beyond the fourth day of first administration.
• Recent streptococcal infection.
• Large anterior infarcts if presenting within 4 h.
• Hypotension: systolic pressures <100 mmHg.
• Probable need for temporary pacing (tPA has shortest half-life).

Reperfusion
This occurs spontaneously in about 20% of untreated control patients. Reperfusion occurs in approximately 30–60% of patients who receive thrombolysis within 4 h of pain onset. The greatest improvement occurs in patients treated within 2 h. It has also been shown that fibrin-specific thrombolytic agents (e.g. rtPA) are superior to streptokinase in producing reperfusion, but only margin-

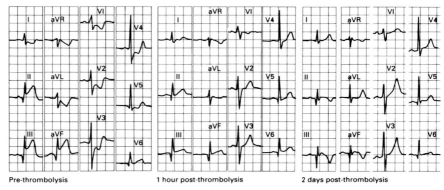

Figure 5.20 Rapid evolution of ST segment changes with thrombolysis. Acute inferior infarction in a 47-year-old man receiving 1.5 MU streptokinase within 2.5 h of onset of chest pain. Left panel: marked inferior ST-segment elevation with reciprocal ST depression in anteroseptal leads. Middle panel: there is rapid improvement in the ST segments within 1 h of completing streptokinase. Right panel: by 2 days the ST segments are isoelectric.

ally superior in reducing overall mortality. Early reperfusion reduces infarct size and helps preserve LV function. In the large majority of patients who receive intravenous therapy, successful reperfusion is marked by a rapid improvement in chest pain and a fall in ST segment (Figure 5.20). Occasionally reperfusion arrhythmias occur as a result of washout of toxic metabolites. They are not an indication to stop the thrombolytic agent. The most common is a short run of accelerated idioventricular rhythm but VT or VF may occur (as they may after successful primary PCI). Washout also results in a brisker rise in CPK levels. Peak CPK levels may be higher than in non-thrombolysed patients but the total area under the CPK/time curve (a measurement of total myocardial damage) will be less.

Myocardial stunning occurs after reperfusion. It is delayed functional recovery. Poor LV function post-thrombolysis may not be permanent.

Failed Thrombolysis

This occurs in approximately 40% of patients receiving thrombolysis and is more likely in patients who receive their thrombolytic agent late after symptom onset (>3 h). Failure of the ST segments to fall by >50% plus continuing chest pain indicate failed thrombolysis. The only management strategy that has been shown to be of value in this situation is a rescue PCI and the patient should be transferred urgently to an angioplasty centre if not already in one. The REACT trial showed that, at 6 months, 15.4% of patients who had had a rescue PCI reached a primary composite endpoint of death, reinfarction, CVA or CCF, compared with 31.3% patients who had a second dose of thrombolytic and 29.9% of those who were managed conservatively with just heparin.

Heparin or a repeat dose of thrombolytic is valueless. A rescue PCI is mandatory for failed thrombolysis.

Re-occlusion

Exact rates of re-occlusion are unknown, because coronary angiographic data are not available in large numbers. It is probable that 25% of patients re-occlude within 3 months of thrombolysis unless the residual stenosis is dealt with by angioplasty.

Complications

Haemorrhage

This is by far the biggest problem. It affects 7–10% of patients receiving strep-tokinase. Bleeding from drip sites and intramuscular injection sites is common and a large intramuscular haematoma can develop from simple intramuscular analgesic injections. Transfusion is occasionally required. General practition-ers and A&E physicians should be encouraged to give analgesic injections intravenously to patients who are likely to be candidates for thrombolysis. More serious bleeding complications include haematemesis and melaena from occult peptic ulcers and cerebral haemorrhage.

Bleeding from a drip site is treated with local pressure. More severe bleed-ing complications require transfusion, and possible FFP or cryoprecipitate. Very rarely the streptokinase can be reversed by slow intravenous infusion of tranexamic acid 10 mg/kg body weight.

Allergic Reactions

These are common with streptokinase. A low-grade fever and rash are common. Nausea, vomiting, headaches and flushing are also reported after a few days. One of the advantages of fibrin-specific agents (e.g. rtPA) is that it does not cause allergic reactions and is the agent of choice in patients who have had a course of streptokinase in the past.

Systemic Emboli

Lysis of preformed thrombus within the left atrium, left ventricle or great vessels may result in systemic embolism. Aortic aneurysm and LV aneurysm containing thrombus, however old, are contraindications to thrombolysis (see Figure 5.19).

Cerebrovascular Bleeds

Thrombolysis results in a slight increase in the incidence of intracerebral bleeds. The risk is 0.3% for streptokinase and 0.6% for tPA. The risk is small and should not influence the use of thrombolytics even in elderly people.

Early Hazard

This is the definite but slight increase in mortality in the first day of patients receiving thrombolysis. It probably results from cardiac rupture causing pulseless electrical activity. It is common in elderly people, those receiv-ing thrombolysis late and patients who have had previous infarctions. β Blockade possibly reduces cardiac rupture, but a trial of thrombolysis with and without β blockade has not been performed.

Subsequent Management

After successful thrombolysis, patients who need PCI must be identified. This requires exercise testing in those patients who are pain free. Patients who continue to get angina after thrombolysis, or who have positive exercise tests at low workload, need coronary angiography. The proportion of patients who are likely to need PCI after thrombolysis is probably >30%. The exact timing of PCI after successful thrombolysis remains controversial. The increase in thrombolysis will put a greater burden on cardiac catheter laboratories, and facilities for performing PCI may not be available close to the district hospital.

Future Trends

Speeding up Administration

Unfortunately research has been directed at finding newer and better thrombolytic agents with only marginal benefit over agents already available rather than directing attention at the real problem of getting patients treated within less than 90 min of symptom onset. This could be achieved by the following:

• More out-of-hospital thrombolysis will reduce time to administration. This involves education of the general public to recognize their symptoms plus the establishment of a rapid response and highly trained ambulance team. This is now happening in almost all ambulance trusts in England and Wales with a rate of 250 cases/month. It is particularly of value in rural communities where a primary PCI centre may be far distant. Drugs that can be given as a bolus – reteplase and tenecteplase – are the agents of choice in this situation.

• A shorter door-to-needle time for those patients brought into A&E who have not received thrombolysis in the community. This should be <15 min in A&E with a fast-track system for definite infarcts. The thrombolytic should be administered in A&E rather than waiting for the patient to be transferred to the CCU. Specialist triage nurses are effective in helping to achieve this.

Newer Pharmacology

• *Lanoteplase*: nPA or novel plasminogen activator – two domains deleted from wild-type rtPA. This has a longer half-life than rtPA (37 min). Single bolus administration. There are few comparative data yet. The 30-day mortality is similar to that of tPA but with higher bleeding rates in the InTIME II trial.

• *Recombinant staphylokinase*: this is more fibrin-specific than streptokinase and causes less fibrinogen depletion.

• *Vampire bat plasminogen activator*: half-life 2.8 h, could be single bolus. Under study. Probably immunogenic.

• *Platelet IIb/IIIa receptor antagonist combined with lower dose fibrinolytic*: initial hopes were that this combination might produce the best reperfusion figures of all. In the TIMI 14 trial a combination of abciximab plus low-dose tPA resulted in a 71% TIMI 3 flow (normal coronary flow) at 90 min. However, the larger GUSTO V trial failed to show any survival benefit with this combination.

• *Thrombin inhibitors*: the search continues for a better antithrombotic agent than heparin. Hirudin has been shown to be of no benefit over heparin. The addition of argatroban (a direct thrombin inhibitor) to streptokinase as adjunctive therapy has not been shown to carry any benefit at 30 days post-infarct. Attempts to increase the heparin dose in several trials have resulted in increased bleeding. The latest hirudin analogue, bivalirudin, can inhibit fibrin/clot bound thrombin *in situ*. It has proved superior to unfractionated heparin during PCI – causing fewer bleeding complications – and may prove to be better than heparin as adjunctive treatment after thrombolysis.

5.9 Percutaneous Coronary Interventions (PCI)

First performed in humans in 1977, this has now become a standard technique in cardiology offering some patients a real alternative to conventional CABG surgery.

PCI is performed in the catheter laboratory under local anaesthetic and sedation only. The technique is illustrated in Figure 5.21 and can be performed via the femoral, brachial or radial artery route. Rapid advances in equipment design have enabled cardiologists to attack more difficult and more numerous lesions. Initially the technique was applied to single-vessel disease but multivessel dilatation is now routine.

In the UK in 2005, the PCI rate was 1165 per million population as against a minimum NSF (National Standard Framework) recommended target of 750/million. Some 83 centres now perform PCI. The PCI rate has doubled in 5 years, but only 6.6% were primary PCI procedures for acute MI. These figures are still much lower than those of many European countries, probably as a result of a lack of staff and facilities, as well as perhaps the conservative views of some community physicians. Most centres are now implanting stents in > 93% cases, with drug-eluting stents being used in 65% cases.

Many trials have now compared PCI with CABG, all showing similar results. PCI is as effective as surgery initially in relieving angina. Both mortality and morbidity are lower with PCI than with CABG, and the patient returns to work sooner. Overall costs are still cheaper with PCI. However, the need for re-investigation or re-intervention was much higher with PCI (38% in the UK RITA trial) as a result of restenosis. All these comparative trials were in the pre-stent era. Unfortunately trials in the post-stent era (e.g. ARTS, SOS trials) still have the same message. Even though restenosis has fallen sharply with stenting, re-intervention rates after PCI are still higher than after CABG. Registry data from the British Cardiovascular Intervention Society show that the re-intervention rate for restenosis after PCI continues to fall and, in 2005, only 3.8% of 70 142 procedures were performed for restenosis. The results of the SYNTAX trial, a real-world trial comparing CABG with modern PCI (three-vessel and left main stem disease), are awaited with interest.

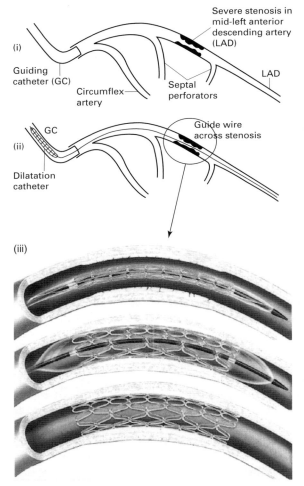

Figure 5.21 Stages in coronary angioplasty: pre-dilatation for very tight lesions. (i) The guiding catheter (GC) is positioned in the ostium of the left coronary artery (LCA). Angiography shows a severe stenosis in the mid-anterior descending artery. (ii) A guidewire (0.014 inch) is positioned across the stenosis. (iii) The balloon is advanced across a pre-dilated stenosis with the stent premounted on the balloon. The balloon is inflated, expanding the stent and compressing it into the arterial wall. In the bottom panel, the balloon and wire are withdrawn leaving the stent fully expanded. In many lesions pre-dilatation is not necessary and the low-profile stent can be advanced directly across the lesion.

Indications for PCI
- Anyone being considered for CABG: are their lesions suitable for PCI?
- Patients with refractory angina who are not fit for CABG because of other medical reasons (e.g. renal failure, severe lung disease)
- Elderly people

• Patients who have already had CABG: stenosis in a native vessel, internal mammary artery or vein graft
• Severe varicose veins
• Lack of or unsuitable arterial conduits
• Major clotting disorders
• Very poor LV function
• Intolerance to medical therapy
• Post-thrombolysis: in patients with severe stenoses, symptoms or positive stress tests
• Acute MI if catheter laboratory immediately available (see Section 5.7).

The recent COURAGE trial claimed that PCI carries no benefit in prevention of long-term cardiovascular events in patients with stable angina when compared with medical therapy alone. However, a third of the patients in the medically treated arm crossed over for revascularization (mostly PCI) and this has devalued the trial in the eyes of the interventionists. Nevertheless PCI should mainly be considered where drug therapy is not controlling symptoms adequately and in ACSs.

Relative Contraindications

None of these is absolute; they depend on the skill and experience of the operator, together with the patient's wishes and medical condition. Generally the following problems would make a cardiologist think twice before proceeding to angioplasty:
• Unprotected left main stem disease (no grafts to the left coronary artery), particularly if the stenosis is at the distal end of the main stem involving the origin of the LAD and circumflex vessels
• Very tortuous coronary vessels
• Multiple restenoses at the same site
• Diffuse proximal coronary disease with bypassable vessels
• Total occlusion of an important vessel for >6 months
• Three previous PCIs
• Patients with diabetes and multivessel disease: the BARI trial showed that these patients were best managed surgically
• Very poor LV function without IABP back-up (see Section 6.14)
• Single remaining coronary artery
• Massive fresh thrombus in a bypass graft
• Heavily calcified vessel.

Suitable Lesions

Some lesions are definitely easier than others and Table 5.14 outlines characteristics that make lesions easy or difficult, lower risk or higher risk.

Risks and Complications

In experienced hands the mortality risk of PCI is lower than that of CABG surgery. The risk is slightly higher for multivessel disease (MVD) than

Table 5.14 Lesion morphology and PCI risk

Easier lesions: lower risk	More difficult lesions: higher risk
Single-vessel disease	Multivessel disease
Good LV function	Poor LV function
Young patient	Old patient
Short history of angina	Long history of angina
Discrete	Longer stenosis
Smooth concentric stenosis	Rough ulcerated eccentric stenosis
Non-calcified	
Proximal part of vessel	Calcified distal part of vessel
No side-branch involved	Side branches involved or bifurcation stenosis
Left anterior descending artery	Right or circumflex vessels

(Softer lesions bracket groups: Young patient, Short history of angina, Discrete, Smooth concentric stenosis, Non-calcified)

(Rougher harder lesions bracket groups: Old patient, Long history of angina, Longer stenosis, Rough ulcerated eccentric stenosis)

single-vessel disease (SVD) and slightly greater still in patients with unstable angina. PCI is already having a substantial effect on lowering the mortality in cardiogenic shock. Table 5.15 shows the present risks from the audit of the British Cardiovascular Intervention Society 2005.

Mortality (see Table 5.15)
Overall this is approximately 1 in 200 or 0.5%. (all cases including shock).

Acute Coronary Occlusion
This results from acute dissection or thrombus or both. Direct use of the coronary stent at first inflation, and the use of glycoprotein IIb/IIIa receptor blockers, have considerably reduced the problems of acute occlusion. Stenting has lowered the acute referral rate for coronary bypass surgery dramatically over the last few years to 0.12% (1 case in 833 procedures).

Damage to Coronary Artery at Site Other than Dilatation Site
For example, ostial dissection with guiding catheter.

Perforation of the Coronary Artery
This is very rare but may be caused by the guidewire or use of a stent with too big a diameter. This may be dealt with by implantation of a covered stent, or

Table 5.15 UK PCI risks for the year 2005

	Elective (all cases)	Unstable angina	Primary PCI	Cardiogenic shock	Overall
Death (%)	0.14	0.64	3.2	24	0.59
Emergency CABG (%)	0.1	0.13	0.3	0	0.12
MI (new Q-wave MI) (%)	0.4	0.6	N/A	N/A	0.24

inflating an occlusion balloon proximal to the perforation. Emergency surgery may be necessary if paricardial aspiration fails to control the situation.

Guidewire Fracture
Distal fragment has to be removed surgically.

Side-branch occlusion
This may reverse spontaneously. Risks of this can be reduced using a 'two-wire' technique, or a pair of balloons: the kissing balloon technique.

Distal Vessel Emboli
This is probably much more common than is generally realized, involving microemboli into tiny distal vessels. More serious occlusion of the larger vessels can occur as a result of distal movement of thrombus or atheromatous material. Vigorous heparinization during the procedure is mandatory. PCI of acutely embolized vessels may be necessary. Ingenious distal vessel protection devices are now available, but do not reduce major adverse events.

Complications of Arterial Catheterization
The guiding catheter is slightly larger than a conventional coronary catheter. Haematoma and false aneurysm formation at the femoral puncture site may occur. More serious is the possibility of systemic emboli from within the guiding catheter itself if heparinization is inadequate.

Successful PCI
This is judged primarily angiographically, and a reduction in the stenosis by >20% was judged by Gruntzig as a primary success. Most PCI procedures using coronary stents reduce the stenosis by considerably more. In small arteries (<2 mm) the vessel may look slightly shaggy after balloon dilatation alone, but the vessel quickly remodels and provided that there is a good lumen, with a good perfusion pressure, there is usually no problem. Remodelling occurs in the subsequent 3 months. The advent of coronary stents has largely solved problems of dissection flaps, etc. seen in the past with stents now available for vessels down to 2.25 mm (Figures 5.16 and 5.17).

Preparation of the Patient
The operator must explain the entire procedure to the patient. Most patients will already be familiar with the catheter laboratory, having had previous coronary angiography. Diagrams (e.g. Figure 5.21) help in the explanation. Important points that should be included are listed:
• The procedure takes a little longer than coronary angiography, but in many respects is very similar. There will be no hot flush (no need for repeat LV angiography). There is no need for a general anaesthetic. A sheath may be left in the patient's groin for a few hours after PCI but most centres now remove it immediately at the end of the procedure using a femoral artery closure device.

- The patient should expect angina during balloon inflation and should tell the operator if he or she gets it.
- There is a possible need for emergency coronary bypass surgery (0.12%).
- The very small mortality risk (<0.5–0.6% overall, but much lower for elective PCI).
- The need for one or more intracoronary stents (90–95% cases). This is particularly likely for PCIs of the LAD and bypass grafts. There is <1% risk of subacute stent thrombosis.
- The possible need to repeat the procedure in the next 6 months. If the vessel is stented re-intervention is probably needed in <4% now (3.8% – UK figure for 2005). The patient may spend the night after the procedure in the CCU. Day-case PCI is now common, particularly if the radial approach is used.
- The operator should obtain the patient's consent on a special consent form documenting the risks.

The house physician must help organize the drug regimen, group and save serum, etc. He or she should have observed coronary angioplasty to answer the patient's questions. A standard regimen is:

- soluble aspirin 75–150 mg daily and clopidogrel 600 mg the day before the procedure if possible or the morning of the procedure (see below).
- oral or intravenous nitrates and a calcium antagonist in standard doses for unstable cases
- for patients with known renal impairment (creatinine >120 µg/l) saline volume loading is necessary to prevent contrast nephropathy. Give 1 l 0.9% saline overnight before the procedure and 1 l over 8 h after it. In addition NAC 600 mg is given for three doses before the PCI if possible. (see Section 16.3)

On the morning of the procedure:

- starve the patient for 4 h before PCI
- group and save serum
- clopidogrel 600 mg orally: clopidogrel is started pre-PCI if possible as well as soluble aspirin 150 mg daily in stent cases. Clopidogrel has been shown in the CLASSICS trial to be superior to and safer than ticlopidine. Onset of action is also faster. Loading dose of clopidogrel is 600 mg followed by 75 mg daily for 1 year for drug-eluting stents. Both drugs inhibit ADP-induced platelet aggregation and platelet serotonin release. The incidence of leukopenia is much lower with clopidogrel than with ticlopidine, and patients no longer have to have a blood count during the course. There is no advantage or need for warfarin over this simple aspirin and clopidogrel regimen.
- premedication as for conventional cardiac catheter for the anxious patient. Additional sedation may be given in the catheter laboratory if necessary.

Management of the Patient after PCI

The patient is monitored overnight in the CCU and can usually go home the next day. Day-case angioplasty is now common for uncomplicated cases:

- Careful monitoring of blood pressure is necessary. It is important to avoid hypotension, with excess sedation, analgesia and nitrates all causing a fall in systemic pressure and hence a drop in coronary perfusion pressure. This could potentiate the development of acute coronary occlusion. A fall in systemic pressure <90 mmHg should be corrected by intravenous saline, Dextran 40 (which may help prevent red cell sludging), Haemaccel or Gelofusine. In addition atropine 0.6–1.2 mg i.v. may be needed if the patient is bradycardic.
- No further heparin is given once the patient leaves the catheter laboratory, except in unusual circumstances where the procedure was complicated by thrombus or unresolved dissection, in which case it may be continued overnight.
- Stent cases: no extra heparin is needed.
- The arterial sheath should be removed at the end of the procedure before the patient leaves the laboratory and an arterial closure device (e.g. Angioseal, Vasoseal) employed. With lower doses of heparin used in the PCI itself (70 U unfractionated heparin/kg) groin haematomas are much rarer than formerly. For the exceptional and difficult case where there is the possibility of reintervention in the few hours post-procedure, the arterial sheath is removed after 4–6 h. If the patient is on heparin this is stopped 2 h earlier. The ACT (activated clotting time) can be checked before sheath removal with a Haemochron and should be <150 s (normal <100 s). Very occasionally with difficult cases the sheaths are removed the following morning. Late sheath removal is painful, because the local anaesthetic will have worn off. Patients may develop an acute vagal episode and it is sensible to premedicate them: atropine 0.6 mg i.v. + Diazemuls 10–20 mg i.v. Some patients develop oozing from the entry site, particularly after the use of glycoprotein IIb/IIIa inhibitors and a Femo-stop device is used to control this.
- A post-PCI ECG is taken as soon as is practical.
- Cardiac markers (CK and troponin) are requested for any case that is not straightforward.
- Acute occlusion of the dilated vessel is suggested by the development of chest pain and rapidly rising ST segments over the relevant leads. This is a medical emergency and is usually managed by transferring the patient back to the catheter laboratory for a repeat PCI procedure as soon as possible. If the first PCI was particularly complex or difficult, the operator may opt for emergency coronary bypass surgery. Intravenous thrombolysis is a rare possibility, because there will be bleeding problems from the arterial puncture site.
- Discharge home: the patient should take soluble aspirin 75–150 mg daily indefinitely, and clopidogrel 75 mg o.d. for 1 year for drug-eluting stents and for 3 months for bare metal stents (see above). β-Blocking agents and calcium antagonists can usually be stopped unless the patient is hypertensive. Follow-up is at 1 month and 6 months. Exercise testing and thallium[201] scanning may be needed for patients who redevelop symptoms and coronary angiography where indicated. Patients must not drive for 1 week post-PCI. Group

2 licence holders (formerly HGV/PCV drivers) must not drive for 6 weeks and then must pass an exercise test (see Appendix 6).

Re-stenosis

Denuded endothelium stimulates platelet accretion, release of platelet-derived growth factor (PDGF) and many other growth factors. These reach the media within 24 h and stimulate smooth muscle cell proliferation. These cells then migrate through into the intima and rapidly cause restenosis. The re-stenotic lesion is thus a result of fibrocellular proliferation and not lipid deposition.

It is recognized that this occurs in 30% of all cases undergoing PCI (balloon only), usually within the first 6 months. This re-stenosis rate has been reduced by the use of coronary stents. Two early stent trials (BENESTENT, STRESS) using the first commercially available Palmaz–Schatz stent showed a reduction in angiographic re-stenosis at 7 months from 32% to 20%. The use of more modern drug-eluting stents plus adjunctive therapy has reduced re-stenosis rates to about 15% of patients, of whom only about 4% actually require re-dilatation. Few centres perform routine repeat coronary angiography and re-stenosis is suggested by the development of angina again or the recurrence of a positive treadmill test.

The only drug regimen found to reduce re-stenosis as assessed by the need for reintervention (CABG or PCI) or MI or death has been the use of a monoclonal antibody to the platelet glycoprotein IIb/IIIa receptor (abciximab) in the EPIC trial. This was tested only in patients with unstable angina or impending infarction and did cause an increased haemorrhagic risk at the time of the PCI. Re-stenosis has not been prevented by any other antiplatelet regimen (including aspirin), calcium antagonists, ACE inhibitors, 5-HT inhibitors, steroids, self-administered subcutaneous heparin, oral anticoagulation, or ω-3 fatty acid or folic acid supplements.

Factors reported to be associated with re-stenosis are:
- inadequate initial dilatation, e.g. balloon undersizing
- high inflation pressures at initial PCI
- male sex
- PCI of vein bypass graft
- smoking
- variant angina
- multivessel disease
- long stenoses
- diabetes
- complex dissection and vessel trauma at first dilatation
- ostial lesions
- proximal LAD lesions.

In addition some trials have suggested that restenosis is more likely with higher plasma ACE levels as found in patients with the DD ACE polymorphism. Unfortunately ACE inhibitors have not been shown to reduce re-stenosis.

Short segment re-stenosis is dealt with by repeat PCI. The lesion may be smoother and not ulcerated compared with the initial dilatation, and the procedure often easier with a lower complication rate.

Coronary Stents

These have revolutionized coronary angioplasty, having been used in 93% of all UK angioplasty procedures in 2005. The stent is delivered to the lesion over a conventional balloon. More than one can be put into the same vessel – in series – and side branches remain patent. High-pressure inflation (16–20 atm) may be employed at stent deployment to ensure good stent strut apposition against the arterial wall. A wide variety of designs (coil or mesh stents) and lengths (6–49 mm) is available. They are stainless steel, cobalt–chromium, tantalum, nitinol or platinum, and are only just visible on radiological screening. Gold has been abandoned as a coating.

Stents are in routine use now for most lesions in vessels >2.5 mm. Smaller sizes (2.25 mm) are available but re-stenosis rates are higher. Stents are particularly indicated for dilatation of the left main stem, LAD, vein graft lesions (Figure 5.22), ostial stenoses (where the re-stenosis rate is so high), and bulky and ulcerated lesions as an elective procedure. As well as compressing plaque, they prevent elastic recoil at the site of dilatation. An example of multiple stenting following rotablation in a small diffusely diseased vessel is shown (Figures 5.23 and 5.24).

Stents coated with silicon carbide have been shown to reduce acute stent thrombosis. Drug-eluting stents are coated with a polymer containing a variety of anti-mitotic agents (Table 5.16). Post-stent management is now much simplified. Anticoagulation with heparin or warfarin is unnecessary once the patient has left the catheter laboratory. Patients just receive aspirin and clopidogrel (see Management above). Aspirin is taken for life and

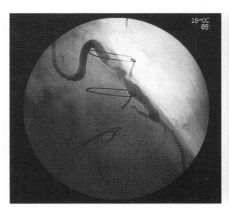 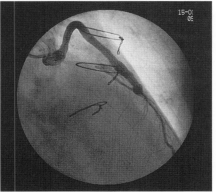

Figure 5.22 Left: 68-year-old lady 13 years after coronary artery bypass grafting. Vein graft to the left anterior descending coronary artery is severely degenerative. Right anterior oblique view. Right: after stent deployment.

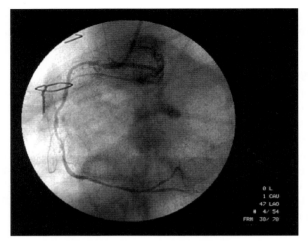

Figure 5.23 Diffuse disease of small right coronary artery in a patient with diabetes: left anterior oblique view. Previous CABG with graft occlusion. Pre-stenting.

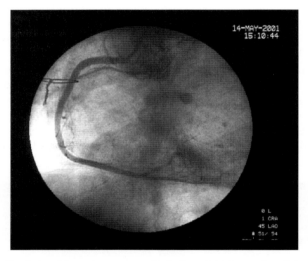

Figure 5.24 Left anterior oblique view: same patient after rotablation and multiple coronary stents.

Table 5.16 Drug-eluting stents

Stent name	Manufacturer	Antimitotic agent
Cypher	Cordis	Sirolimus
Taxus	Boston Scientific	Paclitaxel
Endeavor	Medtronic	Zotarolimus
Xience	Abbot	Everolimus

clopidogrel for a minimum of 1 year. The costs of implementing this are considerable.

Drug-eluting Stents vs Bare Metal Stents

Stents are now either a bare metal stent (BMS), which is usually stainless steel, or a drug-eluting (DES). The DES starts as a basic BMS platform that is coated with a polymer containing an antimitotic drug. These drugs are cell cycle inhibitors similar to tacrolimus, used in preventing graft rejection (Figure 5.25). The drug is released over a period of days, eluted into the coronary artery wall, and inhibits smooth muscle cell division, greatly reducing in-stent restenosis (from about 20% with BMSs to 4% with DESs at 6 months after the implant).

Various DESs are now available (Table 5.16). An example is shown in Figure 5.26.

The polymer that contains the drug itself is also important. Some polymers may provoke an inflammatory reaction, and new developments include the

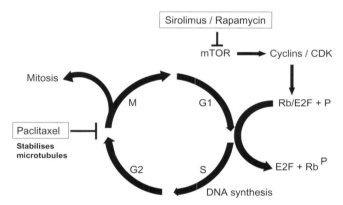

Figure 5.25 Sites of cell cycle inhibition by paclitaxel and sirolimus (rapamycin): mTOR is the mammalian target for rapamycin and it activates the cyclin/cyclin-dependent kinase (CDK) complexes. This in turn phosphorylates (P) the retinoblastoma (Rb) E2F complex which results in the free E2F transcription factor stimulating DNA synthesis. Thus inhibition of mTOR by sirolimus inhibits the cell entering the S (synthetic) phase and induces cell cycle arrest late in G1 phase.

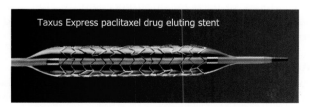

Figure 5.26 Taxus Express drug-eluting stent. (Reproduced with permission of Boston Scientific.)

addition of a second anti-inflammatory agent that is released from the polymer to prevent this.

An early randomized study (the TYPHOON trial) suggests that DESs are superior to BMSs in primary PCI for acute MI.

Five main problems related to stent use remain.

1 Deliverability
The additional stiffness of a stent on a balloon may make it impossible to deliver the stent through a tortuous vessel, even though a balloon alone itself passed easily. Means to help solve this problem include better guidelines to catheter support, the use of stiffer guidewires, further pre-dilatation or rotablation pre-stenting (Figures 5.23, 5.24).

2 Cost
Stents are expensive (approximately £600 each for a DES compared with £250 for a BMS) but have been shown to reduce re-stenosis (see above). In the UK the National Institute for Health and Clinical Excellence (NICE) has issued guidelines that these stents should be used only in patients whose lesions are longer then 15 mm or where the diseased vessel is <3 mm in diameter. As yet NICE has not reported on the use of DESs in MI.

3 Endothelialization
The third problem with stents relates to endothelialization. After stent deployment the native endothelium gradually grows over the metal framework of the stent, completely incorporating it into the vessel wall. Animal and post-mortem studies in humans have shown a pearly white layer of endothelial cells covering the metal struts, through which the stent can be seen. It is felt that vigorous antiplatelet therapy (aspirin + clopidogrel) is necessary after deployment until the stent has been completely endothelialized in this way to prevent subacute stent thrombosis. Clopidogrel can then safely be discontinued, leaving the patient on just aspirin (e.g. after 3 months with a BMS). It is known that the process of endothelialization takes longer with DESs, but as yet we do not know how long. Current recommendations are that after the deployment of a DES the patient should continue aspirin and clopidogrel for 1 year, before stopping the latter. The PCI -CURE trial showed that continued use of clopidogrel up to 9 months post-PCI was of benefit.

If a patient is likely to need major surgery shortly after stenting, BMSs should be used so that the clopidogrel can be stopped earlier and reduce the bleeding problems at operation.

4 Instent Restenosis
Re-stenosis within a stent can also be dealt with by balloon dilatation (for short lesions <13 mm), or by rotablation. For longer in-stent re-stenotic lesions there is a choice of intracoronary radiation (brachytherapy), repeat stenting

(sandwich stenting), referral for CABG or continued medical therapy. Balloon dilatation alone is of little value in this situation (see below).

Several avenues of research in re-stenosis prevention are underway:

• Brachytherapy: transluminal intracoronary radiation after stent deployment. Radioactive seeds deployed down a catheter within the stenosis are then withdrawn at a specific time. They emit β or γ irradiation and completely prevent smooth muscle cell hyperplasia. Few centres in the UK have this facility, but brachytherapy's main place now is in the management of long in-stent restenotic lesions.

• Delivering a gene locally inside a coronary artery using a non-replicating adenoviral vector containing antisense oligonucleotide to proto-oncogenes (e.g. c-*myb*) is now a possibility. Keeping it at the site of the angioplasty is the problem and this technique has not yet proved of value clinically.

• Balloon-only delivery of anti-mitotic agent e.g. in small vessels, instent re-stenosis.

• Biodegradable stents (see below).

5 Late Stent Thrombosis

Recently a meta-analysis of randomized studies has suggested that there is an increased incidence of late stent thrombosis in patients with DESs compared with patients with BMSs. This has caused a major furore in the press, as well as anxiety in the recipients. In some cases the thrombosis appeared to occur after early cessation of clopidogrel. It has been suggested that this may have been the result of prolonged exposure of the stent struts (delayed endothelialization with the antimitotic drug) or suboptimal platelet inhibition by aspirin and clopidogrel (low responders). A hypersensitivity vasculitis may be to blame in some cases who are clopidogrel compliant.

Each of the manufacturers in Table 5.16 has analysed its own data. The conclusions are as follows:

• There is a very slight increase in late stent thrombosis in patients receiving DESs (about 0.5% increase per year).

• This does not reflect any increase in mortality.

• DESs remain safe and effective and have a major advantage over BMSs in reducing the rate of restenosis.

• DESs should continue to be used, particularly in long lesions, small vessels and patients who are likely to have a higher incidence of restenosis (e.g. those with diabetes, renal failure) (see above).

• Clopidogrel should be given for a minimum of 1 year after a DES (FDA recommendation).

• As yet no particular DES is clearly better or worse than any other.

Other Technology

There are various new technologies available to help the interventionist with difficult stenoses or occlusions.

Coronary Angioscopy

This has been used intraoperatively to examine the vessel in unstable angina and the effects of PCI. Angioscopy is now starting in the catheter laboratory and will greatly improve our understanding of the effects of PCI on the vessel wall.

Intravascular Ultrasonography (IVUS)

Special monorail, solid-state, intracoronary catheters are available using 20 or 40 MHz transducers mounted cylindrically in a phased array pattern. They are expensive because they are used for one patient only. Imaging before and after the PCI gives extra information about tissue characterization and dissection not available at angiography, e.g. IVUS often shows more calcification in a lesion than had been suspected at angiography. IVUS has proved useful in coronary stenting – particularly of the left main stem – as it is important to ensure that the stent struts are fully deployed against the arterial wall. This can be detected only with IVUS.

Although routine use of IVUS showed no benefit in 1 year major adverse cardiac events (OPTICUS trial) more recent work from a large registry in Seoul using IVUS in left main stem stenting has shown a substantial advantage in patients stented with IVUS guidance. (The MAIN-COMPARE registry). IVUS is also being used to identify vulnerable plaque with a thin fibrous cap (virtual histology) and the results of the PROSPECT trial in ACS patients are awaited.

Directional Coronary Atherectomy (DCA)

This device is placed across the stenosis via a conventional guidewire and punches out slivers of atheroma, which can be examined histologically and from which smooth muscle cells, etc. can be grown. Atherectomy is used for bulky and eccentric lesions in large vessels (>3.0 mm). It is not suitable for tortuous arteries and the circumflex vessel can be difficult. Unfortunately two trials (CAVEAT and CCAT) have shown that elective atherectomy is inferior to conventional balloon angioplasty, with a higher cost, and greater MI and acute closure rates. DCA remains a possibility for bulky eccentric lesions, particularly in the main LAD, but re-stenosis rates are similar to balloon angioplasty and a subsequent DES would be needed. It is rarely used now with all the advantages of stenting.

Laser Technology

The expense and problems with control of the laser beam have reduced the popularity of this technique. Excimer laser angioplasty can tackle difficult long stenoses, ostial lesions and total occlusions that are not possible with conventional balloon dilatation.

Rotablation

This is a diamond-studded burr rotating at 150 000–200 000 rev./min over a special guidewire (Figure 5.27). It is valuable for long lesions and diffuse

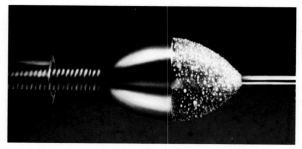

Figure 5.27 Rotablator. (Reproduced with permission of Boston Scientific.)

disease, as well as tough or calcified lesions (see Figures 5.23 and 5.24). It can be used in smaller vessels where stenting is less successful and to deal with in-stent re-stenosis. Pulverized microscopic debris migrates distally and can cause coronary spasm. Patients receive an infusion of nitrates and verapamil to prevent this and temporary pacing is often necessary.

Cutting Balloon
This is a conventional angioplasty designed balloon modified to incorporate a cutting blade for tough or calcified lesions. After successful use one or more stents should be deployed because otherwise re-stenosis rates are high.

Future Stent Technology
Biodegradable stents have been developed made from magnesium. Although theoretically allowing the coronary artery to return to a more elastic vessel, further trials are awaited to see if they really carry any long-term advantage. Early work with a biodegradable DES suggests that late loss and restenosis may be greater than with conventional DESs.

Further studies are also under way with other coatings such as vascular endothelial growth factor (VEGF)-coated stents in chronic total occlusions to try to induce angiogenesis. Studies are progressing using stents coated with endothelial cells or endothelial progenitor cells to try to reduce late stent thrombosis.

Choice of PCI or Surgery (CABG) for Stable Angina
The RITA trial has shown that both forms of treatment are very successful in relieving angina with very low rates of mortality or MI. However, patients treated with PCI are more likely to get angina again, need antianginal medication and require further hospital admission for repeat coronary angiography and/or repeat PCI. Assuming that some form of intervention is needed; generally patients with single-vessel disease are managed with PCI if possible. Patients with two-vessel disease can be managed with either technique, depending on the nature of the lesions, and patients with three-vessel disease or long-standing occlusions are managed with coronary bypass surgery. In

Table 5.17 The choice between redo CABG and PCI

Favours redo CABG	Favours PCI
Late restenosis > 5 years	Earlier restenosis
Diffuse graft disease	Discrete graft lesions
LIMA not previously used	Patent LIMA to LAD
Poor LV function	Normal LV function
Good distal vessels	Poor distal vessels
Multiple new lesions	Single new lesions
Long-standing total occlusion	Recent total occlusion (<6 months)

the ARTS trial event-free survival at 1 year in patients with multivessel disease was higher in the surgical group than in the PCI group (87.3% vs 73.3%) because of the need for reintervention in the stented patients (restenosis). The UK-based SOS (stent or surgery) trial has confirmed these findings.

Diabetic patients

There is a trend to refer patients with diabetes for CABG rather than PCI because the reintervention rates are higher with PCI.

Particular indications for CABG in patients with diabetes are:
- multivessel disease
- proteinuria (indicating microvascular disease)
- restenosis.

However, the use of abciximab in patients with diabetes undergoing PCI has reduced the mortality and the need for reintervention (EPISTENT trial, see Section 11.8).

Redo CABG

Redo CABG must be considered in about 10% patients at 10 years and 25% at 20 years from their first CABG operation. The mortality rate for first-time CABG in all patients in the UK is 1% but redo CABG carries a 7% mortality rate and second redo about a 10% mortality risk. Factors to consider in the choice of redo CABG vs PCI are given in Table 5.17.

The decision is a joint one between a cardiologist and a cardiac surgeon.

Assessment of Surgical Risk

The decision to operate on a patient with coronary disease involves assessing the operative mortality risk. The most widely used scoring system is the European system for cardiac operative risk evaluation or EuroSCORE (Table 5.18). This has superseded the original American Parsonnet scoring system because this earlier system allowed subjective scoring of some variables and tended to exaggerate the operative risk.

The predicted percentage mortality risk is obtained by summing the points in Table 5.18 for the relevant variables.

Table 5.18 EuroSCORE

Factor	Definition	Score
Age	Per 5 years or part thereof over 60	1
Gender	Female	1
Chronic pulmonary disease	Long-term use of bronchodilators or steroids	1
Extracardiac arteriopathy	Any one or more of the following: claudication, carotid occlusion or >50% stenosis, previous or planned surgery on the abdominal aorta, limb arteries or carotids	2
Neurological dysfunction	Disease severely affecting ambulation or day-to-day functioning	2
Previous cardiac surgery	Previous surgery requiring opening of the pericardium	3
Serum creatinine	>200 µmol/l preoperatively	2
Active endocarditis	Patient still on antibiotic treatment for endocarditis at the time of surgery	3
Critical preoperative state	Ventilation before arrival in the anaesthetic room, preoperative inotropic support, intra-aortic balloon counterpulsation (IABP) or preoperative acute renal failure (anuria or oliguria <10 ml/h)	3
Unstable angina	Angina requiring intravenous nitrates until arrival in the operating room	2
LV dysfunction	Moderate (LVEF 30–50%)	1
	Poor (LVEF <30%)	3
Recent myocardial infarct	<90 days	2
Pulmonary hypertension	Systolic PA pressure >60 mmHg	2
Emergency	Carried out on referral before the beginning of the next working day	2
Other than isolated CABG	Major cardiac operation other than or in addition to CABG	2
Surgery on thoracic aorta	Ascending, arch or descending aorta	3
Post-infarct septal rupture		4

Refractory Angina

A few patients remain severely symptomatic in spite of two or more CABG operations and several angioplasty procedures. They continue to get bad angina interfering with any quality of life. They are a considerable management problem. Possible options in order are:

• Further adjustments to medical therapy: nocturnal angina can be helped by taking a long-acting nitrate on going to bed rather than in the morning. An additional β blocker or slow-release calcium antagonist may help. Angina provoked by lying flat is caused by increased LV wall stress and this may be reduced by taking a diuretic at about 6 pm, or by propping the head of the bed up. Aim for long-acting or slow-release preparations. Many patients do not take their GTN spray prophylactically. Blood pressure control must be

optimal and ACE inhibitor therapy maximized. Consider addition of newer drugs (see above).
• Second opinion on latest angiogram: is there in fact a further angioplasty or surgical option?
• TENS device: a few patients are helped by this transcutaneous nerve stimulator, which can usually be tried initially from the physio-therapy department. It is not suitable for patients with permanent pacemakers.
• Left stellate ganglion block: performed by an anaesthetist or pain management consultant. This can be remarkably successful with symptom relief up to 6 months before it needs repeating.
• Spinal cord stimulator (SCS): introduced in 1987 in Australia this involves the passage of an electrode epidurally up to the C7–T2 region. The electrode is then tunnelled subcutaneously according to the severity of the anginal attack. Implantation must be performed on the conscious patient lying prone. The position of the electrode is critical. Once in place the electrode is tested. An implanted stimulator can be programmed externally by the patient with a hand-held portable programmer. The intensity of the stimulation can be varied by the patient; the patient should experience warm paraesthesiae across the chest once the stimulator has been activated.

Trials with this device have shown increased work capacity, reduction in opiate consumption, increased time to angina on the treadmill and less ST depression. It will not mask very severe ischaemic/infarct pain. There is some evidence that it may increase coronary blood flow.

5.10 Complications of MI

See separate sections for:
• Recurrent unstable angina (see Section 5.6)
• Bradycardias or heart block requiring pacing (see Sections 7.1 and 7.4)
• Tachyarrhythmias, atrial or ventricular (see Chapter 8)
• Cardiac arrests (see Section 6.16)
• LV failure (see Section 6.1).

Sudden Death
This can occur at any time after an infarct and is usually the result of:
• acute cardiac rupture
• VF or fast prolonged VT degenerating to VF
• massive pulmonary embolism
• left main stem embolism from mural thrombus (rare).

Acute cardiac rupture occurs usually from about the fourth to the tenth day post-infarction. Pulseless electrical activity (Electromechanical dissociation) is typical (good ECG with no output at all). Very occasionally it is contained by the pericardium (see Tamponade, Section 10.2). Analysis of the causes of death in β-blocking trials and myocardial infarcts suggests that β blockers reduce mortality in infarction by reducing the incidence of cardiac rupture, but the drug has to be given early – within the first 2 days.

Massive pulmonary embolism may also show pulseless electrical activity (PEA) on the ECG.

RV Failure

This is less common than LV failure but is very important because usually it is either missed or wrongly treated.

It occurs primarily after inferior infarction and is usually transient. RV infarction is probable if the V4R lead on the ECG shows ST-segment elevation.

Persistent RVF presents with high neck veins and hepatic congestion. In the acute stage in severe cases, Swan–Ganz monitoring is required and may show low left-sided filling pressures with high right-sided pressures. Cardiac output may be improved by plasma expansion in carefully regulated amounts, rather than diuretic therapy, which may make the situation worse.

The differential diagnosis is pulmonary embolism (see Section 13.2).

Pericarditis

This is often acute (within the first few days) and transient. It may occur with anterior or inferior infarcts. Pain is typically cardiac in distribution and relieved by sitting up or leaning forward. It is worse when lying flat. Inferior/diaphragmatic involvement may cause shoulder-tip pain. A pericardial or pleuropericardial rub may be heard, but the pain is so typical in character that it should be suspected with the history alone. The ECG shows transient T-wave changes or 'saddle-shaped' ST-segment elevation (see Chapter 10, Figure 10.1 and 16.10).

Treatment is with non-steroidal anti-inflammatory agents (e.g. soluble aspirin, indometacin, ibuprofen). Echocardiography should be performed frequently to check for an enlarging effusion. The ECG with an enlarging effusion shows progressive voltage reduction and sometimes electrical alternans (see Chapter 10, Figure 10.2).

Systemic Embolism

Systemic embolism from mural thrombus is more frequent after large infarctions and generally occurs 1–3 weeks post-infarct. Patients with large infarctions should be heparinized until fully mobile (e.g. for first week), but the evidence that anticoagulants improve mortality figures from acute infarcts is small and possible only with pooled trials.

Peripheral limb emboli may be removed surgically (e.g. Fogarty technique). Large mesenteric emboli are generally fatal. Coronary emboli may account for a small number of reinfarctions.

Pulmonary Embolism (see Section 13.2)

This occurs as a result of a combination of:
• low cardiac output, poor peripheral flow and venous stasis if venous pressure is high
• prolonged bed rest

- haemoconcentration with diuretic therapy
- increased platelet stickiness.

Patients are thus mobilized early – within 48 h of uncomplicated infarction to avoid pulmonary emboli – and discharged early. Patients who are likely to require several days' bed rest should be heparinized until they are fully mobile.

Tamponade (see Section 10.2)

This occurs after subacute cardiac rupture in which the pericardium acts as a barrier. A false aneurysm may follow if the patient survives (Figure 5.28).

Examination may reveal raised neck vein filling on inspiration, with systolic 'x' descent. There is a small-volume pulse possibly with pulsus paradoxus (see Figure 10.4). There are soft muffled heart sounds.

The cardiac rhythm quickly becomes slow, idionodal or ventricular bradycardia with no output (pulseless electrical activity).

Diagnosis can be confirmed by echocardiography. Needle aspiration may be of temporary benefit, but in the acute stage the condition is usually fatal unless urgent surgical repair is possible. (The false aneurysm has a narrow neck and can be repaired occasionally in the acute stage.)

Acute cardiac rupture is a common cause of sudden death after an MI.

Mitral Regurgitation (see Section 3.3)

Mild subvalvar mitral regurgitation is common after inferior or posterior infarction, as a result of papillary muscle dysfunction. It is often transient. The murmur is ejection in quality, often mid- or late systolic, and heard at both apex and left sternal edges.

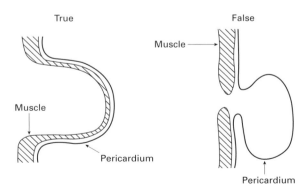

Figure 5.28 Ventricular aneurysm: shows the difference between a true and a false ventricular aneurysm. The true aneurysm is lined by a thin layer of a muscle/scar tissue as well as pericardium. The false aneurysm is subacute cardiac rupture with only pericardium lining the aneurysm. It tends to have a narrower neck than a true aneurysm.

Severe mitral regurgitation is caused by chordal rupture or papillary muscle infarction and rupture. Pulmonary oedema occurs rapidly, often with a small left atrium.

Physical Signs

There is a loud pansystolic murmur at apex or left sternal edge with a possible thrill. Systolic expansion of the left atrium may be confused with an RV heave.

Echocardiography may show chaotic movement of the posterior leaflet with anterior movement during diastole and fluttering.

Treatment depends on the patient's condition (see LVF, Section 6.4). Diuretics and vasodilator therapy (nitroprusside) may hold the situation before mitral valve replacement, which may be life-saving in the acute stage.

Acquired VSD

Physical signs may be very similar to acute mitral regurgitation; however, acute pulmonary oedema is less prominent and right-sided signs predominate in the early stages, with very high venous pressures. A VSD may occur with an anterior or an inferior infarct. Without echocardiography it may be impossible to differentiate acute VSD from mitral regurgitation. Table 5.19 is a general guide only.

Swan–Ganz catheterization will confirm the diagnosis with a step-up in saturation in the right ventricle.

Echocardiography

This is proving very valuable in diagnosis. Pulsed or continuous wave Doppler ultrasonography is necessary. The sample volume is scanned up the RV border of the septum in the four-chamber view and the Doppler signal is picked up at the site of the VSD. This technique may avoid the need for Swan–Ganz catheterization. There may be multiple defects – 'Swiss-cheese defect'.

Table 5.19 Acute mitral regurgitation vs VSD in MI: clinical differences

	Mitral regurgitation	VSD
Infarct site	Inferior/posterior	Anterior
Chest radiograph	Acute pulmonary oedema	Pulmonary plethora
Dyspnoea	Severe orthopnoea and PND	Less dyspnoeic
JVP	May be normal	Raised

But: Both may have pansystolic murmur and thrill at left sternal edge, parasternal heave (RV or LA+) Both may be in cardiogenic shock

Treatment

Earlier attempts to control the situation with medical treatment for as long as possible are now considered inappropriate. Instead surgery is recommended as early as possible. A double-patch technique either side of the septum may be needed to close the Swiss-cheese defect. Recurrence of a small VSD postoperatively is not uncommon. Posteroinferior VSDs carry a higher mortality than anteroapical VSDs. RV function is an important predictor of survival. This is a high-risk condition: 50% mortality within the first week and 80% within 4 weeks.

Device Closure

This is a possibility using an Amplatzer device with the internal jugular vein being a useful entry site. It is important to choose a device that is 6–8 mm larger than the estimated defect size to ensure adequate overlap.

LV Aneurysm

Anterior

This is suspected clinically if the high paradoxical apex of an anterior infarct persists. The ECG shows persistent elevation of ST segments after 4–6 weeks.

The patient may have no symptoms. The diagnosis can be confirmed by:
- enlarging heart on the chest radiograph (Figures 5.29 and 5.30)
- echocardiography
- MUGA scanning
- LV angiography.

Symptoms are commonly LV failure or angina refractory to medical treatment. Occasionally patients develop recurrent VT or systemic emboli.

Symptomatic patients are investigated with a view to LV aneurysmectomy (Figures 5.31–5.34) if the residual contractile segment function is adequate and if medical treatment fails to control symptoms.

Inferior/Posterior

This is less common than anterolateral aneurysm. It may be associated with considerable mitral regurgitation. False aneurysm may also occur inferoposteriorly.

Physical signs are less obvious, because there is no paradoxical apex. Persistent ST elevation occurs on inferior leads. The inferior aneurysm bulges downwards (Figure 5.35) and may be missed on the chest radiograph, which may fail to show progressive cardiac enlargement unless there is additional mitral regurgitation.

Investigation and indications for surgery are as with anterior aneurysms, but additional mitral valve replacement may be necessary. Surgical mortality is higher in this group.

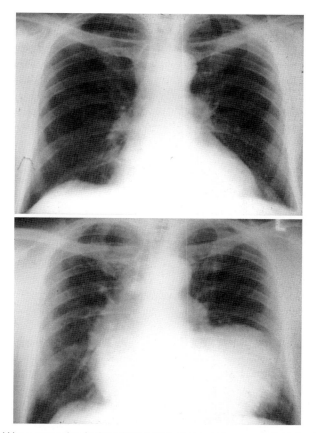

Figure 5.29 LV aneurysm developing within 1 year of an anterior myocardial infarct.

Late Malignant Ventricular Arrhythmias

Occurring 1–3 weeks after an MI, often at about 10 days, these are the cardiologist's nightmare: the patient having made an uneventful recovery, about to return home, suddenly collapses with VF.

Fortunately the problem is uncommon; even so patients with large infarcts should have 24-hour monitoring before discharge. Early exercise testing may point to patients at risk. Recently signal averaging of the standard 12-lead ECG has shown that patients at risk of late ventricular arrhythmias may show late or after-potentials. Signal averaging of ECGs is expensive and not generally available yet (see Risk Stratification, Section 5.7).

The most easily avoidable cause is hypokalaemia from excessive diuretic therapy. Digoxin should be avoided in infarcts unless the patient is in AF.

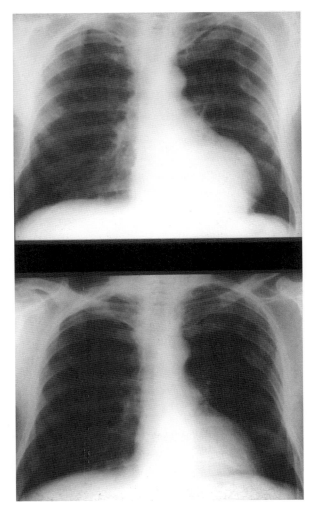

Figure 5.30 Chest radiograph before and after LV aneurysm resection.

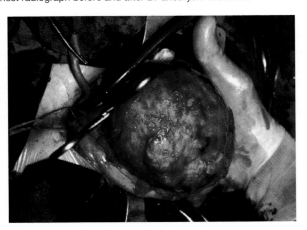

Figure 5.31 LV aneurysm at surgery.

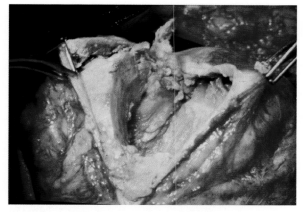

Figure 5.32 LV aneurysm opened to show laminated thrombus.

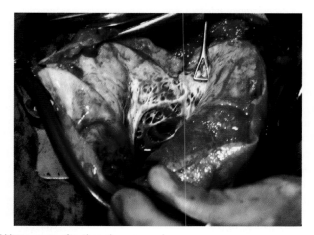

Figure 5.33 LV aneurysm after thrombus removal.

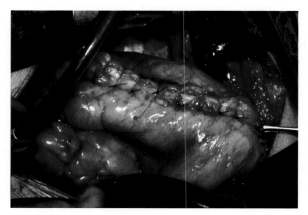

Figure 5.34 LV aneurysm: completed resection.

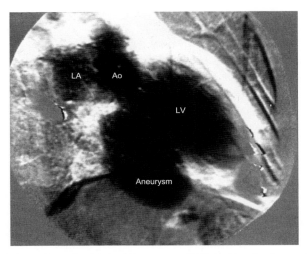

Figure 5.35 LV cineangiography: inferior LV aneurysm. Digital subtraction image of end-diastolic frame. Right anterior oblique view. There is additional moderate mitral regurgitation into the left atrium (LA).

Dressler's Syndrome

Described in 1956, this is a syndrome of recurrent pericarditis, pleural effusions, fever, anaemia and high ESR. It occurs in about 1–5% of infarcts, usually 1–4 weeks after an MI. It is thought to result from an autoimmune reaction to exposed myocardial antigens after infarction (and a similar illness may occur after cardiac surgery – also called the postcardiotomy syndrome). Anti-heart antibodies have been demonstrated, but are not useful clinically.

It is a chronic condition. Treatment in the first instance is with non-steroidal anti-inflammatory agents, or steroids in more severe or refractory cases. Steroids are said to increase the likelihood of LV aneurysm development, but the evidence for this is anecdotal.

Treatment may have to be continued for several months and patients observed when treatment is stopped or weaned off, because the syndrome may recur. Tamponade is rare.

Shoulder–Hand Syndrome

This is now rare after an MI, probably as a result of early mobilization. It develops from 2 weeks to 2 months post-infarct as stiffness and pain in the shoulder (usually the left), and pain and swelling of the hand (becoming puffy and mottled).

A few late cases develop wasting of small muscles of the hand with irreversible contractures forming (such as Dupuytren's contractures).

Treatment is with mobilization, physiotherapy of the hand and shoulder and analgesia. Hydrocortisone injections into the subacromial bursa may help. Systemic steroids are not used.

Depression and Anxiety

A psychological assessment using the Hospital Anxiety and Depression (HAD) scale shows that at least 25% of patients have raised scores, with anxiety being more prevalent than depression. In a service that concentrates on shorter and shorter length of stay for infarct patients, this aspect of their care is easily overlooked. Depression after an infarction may result in denial of symptoms, with the patient being too frightened to admit to any problems. It can be largely prevented by the following:

• A sensible encouraging approach from the doctor: worried doctors produce worried patients
• Early mobilization
• Pre-discharge advice about work, driving, sex, travel, etc.
• Exercise programme and follow-up to check that the patient is considering returning to work
• Avoidance of antidepressant drugs if possible; if absolutely necessary mianserin, doxepin or lofepramine are said to have fewer cardiac effects than earlier tricyclics (amitriptyline or imipramine)
• Cardiac rehabilitation course: there is renewed interest in this aspect of cardiac care. There is no doubt that cardiac rehabilitation provides motivation, company, reassurance and carefully graded and medically supervised exercise.

5.11 Management of Hyperlipidaemias

Several large trials have confirmed that active reduction of serum cholesterol reduces the risk of death, MI, the need for coronary intervention and stroke in patients with hypercholesterolaemia (Table 5.20). The risk of fatal or non-fatal MI in the primary prevention (WOSCOPS) trial was reduced by about 30%. The reduction in the secondary prevention trials (4S and CARE studies) is similar. There was no increased risk of cancer or suicide in the treated groups. Meta-analysis of these trials has suggested that a 10% reduction in serum cholesterol results in a 20% reduction in mortality from cardiac disease and a 17% reduction in incidence of MI. Aggressive lowering of cholesterol has also been shown to reduce the progression of disease in coronary vein grafts.

Reduction of triglycerides is important in reducing episodes of pancreatitis and peripheral neuropathy in relevant cases, but has not yet been shown to reduce coronary risk in large trials.

Motivation of patients is important. The diet is unpleasant and rigid. Some drugs may have unpleasant side effects and patients rarely feel better on medication. In addition the doctor rarely sees any immediate benefit and therapy is expensive. Patient compliance will be a problem.

Screening

Fasting blood is needed only for estimation of triglycerides. Patients should also avoid alcohol for 24 hours before the test. A random test is suffi-

Table 5.20 Results of three large cholesterol-lowering trials

Trial	Drug	Number	Time (years)	Reduction in total serum cholesterol (%)	Reduction in fatal or non-fatal MI (%)	Reduction in CVAs (%)	Reduction in need for CABG/PCI (%)
4S	Simvastatin 20–40 mg once daily	4444	5.4	28	37	35	34
CARE	Pravastatin 40 mg once daily	4159	5	20	24	31	27
WOSCOPS (Men only)	Pravastatin 40 mg once daily	6595	4.9	20	31	11	37

For references, see Appendix 4.

cient for cholesterol alone. The following groups of patients should be screened:
- A family history of coronary disease, especially if <50 years
- A family history of hyperlipidaemia
- Xanthomas (see Figures 1.2, 1.3, 1.5)
- Xanthelasma or corneal arcus <40 year, as these signs are less specific than xanthomas, except in younger age groups (see Figure 1.4)
- Obesity
- Hypertension
- A history of myocardial infarct, CVA or intermittent claudication and aged <60 years
- Patients with conditions likely to cause secondary hyperlipidaemia (Table 5.21).

Finger-prick-testing kits are now available. They can be used in outpatients with the results available immediately. Care is required in sampling in order to get accurate results, and the reagent strips are not cheap. If a random test is performed and a total cholesterol level >6.5 mmol/l is found, the test is repeated under fasting with estimation of both low-density lipoprotein (LDL)- and high-density lipoprotein (HDL)-cholesterol and triglycerides. The ratio HDL:LDL-cholesterol is often calculated. A ratio <0.2 is considered a risk factor for coronary disease.

Table 5.21 Conditions likely to cause secondary hyperlipidaemia

Dietary
Excess dietary fat or calories
Excess alcohol
Anorexia nervosa
Drugs
Steroids
Oral contraceptives
Thiazide diuretics
Protease inhibitors (HIV)
Isotretinoin (acne)
Endocrine
Hypothyroidism
Poorly controlled diabetes
Intestinal
Biliary obstruction
Acute pancreatitis
Renal
Nephrotic syndrome
Chronic renal failure
Long-term dialysis

The drugs listed in Table 5.21 also cause a rise in plasma triglycerides. HDL-cholesterol rises with thiazides and the contraceptive pill, but falls with isotretinoin and non-selective β blockers. Women with a history of hyperlipidaemia coronary or cerebrovascular disease should not take the oestrogen-containing pill. Protease inhibitors cause hypercholesterolaemia, insulin resistance and hyperglycaemia.

Types of Lipid Measured (in Decreasing Order of Size)

Chylomicrons
This is the largest lipid particle with a size >80 nm. It is formed in the small bowel mucosal cells and carried in the lymphatics and plasma; it consists mainly of triglyceride. This is removed in the peripheral tissue by the action of lipoprotein lipase. The remnant particles are reabsorbed by the liver.

VLDLs
These are very-low-density lipoproteins of size 30–80 nm. It is synthesized in the liver from endogenously synthesized triglyceride. VLDLs are broken down by lipoprotein lipase to smaller LDL particles.

LDLs
These are of size 20 nm. They are a major carrier of cholesterol in the plasma, and derived from intravascular breakdown of VLDL particles. LDL is primarily removed by the liver from the circulation. Its removal depends on the available number of LDL receptors on the liver and peripheral cells. The receptors available depend partly on the need for intracellular cholesterol and partly on a genetic factor. Thus a reduction in the intrahepatic cholesterol pool (e.g. by bile acid depletion with cholestyramine) increases the number of LDL receptors on the hepatocyte membrane, resulting in an increased uptake of LDL by liver and peripheral cells and a fall in plasma LDL-cholesterol. High levels of LDL-cholesterol are associated with coronary disease (e.g. LDL >5 mmol/l). The main carrier is Apo-B lipoprotein.

HDLs
These are of size 10 nm. It is the smallest lipoprotein rich in phospholipid and carries about a quarter of the total cholesterol. It is secreted by the liver and also produced from chylomicron metabolism. Low levels of HDL are associated with coronary disease (e.g. <1 mmol/l). Regular exercise increases HDL levels. The main carrier is Apo-A1 apoprotein.

Apoproteins
There are at least 10 different apoproteins that form an essential part of the lipoprotein particle. Each is specific for a type of lipoprotein or involved in lipid transport, enzyme activation, or cellular uptake and receptor recognition.

Raised levels of some apoproteins have been shown to be better discriminators for the presence of coronary disease than their respective lipoproteins, e.g. raised levels of Apo-A1 and Apo-B. Patients with levels of Apo-B > 125 mg% are at risk of coronary disease. Lipoprotein(a), known as Lp(a), is an LDL-like particle containing Apo-B100 and Apo(a). Levels are raised in patients with coronary disease. The ratio Apo-B : Apo-A1 was one of the nine discriminating variables of cardiovascular risk in the INTERHEART study (see Section 5.7).

Normal Lipid Levels

Plasma lipid levels rise with age. These figures are a guide to patients aged under 70 years:

- Total cholesterol: 4.0–6.5 mmol/l (150–250 mg/100 ml); mean 5.6 mmol/l
- HDL-cholesterol: 0.8–2.0 mmol/l
- LDL-cholesterol: <4.9 mmol/l
- Triglycerides: 0.8–2.0 mmol/l (70–170 mg/100 ml).

The aim of treatment is to reduce the cholesterol to <4.0 mmol/l and the LDL to <2.0 mmol/l in high-risk patients. In low-risk patients the initial targets are 5.0 mmol/l and 3.0 mmol/l respectively. Vigorous reduction in saturated fat intake will reduce the plasma cholesterol only by a maximum of 15%. Patients with cholesterol levels >6.5 mmol/l who are already on a low-cholesterol diet and who are aged under 70 years should be considered for additional drug therapy. Top dose of statin therapy should lower total serum cholesterol by at least 30%.

Treatment

Diet

Weight reduction, cutting back on alcohol intake and a low-fat diet are the first stage in treatment. This means avoiding: egg yolks, butter, cream, lard and fatty meats. Reduce cheese intake, but cottage cheese is allowed.

- Substitute margarine for butter, vegetable oils for lard, chicken and turkey for red meat
- Encourage fish intake (avoid fish roe), vegetables and fibre
- Reduce red meat intake to 3 oz/day.

This diet will reduce both cholesterol and triglycerides. The benefit of a low-fat diet depends on whether the patient is a high absorber or a high synthesiser of cholesterol. Even the most stringent low-fat diet will not usually lower total cholesterol by >15%.

Drug Therapy for Hypercholesterolaemia

Several drugs below may be needed in combination.

1 The first choice is the statins. Five statins are available in the UK (Table 5.22). Cerivastatin was withdrawn after fatal cases of rhabdomyolysis (some

Table 5.22 Currently available statins in the UK

Drug	Daily dose range (mg)
Atorvastatin (Lipitor)	10–80
Fluvastatin (Lescol)	20–80
Pravastatin (Lipostat)	10–40
Rosuvastatin (Crestor)	5–20
Simvastatin (Zocor)	10–80

in combination with gemfibrozil). In addition lovastatin (Mevacor) is prescribed in the USA (dose 10–40 mg twice daily).

These drugs inhibit hepatic cholesterol synthesis by inhibiting hydroxymethylglutaryl coenzyme A (HMG-CoA) reductase. The resulting upregulation of hepatocyte LDL receptors causes increased uptake of LDL in the liver and a reduction in the serum by up to 50%. Hepatic LDL receptors are increased, HDL-cholesterol is increased and triglycerides reduced slightly. They are safe in renal disease (biliary excretion only). They are well-tolerated drugs and by far the most palatable in hypercholesterolaemia. The drugs vary in potency and cost and there are few back-to-back trials. Fluvastatin is probably the weakest but is cheap compared with rosuvastatin, which is probably the most potent available but also the most expensive at top dose.

Side effects. These are both idiosyncratic and dose-related. There is a minor elevation in liver transaminases, which is rarely a problem. Stop the statin if liver enzymes exceed three times normal or if the patient develops muscle pain. Muscle pain is a class effect and is likely to recur even if the statin is switched to a different brand. Rhabdomyolysis with greatly raised CPK levels is fortunately rare, but the risk is increased slightly if the statin is combined with a fibrate or nicotinic acid. If the drugs are combined, start with low doses of both (preferably using fenofibrate) and follow up closely. Patients should be told to discontinue the combination should they get unexplained muscle pains. The combination of a statin with gemfibrozil should be avoided.

Low-dose statins should be used initially in:
- South Asians (tend to have higher plasma levels)
- Those aged >70
- Hypothyroidism
- Moderate renal impairment: creatinine clearance <60 ml/min
- Concomitant use of fibrates (avoid gemfibrozil use)
- Personal or family history of hereditary muscle disorders.

Avoid statins in the following: liver disease, alcoholism, pregnancy, lactation, immunosuppression with ciclosporin (rhabdomyolysis risk), patients on gemfibrozil.

Dose. Starting dose is 10 mg at night for most statins. Rosuvastatin can be started at 5 mg (cholesterol synthesis is said to occur predominantly at night). Maximum effect is seen in 4–6 weeks (for maximum doses, see Table 5.22). They are not identical drugs, however. Pravastatin does not interfere with the cytochrome P450 system. At high doses simvastatin causes a slight increase in Apo-A1 and HDL whereas atorvastatin causes a slight decrease.

In mixed hyperlipidaemia with both cholesterol and triglycerides raised, use a double statin dose.

2 The second choice is ezetimibe (Ezetrol, Vytorin). This inhibits cholesterol absorption in the small bowel and reduces LDL-cholesterol by 15–25%. The dose is 10 mg o.m. Larger doses are of no extra benefit. The exact gain in LDL reduction depends on whether the patient is a high absorber (responds best to ezetimibe) or a high synthesizer of cholesterol (responds best to a statin). A combined preparation with simvastatin (20 mg or 40 mg) is available: Inegy (Zetia) – a highly potent reducer of LDL-cholesterol that avoids the need for a high-dose statin and the risk of rhabdomyolysis.

Ezetimibe is very well tolerated with minimal or no side effects. It can be used as monotherapy, or combined with a statin (see above) or with fenofibrate. It is the drug of choice in statin-intolerant patients. It can be used in pregnancy but is excreted in breast milk.

3 The third choice is fibrates: primarily drugs for hypertriglyceridaemia. They activate lipoprotein lipase and increase the number of hepatic LDL receptors. They partly inhibit HMG-CoA reductase also. HDL levels are increased slightly:
• Bezafibrate (Bezalip): 200 mg three times daily after meals, or monopreparation (Bezalip mono) 400 mg once daily.
• Gemfibrozil (Lopid): 600 mg twice daily (best to avoid in combination with a statin). Shown to increase HDL and reduce coronary risk by 22% in one trial.
• Fenofibrate (Lipantil): 100–200 mg once daily.
• Clofibrate (Atromid-S): 500 mg three times daily after meals. Hardly used now except for hypertriglyceridaemia with pancreatitis risk.
  The problems with fibrates are:
• nausea, abdominal discomfort occasionally
• risk of gallstones as a result of increased excretion of cholesterol in bile
• they potentiate warfarin, so reduction in warfarin dose necessary
• need to avoid in liver or renal disease
• a risk of rhabdomyolysis if combined with statins (gemfibrozil).

4 The fourth choice is nicotinic acid: dose 100 mg three times daily, gradually increasing to 1 g three times daily. Reduces hepatic VLDL synthesis and inhibits release of FFA from fat cells. Reduces LDL synthesis by reducing synthesis of Apo-B in the liver.

The following side effects may limit its use:
• Flushing soon after taking the drug (reduced by adding small dose of aspirin); less of a problem with a slow-release preparation
• Nausea, abdominal discomfort, diarrhoea
• Rarely, itching, hyperpigmentation, acanthosis nigricans, macular oedema
• Rise in serum alkaline phosphatase, liver enzymes, uric acid and glucose.
Avoid nicotinic acid in liver disease, gout, history of recent peptic ulcer.

5 The fifth choice is anion exchange resins: cholestyramine 4–8 g three times daily; colestipol 5–10 g three times daily. These bind the bile acids in the small bowel, preventing their reabsorption in the distal 200 cm of the terminal ileum. The intrahepatic bile salt pool is reduced, there is an increase in LDL receptors on the hepatocyte and more cholesterol is absorbed from the plasma to synthesize more bile salts.
The following are the side effects:
• Constipation, bloating, flatulence, haemorrhoids, even intestinal obstruction
• Fat-soluble vitamin supplementation may be needed (i.e. vitamins A, D, E, K)
• Drug absorption reduced, e.g. digoxin, thyroxine, warfarin; dose may need to be increased.
New more powerful bile acid sequestrants are under development.

6 The sixth choice is drugs rarely used now: D-thyroxine, probucol, neomycin.

The following are other terms commonly used to describe subtypes:
• Type I: familial hypertriglyceridaemia or chylomicronaemia. Lipoprotein lipase deficiency.
• Type II: familial or primary hypercholesterolaemia. This may be homozygous presenting in childhood with angina, MI or aortic stenosis. More commonly it is heterozygous (1 in 500 of the population) presenting in early adult life.
• Type IIb or IV: familial combined hyperlipidaemia.
• Type III: broad B hyperlipoproteinaemia.
• Type IV: endogenous hypertriglyceridaemia.

Drug Therapy for Hypertriglyceridaemia (e.g. Types I, III, IV and V)
(Table 5.23)
• *First choice*: fibrates (see above): the best single drug type for high triglycerides.
• *Second choice*: nicotinic acid (see above).
• *Third choice*: marine oil supplementation. Inhibit hepatic VLDL synthesis. Fish oils providing 5–20 g ω-3 fatty acids daily lower triglycerides. They are expensive (approximately £40 per month on low dosage).

Table 5.23 Frederickson classification of primary hyperlipidaemias

Type	Frequency	Lipoprotein abnormality	Triglyceride and cholesterol	Clinical features
I	Rare	Chylomicrons+++ Plasma lipaemic LDL ↓ VLDL →	Triglyceride+++ Cholesterol+	Abdominal pain Hepatosplenomegaly Pancreatitis Eruptive xanthomas
IIa	Common	LDL+++ VLDL →	Cholesterol+++	Premature atheroma Tendon xanthomas
IIb	Common	LDL++ VLDL+	Cholesterol++ Triglyceride+	As in type IIa
III	Uncommon	VLDL+ Remnants+ Abnormal apolipoprotein E	Cholesterol++ Triglyceride+++	Diabetes, gout Premature atheroma Orange palmar crease Eruptive xanthomas

IV	Common	VLDL+
		LDL →
			Triglyceride++	May have diabetes, gout,
				  obesity, premature
				  vascular disease

V	Uncommon	VLDL++ Chylomicrons++ Plasma lipaemic LDL ↓	Triglyceride++ Cholesterol+	Pancreatitis Hepatosplenomegaly Diabetes, gout, eruptive xanthomas

• *Fourth choice*: consider low-fat diet with MCT (medium-chain triglyceride) supplementation.

Other Forms of Treatment for Hypercholesterolaemia
In patients with homozygous hypercholesterolaemia high levels of cholesterol (15–30 mmol/l) may not be reduced satisfactorily on diet and combination drug therapy. These patients are usually children and further options to be considered are the following:
• Plasma exchanges every 2–3 weeks
• Plasma exchange using an LDL immunoabsorber column
• Surgery: resection of distal 200 cm of ileum or bypassing this segment, preventing reabsorption of bile acids. Portacaval shunt; liver and heart transplantation. The liver transplant provides new LDL receptors and the heart transplant is necessary because severe premature coronary disease develops in the first few years of life. These are highly specialized procedures requiring referral to a specialist centre.
• Gene therapy: recently three patients have been treated with a gene for the LDL receptor transfected into cultured hepatocytes (the hepatocytes cultured from the patient's own left hepatic lobe). This in time may prove the most effective form of treatment.

Regression of Coronary Lesions on Treatment

Theoretically, getting lipid out of coronary plaques should make them more solid – reducing their growth and making them more stable. There is growing clinical evidence that this is the case. Vigorous therapy to lower serum LDL-cholesterol with either drugs (e.g. with lovastatin and colestipol, or niacin and colestipol – the FATS study) or partial ileal bypass (the POSCH study) in six separate trials has been shown to delay progression of coronary lesions on angiography, or reduce clinical events. In some cases regression of coronary lesions was seen. In the ileal bypass trial (POSCH) there was a highly significant reduction in non-fatal coronary events, and the need for PCI or CABG in the ileal bypass group compared with controls. Although combination therapy trials have shown a fall in LDLs they have produced a mean stenosis regression of only 1–2%. High-intensity statin therapy (e.g. with rosuvastatin in the ASTEROID trial) results in a small but significant reduction in atheroma volume on coronary IVUS. In contrast, there has been a striking reduction in statin trials in cardiovascular events such as MI, death or the need for revascularization by >50%.

As well as changing the plaque composition, reducing the number of foam cells, thickening the fibrous cap, etc., cholesterol lowering can improve endothelial function and EDRF release. Studies of coronary flow in patients who have had successful lowering of their cholesterol have shown a reduction or loss of a vasoconstrictor response to acetylcholine in the epicardial coronaries. Lipid lowering improves endothelial vasomotor function. In addition pravastatin and lovastatin appear to have an anti-inflammatory effect and have been shown to reduce CRP levels. Statins also inhibit leukocyte integrin ($\alpha_1\beta_2$), which binds to the intercellular adhesion molecule (ICAM).

Summary of Pleiotropic Effects of Statins (other than LDL Lowering)

- Prevent plaque progression
- Plaque regression at high statin (atorvastatin, rosuvastatin) dose
- Improve endothelial function
- Anti-inflammatory action.

The Heart Protection Study (MRC/BHF-HPS)

This was the largest cholesterol-lowering trial ever undertaken at a cost of £21m. Between 1994 and 1997, 20536 patients in 69 hospitals in the UK were randomized to receive simvastatin 40mg once daily, an antioxidant regimen, either, both or placebo on a factorial design. The antioxidant regimen was vitamin E 600mg, vitamin C 250mg and β-carotene 20mg once daily. To be included patients had to be aged 40–80, their total cholesterol had to be >3.5mmol/l and they had to be thought to be at increased risk of death from coronary heart disease as a result of previous MI or known CAD, diabetes or treated hypertension.

Five years of simvastatin treatment lowered total cholesterol by an average of 1.3mmol/l and LDL-cholesterol by 1.0mmol/l. Major vascular events were reduced by simvastatin by one-third. Five years of statin therapy was found to prevent major vascular events in:

- 1 in 10 people who have had a previous MI
- 8 in 100 people with angina or signs of coronary disease
- 7 in 100 people who had ever had a stroke
- 7 in 100 people with diabetes.

A reduction in LDL by 1 mmol/l reduced the relative risk of vascular events (CHD and stroke) by 25%. All ages benefited, as did both women and men. Patients with low cholesterol levels also benefited. This trial shows conclusively that any patient with a history of previous MI or stroke, peripheral vascular disease or diabetes should be on a statin (whatever their level of cholesterol – even if it is 'low' by conventional standards).

The antioxidant regimen was valueless but harmless.

High-density Lipoprotein (HDL)

The vast majority of lipid trials have concentrated on lowering LDL-cholesterol, and from these trials the 'lower the better' philosophy has arisen. Small increases in HDL with statin therapy have been noted and were thought to be of additional benefit.

Analysis of the Framingham data showed a 2–3% reduction in risk of cardiovascular disease with every 1 mg/dl increase in HDL level. In addition transfection into mice of the human Apo-A1 (the main carrier of HDL) gene or infusion of HDL substantially reduces atherosclerosis. In addition the mutant form of Apo-A1 (Apo-A1 Milano), which is found in residents of Limone on Lake Garda in Italy, have remarkable longevity. The effect of infusions of recombinant Apo-A1 Milano in patients with ACSs has been shown to reduce atheroma volume by 14% on intravascular ultrasound studies (Nissen).

All this work suggested that high levels of HDL (and Apo-A1) were protective of cardiovascular disease. There have been several trials attempting to increase HDL, but these have met with nothing like the success of the LDL-lowering trials.

Fibrate Trials

One Veterans Affairs trial (VA-HIT) with gemfibrozil showed a 22% reduction in death from coronary disease. There was a 6% increase in HDL at 1 year and a 31% fall in triglycerides. However, a trial with fenofibrate (FIELD trial) was negative.

Cholesterol Ester Transport Protein (CETP) Inhibitors

This protein facilitates the transfer of HDL-cholesterol to Apo-B lipoproteins (LDL), and CETP inhibition increases HDL levels. Trials with a new CETP inhibitor torcetrapib have proved ineffective. Although torcetrapib increased HDL-cholesterol by 61%, it had no significant effect on atheroma volume measured by intracoronary ultrasonography (ILLUSTRATE trial). In addition one trial (ILLUMINATE) with this drug was stopped early as a result of an increase in vascular events in the torcetrapib arm. Trials with other CETP inhibitors are under way, and it is not clear why torcetrapib was not antiatherogenic. Perhaps the increased HDL was non-functional. The drug itself caused an increase in systolic blood pressure of 4.6 mmHg.

HDL: Future Directions

Synthetic residues of Apo-A1 containing only 10 amino acids have been shown to reduce atheroma volume in mice, and have antioxidant properties. Clinical trials are also under way. A study with a new PPAR-α agonist that increases HDL has reported, but so far results are disappointing.

CHAPTER 6

6   Cardiac Failure

Cardiac failure occurs when cardiac output and blood pressure are inadequate for the body's requirements. The incidence increases with age and carries a poor prognosis. The average age at diagnosis is 76 years. In the USA it probably affects 3 million patients with 200 000 deaths annually. The annual incidence is 1–4/1000 population. In the Framingham study the 5-year mortality rate was 62% for men and 42% for women. No patient in the CONSENSUS 1 trial of grade IV heart failure patients published in 1987 is still alive. The mean survival from diagnosis in the London Heart Failure Study was 3 years. About 33% die in the first year from diagnosis, then a further 10%/year. In the UK cardiac failure accounts for 5% of all hospital admissions, with an estimated cost to the NHS in 2000 of £628m annually, of which drug costs were £54m.

Left and right ventricular failure may occur independently or together as CCF. The terms 'forward' and 'backward' failure refer to symptoms and signs relating to a poor cardiac output (forward failure) or venous congestion (backward failure). The normal cardiac index is 2.5–4.0 l/min per m². In CCF this may fall to ≤1.0 l/min per m².

Some patients may have the symptoms and signs of CCF but preserved systolic function and a normal LVEF on echocardiography. This is diastolic heart failure (see Section 6.11).

High-output failure is an uncommon condition in which a high cardiac output (often >10 l/min) is associated with failure symptoms and signs such as pulmonary oedema. It may occur in sepsis, thyrotoxicosis, large AV fistula, chronic anaemia, beri-beri and severe Paget's disease of bone.

6.1 Aetiology

- Coronary artery disease
- Hypertension

Swanton's Cardiology, sixth edition. By R. H. Swanton and S. Banerjee. Published 2008 Blackwell Publishing. ISBN 978-1-4051-7819-8.

- Valve disease
- Cardiomyopathy: dilated > hypertrophic
- Infiltrative, e.g. amyloid, sarcoid, iron, rarely malignant
- Infective, e.g. viral myocarditis, rheumatic myocarditis, sepsis, infective endocarditis with myocarditis
- Collagen vascular disease
- Drug induced, e.g. doxorubicin (Adriamycin), daunorubicin, 5-fluorouracil
- Metabolic and endocrine, e.g. myxoedema, thyrotoxicosis, acromegaly, phaeochromocytoma
- Toxins, e.g. alcohol
- Radiation, e.g. myocardial fibrosis after radiotherapy for breast carcinoma
- Nutritional, e.g. beri-beri, kwashiorkor, pellagra
- Inherited, e.g. Fabry's disease, muscular dystrophies, Friedreich's ataxia, glycogen storage diseases
- Hypersensitivity, anaphylactic shock
- Cardiac transplant rejection
- Incessant tachycardia
- Miscellaneous: trauma, etc.

By far the most common causes in the western world are coronary disease and hypertension. Several of the insults listed above also affect the pericardium at the same time, e.g. radiation, and viral, bacterial and rheumatic carditis. Ventricular dilatation will lead to functional mitral and/or tricuspid regurgitation.

6.2 Symptoms

These depend on which ventricle is primarily affected, the severity of the damage and the aetiology.

LV Failure
- Fatigue and increasingly limited exercise tolerance, exhaustion after even minor tasks, dyspnoea in all its stages (see Section 1.1), orthopnoea and paroxysmal nocturnal dyspnoea
- Dry nocturnal cough, cold peripheries, palpitation, angina, giddiness or syncope on effort; leaden sensation in legs on walking
- Systemic embolism
- Nocturia and reversed diurnal rhythms
- Weight loss, muscle wasting and eventual cachexia.

RV Failure
- Peripheral oedema increasing to thigh and sacral oedema, ascites and anasarca
- Abdominal distension with ascites

- Hepatic pain, especially on effort
- Nausea and anorexia
- Facial engorgement
- Pulsation in face and neck (tricuspid regurgitation)
- Distended and even pulsatile varicose veins
- Epistaxes.

Note that to all these should be added the common side effects of treatment, e.g. nausea and anorexia (digoxin), gout, impotence, diabetes mellitus, hypokalaemic weakness (thiazide diuretics), postural hypotension (diuretics and all afterload-reducing agents), dry nocturnal cough and abnormal taste (ACE inhibitors), headache and migraine (nitrates).

Psychological

Depression is very common. Many patients have to give up work and may get into financial difficulty at a time when they feel too ill to cope with their problems. All sports, hobbies such as gardening and often sex have to be abandoned. Impotence is common even in the absence of thiazides. Foreign travel becomes difficult and can be hazardous. It is hardly surprising that patients get depressed.

Predictors of Death in Cardiac Failure

- Low serum Na^+
- Wide QRS on ECG
- High noradrenaline levels
- Low LVEF
- High BNP level >300 pg/ml
- Microvolt T-wave alternans
- Cardiac cachexia with >7.5% body weight loss.

Signs to Look for

- An exhausted, ill-looking patient; dyspnoeic at rest or after minor effort.
- Cool hands and feet with peripheral cyanosis; muscle wasting.
- Blood pressure: low systolic pressure with low pulse pressure. Check no paradox.
- Raised JVP. Prominent systolic wave of TR. Kussmaul's sign should be negative. Prominent 'x' and 'y' descents in restrictive cardiomyopathy. Prominent veins over shoulders, chest, abdomen and legs.
- Low volume pulse. Resting tachycardia. Possible pulsus alternans (Figure 6.1). May be in fast AF. Check for possible anacrotic pulse in occult aortic stenosis.
- Displaced apex with LV dilatation. Thrusting apex of hypertensive heart failure. May have high diffuse paradoxical apex of LV aneurysm. Systolic apical thrill in ruptured mitral chordae. Double apex of LV hypertrophy in sinus rhythm.

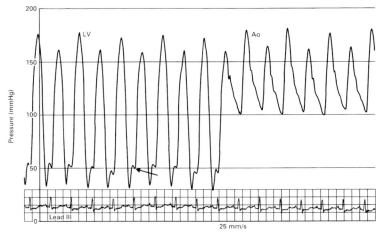

Figure 6.1 Catheter withdrawal from left ventricle (LV) to aorta (Ao) in a patient with LV failure. There is a very high left ventricular end-diastolic pressure (LVEDP; arrowed) of 50 mmHg. There is also pulsus alternans in the peak LV pressure and the aortic pressure trace.

- RV heave in pulmonary hypertension or with TR. Severe MR may produce a sensation similar to an RV heave as a result of systolic expansion of the LA.
- Auscultation: S3 gallop is the most important sign of all. Signs of organic aortic or mitral valve disease. May just have functional mitral and/or tricuspid pansystolic murmurs. In low-output states, murmur of severe aortic stenosis may not be heard. Loud honking systolic murmur of torn mitral xenograft or diastolic murmur of torn aortic xenograft. More continuous murmur of ruptured sinus of Valsalva.
- Smooth hepatomegaly. Pulsatile liver with TR.
- Ascites with TR and RVF.
- Leg oedema. Check sacral pad. Oedema is more easily seen round the lower back than on anterior abdominal wall.
- Ventilation pattern: hyperventilation if in acute pulmonary oedema. Cheyne–Stokes ventilation in a sedated patient with a very low-output state.
- Chest: bilateral basal effusions. Expiratory wheeze. Bubbly cough. Fine basal crepitations are an unreliable sign of pulmonary oedema. In addition check for signs of possible infective endocarditis (see Chapter 9).

Differential Diagnosis

Pulmonary Oedema (Figure 6.2)
Mitral stenosis, cor triatriatum and atrial myxoma may all present in pulmonary oedema with perfectly normal ventricular function. The murmurs may

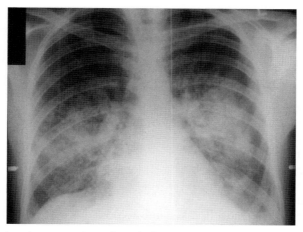

Figure 6.2 Acute pulmonary oedema: 'batswing' appearance. Note small heart. Restrictive cardiomyopathy.

be very difficult to hear in an acutely breathless patient. Echocardiography is diagnostic.

Pulmonary oedema may occur with low LA pressures with sepsis, noxious gas inhalation, severe myxoedema, hypoalbuminaemia, head injury, subarachnoid haemorrhage or adult respiratory distress syndrome.

RV Failure

The most important differential is from pericardial constriction. This is covered in Section 10.3. Also consider SVC obstruction (non-pulsatile neck veins), malignant ascites with liver secondaries, nephrotic syndrome and pelvic nodes causing lymphatic obstruction, and leg oedema.

6.3 Concepts of Treatment

Neuroendocrine Activation

The concept of treating both acute LV failure and chronic CCF with afterload reduction is now firmly established. In heart failure there is an inappropriately raised systemic vascular resistance caused by a combination of sympathetic overdrive and activation of the renin–angiotensin system. Neuroendocrine activation results in raised levels of angiotensin II, noradrenaline and arginine vasopressin (antidiuretic hormone, ADH). Endothelin levels (released from vascular endothelium) are also raised in heart failure, contributing to the vasoconstriction. The use of inotropes on top of this vasoconstriction may increase afterload and cardiac work still further.

On top of this there is an increased cytokine release and raised levels of TNF-α contribute to cardiac cachexia. There is a reduction in fibrinolytic activity, plus myocyte starvation and increased apoptosis.

Natriuretic Peptides

Raised levels of atrial natriuretic peptide (ANP) and brain natriuretic peptide (BNP) also occur in heart failure. They promote a natriuresis and arterial and venous dilatation, and inhibit ADH and aldosterone release. However, their effects are overwhelmed by the other neuroendocrine activation mechanisms described above. B-type natriuretic peptide is synthesized by myocardial cells in response to raised ventricular filling pressure.

Levels are raised in heart failure, but false positives may occur in:

- AF
- LV hypertrophy
- pulmonary emboli
- acute coronary syndromes
- renal failure.

The clinical picture must be taken into account. Levels >100 pg/ml indicate heart failure and this cut-off level is a very sensitive (90%) and specific (76%) test, helping to differentiate pulmonary from cardiac causes of dyspnoea. In severe heart failure levels are much higher. High BNP levels carry a poor prognosis (e.g. >300 pg/ml), particularly if levels do not fall on treatment.

BNP has been found to be better than peak Vo_{2max} at predicting adverse cardiac events.

6.4 Cardiac Failure Treatment

The use of inotropes to flog a failing heart raises problems other than increasing cardiac work:

- No oral agent other than digoxin has been shown to be safe and effective in long-term trials
- Increased myocardial oxygen consumption
- Possible increase in infarct size
- Arrhythmias with increased myocardial excitability (β_1 effect)
- Increased heart rate with shorter diastolic coronary flow
- Possible vasoconstrictor effect on coronary arterioles (α effect)
- Central-line administration needed with most drugs.

In view of these, heart failure is managed with bed rest, diuretics and vasodilating agents. Vasodilators are divided into three groups.

1 *Venodilators*: reduce preload by dilating venous capacitance vessels, e.g. nitrates, some diuretics. They lower filling pressures without initially much improvement in stroke volume. At higher doses they also become arterial dilators.

2 *Arterial dilators*: reduce afterload. Dilate arterial resistance vessels, e.g. hydralazine. They improve stroke volume without much reduction in filling pressure or pulmonary venous pressure.

3 *Combined arterial and venous dilators*: drugs such as nitroprusside and α-blocking agents. These improve stroke volume and reduce filling pressure. They are very useful in LVF.

A wide variety of vasodilating drugs are now available (Table 6.1).

Table 6.1 Vasodilating drugs in heart failure

Drug	Arterial dilator	Venous dilator	Oral dose (mg)	Intravenous dose (adult) (mg)	Side effects other than hypotension
Captopril	++	+	6.25–50 three times daily	–	Dry cough, loss of taste, abdominal pain, stomatitis, leukopenia, proteinuria, hyperkalaemia, rashes
Diazoxide	++	+	100 three times daily	150 at 5- to 10-min intervals	Diabetes mellitus, action intravenous not sustained, fluid retention
Hydralazine	+++	–	25 three times daily to 150 four times daily	20 over 5 min (0.3 mg/kg)	Lupoid reaction (>200 mg/day), fluid retention, tachyphylaxis
Isosorbide dinitrate	(+)	+++	10 6-hourly to 30 4-hourly	1–7 mg/h	Headaches, nausea
Minoxidil	++	+	2.5 twice daily to 10 three times daily	–	Hirsutism, gut disturbances, fluid retention, breast tenderness
Nitroprusside	+++	+++	–	1–6 µg/kg per min	Cyanide toxicity, metabolic acidosis, hypothyroidism
Phentolamine	+++	+	50 mg four times daily	5–10 i.v. stat 10–20 µg/kg per min	Diarrhoea, flushing, tachycardia
Phenoxybenzamine	+++	+	10 mg at night to 30 mg twice daily	10–40 slowly i.v.	Paralytic ileus – dry mouth, impotence
Prazosin	++	++	0.5 mg test dose 1–10 mg three times daily	–	First-dose syncope, drowsiness, impotence, tachyphylaxis
Salbutamol	+	(+)	4–8 mg three times daily	10–40 µg/min	Tremor, hyperglycaemia, apparent hypokalaemia
Trimetaphan	++	+	–	3 mg/min	Tachycardia

Choice of Vasodilators

LV Failure (Acute) with Pulmonary Oedema and Normotension

Examples are acute mitral regurgitation, septal infarction with VSD; acute infarction in normotensive patient:
• nitroprusside: if full haemodynamic monitoring available, with intravenous furosemide.

If no monitoring facilities available other than ECG:
• furosemide i.v. + isosorbide dinitrate or glyceryl trinitrate i.v., then
• oral isosorbide dinitrate + ACE inhibitor + oral diuretic as the patient improves.

The great majority of patients with LVF can be managed with this regimen without the need for arterial pressure monitoring.

Low-output States

Hypotensive, cool, oligaemic patients (so-called 'forward failure'):
• Dopamine (see Inotropes, Section 6.9), monitoring haemodynamics. Once normotension is restored, addition of nitroprusside may be beneficial. Alternatively dobutamine if urine output satisfactory.

Chronic CCF (Oral Therapy Only) in Combination

• Furosemide (+ amiloride or spironolactone) if hypokalaemic
• ACE inhibitor, especially if hypertensive
• Long-acting nitrate once or twice daily
• Digoxin if in AF, large heart on chest radiograph or audible S_3
• Warfarin if large heart or in AF
• No added salt to food (allow a little for cooking in most cases).

The systolic arterial pressure and renal function will dictate the dose of ACE inhibitor possible and whether the patient will tolerate other vasodilators such as nitrates. The aim should always be to maximize the vasodilator therapy and to use the minimal amount of diuretics possible. However, some patients will need quite vigorous diuretic therapy to cope with systemic oedema. Spironolactone 25–50 mg three times daily is very useful in this situation. Start with 25 mg once daily if the patient is already on an ACE inhibitor (see Section 6.6).

For refractory oedema not responding to increasing doses of intravenous furosemide, consider:
• two-dimensional echocardiography to exclude pericardial collection or constriction
• fluid restriction to 1500 or even 1000 ml daily
• a furosemide infusion at 0.5–1 mg/min for 4 h
• oral metolazone 2.5 mg up to 10 mg daily
• spironolactone 25–50 mg two to three times daily, or eplerenone 25 mg once daily
• low-dose dopamine through a central line: 5–10 µg/kg per min
• haemofiltration/ultrafiltration.

Prazosin has not been included because of its tachyphylactic problem and hypotensive first-dose effect. Hydralazine is less used now, because tachyphylaxis is also a problem, the lupus syndrome may occur in doses >150 mg/day (see Section 6.7), and ACE inhibitors have been shown to be superior in the VHeFT II study. Calcium antagonists should be avoided. The ACE inhibitors have revolutionized the treatment of chronic CCF following the demonstration of reduced mortality in the CONSENSUS trial in patients taking enalapril.

Peripheral Ultrafiltration

Ultrafiltration was first used by Lunderquist in 1952 to treat excessive oedema. It is now possible using portable equipment for up to 8 h only, needing peripheral venous cannulation with minimal dead space (e.g. 33 ml). This is an efficient way of gradually removing fluid in patients who are diuretic resistant. Renal function need not deteriorate, the risks of central venous cannulation can be avoided and hospital stay can be reduced.

6.5 Drugs in Acute LVF

Intravenous Nitrates
See Section 5.4.

Intravenous Sodium Nitroprusside (SNP)

Controlled infusion of nitroprusside is of great value in the treatment of acute LVF (e.g. ruptured chordae), the management of hypertensive crises and the post-cardiac surgical control of hypertension. It can be used to lower blood pressure in aortic dissection before surgery.

Its great advantage is its rapid onset and equally rapid cessation of action on switching the infusion off. A computerized feedback technique is available in which automatic control of the SNP infusion rate is governed by the arterial pressure.

It is a potent dilator of arteries and veins by acting locally on vascular smooth muscle. Infusion preparations include the following.

Weak Solution
• Dissolve 50 mg SNP (Nipride) in 2 ml 5% dextrose; add this to 500 ml 5% dextrose. Infusion strength 100 mg/l (100 µg/ml). Start at 1 µg/kg per min (40–70 µg/min usually). Maximum infusion rate 400 µg/min.
• Wrap infusion bottle/paediatric giving set/infusion line in aluminium foil to protect from light.
• Renew infusion every 4 h. Must be in a separate line from bicarbonate.

Strong Solution
This is often easier to manage clinically and involves smaller volume load:
• Add 50 mg SNP to 100 ml 5% dextrose solution (in paediatric giving set) = 500 µg/ml.

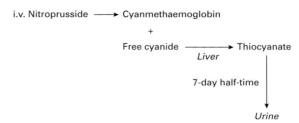

Figure 6.3 Nitroprusside metabolism.

• Then 6 drops/min (paediatric microdrops) = 50 μg/min; 12 drops/min = 100 μg/min; 30 drops/min = 250 μg/min, etc.

Cyanide Toxicity
Over 90% of cyanide released from nitroprusside is bound by erythrocytes. Cyanide free in plasma is freely diffusible and causes a cytotoxic hypoxia by inhibition of cytochromic oxidase. Cyanide is slowly metabolized to thiocyanate (Figure 6.3):
• Toxicity is related more to the rate of infusion than to total dose, but care must be taken once a total dose of 50 mg is exceeded.
• Plasma cyanide or thiocyanate levels are not necessarily a reliable guide to toxicity.
• A metabolic acidosis (arterial lactate from anaerobic metabolism) occurs with cyanide toxicity, but may not necessarily be caused by it. However, it is the easiest guide to nitroprusside dose and usually reverses quickly when the infusion is stopped.

Summary of Nitroprusside Infusion
• Monitor arterial and preferably PAW pressure
• Frequent measurement of acid–base balance
• Keep levels as below (if assays available):
  – plasma cyanide <3 μmol/l
  – plasma thiocyanate <100 μg/ml
  – red cell cyanide <75 μg/100 ml.
• Maximum infusion rate <400 μg/min (approximately 5–6 μg/kg per min in adults).
Toxic levels of thiocyanate may cause hypothyroidism. If possible, nitroprusside infusion should not be used for >48 h.

Hydroxycobalamin infusion given at the same time as SNP infusion reduces plasma cyanide levels (forming cyanocobalamin). This infusion also has to be protected from light. Dose of vitamin B_{12} = 25 mg/h (mixture of 100 mg vitamin B_{12} in 100 ml 5% dextrose).

Emergency Treatment of Cyanide Toxicity
• Amyl nitrite inhalation or isosorbide dinitrate i.v. (increase methaemoglobin)

- Sodium thiosulphate injections
- Bicarbonate for lactic acidosis
- Hydroxycobalamin infusion.

6.6 Drugs in Chronic CCF

ACE Inhibitors (Table 6.2)

These are a group of drugs that inhibit the conversion of inactive angiotensin I to the powerful vasoconstrictor angiotensin II. At present there are 10 ACE inhibitors available in the UK, but there will be many more in the next few years. The profound vasoconstrictor effect of angiotensin II is reduced. They work in CCF where other drugs have failed and have a sustained action. They may be useful even when plasma renin activity is low. This may be mediated by reduction of bradykinin degradation and activation of prostaglandin production.

Some are prodrugs converted in the liver to the active metabolite (e.g. enalapril, cilazapril) and this may delay onset of action after an oral dose. At present there seems little to choose between all these long-acting drugs.

Starting Therapy with ACE Inhibitors

Hypertensive patients can be safely started on ACE inhibitors as outpatients with the first dose taken on going to bed at night. They should be warned of possible initial postural hypotension. A small dose of a long-acting ACE inhibitor (e.g. enalapril 2.5 mg or lisinopril 2.5 mg) can be used safely.

Patients with CCF are best started on ACE inhibitors under close supervision in hospital. Again the first dose is given at night and captopril, the only short-acting drug, should be used. It is important that the patient is not hypovolaemic, and if on diuretics with invisible neck veins the diuretic should be stopped for 48 h before starting the captopril. Once the patient is comfortably established on captopril, the drug can be switched to a longer-acting agent.

Problems and Side Effects with ACE Inhibitors

- *Hypotension*: this is the most common problem, especially with the first dose. Severe hypotension can result in a neurological deficit or renal failure. It is important to make sure that patients are not hypovolaemic or severely hyponatraemic (excess diuretics) before starting treatment. May need intravenous physiological (0.9%) saline.
- *Chronic cough*: this is the most common and most irritating side effect of ACE inhibitors and possessed by all the drugs. It is one of the chief reasons for dose limitation. It is probably a result of bradykinin levels being increased by ACE inhibition. It responds to a reduction in dose, but not often to cough suppressants. One trial has suggested that low-dose oral iron therapy (e.g. ferrous sulphate 200 mg once daily) is of benefit.
- *Loss of taste*: this or abnormal taste (dysgeusia) may be due to the –SH (sulphydryl) group in some drugs. Aphthous ulcers may develop.

Table 6.2 ACE inhibitors

Drug (proprietary name(s)	Starting dose (mg)	Maximum dose (mg)	Doses daily	Pro-drug	Half-life (h)	Metabolism and excretion
Captopril (Capoten, Acepril)	6.25 three times daily	50 three times daily	3	No	3	Has –SH group. Liver and kidney. Rapid onset action
Enalapril (Innovate)	2.5 once daily	40 once daily	1	Yes	6	No –SH group. Liver to active enalaprilat
Lisinopril (Carace, Zestril)	2.5 once daily	40 once daily	1	No	12	No –SH group. Renal excretion only, unchanged
Cilazapril (Vascace)	0.5 once daily	5 once daily	1	Yes	9	Liver to active cilazaprilat. Renal excretion only unchanged
Fosinopril (Staril)	10 once daily	40 once daily	1	Yes	11	Liver to active fosinoprilat. Liver and kidney excretion
Moexipil (Perdix)	7.5 once daily	30 once daily	1	Yes	14	Liver to active moexiprilat. Renal and faecal excretion
Perindopril (Coversyl)	2 once daily	8 once daily	1	Yes	25	Liver to active perindoprilat. Renal excretion
Trandalopril (Gopten Odrik)	0.5 once daily	4 once daily	1	Yes	16–24	Liver to trandaloprilat. Renal and faecal excretion
Quinapril (Accupro)	2.5 once daily	40 once daily	1	Yes	4	Liver to active quinalprilat
Ramipril (Tritace)	1.25 once daily	10 once daily	1	Yes	15	Binding to tissue ACE ++. Renal and hepatic excretion

• *Hyperkalaemia*: this results from a reduction in aldosterone. Care is needed with potassium-retaining diuretics.
• *Deteriorating renal function*: this may be caused by hypotension and 'prerenal failure'. In hypertensive patients with pre-treatment normal renal function, who suddenly deteriorate on ACE inhibitors, consider renal artery stenosis. Deteriorating renal function is the most common long-term reason for restricting or reducing the dose. Careful monitoring of blood urea and creatinine is needed.
• *Urticaria and angioneurotic oedema*: ACE inhibitors should be avoided if there is a history of angio-oedema from any cause.
• *Rarely*: proteinuria, leukopenia, fatigue, exhaustion.
• *False-positive urine test for ketones* (captopril).

There is little evidence to suggest that ACE inhibitors without the –SH group (e.g. enalapril and lisinopril) may have fewer side effects, e.g. with taste problems, than captopril. There is no rebound hypertension on stopping ACE inhibitors.

Contraindications to ACE Inhibitor Treatment
• Severe renal failure, serum creatinine >300 μmol/l
• Hyperkalaemia
• Hypovolaemia
• Hyponatraemia
• Pregnancy or lactating mothers
• LV outflow obstruction
• Hypotension, peak systolic pressures <90 mmHg
• Cor pulmonale
• Renal artery stenosis.

Use with Other Drugs

Digoxin and Diuretics
ACE inhibitors can be safely used with digoxin and diuretics (care with volume and sodium depletion).

Aldosterone Antagonists: Spironolactone and Eplerenone
Spironolactone 25 mg daily can be used with ACE inhibitors and the risk of hyperkalaemia is small but must be checked. The dose of spironolactone can be increased to 50 mg daily watching the plasma K^+ level. The combination has proved very effective in heart failure with a 27% reduction in annual all-cause mortality in the RALES trial. ACE inhibitors may be used in combination with other hypotensive agents if necessary, e.g. nitrates and β blockers. The effect is synergistic.

A newer selective aldosterone blocker, eplerenone 25–50 mg daily, has also been shown to reduce mortality, or hospitalization in patients developing LVF after a myocardial infarct (EPHESUS trial). Eplerenone selectively blocks the mineralocorticoid but not the glucocorticoid receptor, and hence does not cause the gynaecomastia and impotence associated with spironolactone. Both drugs should be avoided in severe renal failure.

Spironolactone is generic and is much cheaper than eplerenone; eplerenone should be tried only if side effects are a problem.

Angiotensin II Receptor Antagonists (AIIRAs)

Dual blockade with an ACE inhibitor and an AIIRA blocker is of added benefit in CCF. Regular checks for possible hyperkalaemia are needed and volume depletion with diuretics may produce hypotension. In people with diabetes dual blockade has been shown to reduce proteinuria, improve BP control and reduce progression to end-stage renal failure.

The CHARM added trial showed a 15% further risk reduction when candesartan was added to conventional ACE inhibitor therapy in patients with cardiac failure. However, there was no benefit in the ValHEFT study when valsartan 160 mg once daily was added to conventional treatment. This may have been a result of inadequate dosing with valsartan, but a class effect cannot be assumed with ARBs.

Management of Hyperkalaemia

• Discontinue potassium-sparing diuretics, potassium supplements, ACE inhibitors, AIIRAs, non-steroidal anti-inflammatory agents and salt substitutes.
• Restrict intake of fresh fruit, fruit juice and vegetables (rich in potassium).
• Add 12 units soluble insulin (Actrapid) to 50 ml 50% glucose and infuse over 15 min. This should temporarily lower the serum K^+ by 1 mmol/l for about 2 h. If K^+ is still >6.5 mmol/l repeat the regimen and contact the renal team.
• Check arterial blood gases for a metabolic acidosis. If base excess >5 give 50 ml sodium bicarbonate 8.4% slowly intravenously, and repeat blood gases. Dose may need repeating.
• If ECG changes of hyperkalaemia present (see Section 16.1) give 10 ml 10% calcium chloride slowly intravenously but not in the same line or vein as sodium bicarbonate.
• Consider calcium resonium 15 g three times daily orally or 30 g enema (8% w/w calcium). This causes constipation and a laxative, e.g. co-danthramer, must also be given.
• Severe unresponsive cases may need haemafiltration.

ACE Inhibitors with Normal LV Function

The HOPE trial has shown an improved outcome for high-risk patients with known vascular disease or diabetes plus one other risk factor for coronary disease who were given ramipril 10 mg daily for 5 years. These patients were not known to have LV dysfunction. Ramipril reduced cardiovascular deaths from 8.1% to 6.1% (absolute risk reduction 2%, relative risk reduction 26%), and similarly reduced myocardial infarcts, strokes, deaths from any cause, revascularization procedures and diabetic complications. The beneficial effects of ramipril were thought not just to be the result of its action of lowering blood pressure but also possibly the result of long-term changes in the vessel wall inhibiting tissue ACE.

Drugs in Asymptomatic LV Dysfunction

ACE inhibitors started in asymptomatic patients with mediocre LV function (LVEF <35%) help prevent the development of clinical heart failure and reduce long-term mortality slightly (8% in the SOLVD trial using enalapril). Patients with large hearts on the chest radiograph or poor ejection fractions should be started on ACE inhibitors whether or not they have symptoms.

Angiotensin Receptor Antagonists (AT$_1$-receptor Antagonists, ARBs, AIIRAs) (Table 6.3)

Figure 6.4 shows the difference in site of action of these drugs compared with ACE inhibitors. Bradykinin is a vasodilator and thought to be responsible for the ACE inhibitor cough. Its degradation is not inhibited by AT$_1$-receptor antagonists. Hence, theoretically these drugs might not be quite as effective as ACE inhibitors in heart failure. Losartan has been shown to improve haemodynamics in CCF and was not superior to captopril in the ELITE II trial. There is no evidence yet that this class of drugs is superior to ACE inhibitors in heart failure management. More trials are needed.

ARBs should be used in CCF:
- when patients are unable to tolerate the ACE inhibitors cough
- when patients are intolerant of β blockers; use an ACE inhibitor in combination with ARAs.

Table 6.3 Angiotensin II receptor antagonists available in the UK

Drug	Trade name	Starting daily dose (mg)	Maximum daily dose (mg)	Tablets available (mg)
Candesartan cilexitil	Amias	2 once daily	32 once daily	2, 4, 8, 16
Eprosartan	Teveten	300 once daily	800 once daily	300, 400, 600
Irbesartan	Aprovel	75 once daily (age >75)	300 once daily	75, 150, 300 150 once daily (age <75)
Losartan potassium	Cozaar	25 once daily	100 once daily	25, 50, 100
Olmesartan medoxomil	Olmetec	10 once daily	40 once daily	10, 20, 40
Telmisartan	Micardis	20 once daily	80 once daily	20, 40, 80
Valsartan	Diovan	40 once daily	160 twice daily	40, 80, 160

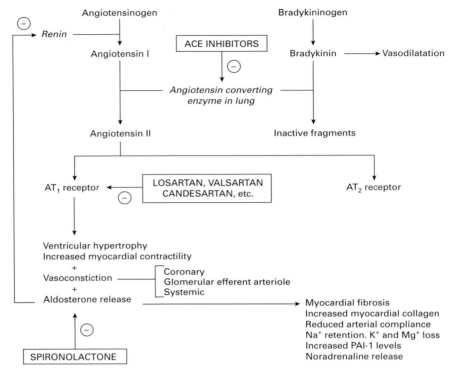

Figure 6.4 Angiotensin actions and sites of drug inhibition.

• patients remaining symptomatic when already on optimum doses of ACE inhibitor and β blockers.

For details of use in combination with ACE inhibitors, see above.

6.7 Drugs of Second Choice in Heart Failure

Hydralazine

This drug causes arteriolar vasodilatation and a rise in stroke volume. Its inotropic effect may be primary or secondary to vasodilatation. It does not reduce PCWP or systemic venous pressure to any great extent. In heart failure a compensatory reflex tachycardia does not necessarily occur. It has potent antioxidant effects by inhibiting NADPH oxidase.

Starting oral dose is 25 mg three times daily (half-life 2–8 h). It is acetylated in the liver and excreted in the urine.

The Lupus Syndrome

This is more likely to develop in patients who:

• receive >200 mg daily (check ANF and LE cells)
• are slow acetylators
• have histocompatibility locus DR4.

However, the lupus syndrome may occur on doses <200 mg daily. Positive ANF is not an indication to stop the drug, because it occurs in 30–60% patients receiving hydralazine for ≥3 years, but lupus occurs in only 1–3%. The lupus syndrome is less common in black patients. It is fully but slowly reversible on stopping the drug.

Tachyphylaxis
Unfortunately, recent reports suggest that long-term tolerance to the drug occurs, possibly as a result of reduction in the number of receptor sites in the arterial wall, or of a change in the receptor itself.

Benefit from acute administration may not persist and a change of drug may be necessary. The drug may cause fluid retention and should be used with a diuretic.

Parenteral Administration
This is possible in emergency situations (e.g. severe hypertension, pre-eclampsia). The drug can be given intramuscularly (20 mg) or slowly intravenously (20 mg slowly over 5 min).

A-HeFT trial
Recently a combination of hydralazine and isosorbide dinitrate has been shown to be particularly beneficial in black patients with grade III or IV heart failure. After a mean follow-up of 10 months in 1050 patients in the A-HeFT trial, all-cause mortality was reduced from 10.2% to 6.2% in patients receiving this combination when compared with standard treatment. Although this drug regimen has a relatively short follow-up period it should be considered in refractory heart failure.

Prazosin
This acts on α_1-receptors in the vessel wall and causes arterial and venous dilatation. Unfortunately tachyphylaxis is a problem.

The initial dose is 0.5 mg taken on going to bed. In spite of this a few patients develop first-dose syncope, which limits its use. If the test dose is taken satisfactorily, then the patient is started on 1 mg three times daily.

The drug is well absorbed after oral administration (half-life 3–4 h). It is probably more useful in hypertension than chronic heart failure.

Care should be taken in using nitrites with prazosin, as both are powerful venodilators and may cause syncope when taken together. Although prazosin reduces systemic vascular resistance, renal plasma flow is reduced and fluid retention may result.

Salbutamol
This β_2 agonist causes arterial dilatation, an increase in stroke index and also an increase in heart rate. It does not restore normotension in the hypotensive patient with LVF. It is not suitable for the patient in acute pulmonary oedema.

It causes tremor. It shifts potassium into the cells and causes an apparent hypokalaemia. It causes restlessness and insomnia.

α-Blocking Agents

Phenoxybenzamine, Phentolamine

These drugs can be used in the management of acute LVF, but nitroprusside is better because of its more pronounced venodilating properties.

They are more useful in hypertensive crises or management of phaeochromocytoma. Phenoxybenzamine may be of some use in coping with severe Raynaud's phenomenon.

Of these two drugs, phentolamine may be the more useful in heart failure by having a weak inotropic effect (noradrenaline release) as well as α-blocking properties.

Diazoxide

This is rarely used now in hypertension or LVF. Acute intravenous administration (150–300 mg) causes a sudden fall in blood pressure, but the fall is not sustained and the dose needs to be repeated in 10–15 min. Chronic use causes diabetes mellitus. It also causes fluid retention. Infusion of diazoxide is not as hypotensive as bolus administration.

Minoxidil

This drug causes salt and water retention and is not suitable for chronic heart failure. It is more useful in hypertension and must be given with a diuretic. Hirsutism limits its use to men. Reflex tachycardia requires additional β blockade. The drug has a long half-life (1–4 days) and can be given as a single oral dose daily (starting 5 mg once daily) initially.

6.8 Digoxin

Controversy about the value of digoxin in patients with cardiac failure continues even 210 years after its discovery by Withering. The large DIG mortality trial showed that digoxin reduced hospital admissions caused by heart failure but did not reduce overall mortality in a randomized trial against placebo of 7700 patients in whom digoxin levels were measured. In the RADIANCE trial patients with heart failure already on an ACE inhibitor fared worse if their digoxin was withdrawn, with more hospital readmissions. The benefit of digoxin appears to be on symptomatic improvement rather than mortality reduction. It is, however, the only inotrope that has not been shown to increase mortality in the long term in patients with heart failure.

Action

Digoxin is thought to inhibit the action of sarcolemmal membrane Na^+/K^+ ATPase, inhibiting the sodium pump. This allows greater influx of sodium and displacement of bound intracellular calcium. The increase in calcium availability exerts the inotropic effect. Other effects of digoxin are:

- AV node refractory period prolonged
- AV node conduction slowed
- mild peripheral vasoconstriction (arteries and veins)
- vagotonic effect
- automaticity increased (myocardial excitability)
- possible acceleration of bypass conduction in WPW syndrome.

Its inotropic effect is much weaker than that of sympathomimetic inotropes.

Indications

CCF with AF
This is the classic situation for digoxin. Its effect on the AV node slows ventricular response to fast AF, and its positive inotropic effect helps the dilated failing left ventricle increase its stroke volume.

Control of Chronic AF (e.g. Mitral Valve Disease)
The drug is used for its effect on the AV node; however, in some cases additional therapy with a β blocker or verapamil may be needed.

Management of Paroxysmal AF
Digoxin is of no value in the management of paroxysmal AF unless the episodes are frequent and prolonged, when it may help control ventricular rate when it occurs. The most effective drug is amiodarone, but side effects limit its use. Flecainide or propafenone should be considered as alternatives and are effective at reducing frequency and length of episodes. Quinidine is rarely used now (see Section 8.9).

Heart Failure in Children
Digoxin is still the mainstay of therapy.

CCF and Sinus Rhythm
Several studies have claimed that digoxin is of benefit in this situation and that the effect is sustained. The presence of a third sound is a strong correlate of a good response to digoxin. However, not all patients benefit from digoxin and, in a group of patients already on the drug, about a third deteriorate when it is withdrawn. Two digoxin withdrawal trials (RADIANCE and PROVED) showed that patients who remained on digoxin had fewer readmissions for heart failure.

Thus, digoxin is not the drug of first choice in CCF with sinus rhythm. If bed rest, diuretics and vasodilators do not achieve or maintain an improvement, digoxin should be tried. It is likely to help in patients who:

- have a third sound with a large heart
- do not have valvar obstruction.

Once heart failure has been controlled and the heart is smaller, digoxin may be withdrawn under supervision.

The following are conditions for which digoxin is no longer the drug choice:
- SVT: this is better managed with intraveous verapamil or adenosine.
- Sinoatrial disease: this is probably better managed with β blockade, amiodarone and/or pacing.
- Cor pulmonale: there are no studies to show that it helps. The side effects of digoxin could be dangerous. It can be used only if the patient is in AF.
- MI, unless the patient is in AF.
- Valvar or subvalvar aortic stenosis, unless the patient is in uncontrolled AF. Digoxin will increase the gradient in muscular subaortic obstruction (HCM).
- Hypertensive heart failure: this is better managed with afterload reduction.

Contraindications
- WPW syndrome
- HCM, unless in AF with end-stage LV dilatation
- Second- or third-degree AV block: chronic first-degree AV block is not a contraindication to digoxin, although acute prolongation of the PR interval (e.g. MI, infective endocarditis) is more dangerous and patients should be monitored carefully
- Patients with recurrent ventricular arrhythmias.

Avoiding digoxin toxicity is particularly important in the following situations:
- Before DC cardioversion
- Severe renal failure (creatinine clearance <10 ml/min)
- Cardiac amyloidosis.

Digitalization

Acute Intravenous
This is not often necessary and the patient should be normokalaemic. Use digoxin 0.25 mg i.v. 2-hourly until effect is achieved; usually 0.75–1 mg is required. Using intermittent doses of 0.25 mg i.v. is safer than a bolus dose of 0.75–1 mg over 30 min. After control of the fast AF, the patient is maintained on 0.125 mg i.v. as required 4-hourly.

Oral
The loading dose depends on lean body mass, because skeletal muscle binds digoxin. It is necessary only if a rapid result is required. Often patients can be started on the maintenance dose. Loading dose is 1.0–1.5 mg orally for a 70 kg adult; maintenance dose depends on renal function and is 0.25 mg.

Larger doses (≤0.5 mg daily) may be required, but care must be taken and, with larger doses, plasma levels are helpful.

A useful compromise in the absence of an emergency is to use digoxin 0.25 mg twice daily for 2 days then 0.25 mg once daily. Digoxin can be given intramuscularly if necessary, but not subcutaneously (very irritant).

Plasma Levels

Normal level for satisfactory therapeutic effect is 0.8–2 ng/ml (1–2.5 nmol/l). Blood is taken 6–8 h after an oral dose. Serum half-life is 30 h. However, the level should never be used as more than a guide and the clinical effect must be taken into consideration, i.e. levels >2 ng/ml do not necessarily mean digoxin toxicity unless the patient's condition or ECG is consistent with this.

Very high plasma levels are associated with acute intravenous administration (e.g. ≤100 ng/ml), but these levels are transient and not toxic.

If the required effect is not achieved with plasma levels of 3–4 ng/ml then additional therapy with β blockade or verapamil should be used.

Approximately 20–40% of digoxin is bound to plasma proteins. Most digoxin is excreted unchanged by the kidney by both filtration and active tubular secretion. About 10% is excreted in the stools, and a smaller percentage metabolized in the liver.

Reduction in Digoxin Dose

This is required in the following situations:

• Symptoms of digoxin toxicity: anorexia, nausea, vomiting, xanthopsia (very rare), neurological symptoms (paraesthesiae, fits, mental confusion), gynaecomastia, etc.

• ECG changes: functional bradycardia, ventricular bigeminy, salvos of ventricular ectopics or paroxysmal VT. Second- or third-degree AV block. Paroxysmal atrial tachycardia with varying block (PATB) may be a sign of digoxin toxicity in patients who are fully digitalized. The digoxin effect on the ECG is not an indication to reduce the dose.

• Other drug therapy: several drugs increase plasma digoxin levels, possibly by protein displacement, reduced renal clearance or diminished distribution to the tissues. In several cases the cause is unknown.

Drugs increasing plasma digoxin are:

• quinidine
• captopril: reduced renal clearance
• amiodarone
• propafenone
• verapamil
• nifedipine
• nitrendipine: displacement from protein binding
• erythromycin
• tetracycline: reduction in gastrointestinal bacteria which convert digoxin to inactive dihydrodigoxin.

Patients on any of these drugs should be on half the expected digoxin dose:
• Development of renal failure: plasma digoxin levels may help. Digitoxin does not need dose reduction in renal failure. If creatinine clearance <10 ml/min, it is probably better to avoid digoxin altogether. Dose 10–25 ml/min, 0.0625–0.125 mg daily; 25–50 ml/min, 0.125 mg/0.25 mg alternate days; 50 ml/min, 0.25 mg daily. Cardiac glycosides are not removed by dialysis.
• Elderly people require a smaller dose of digoxin. The paediatric 0.0625 mg tablets are small and blue and are easily recognizable. If digoxin is necessary, they can usually be managed on 0.0625–0.125 mg/day.
• Increased sensitivity to digoxin occurs in the following conditions and dose reduction may be necessary: hypokalaemia, hypercalcaemia, hypoxia, chronic pulmonary disease, hypomagnesaemia (e.g. chronic diarrhoea or prolonged diuresis), hypothyroidism.

Increase in Digoxin Dose
This may be needed in patients taking:
• cholestyramine: binds digoxin to the resin
• phenytoin
• rifampicin: increased hepatic metabolism
• sulfasalazine
• neomycin
• malabsorption syndromes: delayed absorption
• cancer chemotherapy: damage to gut mucosa may delay absorption.

Children
Paediatric digoxin elixir (lime flavour) contains 0.05 mg/ml. Children tend to need more digoxin than their small weight would suggest. Digitalizing dose is 0.01 mg/kg 6-hourly until therapeutic effect is obtained; maintenance dose is 0.01 mg/kg per day. Toxicity in children: sinus bradycardia, vomiting, drowsiness. AV block is not as common as in adults.

Digoxin Overdose
The development of digoxin antibodies has made a great difference to the therapy of digoxin overdose. Infusion of the antibody fragment Fab (raised in sheep) rapidly reverses the toxic effects of digoxin. The dose is calculated from the plasma digoxin concentration assuming an interval of >6h from ingestion.

Digoxin load (mg) = Plasma concentration (ng/ml) × Body weight (kg) × 0.0056

Antibody load needed (mg) = 60 × Digoxin body load.

If digitoxin has been ingested the factor 0.00056 is used not 0.0056. The Fab fragments are excreted in the urine (half-life 16h). With reduction in serum digoxin, hypokalaemia may result as potassium goes back into the cells. Hypersensitivity and anaphylactic reaction are a theoretical possibility because this is a sheep protein. Drug trade name: Digibind –40 mg of Fab fragments/vial.

6.9 Inotropic Sympathomimetic Drugs

Most inotropic drugs work by increasing the level of intracellular cAMP, which with intracellular calcium promotes contractility. The increase in cAMP may be achieved by:
- stimulation of β-receptors, i.e.
  - β_1: isoprenaline, dobutamine, dopamine, ibopamine
  - β_2: salbutamol, terbutaline, pirbuterol, prenalterol, dopexamine
- stimulation of glucagon receptor: glucagon
- stimulation of H_2-receptor: histamine
- inhibition of phosphodiesterase, the enzyme that converts cAMP to inactive 5'-AMP; there are many drugs in this group, e.g.
  - bipyridines: amrinone, milrinone
  - imidazoles: enoximone, piroximone, imidazopyridine, sulmazole
  - xanthine derivatives: caffeine, aminophylline.

Other Inotropes That Do Not Work by Increasing cAMP
- Digoxin (see Section 6.8)
- α Agonists: stimulate postsynaptic α-receptors in the myocardium without increasing cAMP: noradrenaline, adrenaline, high-dose dopamine (via noradrenaline)
- Calcium sensitizers: increase the sensitivity of troponin to calcium: pimobendan, levosimendan
- Enhancing sodium influx, resulting in increased delivery of calcium to the myofilaments: vesnarinone.

Many of these drugs are under development. A few have been tried as oral agents in some countries in the long-term management of cardiac failure, e.g. xamoterol(now withdrawn in the UK), ibopamine, enoximone, milrinone.

Dopamine
The precursor of noradrenaline, dopamine has become a standard drug in the management of cardiogenic shock and low-output LV failure secondary to MI. It is also used in septic shock and postcardiac surgery.

It acts on several different receptors with activity changing with increasing dose.

Dose 1.0–5.0 μg/kg per min
Dopaminergic (DA_1) receptors are activated, resulting in dilatation of coronary, renal, cerebral and splanchnic beds. This is called the 'renal' dose of dopamine. Other sympathomimetics increase renal blood flow only by increasing cardiac output. Dopamine has this unique action on the renal

vascular bed. Dopaminergic (DA_2) receptors are activated in the periphery, which inhibit presynaptic release of noradrenaline, causing vasodilatation.

Dose 5.0–10.0 μg/kg per min
β-Receptors are activated. This is the inotropic dose. $β_1$ Activation increases contractility. Heart rate is increased probably more than by dobutamine. $β_2$ Activation helps vasodilatation. Doses >10 μg/kg per min are likely to cause arrhythmias.

Dose >15.0 μg/kg per min
α-Receptors are activated. The drug also releases noradrenaline from myocardial adrenergic nerve terminals. Vasoconstrictive doses of dopamine are not beneficial. Renal blood flow falls. Addition of nitroprusside or an α-blocking agent helps prevent this.

Precautions
As with all sympathomimetic agents except dobutamine, the drug must be given by a central line. Peripheral administration causes vasoconstriction and skin necrosis. This can be reversed by injections of subcutaneous phentolamine (5–10 mg phentolamine in 10–15 ml saline).
• The drug is inactivated by bicarbonate or other alkaline solutions.
• Dopamine is metabolized by β-hydroxylase and monoamine oxidase (MAO). It is contraindicated in patients on MAOIs.
• It is contraindicated in phaeochromocytomas and ventricular arrhythmias.
• Although it may promote a diuresis, it does not offer nephroprotection and dopamine has not been shown to improve prognosis in shock.

Dopamine Infusion Preparation (Table 6.4)
Four ampoules of dopamine (Intropin) each of 200 mg are added to 500 ml 5% dextrose. Using paediatric giving set (60 microdrops = 1 ml) infusion strength: 1 microdrop = 26.7 μg dopamine.

Table 6.4 Dopamine Infusion rate chart (microdrops/min)

Weight of patient (kg)	Dopamine dose (μg/kg per min)				
	2	5	10	15	20	25
30	2	6	12	18	23	29
40	3	8	16	23	31	39
50	4	10	20	29	39	49
60	5	12	23	35	47	58
70	5	14	27	41	55	68
80	6	16	31	47	62	78
90	7	18	35	53	70	88
100	8	20	39	58	78	97

Dobutamine

This synthetic inotrope is structurally similar to dopamine, but differs from it in several respects (Table 6.5). It does not activate dopaminergic receptors and does not cause local release of noradrenaline from myocardial stores. Its advantage over dopamine is its lack of chronotropic effect at low doses, where it seems to be an exclusive inotrope. In addition, dobutamine can be given via a peripheral line if there is no central line available. Dopamine must never be given via a peripheral line.

Dobutamine is a racemic mixture of L- and D-dobutamine. D-Dobutamine is a potent β_1 agonist, and L-dobutamine a potent α agonist with weak β_1 and β_2 action. As with all β_1 agonists, dobutamine may be susceptible to down-regulation and tachyphylaxis is a concern. The PCWP may fall initially and then gradually rise again. Splanchnic flow is reduced.

Both dopamine and dobutamine have their advocates. Crossover studies have suggested:

- heart rate lower with dobutamine for same increase in cardiac output
- PWP lower with dobutamine
- fewer ventricular ectopics
- more sustained action over 24 h.

Its α effects are less than those with noradrenaline and its β_2 effects less than those with isoprenaline.

Precautions are the same as for dopamine. Both drugs have a very short half-life (e.g. dobutamine approximately 2.5 min). Of the two drugs, dobutamine and dopamine, the former is probably the superior inotrope.

Dobutamine Dose

Ampoules 20 ml are available containing 12.5 mg/ml: total in ampoule 250 mg. Dilute a 20 ml ampoule to 50 ml with 0.9% saline or 5% dextrose in a syringe driver: 1 ml = 5 mg. Inotropic dose is 2.5-10 μg/kg per min. Assuming a 70 kg patient, initial dose of 2.5 μg/kg per min is 10.5 mg/h = 2.1 ml/h.

Second-line Sympathomimetic Drugs

Isoprenaline

This is rarely used as an inotrope now unless an increase in heart rate is required. Junctional bradycardia, transient second-degree AV block or sinus bradycardia unresponsive to atropine after an MI or cardiac surgery will be helped by isoprenaline, and may obviate the need for temporary pacing. However, the risk of increased myocardial excitability must be considered. It reduces systemic vascular resistance and dilates skeletal and splanchnic vessels (β_2 effect), which is not where the flow is needed.

Dose and infusion preparation (various strengths available, e.g. 0.1 mg/ml, 1 mg/ml): add 2 mg isoprenaline to 500 ml 5% dextrose: mixture strength = 4 μg/ml. Start infusion at 1 μg/min = 15 microdrops/min. Increase dose as required, generally up to 10 μg/min.

Table 6.5 Inotropic sympathomimetic drugs

Drug and receptor affected	Increase heart rate (β_1 effect)	Myocardial release of noradrenaline	Peripheral vasoconstriction (α effect)	Peripheral vasodilatation (β_2 effect)	Renal blood flow (dopaminergic)	Intravenous dose
Dopamine Dopaminergic, β_1 α at high dose	++	++	− to ++	++ Low doses	++	Renal dose: 1–5.0 µg/kg/min Inotropic dose: 5.0–10 µg/kg/min Constricting dose >15 µg/kg/min
Dopexamine DA_1 and β_1 (β_2 small)	++	+	−	++	++	0.5–6.0 µg/kg/min
Dobutamine β_1 (β_2 small)	+	−	− to +	++	−	2.5–15.0 µg/kg/min Low dose – inotropic High dose – inotropic + chronotropic
Salbutamol β_1 (β_2 small)	++	−	−	++	−	10–40 µg/min (≤0.5 µg/kg/min)
Isoprenaline β_1 and β_2	+++	−	−	+++	−	1–10 µg/min
Adrenaline $\beta_1 > \beta_2$ (α small)	+++	+	+	−	−	1–12 µg/min
Noradrenaline α (β small)	− or +	++	+++	−	−	1–12 µg/min

Adrenaline

There is still a place for adrenaline infusion when other inotropes have failed. It has a mixed β- and α-receptor activity.

Infusion preparation: 5 ml 1:1000 adrenaline (= 5 mg) in 500 ml 5% dextrose; mixture = 10 μg/ml. Start at 1–2 μg/min (6–12 paediatric microdrops/min).

Glucagon

This activates adenylyl cyclase by a mechanism separate from the $β_1$-myocardial receptor. It can be used in β-blocked patients. It is not a powerful inotrope, does not have a sustained effect, and causes hyperglycaemia, hypokalaemia and nausea. It is expensive and of little value in LVF or cardiogenic shock. It is of more use in treating hypoglycaemia.

Dose 1–5 mg i.v. slowly repeated after 30 min. Infusion rate is 1–7.5 mg/h.

Choice of Parenteral Inotrope

In low-output states with oliguria (<30 ml/h) low-dose dopamine is the drug of choice. If urine output is >30 ml/h then dobutamine is preferable. In hypotensive states with pulmonary oedema, a combination of dopamine or dobutamine with nitroprusside should be tried. Dopamine and dobutamine may be employed together using the 'renal' dose of dopamine and dobutamine as the inotrope (Table 6.5).

Other Inotropes

Dopexamine

An alternative to dopamine but also only available as an intravenous preparation. Stimulates DAB dopamine receptors (renal vessels dilate). It is a strong $β_2$ agonist and weak $β_1$ agonist. It also inhibits noradrenaline release (DA_2 receptor). It is thus a potent vasodilator plus the effects of dopamine. Dose: start at 0.5 μg/kg per min. Try to avoid doses >4 μg/kg per min, because tachycardia and hypotension occur at high doses.

Ibopamine

This is the only oral inotrope available that is related to dopamine. It is hydrolysed in plasma to epinine (methyldopamine). There is little increase in heart rate at standard doses. There is a diuretic effect with DA_1- and DA_2-receptor activation, i.e. the drug is a renal and peripheral vasodilator. Dose 50–100 mg three times daily (becoming inotropic at >800 mg daily). The multicentre European trial (PRIME II) of ibopamine 100 mg three times daily versus placebo in heart failure was terminated early as a result of more deaths in the ibopamine group. The adverse effect was particularly noted in severe heart failure or in those patients on amiodarone therapy. There seems to be nothing to recommend this drug in heart failure.

Enoximone

This is a phosphodiesterase (PDE) inhibitor, once available as an oral preparation in some countries. Preliminary trials showed a sustained benefit in LVEF, exercise tolerance and symptoms. However, one small trial showed a high withdrawal rate and only a transient improvement. The concern of a proarrhythmic effect, as with other PDE inhibitors, remains (see Milrinone below). It can be used as an intravenous preparation with dobutamine. The oral preparation has been withdrawn. Parenteral dose: 90 µg/kg per min over 30 min, then 5–20 µg/kg per min. Dose not to exceed 24 mg/kg over 24 h.

Milrinone

This is a PDE inhibitor, much more potent than amrinone and available orally. In one trial it was found to be inferior to digoxin and in the PROMISE trial, treating patients with severe heart failure, the mortality rate with milrinone was 28% higher than with placebo and the trial was stopped early.

Pimobendan

This inotrope works by sensitizing the myofibril to cytosolic calcium and it is also a modest PDE inhibitor. It prolongs contraction and delays relaxation more than levosimendan. In a multicentre European trial exercise duration was increased slightly after 24 weeks' therapy but functional status, quality of life or VO_2max was not improved. There was a trend to an increased mortality in the pimobendan group – particularly in patients on digoxin. This drug has been withdrawn in Europe but is still in use in Japan.

Levosimendan

This is a calcium sensitizer and K^+ ATP channel opener with minimal effect on relaxation. Intravenous infusion reduces PCWP, increases stroke volume and acts as a vasodilator. In the LIDO trial it appeared to be better than dobutamine with greater acute increase in cardiac output (at 24 h) and better survival at 180 days. An oral preparation has been tried in a phase II study weaning patients with severe cardiac failure off intravenous inotropes, but ventricular arrhythmias and hypotension were a problem.

Choice of Inotropes

In the short-term management of acute LVF the use of PDE inhibitors remains valuable. Combination therapy is now being tried. Enoximone plus noradrenaline is very useful. The inotropic effect of enximone is used with the α effect of low-dose noradrenaline to maintain systolic pressure by preventing the marked vasodilatation induced by enoximone. The degree of vasodilatation varies from patient to patient and it is necessary to fine-tune the noradrenaline dose to maintain a mean systolic pressure of 90 mmHg.

Enoximone has also been tried with a β blocker (e.g. metoprolol plus enoximone). Once a patient is established on this combination it may be possible gradually to withdraw the enoximone in time.

Levosimendan looks to be a promising drug, certainly in the short term intravenously. Low-dose β_1 agonists must be reserved for the severely hypotensive (peak systolic pressure <90 mmHg) and oliguric patient.

On present evidence PDE inhibitors cannot be recommended for the long-term management of cardiac failure with their possible proarrhythmic effect. The long-term results of other oral inotropes are awaited, but for the moment we continue with digoxin, vasodilators, ACE inhibitors and the gradual introduction of β blockade.

6.10 Downregulation of β-Receptors and β Blockade in Heart Failure

The normal myocardium contains both β_1- and β_2-receptors in a ratio of about 4:1. In heart failure this ratio is reduced or reversed because the number of β_1-receptors falls by at least 50%. This may be a result of chronic high levels of circulating noradrenaline, and these high levels are known to increase apoptosis. Both circulating catecholamines and administered β_1 agonists have less effect (desensitized) and treatment with β_2 agonists should theoretically assume more importance. Unfortunately β_2 agonists have not proved of much help either in heart failure, perhaps because the β_2-receptors become partially uncoupled.

Attempts with low-dose β-blocking agents that partially block the β_1-receptor have been tried in patients with heart failure to try to overcome this downregulation. Xamoterol, a drug with intrinsic sympathomimetic activity, caused a deterioration in moderate or severe heart failure and was abandoned. Since then several β-blocking agents have proved highly successful in the long-term management of heart failure.

β_1 Blockade in Heart Failure

β_1 Blockade has been conclusively shown in several trials to improve survival, reduce hospital admissions, and improve symptoms and quality of life in patients with heart failure when used in combination with standard diuretic and ACE inhibitor therapy (Table 6.6). This is not a class effect because a trial with bucindolol did not significantly reduce all-cause mortality (BEST trial). The three drugs with the best evidence are carvedilol, metoprolol and bisoprolol. The antiarrhythmic effect of β blockade contributes to the mortality reduction (reducing sudden cardiac death).

β Blockade should be attempted only on an outpatient basis in patients with mild or moderate heart failure (NYHA class II or III) in patients who are already established on a diuretic and preferably an ACE inhibitor. The lowest dose possible is started (Table 6.6) and the dose only increased once every 2 weeks. There is no rush, and any tolerated dose of a β blocker is better than

Table 6.6 β-Blocking trials in heart failure

Drug	Starting dose (mg)	Target dose (mg)	Trials tested	Year	Patients tested	Percentage reduction in mortality[a]
Bisoprolol	1.25 once daily	10 once daily	CIBIS I	1994	IHD/DCM	20
			CIBIS II	1999	IHD/DCM	32
Carvedilol	3.125 twice daily	25 twice daily	US-HF	1997	IHD/DCM	65
			ANZ-HF	1995	IHD	NS
			COPERNICUS	2001	Severe HF	35
			CAPRICORN	2001	Post-MI	23
Metoprolol	12.5 once daily	50 three times daily	MDC	1993	DCM	34
			MERIT-HF	1999	IHD/DCM	49

See Appendix 4 for trial references.
[a]This is percentage relative risk reduction in all-cause mortality.

none. Patients with grade IV heart failure should be admitted to hospital for a trial of therapy because even these severely ill patients may benefit from β blockade (COPERNICUS trial). The beneficial effects may take several months to be achieved. They have been shown to reduce LV volumes about 6 months after an MI, i.e. they help prevent remodelling.

Reasons to Halve the Dose of β Blocker
- Heart rate <50/min, but check for other drug therapy that might exacerbate this, e.g. diltiazem, digoxin, amiodarone
- Marked fatigue, increasing dyspnoea, provocation of asthma or disabling claudication
- Weight gain >2 kg over 2 days if doubling diuretic does not work
- Symptomatic hypotension (not necessary if patient is asymptomatic)
- Second- or third-degree heart block.

It is important that patients are instructed to weigh themselves daily. If weight gain exceeds 2 kg then the diuretic dose is doubled. If this fails to reverse the weight gain the β blocker is halved, but must not be stopped suddenly. There are concerns about rebound ischaemia and/or arrhythmias on suddenly stopping β blockers.

Choice of β Blocker
There is not enough evidence yet to determine if any of the three drugs listed is superior in heart failure. Metoprolol and bisoprolol are both cardioselective (β_1 blockade only), whereas carvedilol is non-selective but also blocks α_1-receptors and has antioxidant properties. One small study suggested that carvedilol was superior to metoprolol.

ACE Inhibitor or β Blocker First?

The CIBIS III trial suggested that starting either group of drug first followed by the other was equally effective. Conventionally in the UK the ACE inhibitor is started first. Generally there is a low use of β-blocker therapy in the UK in elderly people.

6.11 Diastolic Heart Failure (Heart Failure with Preserved Systolic Function)

Some patients may have all the symptoms of cardiac failure but a normal LVEF on echocardiography (>50%) and a normal size heart on the chest radiograph. A wide variety of cardiac conditions may cause this picture:

- Incorrect assessment of LVEF
- Valvular heart disease (e.g. aortic stenosis, acute mitral regurgitation)
- Restrictive cardiomyopathy (see Section 4.3 and 11.3)
- Pericardial constriction (see Section 10.3)
- Systemic hypertension
- IHD
- Atrial myxoma (see Section 11.6)
- Idiopathic diastolic dysfunction.

Essentially in most of these hypertrophy, infiltration or fibrosis results in a stiff myocardium, causing effort dyspnoea and possible pulmonary oedema. Congestive symptoms are more related to diastolic than to systolic function. Diastolic function declines with age and patients with diastolic heart failure tend to be in the older age group. Two recent longitudinal studies have shown that long-term survival (65% 5-year mortality rate in one series) is only marginally better than in patients with classic systolic heart failure. Diastolic heart failure is an equally lethal condition.

Cardiac Catheterization

At cardiac catheterization LVEDP and PAW pressures are elevated but systolic function is preserved. The diastolic pressure–volume curve is shifted upwards and to the left (higher LVEDP at lower end-diastolic volume). Ventricular relaxation is delayed and incomplete. Measurements of chamber stiffness show that this is increased.

Echocardiography

Echocardiographic features are characteristic but transmitral flow velocity patterns must be interpreted with caution (see Section 17.3).

Abnormal E:A ratio: there is a smaller E wave and a larger A wave initially when diastolic dysfunction is mild. As the condition progresses and LA pressure rises the E:A ratio pseudonormalizes. With severe diastolic dysfunction E wave velocity increases as a result of a high transmitral pressure gradient in early diastole from a stiff LV. This severe stage is called the restrictive pattern having originally been described in restrictive cardiomyopathy:

- A deceleration time <70 ms
- E deceleration time <140 ms or >300 ms
- Blunted systolic forward flow in pulmonary veins
- Increased flow reversal in pulmonary veins during atrial systole.

Management
- Management of these cases depends on the aetiology of the stiff ventricle.
- Vigorous control of hypertension is important.
- Diuretics, salt restriction and ACE inhibitors are helpful for symptom control.
- Maintenance of sinus rhythm is important because atrial transport helps maintain cardiac output and rapid deterioration occurs with the development of AF. Urgent DC cardioversion may be needed, and also amiodarone and an electrophysiological opinion. If the LA <6.0 cm on echocardiography RF ablation of the AF may be a possibility.
- Revascularization may be needed for the ischaemic left ventricle.
- Slow-release verapamil may be helpful in idiopathic cases.

Drug Compliance in Cardiac Failure
This is a crucial problem, often ignored in busy clinics. Patients are often frail and elderly with memory difficulties. The use of a segmented plastic pillbox with a tabulated regimen helps. Nausea induced by drugs or hepatomegaly also causes non-compliance. Adherence by the patient to a standard heart failure regimen definitely improves outcome. In addition adherence by physicians and cardiologists to guidelines of heart failure therapy is also a strong predictor of outcome.

Anaemia in Cardiac Failure
Anaemia is a common problem in cardiac failure. It is often ignored but contributes to the symptoms of fatigue and dyspnoea, as well as reducing myocardial oxygen delivery. The anaemia is probably multifactorial: nutritional deficiencies from anorexia, secondary to marrow suppression from prerenal failure and possibly caused by occult blood loss from a congested gastrointestinal tract in an anticoagulated patient. Iron and folate supplements may be needed as well as erythropoietin (EPO) injections for the anaemia of renal failure.

The Importance of Maintaining Sinus Rhythm
Atrial systole may contribute up to 25% of the cardiac output and the loss of SR in a patient with poor LV function usually leads to a symptomatic and clinical deterioration. Atrial stretch results in AF. The loss of atrial transport results in a fall in cardiac output, a further rise in LA pressure and possible pulmonary oedema. In addition the resultant tachycardia may contribute to a tachycardia cardiomyopathy.

Possible attempts to overcome these problems include:
• Amiodarone: the only antiarrhythmic drug that can be used in this situation (no negative inotropic effect). May help preserve SR for a time, but unlikely to in the long term.
• AV node ablation and permanent RV pacing: although this restores a sensible rate RV pacing alone may have a deleterious effect as a result of interventricular dyssynchrony. Atrial transport is lost as AF remains.
• AV node ablation and biventricular pacing: atrial transport again is lost but biventricular pacing overcomes interventricular dyssynchrony and has been shown to produce a haemodynamic and clinical improvement.
• RF ablation of AF: recently Haissaguerre's group have had remarkable success in ablating AF in patients with CCF and an LVEF <45%. Significant improvements in LVEF were seen: 73% were maintained in SR at 1 year. If RF ablation is going to be considered it should be performed early in the course of the disease while there is still a relatively small left atrium (<6.0 cm if possible).

6.12 Possible Future Directions in Pharmacology

Endothelin-receptor Antagonists

Endothelin, a potent vasoconstrictor peptide, was discovered in 1988 and plasma levels of endothelin-1 are elevated in heart failure. It acts through type A receptors (constrictor) and type B (mediated via generation of nitric oxide and prostacyclin – dilators). Antagonists to the type A receptor, or to both type A and B (e.g. bosentan), have been developed. Preliminary work with bosentan in heart failure shows an increase in cardiac output and a fall in PVR and SVR on chronic oral therapy. Early dosing schedules caused a rise in liver enzymes. It may also in time be used for pulmonary or systemic hypertension and after subarachnoid haemorrhage. Trials with intravenous tezosentan (a dual endothelin antagonist) in class III–IV heart failure also look hopeful.

New Sympathetic Antagonists

Moxonidine, similar to clonidine, acts centrally on I_1 imidazoline receptors in the medulla, reducing sympathetic outflow and reducing SVR. Used in hypertension, it may also prove useful in heart failure.

Dopamine β-Hydroxylase Antagonists

Acting peripherally, these agents should reduce noradrenaline levels and increase peripheral dopamine levels and hence renal blood flow.

Vasopeptidase Inhibitors

These drugs inhibit both angiotensin-converting enzyme and neutral endopeptidase (NEP), which breaks down ANP and BNP. ANP and BNP are released from stretched myocytes and promote diuresis and natriuresis. Theoretically adding additional ANP and BNP activity to ACE inhibition should prove of benefit in heart failure. However, the OVERTURE study comparing omapatrilat (a vasopeptidase inhibitor) with enalapril did not show a reduction in the primary endpoint of death or hospitalization for worsening heart failure in the omapatrilat arm. In addition there was an increase in angio-oedema in patients taking omapatrilat compared with enalapril.

Other Possibilities

B-type Natriuretic Peptide Infusion

Nesiritide, a BNP, infusion for 6 h at 0.015–0.03 μg/kg per min improved symptoms and reduced PCWP in patients hospitalized for heart failure. These improvements were maintained for a week. This approach may be of help in the acute management of heart failure. There are concerns over its long-term use.

TNF-α Inhibitors

Tumour necrosis factor α (cachectin) is a proinflammatory cytokine that is released from activated macrophages. Levels are raised in heart failure and, experimentally, TNF-α causes a cardiomyopathy and pulmonary hypertension. One study in patients with DCM using pentoxyfilline, which inhibits TNF-α production, showed an improvement in functional class in patients receiving it. Studies are also under way with etanercept, which binds TNF-α irreversibly.

Carnitine Palmitoyl Transferse 1 (CPT1) Inhibitors

CPT1 is the enzyme getting free fatty acids into the mitochondria and inhibition of CPT1 reduces β oxidation (metabolic switching agents; see Chapter 5, Section 5.5). In heart failure there is as increase in fatty acid utilization as a result of endogenous catecholamine drive. In a small uncontrolled study, perhexiline was shown to increase peak Vo_2 in patients with dilated cardiomyopathy, and to improve the LVEF. Phosphocreatine levels increased on treatment and there was an insulin-sensitizing effect. Toxicity of perhexilene is related to phospholipid accumulation (peripheral neuropathy, hepatitis). Another study has shown an improvement in LVEF with the CTP1 inhibitor etoxomir.

Other experimental ideas for inotropes acting on intracellular pathways include drugs to inhibit phospholamban, enhance SERCA (lower levels in heart failure) or stabilize the ryanodine receptor.

6.13 Non-pharmacological Approaches to Cardiac Failure

Exercise Training in Chronic Heart Failure

Inactivity in patients with chronic heart failure contributes to skeletal muscle weakness and wasting. A programme of supervised cycling 3 days a week has been shown on several small studies to improve symptoms, 6-minute walking distance and peak oxygen consumption. A meta-analysis of nine trials (ExTraMATCH) has shown that exercise training reduces mortality and hospital admissions compared with conventional therapy.

Cardiac Resynchronization Therapy or CRT (Biventricular Pacing)

QRS duration prolongation is frequently found in patients with cardiac failure and most studies have found that prolongation is associated with a worse prognosis. In addition QRS prolongation results in ventricular dyssynchrony with:

• presystolic mitral regurgitation caused by delayed activation to the stretched papillary muscles
• reduced diastolic filling
• paradoxical septal motion: the septum moves away from the lateral wall in systole acting as part of the right ventricle and reduces the septum's contribution to LV stroke volume (see Section 7.9).

These abnormalities can be partly corrected by the use of atrial biventricular pacing and is particularly indicated for patients still in SR and with very wide QRS (>150 ms). This procedure has been shown in the MUSTIC trial to increase the 6-minute walk distance, peak Vo_2, LVEF and quality of life. Hospitalizations with heart failure are reduced but there are no long-term mortality data as yet. The technique is still of some benefit in patients with permanent AF (no atrial wire). Unfortunately up to 30% patients do not respond to biventricular pacing and selection of patients with echocardiography needs to be further refined.

For technical details see the pacing section (Section 7.9).

Implantable Cardioverter Defibrillator (ICD)

Mortality in cardiac failure can be reduced by implanting an ICD in patients with an LVEF <35%. The SCD-HeFT trial (sudden cardiac death in heart failure trial) showed that using an ICD in addition to conventional therapy reduced the 5-year mortality rate by 23%. The mortality rate in the placebo group at 5 years was 35.8% and 28.9% in the ICD group. Amiodarone used in a third arm of the trial was unfortunately no better than placebo (5-year mortality rate 34.1%).

This trial has huge cost implications. Thus use of a biventricular ICD should produce both symptomatic and prognostic benefit in patients with heart failure and low LVEF. Although we are nowhere near implementing these data in the UK, the SCD-HeFT trial has certainly lowered the threshold for device implantation in these patients.

Surgery for Cardiac Failure

There is increasing interest in surgical options for patients in cardiac failure because the long-term prognosis on medical treatment is so poor. Surgeons have been ingenious in this desperate situation.

CAB surgery

Reserved for patients who have demonstrable hibernating myocardium on PET, thallium scanning or stress echocardiography. Additional mitral valve surgery may be required.

Reducing Mitral Regurgitation

There are three main options in these high-risk patients:
1 Mitral annuloplasty
2 Alfieri stitch: a stitch holding the centre of the two mitral leaflets, together resulting in a bow-tie shaped mitral valve; the results are unpredictable
3 Mitral valve replacement.

Reducing LV Volume

LV aneurysmectomy (excision of scar tissue) (see Section 5.10)

Batista operation (partial ventriculectomy)
This involves resection of a segment of the free wall of the left ventricle. It differs from an aneurysmectomy in that living ventricular muscle is excised to reduce the LV volume and hence wall stress.

The operative mortality rate is said to be 15%. Results of trials are awaited but unlikely because few centres have much experience of this procedure. The Cleveland Clinic experience is not encouraging. Only patients with class IV heart failure caused by dilated cardiomyopathy are considered. LVEDD must be >70 mm; 20% patients require an LVAD and at 1 year only 60% patients are alive and not back on the transplant waiting list.

Dor Procedure
This operation involves the insertion of an endoventricular patch within the left ventricle to reduce its volume and to develop a more elliptical shaped ventricle. NYHA class improves although haemodynamic improvement has not been demonstrated. Secondary mitral regurgitation may be induced.

Reducing Continued Cardiac Dilatation: Dynamic Cardiomyoplasty
Devised by Carpentier, this is not suitable for grade IV heart failure patients. The left latissimus dorsi is mobilized, keeping its vascular pedicle intact and transposed into the thorax through partial resection of a rib. The muscle flap is wrapped around the ventricles. A specially designed pacemaker/electrical stimulator is implanted in the rectus sheath and attached to the heart via a sensing electrode and stimulating intramuscular electrodes.

After 2 weeks' rest, the latissimus dorsi is gradually transformed from a fast- to a slow-twitch fatigue-resistant muscle by a series of electrical stimuli synchronized with systole.

The operative mortality rate is approximately 10% and ventricular arrhythmias are the main problem. IABP is used perioperatively.

There is still debate about how the operation works. Systolic augmentation helps but the main effect is probably the muscle wrap preventing further LV dilatation. Collateral blood flow from the muscle wrap to the left ventricle itself may help. Although the vascular pedicle of the latissimus dorsi is preserved, parts may become ischaemic and fibrotic, reducing its contractile potential. This operation has largely been abandoned with its perioperative morbidity and lack of long-term benefit.

LV Assist Device

This has proved a more effective bridge to transplantation than the artificial heart. Some patients who have an LVAD and are waiting for transplantation have been managed at home. The device is implanted in the abdomen with the inflow conduit in the apex of the left ventricle and the outflow conduit in the ascending aorta, incorporating two xenograft valves. Maximum pump output is 11 l/min, and power is supplied by an electrical pack (requiring recharging every 12 h) or bedside console. The LVAD takes all the mitral flow so that the aortic valve does not open significantly and it is thought to be contraindicated in patients with an aortic valve prosthesis with thrombotic risk. Disadvantages of the system are that it still involves a transcutaneous electric cable. Tunnelling this driveline helps reduce the infection risk. The Heartmate LVAD incorporates a textured titanium surface, encouraging neointima formation and reducing the thromboembolism risk. The units are noisy and quite bulky (approximately 800 g).

The LVAD unloads both left and right ventricles and allows some recovery of LV function with regression of LV hypertrophy and myocyte recovery. They have been used in patients unsuitable for transplantation as a 'bridge to recovery' and there have been patients with a dilated cardiomyopathy in whom it has been possible to remove the LVAD after 3–6 months. The LVAD seems to rest the heart with the potential for myocyte recovery.

Jarvik 2000

Successful long-term survival (>1 year) has now been achieved with surgery using the Jarvik 2000 rotary pump implanted in the apex of the left ventricle with a conduit to the descending aorta. It is a small device employing an Archimedes' screw (axial flow impeller pump). The continuous pump renders the patient pulseless and cardiac output can be increased before exercise by increasing the rotation rate (8000–18000 rev./min). Haemolysis does not appear to be a problem. Heart sounds are replaced by a continuous hum. The power cable is tracked up the neck subcutaneously and is mounted on the skull by a titanium pedestal, which is resistant to infection.

In time this device may not only be used as a bridge to transplantation but also replace it as the treatment for end-stage heart failure.

Cardiac Transplantation (see Section 6.15)

Cardiac Allograft Transplantation

Donor hearts are the rate-limiting factor. Generally patients must be under 60 years old; the 1-year survival rate is approximately 85% and the 5-year survival rate is 50%. More recently, a variety of other surgical options has been tried but they are all still under assessment and not generally available.

Xenograft Transplantation

The theoretical use of a pig heart in humans has come a step closer to reality with the development of pigs expressing a human gene for complement regulatory factors. This would prevent acute hyperimmune rejection but not subsequent cellular immune rejection. There is the added worry of transfer of retroviruses from pigs to humans and to date this operation has not been sanctioned in the UK. Again, cost will be a major problem. Shumway – the Stanford pioneer of cardiac transplantation – used to say 'xenografts are the future of cardiac transplantation … and always will be'.

The Artificial Heart

Major problems with a continuous power source, infection, thrombosis and haemolysis have hindered this as a long-term option. The first was the Jarvik 7 (1982), which has been successfully used as a bridge to transplantation. The Abiocor (2001), a 900 g titanium and plastic heart, has been implanted successfully in humans. Power wires are avoided, with the device charged transdermally using a portable battery pack worn externally.

6.14 Cardiogenic Shock

This is a syndrome of inadequate blood supply to vital organs, with failure of elimination of metabolites resulting in their functional and structural disturbance. Clinically this amounts to a hypotensive patient with cool, pale, moist skin, low-volume rapid pulse, oliguria (<30 ml/h) and obtunded consciousness. It usually results from massive MI with >40% of the myocardium involved. The mortality rate is approximately 85% unless urgent revascularization (CABG or PCI) is available.

Pathophysiology

Reduction in cardiac output after an MI results in sympathetic adrenal discharge and vasoconstriction. Shunting may occur as a result (e.g. lungs) and decreased tissue flow causes tissue hypoxia, anaerobic metabolism and lactic acidosis. Precapillary dilatation and postcapillary constriction may cause fluid extravasation. Stasis, sludging of red cells, further reduces flow. Mitochondrial damage, lysosome release and cell death result. Shunting may cause the wrong organs to get the small output (e.g. splanchnic bed) at the expense of renal, coronary and cerebrovascular beds. Oxygen utilization by the tissues is impaired and attempts to increase oxygen delivery by increasing cardiac output may not achieve much. The following are common causes are:
- MI causing pump failure
- VSD
- Prosthetic valve dysfunction: acute obstruction or severe regurgitation

- Acute mitral regurgitation
- Massive pulmonary embolism
- Aortic dissection
- Cardiac tamponade
- Acute myocarditis.

It is vital to establish as soon as possible whether shock is the result of acute MI: if this is the case urgent PCI is required and the patient should be transferred directly to a catheter laboratory with experienced personnel. If PCI is unavailable or shock result from other causes, the steps below should be followed.

Examination

This should be quick and thorough. Examples of signs to note are as follows:
- General condition: state of consciousness, dyspnoea, peripheral cyanosis, xanthomas. Flows are more important than blood pressure.
- Blood pressure in both arms.
- Pulse: volume, rhythm, ? anacrotic, ? pulsus paradoxus, ? pulsus alternans. Check all peripheral pulses. Auscultate carotids and subclavian arteries.
- Venous pressure: no guide to LV filling pressure. May be normal in anterior infarction. High in RV infarction or pulmonary embolism. Systolic ('x') descent in tamponade rising with inspiration.
- Apex beat: position and quality, ? high apex beat of anterior infarction, paradoxical one of LV aneurysm; ? hyperdynamic of acute MR; ? double apex of high LVEDP (prominent 'a' wave); absent in tamponade; ? RV heave of acute pulmonary embolism.
- Thrills: ? apical with ruptured chordae, retrosternal with VSD or mitral regurgitation, in end-stage aortic stenosis with low flows, thrills and murmurs which may disappear.
- Auscultation: ? S_3 gallop, ? left or right, ? pansystolic murmur of acute VSD or MR.

The murmur of these two conditions may be identical, and both may be heard loudest at the left sternal edge. Consider VSD in anterior infarction with the patient lying fairly flat. Consider mitral regurgitation in inferior or posterior infarction with the patient sitting up in acute pulmonary oedema.

Management

The most important factor in cardiogenic shock is time. If >6 hours have elapsed from the onset of shock, it is unlikely that any intervention will make any difference. Several medical personnel will probably be needed to perform the necessary monitoring requirements. Early coronary angiography is needed to identify those patients suitable for early revascularization.

Stage 1: General Measures
- Analgesia
- Oxygen via MC mask or ventilation if necessary

- ECG monitoring
- 12-lead ECG
- Urinary catheter
- Skin (toe) and core (rectal) temperature measurement
- Bloods for FBC, U&Es, LFTs
- Cardiac enzymes
- Blood gases
- Fingertip pulse oximetry.

Endotracheal Intubation and Ventilation
This may be necessary at the outset for patients in severe pulmonary oedema, or an unconscious patient with an unprotected airway.

Insertion of Monitoring Lines
- Radial artery pressure (acid–base status and arterial gases also)
- CVP lines × 2 (may be used for drug administration).

Swan–Ganz Catheter
Consider possible insertion of this catheter (see below).

Initial Chest Radiograph
This is performed if Swan–Ganz catheter has been inserted to check its position and to exclude a pneumothorax. It is also used to check the following: heart size, lung fields, size of aortic root and upper mediastinum, position of endotracheal tube if patient is ventilated.

Echocardiogram
This should be carried out as soon as possible to exclude pericardial effusion. It provides information about LV size and function, and on a two-dimensional machine it may show an LV aneurysm. Ruptured chordae will be seen on M-mode echocardiography as chaotic mitral valve (anterior or posterior leaflet) movement. VSD resulting from septal perforation can be diagnosed reliably by Doppler echocardiography. A double aortic wall suggestive of dissection may be visualized, but transthoracic echocardiography cannot be relied on. Transoesophageal echocardiography, if available, is much better at visualizing dissection.

Swan–Ganz Monitoring
The measurement of LV filling pressure can be performed by right heart catheterization using a balloon flotation catheter introduced by subclavian vein puncture. It can be shown that, in the absence of mitral valve stenosis or pulmonary vascular disease, LVEDP = mean PAWP.

If a good wedge pressure cannot be obtained, PAEDP = LVEDP. The catheter can be safely left in a PA for >24–48 h if necessary. Serial measurements can be made after drug intervention (or exercise testing in fitter patients).

Thermodilution cardiac outputs can be performed. The catheter can be used for:

- cardiac output
- LVFP/PAW/PAEDP measurement
- PA: O_2 content (e.g. for Fick cardiac output)
- right heart saturations (to check for septal perforation in acute MI)
- central core temperature (thermistor in PA)
- PA systolic pressure: a useful monitor of ventilation
- $\bar{S}vo_2$ or mixed venous (PA) saturation: normally about 75%. May fall to <50% in low-output state. A useful guide of cardiac output.

Technique

The balloon is tested before insertion (usually via subclavian route). Once in the right atrium the balloon is inflated and the catheter gradually advanced until a sudden rise in pressure indicates arrival in the right ventricle. The catheter usually easily floats into the PA. The balloon is deflated in the PA and the pressure recorded. The catheter is advanced until a wedge pressure is achieved. The catheter should not be left in the PAW position for any length of time. The catheter is marked with 10-cm graduation marks to indicate how much has been inserted.

In experienced hands the technique is safe. However, numerous complications have been reported:

- All complications of subclavian puncture (see Section 7.2)
- Ruptured pulmonary artery (by the balloon)
- Damage to pulmonary or tricuspid valves
- Pulmonary infarction
- Septicaemia
- Infective endocarditis
- Arrhythmias, often from RV outflow tract
- Catheter knotting: this may occur with too vigorous a movement of the catheter. The knot should not be pulled out through the subclavian vein. The catheter can be snared from the femoral vein using a Dotter retrieval snare, the catheter is cut at the entry site at the clavicle and the whole catheter pulled out through the femoral vein (Figure 6.5).

There is no evidence yet that, in spite of >30 years of Swan–Ganz monitoring, the technique saves lives. The problem is not the technique itself but the response of the cardiologist to the numbers that it produces. The technique is used now only in highly selected patients.

Stage 2: Correction of Filling Pressure

As soon as the Swan–Ganz catheter is *in situ*, attempts are made to get the filling pressure of the left ventricle (mean PAW or PAEDP) to 16–18 mmHg. This is the optimum filling pressure, assuming a normal plasma colloid oncotic pressure. The optimal filling pressure will be lower where the oncotic pressure is lower (e.g. hypoalbuminaemia) or where capillary permeability is greater (e.g. sepsis, myxoedema).

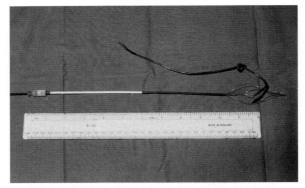

Figure 6.5 Knotted Swan–Ganz catheter removed using a Dotter retrieval snare. The snare is introduced via a sheath in the right femoral vein. Once snared the Swan–Ganz catheter is cut at the skin entry site (subclavian vein) and dragged down and out through the femoral vein.

Filling Pressure too High
- With normotension (mean aortic pressure >90 mmHg) use vasodilators (e.g. nitroprusside), keeping mean aortic pressure >70 mmHg.
- With hypotension use dopamine 5–10 µg/kg per min.

Filling Pressure too Low (Rare)
Give 200 ml plasma and repeat measurement. Vasodilators can always be used if too much plasma is given, and small amounts of plasma may be enough.

Stage 3: Improvement of Stroke Volume
Inotropes are usually required. The choice lies between dobutamine or dopamine (see Section 6.9). Note that the skin temperature gradually warms up as peripheral flows improve.

Although set out in stages, the management of cardiogenic shock depends on many of these procedures being performed quickly and more or less simultaneously.

Stage 4: Further Measures

PCI (see Section 5.9)
This should be considered urgently in patients with acute MI who are going into cardiogenic shock, whether or not streptokinase has been given (see Thrombolysis, Section 5.8). It may still be possible to salvage some myocardium if PCI is performed early enough and there is little to lose in a condition like this with such high mortality. This can be performed with IABP via the other femoral artery or brachial artery. The SHOCK trial showed a reduction in the 6-month mortality rate in those patients aged <75 who received early revascularization (PCI or CABG) within 6 h.

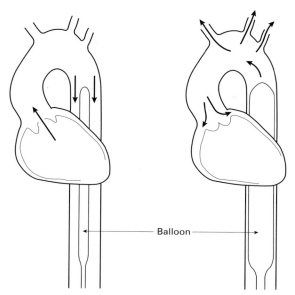

Figure 6.6 Intra-aortic balloon pumping: inflation of intra-aortic balloon in diastole increases cerebral and coronary blood flow.

IABP (Figure 6.6)
The intra-aortic balloon can now be inserted percutaneously without an arterial cut-down procedure and without radiological screening. The R wave of the ECG triggers balloon deflation. The sudden 'sump' effect of balloon deflation acts as afterload reduction, reducing systolic work (Figure 6.7).

The balloon is timed to inflate just after the dicrotic notch of aortic valve closure. Inflation increases coronary and cerebral blood flow. Helium is used as inflation gas.

Patients are fully heparinized while on the balloon. The balloon can be removed percutaneously after deflation and firm pressure over the femoral artery entry site will secure haemostasis. Surgical removal is advised after prolonged use.

IABP quickly settles unstable angina but is rarely necessary now with drug treatment, followed by coronary angiography and possible PCI or coronary bypass surgery. Nevertheless it remains a useful tool in severe unstable angina and conventional coronary angiography can be performed with the balloon *in situ* via the other leg. The main indication for IABP remains the low-output state in the preoperative or postoperative cardiac surgical patient. It is also a useful back-up in patients who are at higher risk for coronary angioplasty.

Glucose/Insulin/Potassium: GIK Therapy
Originally introduced in 1962 by Sodi-Pallares, GIK therapy has never been adequately studied in either acute MI or cardiogenic shock, but a meta-

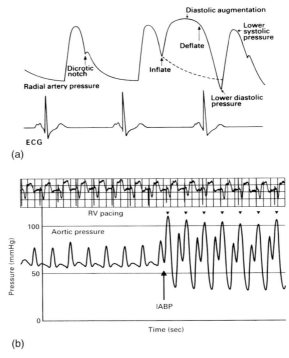

Figure 6.7 (a) Effect of balloon pumping on arterial pressure: shows schematic representation of ECG and radial artery pressure during IABP. The balloon is inflated during the second ECG cycle only to show diastolic augmentation of pressure. The balloon is timed to inflate just after the dicrotic notch, and deflation is triggered by the R wave of the ECG. Note also the lower pressure at end-diastole before the third cycle and the lower systolic pressure of the third cycle. This represents successful afterload reduction by the balloon. (b) Example of IABP in cardiogenic shock as a result of massive inferior infarction. ECG shows RV pacing throughout. Before balloon pumping the aortic pressure is 80/57 mmHg. On starting balloon pumping (large arrow) the peak augmentation pressure is approximately 105 mmHg. Diastolic augmentation is indicated by small arrow heads. The aortic diastolic pressure is much lower at 32 mmHg, with good afterload reduction on balloon deflation. Once IABP had been established, this patient went on to successful right coronary artery reopening and stenting.

analysis of nine trials showed a 28% reduction in mortality in acute MI. It may work by protecting the ischaemic myocardium and lowering free fatty acid levels. It certainly can, in the short term, improve LV function.

Dose: 500 ml 30% glucose + 50 U Actrapid insulin + 80 mmol KCl at a rate of 1.5 ml/kg per h i.v.

Surgery

In cardiogenic shock this is really reserved for urgent mitral valve replacement (e.g. ruptured papillary muscle), repair of acquired VSD or repair of aortic dissection (see Section 14.2). Very occasionally repair of subacute cardiac rupture is possible (see Section 5.10).

6.15 Cardiac Transplantation

About 150 cardiac transplantations are performed in the UK annually and about 10 heart–lung transplantations. Organ availability is the limiting factor and many patients die on the waiting list. There is no absolute age limit for referral but 55 years for ischaemic heart disease and 60 years for dilated cardiomyopathy is a guide. The 5-year survival rate is 65% for heart transplantations and 50% for heart–lung transplantations. The threat in the first year after transplantation is infection or rejection and, in the long term, the development of allograft coronary disease.

Indications
These are usually self-evident:
• Refractory cardiogenic shock
• Dependence on intravenous inotropes for organ perfusion
• Severe ischaemic heart disease not amenable to any other intervention
• Recurrent cardiac failure already on maximal medical therapy
• Recurrent symptomatic ventricular arrhythmias not manageable with an ICD and drug therapy.

Follow-up of Cardiac Transplant Recipients
Early follow-up will be at the transplant centre. Longer-term follow-up at the referring centre will be included. There are many potential problems, particularly detecting signs of early rejection, problems secondary to immunosuppression, prevention of long-term allograft coronary disease, drug interactions and the problem of late malignancy. Close liaison with the transplant centre is essential.

General Advice
Smoking is forbidden. Limited alcohol (e.g. 2–3 units daily) is allowed. A low saturated fat diet is encouraged. Weight gain is common (steroids, inactivity and fluid retention) and, in patients on longer-term steroids, diabetes should be expected. Patients take their own temperatures and weigh themselves daily, contacting the cardiologist if their weight increases by >2 kg over 48 h. Either the patient or the cardiologist should consult the transplant centre with any problems or queries.

Rejection
This is most common in the first year after the transplantation. Activated T cells infiltrate the allograft. If suspected, the patient should be referred back to the transplant centre, if possible, for RV biopsy. Unfortunately early rejection may be asymptomatic with no clinical signs. Suspect it with:
• general malaise, lethargy and fatigue
• dyspnoea and reduction in exercise tolerance
• low-grade fever

- sudden weight gain from fluid retention
- new atrial flutter or AF
- new conduction system abnormalities
- reduction in QRS voltage on ECG.

Many of these are also features of cytomegalovirus (CMV) infection, which itself may provoke rejection and early atherosclerosis of the allograft.

Diagnosis is based on RV endomyocardial biopsy via the right internal jugular vein (developed by Caves in 1973). It is initially performed weekly post-transplantation and then at decreasing intervals over the first 6 months. Generally rejection responds well to early treatment (pulsed methylprednisolone 0.5–1.0 g daily over 3 days). Refractory cases may need antithymocyte globulin (ATG) or monoclonal anti-CD3 antibody (OKT3).

Immunosuppression

Initially, patients are on a combination of steroids, ciclosporin and azathioprine, but after about 3 months many can be weaned off their steroids and maintained on ciclosporin and azathioprine. Steroids may need to be continued with poor renal function or continued rejection. ATG is not used except in acute steroid-resistant rejection because, in the long term, it predisposes to CMV infection and lymphoma and does not improve long-term prognosis.

Patients must be told to report immediately any symptoms that might be a result of oversuppression, e.g. bruising or bleeding, oropharyngeal ulceration or unexplained fever.

Prednisolone

Usual maintenance dose is 10–15 mg daily as a single dose. While patients are on prednisolone they should also take ranitidine for possible peptic ulceration and co-trimoxazole (*Pneumocystis carinii* prophylaxis). Side effects are inevitable: weight gain from increased appetite and fluid retention, sleep disturbance, redistribution of body fat, fragile skin, acne, hypertension, osteoporosis, muscle wasting and proximal myopathy, exacerbation or development of diabetes, and glaucoma and cataracts. More rarely, aseptic femoral head necrosis, benign intracranial hypertension and psychosis occur. Growth retardation will occur in children.

Steroids are weaned gradually after a long course. Acute cessation may result in adrenal insufficiency and also a polymyalgia-like syndrome.

Azathioprine

The maintenance dose is 1–2 mg/kg per day. It causes a dose-related, usually reversible, depression of all elements of the bone marrow. Aim to keep total the white count in the range 4000–6500/mm^3. The total neutrophil count must not fall below 1000/mm^3. Regular blood counts are essential. The drug is generally well tolerated. Hypersensitivity reactions can occur on starting treatment.

The dose of azathioprine must be reduced if allopurinol is started for gout to avoid possible pancytopenia.

Ciclosporin

A cyclic polypeptide originally isolated from fungi now produced synthetically. It inhibits the resting lymphocyte in G0 or G1 phase and prevents the release of interleukin-2 and other lymphokines. Normal maintenance dose is 2–10 mg/kg per day regulated by renal function and drug levels. An oral oily solution (100 mg/ml) is taken once or twice daily in milk or fruit juice. An intravenous form is available if needed (use one-third oral dose).

Impairment of renal function is the most important side effect, particularly with onset of treatment. It responds to dose reduction. Patients may become hirsute (dark hair) and develop gingival hypertrophy (particularly if on nifedipine). Other side effects are tremor, hypertension (see below), liver dysfunction, gastrointestinal disturbances, migraine and peripheral dysthaesiae (burning sensation in hands and feet).

Drug interactions are important with ciclosporin (Table 6.7) because rises in plasma levels resulting from other drugs may rapidly cause deterioration in renal function, or increase the infection risk from oversuppression.

The use of regular ketoconazole or diltiazem with ciclosporin has been used in some centres to cut down the dose (and cost) of ciclosporin, because both drugs inhibit the metabolism of ciclosporin by cytochrome oxidase. Alcohol in moderation is allowed.

Mammalian Target for Rapamycin (mTOR) Inhibitors
(see Chapter 5, Figure 5.26)

Tacrolimus (FK 506). A recently introduced immunosuppressive agent with similar side effects to ciclosporin. It may cause hypertrophic cardiomyopathy in children, and has a long QT interval. Regular echocardiography is needed during treatment. It also may cause hyperglycaemia and CNS disturbances.

Table 6.7 Ciclosporin interactions with other drugs

Drugs increasing ciclosporin levels	Drugs decreasing ciclosporin levels
Ketoconazole	
Diltiazem	Phenytoin
Verapamil	Carbamazepine
Nicardipine	Barbiturates
Propafenone	Rifampicin
Erythromycin	Trimethoprim (intravenous)
Doxycycline	
Oral contraceptives	
Methylprednisolone (high dose)	

Sirolimus (Rapamycin), everolimus. These mTOR inhibitors are being increasingly introduced later in transplantation after successful wound healing. The dose of ciclosporin can then be lowered to preserve renal function.

Hypertension
This is a common problem in heart transplant recipients, induced by steroids, ciclosporin and renal dysfunction. Long-acting nifedipine is tried first. Avoid verapamil and nicardipine (see above). ACE inhibitors are good but renal function needs watching carefully with patients on ciclosporin. β Blockers are unlikely to be tolerated in this group. Avoid thiazides, and care is needed with potassium-retaining diuretics.

Hyperlipidaemia
Lipid levels must be measured regularly. The need to lower serum cholesterol in this group of patients is particularly important to try to prevent late-onset allograft coronary disease:
- HMG-CoA reductase inhibitors have been reported as more likely to cause muscle pains and rhabdomyolysis in patients on ciclosporin. Provided that the patient is warned to report any unexplained muscle pains and a low dose prescribed, these drugs can be used. One report suggests that HMG-CoA reductase inhibitors might help prevent rejection in addition to their cholesterol-lowering properties. Most patients will be on a statin.
- Fibrates: as with HMG-CoA reductase inhibitors. Use in low dose and watch for muscle pains.
- Cholestyramine: should be avoided because it could interfere with absorption of immunosuppressive drugs.

Contraception
Pregnancy should be strongly discouraged because azathioprine is teratogenic. Oral contraceptives may increase ciclosporin levels unpredictably. This seems to be less of a problem with progesterone-only preparations that are the contraceptive of choice if possible. Ciclosporin levels and renal and liver function should be monitored carefully on starting oral contraceptives, and repeated for the first few months.

The intrauterine contraceptive device should be avoided with the infection risk.

Gout
Hyperuricaemia and gout are common in patients on ciclosporin. Non-steroidal anti-inflammatory agents should be used for as brief a time as possible to avoid deterioration in renal function. If allopurinol is used, the dose should not be >100 mg/day, the dose of azathioprine should be halved and blood counts performed every 2 weeks for 6–8 weeks.

Infection and Antibiotics
It is important to take all cultures before treatment (nose, throat, urine, sputum and blood).

Bacterial
Amoxicillin, flucloxacillin, cephalosporins and ciprofloxacin are safe. Aminoglycosides should be avoided if possible (combined nephrotoxicity with ciclosporin). Erythromycin increases ciclosporin levels. Antibiotic prophylaxis should be advised for dental procedures, etc. as if the patient had valve disease (see Section 9.7). Single-dose amoxicillin or clindamycin is the drug of choice. Single-dose erythromycin can be used (see above).

Viral
CMV infection is common in the first 6 months and may follow increased immunosuppression given for rejection. Consider whether the patient has malaise and pyrexia plus additional symptoms of colitis, retinits, pneumonia or even myocarditis.

Ganciclovir is used for acute CMV infection and its continued use in long-term prophylaxis is increasing.

Aciclovir is given orally for herpes simplex infection, but intravenously for zoster infection initially.

Fungal
Oral nystatin is used for oropharyngeal Candida and fluconazole for more severe systemic infection. Aspergillus infection commonly involves the lung. Transbronchial or CT-guided lung needle biopsy may be needed to make the diagnosis. Amphotericin use will be limited by renal function (see Section 9.5).

Protozoal
Pneumocystis carinii pneumonia should be prevented with the use of co-trimoxazole. Toxoplasmosis (transmitted with the allograft into non-immune individuals) should be prevented with an initial 6-week course of pyrimethamine.

Immunization
Live attenuated viral vaccines must be avoided in immunosuppressed patients (Table 6.8). If in doubt consult occupational health centre, professional immunization centre or consultant virologist.

With the exception of hyperimmune γ-globulin, the safe vaccines may not generate an immune response and hence be ineffective. Determined energetic patients may require counselling and encouragement to avoid 'at risk' areas.

Table 6.8 Immunization in immunosuppressed patients

Vaccines to be avoided	Safe vaccines
Oral polio	Polio (killed virus) (intramuscular)
Measles	Influenza
Rubella	Tetanus
Yellow fever	Typhoid
Mumps	Hyperimmune γ-globulin
Hepatitis A or B	Pneumococcal vaccine
BCG	

Allograft Coronary Disease, Transplant Coronary Vasculopathy
This is the most common cause of late death and may occur in all age groups. Coronary arteriograms are usually performed at the end of the second year, then annually thereafter. The disease process is probably a combination of immune-mediated smooth muscle cell hyperplasia and hypercholesterolaemia. Diffuse coronary disease is common but angina rare (denervated heart), patients presenting with symptoms from deteriorating LV function. The process is diffuse and concentric, and may involve the whole length of the artery. It can involve intramyocardial vessels. Coronary angioplasty may occasionally be effective for localized lesions. One study has suggested that sirolimus may reverse angiographic disease in some patients. Re-transplantation may be the only possibility.

The search for effective prevention continues. There are already reports of diltiazem and pravastatin reducing the incidence of new coronary disease.

Malignant Disease
The incidence of malignant disease increases with long-term immunosuppression, and may occur in 10% of long-term survivors of transplantation. About a third of these are squamous cell carcinomas. Patients should be advised to avoid strong sunlight or use barrier creams. Any suspicious skin lesions should be excised. Squamous cell carcinomas may recur and plastic surgery may eventually be necessary.

Another a third of these malignancies are lymphomas (particularly non-Hodgkin's lymphoma). The small tumour mass may respond to high-dose oral aciclovir and a slight decrease in immunosuppression because the non-Hodgkin's lymphoma may be linked to Epstein–Barr virus infection. More extensive lymphomas will require chemotherapy and radiotherapy. Close liaison with an oncology team is essential.

6.16 Cardiac Arrest

Recognition
The recognition of cardiac arrest is based on absent arterial pulsation and an unconscious patient. Spontaneous respiration may continue sporadically for

<1 min after an arrest and the state of the pupils is merely a guide to the time from arrest.

Ideally, the arrest team should consist of at least three medical personnel (one an anaesthetist) trained in resuscitation, who are called to any hospital arrest. Training non-medical personnel to cope with CPR is paying dividends in several cities. The training and equipping of ambulance personnel have improved enormously over the last few years. As well as being trained to intubate and give appropriate drugs, the accuracy of emergency ECG diagnosis has been improved with automated external defibrillators.

New Concepts

The European resuscitation guidelines published in 1992 have changed many long-standing traditions in the management of cardiac arrest. These long-held beliefs were not based on firm evidence. In particular, four precautions were emphasized:

1 Defibrillation at the absolute earliest opportunity with three quick shocks. Every minute that defibrillation is delayed reduces the chances of eventual hospital discharge by 10%.

2 Lidocaine is not given until after several attempts at cardioversion/defibrillation, because this raises defibrillation thresholds. Amiodarone is now the drug of choice.

3 Sodium bicarbonate is not given until very late on in the course of the arrest if at all.

4 Increasing emphasis on effective prolonged cardiac massage.

Management of CPR

Precordial Chest Thump: Check the Clock

A few sharp blows to the mid-sternum may revert ventricular tachycardia. It should be employed only if it is possible within a few seconds of the arrest. Occasionally the thumps may start a rhythm in asystolic patients.

External Cardiac Massage (ECM)

There is a minimal rate of 100/min. Until artificial ventilation (i.e. intubated patient) is under way, pause every 30 beats for 2 breaths: 30 compressions + 2 breaths = 1 cycle of CPR. Aim for 5 cycles in 2 minutes. With good cardiac massage, pressure similar to native pressure can be achieved. Once the patient is intubated cardiac compressions continue without a pause (i.e. no longer in cycles), with the anaesthetist giving 8–10 breaths/min. Check the rhythm every 2 min.

In infants the chest is encircled with both hands and the chest compressed with the thumbs. In children ECM is performed with one hand only.

A hard surface beneath the patient is necessary for effective massage. Correct ECM should not fracture ribs, although this occasionally occurs in elderly people. Massage too near the xiphisternum will not be effective and additionally may damage the liver (Figure 6.8).

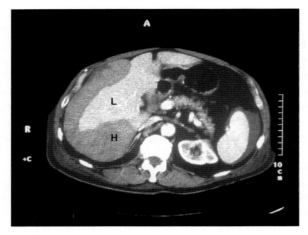

Figure 6.8 Abdominal CT showing a perihepatic haematoma caused by cardiac massage. L, liver; H, haematoma.

Tips for the compressor: try to keep your arms straight and use your body weight from the shoulders. Flexing the arms too much is rapidly tiring. Switch compressors regularly, e.g. every 3 min.

Airway and Artificial Ventilation
The airway should be cleared, dentures removed and vomit aspirated with a sucker. Pillows are removed and the head extended. Initially the patient is ventilated using an oral airway (Guedel), a mask and self-inflating bag connected to an oxygen cylinder. If these are not available a Brooke airway or mouth-to-mouth ventilation is used.

The following should occur when help arrives.

Establish ECG Monitoring
Subsequent action depends on the ECG.

If the Monitor Shows VF or Pulseless VT:
- Precordial chest thump.
- DC shock 200 J/W-s biphasic, 360 J monophasic in an adult: if performed immediately this should defibrillate 90% of adults. If the patient is very heavy, or if the first shock was delayed, greater energy may be needed. The electrodes should be widely separated, nor should they be directly over the sternum (bone has high impedance to electric current). An electrode paste 'bridge' will short-circuit the shock and prove useless.
- Resume CPR immediately: five cycles of CPR.
- *If this fails* repeat shock at 200 J. Resume CPR.
- *If this fails* repeat the shock at 360 J. If the patient is still in VF after three quick shocks the resuscitation is unlikely to succeed. Coarse VF is much more likely to be defibrillated successfully than fine VF.

- *Intubation*: this should be attempted after the first three shocks. It should not be attempted by inexperienced personnel, and ventilation using a mask and self-inflating bag should be continued until experienced help is available. Whatever type of ventilation is established, the chest should be auscultated to check that the lungs are being inflated effectively.
- *Establish intravenous access*: insert a central venous line or preferably two. The internal jugular is safest in an emergency. The subclavian vein is an alternative but a pneumothorax will make resuscitation unlikely to succeed. A peripheral vein may be of temporary help only, but several drugs given through a peripheral line will cause tissue necrosis (e.g. dopamine, adrenaline).
- Give adrenaline 1 mg i.v. and repeat every 3–5 min, vasopressin 40 U i.v. is an alternative for first or second dose of adrenaline.
- Five CPR sequences.
- DC shocks 360 J × 3.

This sequence is a 'loop':

- Repeat the loop twice more.
- Consider: amiodarone 300 mg i.v. is now considered more effective than lidocaine (the ALIVE trial). If amiodarone is unavailable, dose of lidocaine is 100–200 mg i.v.; 10 ml 1% lidocaine contains 100 mg, 10 ml 2% lidocaine contains 200 mg.
- Consider magnesium if torsades de pointes: 1–2 g i.v.
- If this fails, consider another antiarrhythmic agent, e.g. bretylium tosylate 100 mg i.v., and repeat the shock.

Continue massage and ventilation between shocks. The value of good massage cannot be overemphasized and may ride out arrhythmias (other than VF) that are not being successfully managed with drugs. It is also a safer and a better way of correcting an acidosis than bicarbonate (see below). Avoid hyperventilation.

If the Monitor Shows Asystole, Extreme Sinus Bradycardia or PEA

These are all managed similarly. PEA was previously known as electromechanical dissociation (EMD). Continuing electrical activity on the monitor with no palpable pulse is a poor prognostic sign unless it occurs transiently during an arrest (e.g. immediately after defibrillation) or results from a reversible cause.

- Precordial thump; exclude VF on the monitor
- Five cycles of CPR
- Intubate and intravenous access as above
- Adrenaline 1 mg i.v. and repeat every 3–5 min
- Five cycles of CPR
- Atropine 1 mg i.v., up to three doses (maximum 3 mg)
- Check that the rhythm is not shockable; if evidence of electrical activity: emergency pacing; if no evidence of electrical activity: repeat adrenaline 1 mg i.v. or vasopressin 40 U i.v. and CPR
- Consider: large doses of adrenaline, e.g. 5 mg i.v.

Generally the results of resuscitation in asystole are poor unless the patient has gone into complete AV block (with visible P waves), or asystole has just evolved from extreme sinus bradycardia or just after VF defibrillation. It is easy to miss fine VF on a monitor and assume that it is asystole, especially with faulty equipment, artefact or incorrect gain settings.

Intravenous calcium chloride 10 ml of 10% solution has not been included in the above protocol. There is no evidence that it works and calcium loading has been implicated in myocardial cell injury during ischaemia. It may be of benefit in occasional cases, but often this is only transient.

The Search for a Reversible Cause (Table 6.9)

Throughout resuscitation every effort is made to identify a potentially reversible cause for the cardiac arrest. Table 6.9 is easily memorised.

Correction of Acidosis and Sodium Bicarbonate

The use of bicarbonate soon after an arrest is no longer recommended. Effective massage and ventilation should help slow the progression of an acidosis. The measurement of arterial pH and base deficit bears little relationship to the intracellular values, and the inside of the cell may become acidotic (with diffusion of CO_2 into the cell) whereas the extracellular fluid remains alkalotic. Hyperosmolarity with sodium loading occurs, and an alkalosis may be just as dangerous as an acidosis. A single blood gas measurement provides no indication of the rate of acid production.

If in spite of all this after prolonged resuscitation measures have failed, it is reasonable to give 50 mmol sodium bicarbonate i.v. and to repeat the blood gas measurements. A separate central line must be used for bicarbonate because it inactivates catecholamines and precipitates out with calcium chloride or gluconate.

Correction of Hypotension

If the rhythm is reasonably stable but pulse of low volume:
• Check the CVP: this is particularly important in inferior (RV) infarctions where a fluid load may improve the cardiac output. Fluid load should not be

Table 6.9 Potentially reversible causes of cardiac arrest

6 × H	6 × T
Hypovolaemia	Thrombosis: coronary occlusion
Hypo/hyperkalaemia	Thrombosis: pulmonary embolus
Hypoglycaemia	Tension pneumothorax
Hypothermia	Tamponade
Hydrogen ion (acidosis)	Toxins (drugs: iatrogenic or recreational)
Hypoxia	Trauma

attempted without Swan–Ganz monitoring (see Section 6.14). Generally the CVP should be 5–10 cmH$_2$O from the midaxillary line.
• Start dopamine 5 µg/kg per min, increasing to 10 µg/kg per min (for dose regimen, see Section 6.9) via a central line not used for bicarbonate administration.

Correction of Potassium Status
• Hyperkalaemia (K$^+$ >5.0 mmol/l): give 10% calcium chloride 10 ml and check for possible metabolic acidosis. Correction of metabolic acidosis should reduce serum K$^+$ (see also Section 6.6).
• Hypokalaemia: give 20 mmol KCl through central line over 10 min if K$^+$ < 3.0 mmol/l.

Further Measures That May Be Necessary
• Insertion of radial artery and Swan–Ganz catheter in pulmonary artery
• Insertion of urinary catheter
• IPPV continued: in the presence of pulmonary oedema and a reasonable arterial pressure (>100 mmHg) PEEP may help
• Insertion of temporary pacing with screening facilities available
• Echocardiography to exclude pericardial effusion, check LV function, mitral and aortic valve movement and aortic root
• Aspiration of a pericardial effusion if documented
• Pass a nasogastric tube and aspirate the stomach.

Procedures Not Recommended
• *Intravenous dexamethasone*: this does not reduce cerebral oedema if given after the event. It should be used only if the arrest was secondary to an anaphylactic reaction.
• *Intracardiac injections*: with a good central line this is unnecessary. It may damage the anterior or inferior surface of the heart.
• *Attempts to assess neurology during resuscitation*: this is very unreliable. Pupils are affected by a wide variety of drugs used in resuscitation. It is preferable to wait and concentrate on resuscitation.
• *Thrombolysis*: although theoretically most cardiac arrests are thrombus related (MI or pulmonary embolism), thrombolysis has not been shown to improve outcomes in cardiac arrest (TROICA trial).

When to Discontinue Resuscitation Attempts
This depends on many factors, such as the precipitating cause for the arrest if known, other medical conditions and the results of resuscitation measures. Usually resuscitation attempts continue for half an hour and longer if the rhythm is still recognizable VF. In younger patients efforts would continue up to an hour or more if there were recognizable electrical activity.

7 Disturbances of Cardiac Rhythm: Bradycardias, Pacing, the ICD, Biventricular Pacing for Heart Failure

7.1 Indications for Temporary Pacing

AV Block in Acute MI

Complete AV block (Figure 7.1)
In inferior infarction, complete AV block usually results from right coronary artery occlusion. The AV nodal artery is a branch of the right coronary artery. Second-degree AV block (Wenckebach type) does not always represent AV nodal artery occlusion because vagal hyperactivity may play a part. A localized, small inferior infarct may thus cause complete AV block.

In anterior infarction, complete AV block usually represents massive septal necrosis with additional circumflex artery territory damage. The prognosis in complete AV block is dependent on infarct size and site rather than the block itself.

Complete AV block in either type of infarction should be temporarily paced.

Second-degree AV Block (Figure 7.1)
• Wenckebach (Mobitz type I): incremental increases in PR interval with intermittent complete blocking of the P wave. This is decremental conduction at the AV node level. In inferior infarction it does not necessarily require pacing unless the bradycardia is poorly tolerated by the patient. It may respond to atropine. In anterior infarction, Wenckebach AV block should be temporarily paced.
• Mobitz type II AV block: fixed PR interval with sudden failure of conduction of atrial impulse (blocking of the P wave). Often occurs in the presence of a wide QRS because this type of block is usually associated with distal fascicular disease. It carries a high risk of developing complete AV block. It

Swanton's Cardiology, sixth edition. By R. H. Swanton and S. Banerjee. Published 2008 Blackwell Publishing. ISBN 978-1-4051-7819-8.

Types of 2nd degree AV block

Wenckebach 2nd degree AV block

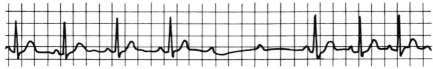

Mobitz type II AV block

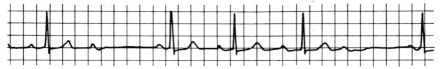

2:1 AV block

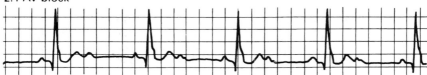

Complete third degree AV block

Congenital: narrow QRS

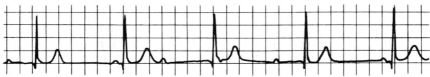

Acquired: broad QRS

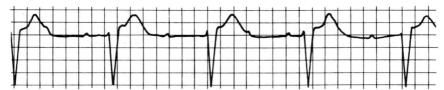

Figure 7.1 Second- and third-degree AV block.

usually occurs in association with anterior infarction, but should be prophylactically paced with either type of infarct.

First-degree AV Block

This does not require temporary pacing, but approximately 40% will develop higher degrees of AV block, and observation is necessary.

Bundle-branch Block (see Chapter 16, Figures 16.7 and 16.8)

This is a more complex group with conflicting evidence from various series. Patients with evidence of trifascicular disease or non-adjacent bifascicular disease complicating MIs should be prophylactically paced, i.e.

- Trifascicular disease
- Alternating RBBB/LBBB
- Long PR interval + new RBBB + LAHB or new RBBB + LPHB
- Long PR + LBBB
- Non-adjacent bifascicular disease: RBBB + new LPHB (see Chapter 16, Figure 16.8).

There is no proof that LBBB with a long PR interval is genuine trifascicular disease without measurements from His bundle studies, but, if it develops in the presence of septal infarction, LBBB is assumed to be LAHB + LPHB. One of the most common bundle-branch blocks complicating anterior infarction is RBBB and LAHB (usually manifest by RBBB + left axis deviation), as these two fascicles are in the anterior septum. In anterior infarction this combination should be paced only if a long PR interval develops. Measurement of the H–V interval is theoretically useful in acute infarction, but involves insertion of an electrode under fluoroscopy and is not generally practical.

Sinoatrial Disease

Profound sinus bradycardia or sinus arrest may occur in acute infarction (typically inferior infarction and right coronary occlusion). The sinus node arterial supply is usually from the right coronary artery. Vagal hyperactivity may contribute and be partially reversed by atropine. However, sinus bradycardia or sinus arrest may need temporary pacing if not reversed by atropine and if poorly tolerated by the patient.

Temporary Pacing for General Anaesthesia

The same principles apply as those in acute infarction: 24-hour monitoring for those thought to be at risk may provide useful information. Notice should be taken of recent ECG deterioration (e.g. lengthening of PR interval, additional LAHB).

Asymptomatic patients with bifascicular block and a normal PR interval do not need temporary pacing. Patients with sinoatrial disease should have 24-hour ECG monitoring before surgery, because vagal influences may produce prolonged sinus arrest.

Temporary Pacing during Cardiac Surgery

Temporary epicardial pacing may be necessary in surgery adjacent to the AV node and bundle of His, e.g.

- aortic valve replacement for calcific aortic stenosis (with calcium extending into the septum)
- tricuspid valve surgery and Ebstein's anomaly

- AV canal defects and ostium primum ASD
- corrected transposition and lesions with AV discordance.

A knowledge of the exact site of the AV node and His bundle can be obtained by endocardial mapping at the time of surgery. Closure of a VSD in corrected transposition or of the ventricular component of a complete AV canal defect may damage the His bundle and permanent epicardial electrodes may be required.

Other Indications for Temporary Pacing

Indications include termination of refractory tachyarrhythmias, during electrophysiological studies and drug overdose (e.g. digoxin, β-blocking agents, verapamil).

7.2 Pacing Difficulties

Failure to Pace or Sense

Wire Displacement

This is the most common reason for failure to pace and is a common problem with temporary wires that have no tines or screw-in mechanisms. To some extent it can be avoided by stability manoeuvres during wire insertion. Positions just across the tricuspid valve tend not to be very stable. Positions in the RV apex are usually more stable but sometimes threshold measurements are not ideal here. Wire displacement requires repositioning in either temporary or permanent systems.

Microdisplacement

If not noticed on chest radiograph this may be overcome by increasing pacing output voltage or pulse width. Otherwise repositioning is necessary.

Exit Block

This may develop in the first 2 weeks as a result of a rise in threshold. As the electrode becomes fibrosed into the endocardium the threshold levels off. With temporary units the threshold is checked daily and the voltage increased if necessary. Occasionally a fibrotic reaction at the pacing tip results in exit block and the lead may have to be removed (Figure 7.2). With programmable permanent pacing units the programmer may be used to increase the output.

During temporary wire insertion a threshold of <1.0 V at 1 ms pulse width is preferable. With permanent pacing the pulse width of the unit to be implanted is used. An acute threshold of <1.0 V is again preferable. If the wire has been implanted for a few months, a chronic threshold of <2.0 V is satisfactory because it is unlikely to rise further. Exit block tends to be more of a problem now with epicardial electrodes. Newer endocardial lead design with carbon porous tip and steroid-eluting leads should reduce the incidence of exit block.

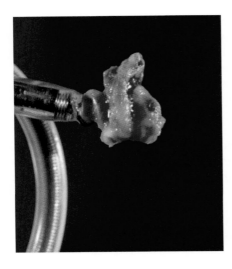

Figure 7.2 Pacing wire removed resulting from failure to pace. Exit block caused by intense fibrotic reaction at wire tip.

Wire Fracture

This may occur as a result of kinking of the wire or too severe looping after implantation. Tight silk ligatures may damage the insulation. Complete fracture may be detected on the chest radiograph (Figure 7.3). Insulation fracture may result in current leakage and pectoral muscle pacing.

Partial fracture results in intermittent pacing, and analysis of the stimulus shows reduced amplitude. A rate drop is not essential with partial wire fracture.

With wire implantation via a direct subclavian puncture there is a rare chance of a pacing wire being crushed between the clavicle and the rib. This

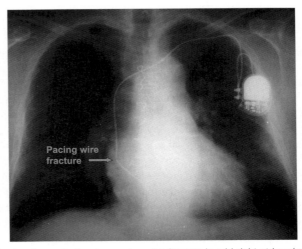

Figure 7.3 Chest radiograph showing pacing wire fracture in mid-right atrium (arrowed).

is a particular possibility with patients who indulge in vigorous arm movements above the head as in the gym or with frequent golf.

Perforation

This is a rare complication of permanent pacing. It sometimes occurs in patients who are temporarily paced for heart block complicating MI (particularly inferior MI affecting the RV). There may be loss of pacing plus signs and symptoms of pericarditis.

The diagnosis can be confirmed by measuring the intracardiac electrogram from the temporary wire. The temporary wire is connected to the V lead of a standard ECG machine. With impaction against the RV wall there should be an endocardial potential of 1.5–8 mV. This is lost with perforation and ST depression and T-wave inversion are recorded (Figure 7.4). Repositioning is necessary.

Battery Failure

Each permanent pacemaker has its own end-of-life characteristics. Premature battery failure has been a problem with some lithium cell designs. Several

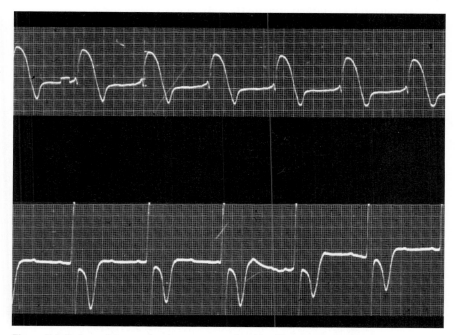

Figure 7.4 Endocardial recording from a pacemaker wire. Top strip shows satisfactory injury current (ST elevation) as wire impacts against RV endocardium. Bottom strip shows loss of injury current as a result of perforation.

factors other than cell design may lead to early battery failure, some of which may be avoided, e.g.:
- low lead impedance with large electrode tip
- wide pulse width
- constant pacemaker use or fast pacing rate
- complex circuitry in automatic pacemakers with two sensing and two pacing circuits (DDD units); recent units have incorporated microprocessors that drain current.

Thus the choice of electrode is important. If a pacemaker with hysteresis mode is available, the takeover rate may be set lower than the basic pacing rate, conserving battery life. Generally the more complex the pacemaker, the shorter the expected battery life.

A pacemaker may have its battery life prolonged by reducing rate, pulse width and output. However, reducing pulse width or output voltage should not be performed until enough time has elapsed from implantation to allow for the establishment of the chronic threshold (e.g. 3 months).

The end of life of most pacemaker batteries is indicated by:
- slowing of the basic pacing rate
- increasing pulse width
- decreasing output voltage.

Regular follow-up at a pacing clinic is necessary to determine the time for elective pacemaker change. Telemetry may help in some areas.

EMG Inhibition (see Figure 7.6)
Electromyographic voltage (e.g. from use of the pectoral muscles) may be of sufficient strength to be sensed by the permanent pacemaker, cause it to be inhibited and hence fail to pace the ventricle. It may exceptionally cause syncope when it is obviously self-limiting. In right-handed patients it is preferable to put the permanent unit on the left side. It is not a problem when a bipolar wire is used and hence does not occur with temporary pacing systems, or most modern permanent pacing systems where bipolar pacing can be programmed. If it does occur in a unipolar system the problem may be overcome by:
- waiting until any effusion around the unit has resolved
- reprogramming the unit to reduced sensitivity VOO (fixed rate ventricular pacing) mode
- placing a non-conducting 'boot' around the pacemaker
- converting the system to a bipolar system with a new wire.

Sensing Failure
The pacemaker fails to notice an intrinsic cardiac impulse and is not inhibited. This may be because the R wave of the intrinsic ECG is too small, the slew

rate is too slow or the pacing unit is too insensitive. In ten
may be a problem in MI (with reduction in or loss of R w;
stimulus-on-T phenomenon. The use of a subcutaneous ind;
as the second pole may help avoid this.

In permanent pacing the sensitivity of the unit may be cha
programmable units (e.g. R-wave sensitivity increased from 2n
A porous tip electrode may offer better sensing capabilities.

False Inhibition (Oversensing) (Figures 7.5 and 7.6)

This is inhibition of the pacemaker by an electrical signal other than by the R
wave. EMG inhibition is an example. It may also occur with spurious signals

Ventricular inhibited pacing

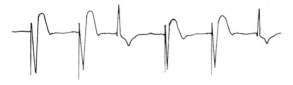

Missing (intermittent failure to pace)

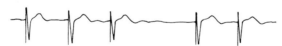

False inhibition (oversensing)

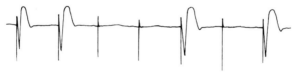

Ventricular triggered pacing

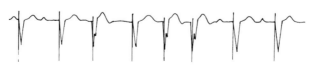

Figure 7.5 Examples of pacing ECGs.

Failure of ventricular capture due to exit block. VVI unipolar system.
Idioventricular rate 36/min

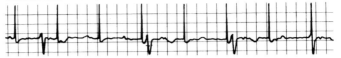

Failure of atrial capture and of atrial sensing with normal ventricular pacing in a
DDD bipolar unit. Unsensed P waves can be seen wandering through the trace

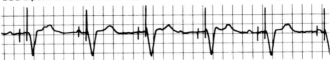

False inhibition (oversensing) in a VVI unit. Lead insulation fracture

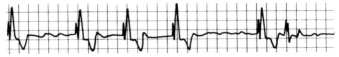

Oversensing and undersensing in a VVI unit programmed to 72/min. Lead
insulation fracture

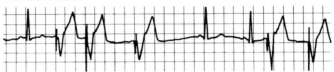

Electromyographic (EMG) inhibition in a unipolar VVI system. Vigorous
pectoral strain produces a signal strong enough to inhibit the unit

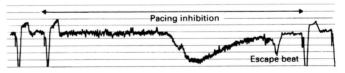

Figure 7.6 Common pacing problems (see also Figure 16.2).

from electrode fracture, or inadequate contacts or bad connections to the internal or external unit. Occasionally, a large T-wave voltage may inhibit the unit. Electromagnetic interference (e.g. leak from microwave ovens) is another possibility. This used to cause false inhibition of early permanent pacing units, but is not a problem now.

Complications of Wire Insertion

Pneumothorax
Following insertion of a pacing wire, the patient should have a chest radiograph to check the wire position and to exclude a pneumothorax.

Infection
Antibiotic prophylaxis is not required for temporary pacing and is indicated only for clinical reasons. After insertion the wire should be anchored with silk sutures to avoid movement and the entry site should be covered with a sterile transparent dressing. If a patient with a temporary wire develops a swinging pyrexia, this is probably the result of a staphylococcal septicaemia. Blood cultures should be taken, the patient started on intravenous flucloxacillin and gentamicin, and the temporary wire removed after a second wire has been put in from the other side (assuming that temporary pacing is still necessary).

Prophylactic antibiotics have been shown to help prevent permanent pacemaker infection. The simplest regimen is to give the patient flucloxacillin 1 g i.v. just before the procedure itself. No further antibiotics are necessary. If the patient has a prosthetic heart valve then the skin may well be colonized by methicillin-resistant staphylococci and teicoplanin 400–800 mg i.v. and gentamicin 80–120 mg should be used (dosage dependent on renal function).

Once a permanent unit has been infected (e.g. extrusion of a corner of a box through ulcerated skin), it should be removed, together with the wire (if possible). There is no point in trying to rescue the situation with antibiotics and resuturing. A new system should be implanted on the other side.

Haemorrhage
This uncommon complication may result from puncture of the subclavian artery with a haemothorax or widening mediastinum features appearing on the chest radiograph. The subclavian artery lies posterior to the vein, and arterial puncture occurs if the entry site is too posterior (supraclavicular approach) or if the needle is directed too posteriorly (supra- and infraclavicular approach). Usually needle puncture of the subclavian artery does not result in complications if the clotting screen is normal. Aspirin and/or clopidogrel should also be stopped if possible 3–4 days before implantation.

In elective permanent pacing, if the patient is on anticoagulants, these should be discontinued where possible to allow the INR/prothrombin time ratio to fall to ≤1.5:1. After box implantation heparin use will cause a haematoma around the box and warfarin should be restarted the evening of the implant rather than continuing with heparin.

Thrombophlebitis, Subclavian Vein Thrombosis

This is usually only a problem with median cubital vein entry site, which should be avoided where at all possible. Temporary pacing from the femoral vein (other than at formal cardiac catheterization) should be avoided because of the risk of infection and deep vein thrombosis. Very occasionally a subclavian vein thrombosis occurs with permanent pacing. Collateral veins develop and dilate around the shoulder and the affected arm may become a little swollen. If caught early enough (within the first 2 or 3 days) thrombolysis given intravenously through the affected arm should be tried followed by formal anticoagulation with heparin and then warfarin.

SVC Stenosis

This is fortunately a rare complication occurring at the junction of the innominate vein to the SVC, caused by the pressure of the pacing wires on the wall of the vessel as they turn the corner into the SVC. It can be dealt with by balloon dilatation (Figures 7.7 and 7.8). Stenting of the SVC has also been

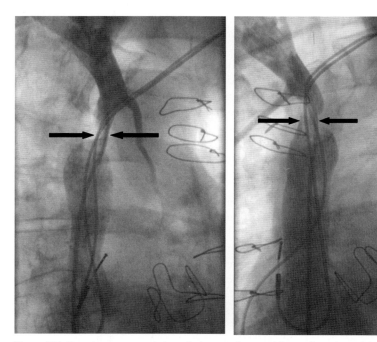

Figure 7.7 Superior vena caval stenosis (arrowed) caused by pacing wires: right anterior and left anterior oblique views. Note no reflux up innominate vein. Previous aortic xenograft valve replacement.

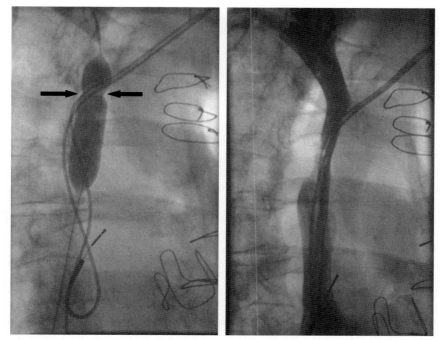

Figure 7.8 Balloon dilatation of superior vena caval stenosis: the tight stenosis indents the balloon even high pressure (arrowed). Right panel: final result. Mild residual tubular narrowing.

successful for this complication and the stent does not seem to harm the wire insulation – possibly because the wires have become endothelialized.

Brachial Plexus Injury

This is rare and occurs also with the entry site being too posterior. If the needle track is kept strictly subclavicular, this will be avoided.

Thoracic Duct Injury

This is rare. The main thoracic duct drains into the junction of the left subclavian and left internal jugular veins. Temporary pacing via the right subclavian vein should therefore be attempted first.

Arrhythmias

Manipulation of the wire in the right atrium may produce atrial ectopics, atrial tachycardia or AF. Manipulation in the right ventricle (especially post-infarction) may produce VT or VF. If the RV is very irritable, a lidocaine infusion should be set up (starting with 100 mg i.v. stat and 4 mg/min). Atrial arrhythmias are usually transient and of less serious consequence, especially if the wire is being inserted for complete AV block.

Pacemaker Box Migration

With modern light generators this is now an unusual complication. Genera-tors can slip from a routine prepectoral position into the axilla and become uncomfortable. In this case repositioning of the unit may be necessary. The problem is avoided by implanting the box beneath pectoralis major in thin people.

Difficulties with Vein Access

Failure to Find a Subclavian Vein

This may be a result of the needle direction being too posterior. A few manoeu-vres may help: keep the needle direction horizontal initially. Try bending the needle at the hub slightly so that the needle points upwards/anteriorly. Remove the patient's pillow briefly to help open the gap between the clavicle and the rib. Ask an assistant to pull on the ipsilateral arm while the subclavian vein puncture is made. Inject dilute contrast through an arm vein to show up the subclavian vein and freeze the image on a slave screen. Finally, if all this fails, wire the subclavian vein retrogradely from the femoral vein and use the wire as a marker.

Upgrading a Pacing System

This can be difficult because the existing lead has already possibly used up the cephalic vein. Subclavian vein puncture is necessary under screening. Keep the needle close to and parallel with the existing wire to access the subclavian. The fear is injury to the existing wire's insulation with the needle, but fortunately this is unusual! If the subclavian or innominate veins is throm-bosed switch to the other side with a new system.

Left SVC Draining into Coronary Sinus

This uncommon anomaly usually comes as an unpleasant surprise after suc-cessful subclavian or cephalic vein cannulation. The wire tracks down the left side of the mediastinum reaching the right atrium via a dilated coronary sinus. If this problem is encountered, switch to a long lead (64cm rather than the conventional 58cm) with an active fixation (screw-in) tip. Once in the right atrium, advance the lead and withdraw the stylet a few inches so that the lead loops over itself into an 'α' formation and the tip can be negotiated down into the RV apex (Figure 7.9).

Pacemaker Implantation in Patients on Anticoagulants

Pacemaker implantation should be performed with the INR <1.5 if possible, and delayed if the INR >2.0. If the patient is taking warfarin only for AF, the warfarin can be stopped 4–5 days before implantation, without the need for additional heparin cover. The warfarin is restarted the night of the procedure.

If the patient is on warfarin for a mechanical valve replacement, heparin cover is advised even though the embolic risk is small for the time

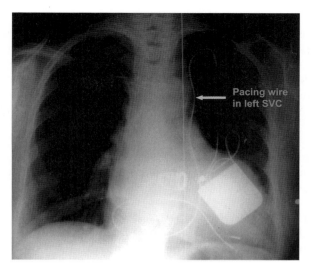

Figure 7.9 Permanent pacing (VVI unit) via left SVC. Previous aortic Starr–Edwards aortic valve replacement and failed pacing via right SVC. The left SVC pacing wire reaches the right atrium via characteristic course down a dilated coronary sinus and is looped over in the right atrium to reach RV apex.

warfarin is stopped. Patients are told to stop warfarin and then admitted for heparin injections once the INR falls below 2.5 (e.g. Fragmin 120 U/kg s.c. twice daily). The low-molecular-weight heparin is stopped the morning of the procedure and warfarin restarted with a loading dose (e.g. twice the maintenance dose) the night of the implantation. Heparin should not be given immediately postoperatively as a wound haematoma is likely. If the INR remains >2.5 48 h after implantation, the heparin could be restarted until the INR rises >2.5.

7.3 Glossary of Pacing Terms in Common Use

Automatic Interval (Basic Interval)
This is the stimulus–stimulus interval during regular pacing.

Bipolar Pacing System
Most temporary wires use a bipolar pacing wire with two ring electrodes. The proximal ring electrode (approximately 1 cm from electrode tip) is the anode, and the distal (tip) electrode the cathode. Sometimes the position of the anode may be higher up the wire (e.g. in the SVC). The pacing spike is small on the surface ECG. Bipolar wires are also available for permanent pacing and are used routinely now. A permanent bipolar system is immune to external signals (see Section 7.9). In addition the bipolar system has the

advantage that the pacing unit will continue to pace the heart when it has been explanted (if still attached to the wire), which greatly facilitates the box change procedure.

Blanking Period
This is the time interval after a pacing impulse during which the pacemaker is insensitive to signals from the heart or from the other channel (avoiding cross-talk).

Chronotropic Incompetence
This is the inability of the heart to increase its rate in response to exercise or metabolic demand.

Committed
This is a dual-chamber pacing system in which the delivery of an atrial stimulus forces the delivery of a ventricular stimulus after a programmed AV delay.

Cross-talk
This happens in DDD units sensing of electronic events from one channel by the other channel, e.g. an atrial stimulus sensed by the ventricular channel resulting in dangerous inhibition of the ventricular impulse. This is avoided by the blanking period (see Figure 7.13).

Demand Pacing (Inhibited)
Unlike the fixed-rate mode, spontaneous cardiac activity is sensed and inhibits the pacemaker, which fires a stimulus only after a pre-set interval if no further impulse is sensed. Thus pacing is inhibited by sensed impulses (atrial or ventricular, see codes in Section 7.5).

Entrance Block
The failure of a pacemaker to sense cardiac events because the sensitivity of the pacemaker is too low, the signals are of too low an amplitude or the lead is fractured (see Figure 7.3).

Epicardial System
This is pacing wires attached to the epicardium either at thoracotomy or by subxiphoid route. The permanent unit is usually intra-abdominal (beneath the rectus muscle and extraperitoneal). It is used in the following:
• Recurrent failure of endocardial systems (infection, exit block, etc.)
• Small children where rapid growth makes transvenous pacing difficult (see Section 7.12)
• Heart block developing during cardiac surgery
• Tricuspid mechanical valve prosthesis; the only exception is a tricuspid Starr–Edwards valve (ball and cage) which can be crossed with a pacing wire

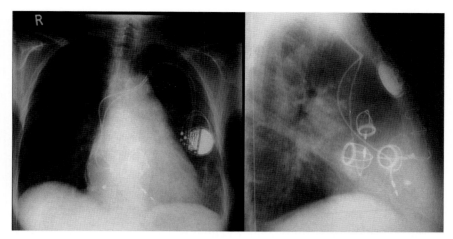

Figure 7.10 Chest radiograph: P/A and right lateral. Triple valve replacement. Starr–Edwards valves. Pacemaker wire through tricuspid Starr valve cage.

(Figure 7.10); the wire obstructs complete ball closure resulting in mild tricuspid regurgitation.

Epicardial systems tend to be less reliable in the long term. Wire displacement and fracture may occur as a result of kinking and vigorous movement. The need for epicardial pacing has diminished with the introduction of LV leads implanted via the coronary sinus. (see Biventricular pacing – Figures 7.17–7.19).

Escape Interval

The interval between a spontaneous cardiac impulse that is sensed and the next pacing stimulus. This is usually the same as the automatic pacing interval unless the pacemaker is programmed to hysteresis mode, in which case the escape interval is longer than the automatic interval.

Exit Block

This is failure of pacing caused by problems at the wire tip such as a fibrotic reaction preventing transmission of the electrical impulse from wire to myocardial cells (see Figure 7.2).

Fixed-rate Pacing

This is constant stimulation of the heart at a fixed rate not influenced by spontaneous cardiac activity.

Hysteresis

This is when the takeover rate of the pacemaker is lower than the pacing rate, e.g. a pacemaker with a pacing rate of 72 beats/min and hysteresis mode set at 60 beats/min will not start pacing until the patient's heart rate falls to <60 beats/min, then the pacing rate jumps to 72 beats/min. Patients may notice the abrupt change in rate, but it conserves battery life.

Lead Impedance

This is a vital factor in battery life. It includes the electrical resistance of the electrode itself plus the impedance of the electrode tip–tissue interface. The size of the electrode tip influences impedance of the wire (the larger the tip, the lower the impedance). Low-impedance wires result in early battery depletion. Average lead impedance is 510 Ω. Development of newer electrodes has resulted in smaller electrode tips (initially 12 or 14 mm^2 now down to 4 mm^2).

Magnet Rate

Application of a magnet over some VVI units converts them to a faster (fixed) pacing rate. This is used to test battery life and satisfactory pacing if there is competition at a slower demand rate.

Missing

This is the term used to denote failure of a pacing stimulus to capture and depolarize atrial or ventricular myocardium. It may be caused by incorrect lead positioning, too low an output voltage or too high a myocardial threshold. Initial management is to increase pacing voltage if a temporary system, and then reposition the wire if this is not successful. Missing with a permanent system cannot be ignored. The unit must be removed, the wire threshold tested and either repositioned or changed.

Mode Switching

This is the ability of a dual chamber pacemaker to switch pacing modes. When a patient with paroxysmal AF or atrial tachycardia goes into AF or SVT the pacemaker switches to VVIR mode, thus avoiding atrial tracking with fast ventricular rates, e.g. rates of >175 for 5–10 cycles or even less in some units will trigger the mode switch. The unit switches back to DDDR mode when sinus rhythm reappears or the atrial rate falls. In patients with regular atrial arrhythmias, some units can mode switch to DDIR mode, thus avoiding atrial tracking.

Myopotential (EMG) Inhibition (see Figure 7.6)

This is an electrical signal from skeletal muscle (usually pectoral), which is sensed by the pacemaker, incorrectly interpreted as cardiac in origin and falsely inhibits the pacemaker impulse.

Non-committed

This is a dual-chamber pacemaker in which the sensing of ventricular activity during the AV interval can inhibit the delivery of a ventricular impulse.

Oversensing (False Inhibition) (see Figures 7.5 and 7.6)

This is inhibition of the pacemaker by non-physiological electromagnetic interference or physiological myopotential signals. In this instance pacemaker sensitivity must be reprogrammed to a lower setting.

Paired Pacing

A double impulse fired in rapid succession to the ventricle results in an increased force of contraction, but a much greater myocardial oxygen consumption and a risk of inducing VT. It is not used in clinical pacing.

Pulse Width/Pulse Duration

This is the duration of the pacing stimulus (usually between 0.5 and 1.0 ms). The broader pulse width may capture the ventricle and pace it when narrower pulse widths fail, but this will drain more current and shorten battery life of permanent units. The same applies to atrial pacing.

Rate-responsive Pacing (Adaptive Rate Pacing)

This is a permanent pacing system in which the pacemaker speeds up and slows down in response to certain physiological stimuli. It may be single-chamber (AAIR or VVIR) or dual-chamber (DDDR) (see Section 7.5).

Relative Threshold

Some pacing units have an analysable threshold once implanted permanently. The relative threshold is the minimum percentage of total available voltage required to pace the heart. Thus a relative threshold of 25% is with maximum unit voltage of, say, 5.2 V is 1.3 V.

Sequential Pacing

This is pacing of the atrium followed at a pre-set interval by pacing of the ventricle. This allows physiological atrial transport (see Section 7.6).

Slew Rate

This is the rate of rise of the endocardial potential (dV/dt). Potentials with a low slew rate may not be sensed.

Telemetry

This is a pacemaker facility to transmit a radiofrequency signal containing information about battery life, programmable functions, frequency of pacemaker use, etc.

Tilt Testing

This is used to provoke syncope in patients with possible cardioneurogenic syncope. Patients lie flat for 20–30 min and are then tilted head-up to 60° for 45 min. Continuous ECG and blood pressure recordings (ideally from a radial artery line) are needed.

Triggered Pacing (see Figure 7.5)

A sensed spontaneous R wave results in immediate pacing stimulus fired into the R wave (the heart obviously refractory and not paced). Triggered pacing units have a built-in refractory period to protect against fast electrical interference inducing VT. Ventricular triggered pacing may be used:

- to avoid EMG inhibition
- when a temporary wire is inserted to cover a failing permanent unit. Stimuli from the failing implanted unit trigger the external unit to fire an impulse. This falls in the absolute refractory period (if the internal unit's impulse depolarized the heart) or alternatively paces the heart if the internal/permanent unit impulse fails to depolarize the heart. It is thus a fail-safe mechanism.

Unipolar Pacing System

The earliest permanent units were unipolar: using the pacing box as the anode (+) and the pacing wire as the cathode (−). The pacing spike was large on the surface ECG. Bipolar pacing leads are now used routinely with a distal tip electrode (cathode) and the anode electrode about 1 cm proximal to the tip. The advantage of this system is that it avoids EMG inhibition.

Voltage Threshold

This is the minimum voltage that will pace the heart.

7.4 Permanent Pacing for Bradyarrhythmias

There has been an enormous increase in pacemaker technology since the first pacemaker was implanted by the Karolinska Hospital team in 1958. Permanent pacing is one of the most cost-effective forms of treatment in the whole of medicine. Numbers of implants are increasing, but the implant rate in the UK is among the lowest in Europe, resulting partly from the lack of pacing centres and partly from the low referral rate for pacing. Data from the HRUK registry (see Appendix 5) show a gradual increase in number of pacemakers implanted in the UK with an increase in dual chamber and rate responsive systems (Table 7.1).

Indications for Permanent Pacing

These vary from country to country, but certain definite categories are recognized.

Chronic Complete AV Block with Stokes–Adams Episodes

This is usually the result of central bundle-branch fibrosis (Lenegre's disease), often with normal coronary arteries in the older group. The QRS complex is wide. Pacing should abolish symptoms and prolong life (1-year mortality rate of 35–50% unpaced, 5% paced). Symptoms other than frank syncope, which may result from AV block, include giddiness, transient amnesia and misdiagnosed epilepsy.

Table 7.1 The changing practice of pacing in the UK

Parameter	1989	1998	2002	2005
Pacing centres (n)	138	177	164	191
Patients paced (n)	10500	24000	27737	36303
Implants/million population (n)	178	406	466	603
VVI units (%)	79	34.9	18	15
VVIR units (%)	2.5	14.1	19	24
DDD units (%)	16	36.9	37	27
DDDR units (%)	1	11.8	25	27
AAIR units (%)	0.36	0.71	1	1

In the younger age group coronary artery disease may be an additional prognostic factor.

Chronic Complete AV Block with No Symptoms
This is a smaller group of patients who should also be paced because life expectancy is increased, and the first Stokes–Adams episode may be fatal: ECG monitoring for 24 hours usually reveals very slow idioventricular rhythm at night (e.g. <20 beats/min).

Congenital Complete AV Block (see Figure 7.1)
In this condition the level of block is higher up in the His bundle or AV node. The QRS complex is narrow and the idioventricular rhythm faster, and it may respond slightly to exercise or other autonomic stimuli. Asymptomatic children may survive into adult life, when a permanent transvenous system is easier to insert. Indications for pacing in congenital complete AV block are:
- development of any rate-related symptoms
- wide QRS
- other cardiac lesions and cardiac surgery
- early presentation
- failure of AV node to respond to exercise ('lazy junction'), etc.
- 24-hour monitoring evidence of functional exit block or paroxysmal tachyarrhythmias
- a daytime mean functional rate <50/min: because this carries a higher long-term risk of syncope and sudden death.

Mobitz Type II AV Block (see Figure 7.1 and Chapter 16, Figure 16.5)
This type of AV block is characterized by a constant PR interval and the sudden failure of conduction of an atrial impulse through the AV node. There is a high incidence of complete AV block developing and patients with this type of AV block should be paced permanently.

It should be noted that Wenckebach type I AV block is not an indication for permanent pacing. It may result from high vagal tone in athletes or children, and may be a transient phenomenon in acute inferior infarction (involving the AV nodal artery). It may result from drug toxicity (digoxin, β blockade, verapamil). Generally it is a benign, transient rhythm disturbance.

Post-MI
After inferior infarction, second- or third-degree AV block is normally transient, and permanent pacing does not need to be considered for 2–3 weeks post-infarct.

After anterior infarction, complete AV block usually represents massive septal necrosis, and mortality from LVF is high. Persistent complete AV block is permanently paced. More difficult is an AV block that regresses during hospital stay. This is still a subject for debate, but 24-hour Holter monitoring may help identify those at risk who need permanent pacing. The ventricular myocardium is often very irritable in the post-infarct period and if possible permanent pacing should be avoided in the first 3–4 weeks.

Chronic Bundle-branch Block
Early work to suggest that His bundle electrograms (Figure 7.16) would identify patients at risk has not been substantiated. Theoretically a prolonged H–V interval in the presence of bifascicular block would indicate the third fascicle at risk. However, this does not seem to be prognostically useful. The incidence of chronic asymptomatic patients with bifascicular block developing complete AV block is low. It does not seem to be precipitated by general anaesthesia. Again 24-hour Holter monitoring may be helpful. Generally, asymptomatic patients with bifascicular block do not merit permanent pacing. Pacing is indicated for patients with symptoms plus bifascicular block, e.g. symptoms plus:
- RBBB + LAHB ⎫ bifascicular disease (see Figures 16.7 and 16.8)
- RBBB + LPHB ⎭

- RBBB with alternating LAHB/LPHB ⎫
- LBBB with alternating RBBB ⎬ 'trifascicular' disease
- LBBB + long PR interval ⎭

Sick Sinus Syndrome
Sick sinus syndrome (SSS) is also known as sinoatrial disease, tachycardia–bradycardia syndrome or generalized conduction system disease. Although primarily involving the sinus node and atrial myocardium, it may develop into a condition including AV node disease, or even be associated with a cardiomyopathy. Systemic emboli are a recognized complication (possibly related to prolonged periods of sinus arrest).

Common ECG abnormalities include the following (often switching from one to another) (Figure 7.11):
- Sinus arrest: chronic or paroxysmal

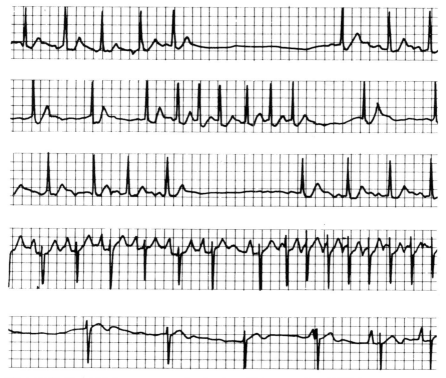

Figure 7.11 Sinoatrial disease: segments of a single 24-hour monitored ECG in a patient with this condition (also known as sick sinus syndrome). The ECG shows episodes of wandering atrial pacemaker and sinus arrest (first line), junctional escape rhythm and AF (second line), sinus arrest (third line), sinus rhythm and supraventricular tachycardia (fourth line) and junctional bradycardia moving into sinus rhythm (fifth line).

- Sinus bradycardia: not necessarily responding to effort or atropine
- Sinus exit block
- Paroxysmal atrial tachycardia, atrial flutter, AF
- Carotid sinus hypersensitivity
- AV block: usually in the older age group, who may have AF with complete AV block and a slow idioventricular rhythm.

Permanent pacing in SSS does not prolong life. The following are the indications for permanent pacing:

- Symptoms with a documented bradycardia
- Symptoms caused by drug-induced bradycardia (used to control the tachyarrhythmias). AAI pacing will maintain atrial transport while AV nodal conduction is still normal. However, the development of AV block may require a change to DDDR pacing (see Section 7.6).

7.5 Pacemaker Codes

With increasing complexity of permanent pacemakers, codes have been developed to enable operators to identify the capabilities of individual units.

The initial three-letter code was introduced by Parsonnet in 1974 and is currently in use on the European Pacemaker card. This has been agreed by the International Association of Pacemaker Manufacturers. The four-letter code is now in general use, but already likely to be superseded by a five-letter code, to cope with facilities available on newer programmable units. A sixth letter may one day be included to cope with telemetric capabilities.

As Table 7.2 shows, the first letter of the code always relates to the chamber paced, the second to the chamber sensed. The third letter indicates the pacemaker response to the sensed impulse. Formerly, this third letter was replaced by a 'fraction', e.g. T/I or TI/I, because the more complex pacemaker responded in different ways to stimuli from atrium and ventricle.

The most frequently used pacemaker in the UK has the code DDD (37% of UK implants in 1998 – see Section 7.6).

Individual Pacing Codes

These are shown diagrammatically with a schematic ECG alongside each.

VOO

This is fixed-rate ventricular pacing only, and is now rarely used, i.e. ventricular pacing, no sensing and no response. The pacemaker is not inhibited by spontaneous ventricular impulses, and there is a small risk of stimulus on T phenomenon causing ventricular tachycardia.

VVI

This is ventricular pacing that is inhibited by sensed ventricular impulses. It is the unit of choice in patients with AV block and AF, and SSS with atrial paralysis.

However, patients with AV block and persistent sinus node function will lose atrial contribution to ventricular filling because often the atria contract against closed AV valves. There will be cannon waves in the JVP, and intermittent reversal of atrial flow. Retrograde AV conduction compounds the problem.

Programmable VVI units may partly overcome this by being programmed to a lower rate, or with hysteresis.

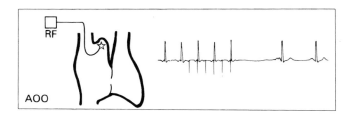

AAI

This is only atrial pacing that is inhibited by sensed P waves. This type of pacemaker is used in patients with SSS who have normal AV node function. (It does not matter if they have retrograde AV conduction.) It may be used in patients with profound sinus bradycardia or in drug-induced sinus bradycardia (in the SSS) (see Figure 16.6). Atrial transport is preserved.

However, this pacing relies on normal AV node function, and patients with SSS may develop abnormalities in AV conduction after the unit has been implanted (≤30% in one series). Also it is obviously unsuitable for patients with SSS and intermittent AF, which may develop after the unit has been implanted.

The are following contraindications to AAI pacing:
- AV block or Wenckebach block with atrial pacing up to 150/min
- Bifascicular block on 12-lead ECG
- Atrial flutter, AF or paralysis
- Carotid sinus syndrome
- H–V interval >55 ms or prolonging with high atrial rates.

Thus His bundle electrograms and atrial pacing studies are necessary before choosing to implant an AAI unit.

AOO

This is asynchronous atrial pacing. Rarely used except in patient-activated bursts to overdrive atrial tachycardias. In using rapid atrial stimulation bursts, it is important to be certain that there is no pre-excitation pathway to the ventricle.

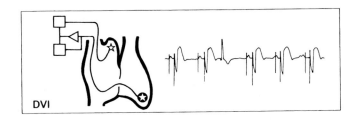

VAT

This is ventricular pacing triggered by a sensed atrial impulse. Two leads are required. This is P-wave synchronous pacing with normal sinus node function. It cannot be used in patients with atrial dysrhythmias, AF or atrial flutter.

Its major disadvantage is that it does not sense ventricular impulses,

and hence will compete with spontaneous ventricular activity. If the patient has frequent ventricular ectopics there is the risk of stimulus-on-T phenomenon.

It is the simplest way of preserving atrial transport in patients with AV block (se Chapter 16, Figure 16.6) but rarely used now.

DVI

This is atrial and ventricular pacing, but only spontaneous ventricular activity is sensed. Spontaneous atrial activity is ignored. Two leads are required. After a spontaneous ventricular impulse is sensed the pacemaker resets to one V–A interval and fires an atrial impulse, followed by a ventricular impulse. Spontaneous P waves occurring within this V–A interval are not sensed.

It can be used in complete AV block or sinus bradycardia. It cannot be used in AF. Although atrial synchrony is maintained at a basal rate, it will not follow an increase in sinus rate with exercise, and competes with atrial rates faster than the pacemaker rate. It is useful in patients with retrograde VA conduction.

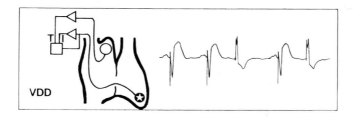

VDD

This is also known as ASVIP or atrially sensed ventricular inhibited pacing. Both chambers are sensed (once two leads were required, but a single pass lead with atrial electrodes is available) and the spontaneous impulse triggers the pacemaker to stimulate the ventricle. Spontaneous ventricular impulses inhibit the pacemaker, which is reset to fire after one standby period.

It is suitable for simple AV block without any evidence of sinoatrial disease. Sinus node function should be normal. If AF develops, the pacemaker reverts to VVI mode. This also occurs if the spontaneous atrial rate falls below the escape rate of the pacemaker.

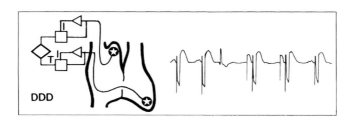

DDD

This is the only fully automatic unit that paces and senses both chambers (two leads required). This unit will either sense the atrial impulse and then pace the ventricle, or pace the atrium and then pace the ventricle if no spontaneous atrial impulse is sensed. It is the necessary advance on the VDD unit because it can be used in the SSS with additional AV nodal disease. If AF develops it also reverts to the VVI mode (mode switching).

KEY TO SYMBOLS

☆ Pacing only   ◯ Sensing only   ◇ Logic function

✪ Pacing and Sensing   I   Inhibited

▢ Pacing output circuit   T   Triggered

◁ Sensing circuit   RF   Radio frequency signal

Table 7.2 Pacemaker codes

Code letter position	First	Second	Third	Fourth	Fifth
Category	Chamber(s) paced	Chamber(s) sensed	Mode of pacemaker response	Programmable functions	Tachyarrhythmia functions
Letters used	V = ventricle A = atrium D = dual *S = single	V = ventricle A = atrium D = dual O = none S = single	T = triggered I = inhibited D = dual R = reverse T/I = atrially triggered and ventricular inhibited T/II = fully automatic	P = programmable (rate and/or output only) M = multi-programmable O = none R = rate responsive	B = burst N = normal rate competition S = scanning E = controlled external (magnet or AF)

*That is, either atrium or ventricle.

7.6 Physiological Pacing and Choice of Pacing Unit

The VVI unit involves a single ventricular pacing lead only, and ignores atrial contribution to cardiac output. Atrial systole may contribute ≤25% of cardiac output in some patients by increasing LVEDV and stroke volume. Utilization of atrial systole by either sensing and/or pacing in synchrony with ventricular pacing has been called 'physiological pacing'. It has many limitations and cannot be strictly physiological at high heart rates. Nevertheless it may improve cardiac output in patients with borderline LV function. It may also help to avoid systemic emboli in patients with SSS by avoiding stagnation in a flaccid left atrium, and may help prevent the development of AF. Table 7.2 details the codes used in describing a pacemakers type, and Table 7.3 summarizes the optimal pacing modes for specific cardiac conditions.

A few patients with AV block may actually do worse with VVI pacing. The AV node may still conduct retrogradely and atrial stimulation may cause atrial contraction against closed AV valves. This has been shown to put up pulmonary wedge pressure: the pacemaker syndrome.

Ideally the choice of a physiological pacing unit should involve knowledge of certain facts, but time rarely allows this degree of investigation:

• The cardiac output should be measured with ventricular pacing and AV synchronous pacing to ensure that the more expensive and sophisticated physiological unit will confer extra benefit to the patient.

• A knowledge of sinus node function: ECG monitoring for 24 hours will provide some information. Tests of sinus node function (sinus node recovery time, sinoatrial conduction time) unfortunately do not reliably predict sinus node function if normal.

• A knowledge of AV conduction, both anterograde and retrograde.

• Does the patient develop SVT or other atrial tachyarrhythmias? ECG monitoring for 24 hours and provocation with atrial extra-stimulus testing may help here.

Sinoatrial Disease with Normal AV-node Function

Single-lead AAI pacing is theoretically adequate. The addition of rate response (AAIR) is an attempt to improve cardiac output on effort in the presence of

Table 7.3 Summary of optimum pacing modes

Condition	Best	Second best	Comments
Sinoatrial disease	AAIR	AAI	AAI may be as good
Sinoatrial disease plus AV block	DDDR	DDD	DDD may be as good
AV block	DDD	VVI	
Chronic AF plus AV block	VVIR	VVI	See text for choice
Carotid sinus syndrome	DDD	VVI	
Malignant vasovagal syndrome	DDD	VVI	

chronotropic incompetence (inability to increase heart rate with exercise). However, it seems to carry little benefit over AAI pacing. Atrial pacing helps prevent systemic emboli and the development of AF.

Although the chance of developing AV block is low, most patients are now paced using a dual chamber system to avoid the difficulties of upgrading the AAI system later. Less than 1% of pacemakers implanted in the UK are currently AAI systems.

Overdrive atrial pacing at night appears to reduce the number of episodes of sleep apnoea in patients with obstructive sleep apnoea.

Complete AV Block with Normal Sinus-node Function

Ideally all patients should have DDD units. Owing to the expense of the units, and the elderly and frail nature of many of the patients presenting with Stokes–Adams attacks, many individuals have been managed and cured with VVI pacing. With these economic problems a reasonable compromise is the provision of DDD units for:

• patients with poor LV function and patients with LV hypertrophy, both having high LVEDP and needing atrial transport to maintain cardiac output
• the younger or mobile elderly patient
• patients with documented retrograde VA conduction
• the development of a pacemaker syndrome with VVI pacing. The older patient with limited mobility can be managed with a VVI unit in most cases.

VVI pacing stood up to DDD pacing unexpectedly well in the UK PACE trial in which patients with complete AV block were randomized to either form of pacing and quality of life determined. One advantage noted on follow-up was a reduction in embolic events in patients with DDD pacing.

Complete AV Block with Additional Sinoatrial Disease

The theoretical ideal is a DDDR system (see above). If the patient exercises, and the sinus node does not follow, there is rate-responsive back-up. A simpler DDD unit will not allow an exercise-induced increase in heart rate if there is background chronotropic incompetence of the sinus node. It has, however, yet to be proved that a DDDR system is superior to DDD in this situation.

Chronic AF with Complete AV Block

A single-chamber rate-responsive system is best (VVIR), allowing some increase in cardiac output on exercise. A VVI unit is a second-best alternative.

Carotid Sinus Syndrome

This is a rare condition with a minimal stimulus to the carotid sinus causing AV block or ventricular standstill (Figure 7.12). Stimuli that may provoke syncope include head turning, shaving, coughing, heavy lifting or Valsalva's

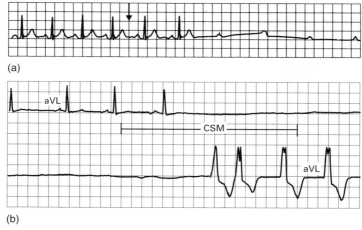

(a)

(b)

Figure 7.12 Carotid sinus hypersensitivity. Normal sinus rhythm is converted to ventricular standstill by the lightest touch on the carotid sinus (arrowed). The sinus node is slowed but there is complete AV block with no ventricular escape. Atropine and a brief period of cardiac massage were required to restore sinus rhythm.

manoeuvre. If a sufferer has a sore throat, even swallowing may provoke syncope. Tight collars must be avoided. Carotid sinus stimulation affects both the sinus node and AV node. Heart rate drop may be sudden and catastrophic (Figure 7.12). DDD or DDDR pacing is necessary.

Neurocardiogenic Syncope (Malignant Vasovagal Syndrome)

This syndrome is incompletely understood. Increased parasympathetic and inhibited sympathetic outflow result in bradycardia (cardioinhibitory response), peripheral vasodilatation (vasodepressor response) or a mixture of both. The drop in heart rate tends to be gradual (in contrast with carotid sinus hypersensitivity). The diagnosis can be made on head-up tilt testing. Hypotension and bradycardia occur, but the problem is only partly relieved by pacing. Treatment involves DDD pacing and drug therapy. Drugs tried have included adenosine blockade (e.g. theophylline), anticholinergics (e.g. transdermal scopolamine or oral disopyramide), β blockade, serotonin reuptake inhibitors (sertraline, fluoxetine) and fludrocortisone. α Agonists may help, e.g. ephedrine, and more recently a new drug, midodrine. Support stockings may help.

Advances in pacing algorithms have allowed some units implanted for this condition to pace at 120/min for 2 min as soon as a sudden rate drop is sensed. This helps abolish an episode before it has time to develop.

Problems with Physiological Pacing Units

Against the obvious advantages of greater cardiac output and higher blood pressure with physiological pacing, there are several disadvantages compared with VVI pacing:

• Two leads generally required except in AAI pacing. The atrial wire positioning can be difficult with both stability and threshold problems, especially in patients who have had cardiac surgery, with no right atrial appendage and often a fibrotic or flabby right atrium. Single-pass leads are available for VDD and DDD pacing with both atrial and ventricular electrodes. Atrial capture may not always be reliable. Temporary pacing with single pass leads can be useful in the ITU.

• Units more expensive.

• Shorter battery life.

• Problems with reliability of complex units and their programming equipment.

• Angina (e.g. SVT developing in VDD pacing causing high ventricular rate).

• Uncertainty at high atrial rates, e.g. episodes of SVT in DDD pacing causing VT. This is dealt with by programming in an upper rate limit (e.g. 140/min), beyond which 2:1 AV block occurs. This rate should be set lower in patients with angina. With frequent atrial tachycardias or atrial flutter where the flutter wave may be interpreted as a P wave, the pacemaker may be programmed to DDI mode (atrial pacing but no atrial tracking). Future units will have automatic programming to DDI mode in this situation, reverting to DDD mode when sinus rhythm resumes.

• Retrograde VA conduction with reciprocating tachycardia (pacemaker-mediated tachycardia). Retrograde conduction occurs in about 70% of patients with normal AV node function and 40% in first-degree AV block. Retrograde conduction of a P wave is sensed by the atrial electrode. It starts an AV interval that is followed by a paced ventricular impulse and a re-entry tachycardia using the pacemaker. This can be prevented by increasing the post-ventricular atrial refractory period or PVARP (see section on basic intervals below). This technique limits the maximum physiological pacing rate, but 150/min is usually considered fast enough. If increasing the PVARP fails to stop the pacemaker-mediated tachycardia, the pacemaker unit should be programmed to DVI (no atrial sensing or tracking) or DDI mode (no atrial tracking).

• Disease progression that limits the pacemaker's potential, e.g. development of AV block in AAI pacing, development of SSS in VDD pacing, development of AF in any DDD system.

Many physiological pacing systems are vulnerable to progression of conduction system disease. DDD units are vulnerable to the development of AF and have to be programmed to VVI mode unless they have an automatic mode switching facility (see Section 7.3).

Basic Intervals in DDD Pacing (Figure 7.13)

AVI
The AV interval starts after the initial atrial pacing stimulus (Ap). The atrial sensing channel is refractory during the AVI.

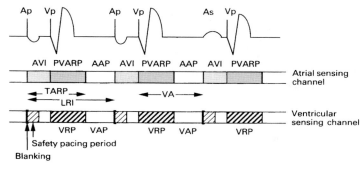

Figure 7.13 Basic intervals in DDD pacing.

PVARP

The PVARP starts after the ventricular pacing stimulus (Vp) during which the atrial sensing channel remains refractory. This helps prevent pacemaker-mediated tachycardia as a result of retrograde VA conduction (see Section above). Both the AVI and PVARP can be programmed. It is rarely necessary to programme the PVARP beyond 400 ms.

TARP

This is the total atrial refractory period = AVI + PVARP. This interval determines at what heart rate 2:1 AV block will occur (upper tracking limit), e.g. AVI of 170 ms and PVARP of 350 ms = TARP of 520 ms and an upper tracking limit of 115/min. Above this, 2:1 block will occur.

AAP

This is the atrial alert period. The atrial channel will sense spontaneous P waves.

LRI

This is the lower rate interval or pulse interval. LRI = AVI + VA interval.

VA

This starts after ventricular stimulus or ventricular sensed beat and ends with either an atrial stimulus or an atrial sensed beat.

Blanking: in the ventricular sensing channel there are two periods when the circuit is closed to external signals. The first is 5–15 ms after the atrial pacing spike and prevents the ventricular channel sensing the atrial pacing output (crosstalk). The second is VRP.

VRP

This is the ventricular refractory period, which is unresponsive to any signal, programmable and begins after a paced or sensed ventricular event.

Safety Pacing Period

This occurs in the AVI just after the blanking period in the ventricular sensing channel. If a ventricular extrasystole falls in this period, it is interpreted as noise and commits the pacemaker to fire in a safety ventricular pacing spike 100–110 ms after the atrial spike. This prevents inappropriate inhibition of ventricular output. A normal VA interval then follows.

VAP

This is the ventricular alert period. The ventricular channel will sense spontaneous ventricular events.

Rate-responsive Pacing (Adaptive Rate Pacing): VVIR

This is a form of physiological pacing that is a useful alternative to dual-chamber pacing. Only one chamber (the ventricle) is paced (as in VVI units), but the pacemaker increases its pacing rate during exercise and slows down physiologically to its basal rate at rest. A variety of biological sensors has been developed that detect a physiological change and signal for an increased (or decreased) heart rate. These must imitate the atrium in physiological terms, and many sensors are still in development. The two most commonly used are QT interval and body activity.

QT interval

This shortens during exercise as a result of catecholamine release; the pacemaker senses the stimulus to T interval (the evoked QT interval). This is the most physiological of all forms of rate-responsive pacing. Early problems resulted from a misconception that the QT interval and heart rate were linearly related. This produced a slow rise in heart rate with effort. The new algorithms have solved this problem.

Body Activity

A piezo-electric crystal is mounted inside the pacemaker can. Vibrations from increased body activity are sensed. However, on some occasions there is little increase in heart rate, e.g. mental activity, isometric exercise and swimming, because there is little body vibration.

Other sensors detect changes in:
- mixed venous oxygen saturation
- RV dP/dt: Intracardiac accelerometer mounted at the tip of the pacing catheter measures peak endocardial acceleration (PEA)
- stroke volume
- temperature
- pH of right atrial blood
- changes in thoracic impedance
- minute volume
- respiratory activity.

Twin Sensors

Some rate-responsive units now contain twin sensors allowing sensor cross-checking and a more physiological increase in heart rate with exercise. Examples are an activity sensor coupled with either a QT sensor or central venous temperature sensor, or the combination of a minute volume and thoracic impedance sensor, with the minute volume sensor taking over at high workloads.

The minute volume sensor pacemaker should be avoided in patients with chronic lung disease. Pacemakers using thoracic impedance as a sensor probably have a shorter battery life. Rate-responsive pacemakers are rapidly increasing in popularity. They allow an increased cardiac output on exercise denied to the patient with a single VVI unit. Their advantages over DDD pacing and their drawbacks are summarized below.

Advantages of VVIR Rate-responsive Pacing Over DDD Pacing
- Single ventricular wire only. Easier and quicker to implant. No problem with unstable atrial wire
- Units cheaper than DDD units
- Possible use in sinoatrial disease or AF

Advantages of DDD Pacing Over VVIR
- The only system to incorporate atrial contribution to cardiac output
- Avoids the pacemaker syndrome
- Of greater benefit in patients with poor LV function and high LVEDP
- Possible reduction in systemic embolic events.

DDDR Pacing
DDDR pacemakers incorporate the best of both systems, i.e. a dual-chamber pacing system with rate-responsive back-up should the patient develop sinoatrial disease (DDDR pacing) or AF (VVIR) pacing. The pacing unit can mode switch between these if paroxysmal AF occurs and telemetry will indicate how many times mode switching has been employed.

7.7 Electrophysiological Measurements and Pacing

Sinus Node Recovery Time (SNRT)

The right atrium is paced at a rate faster than the intrinsic sinus rate for ≤5 min and then pacing is switched off. Rates up to 160 beats/min are used. The SNRT is the longest interval between the last paced beat and first sinus beat. Maximum SNRT is <1.4 s. Corrected SNRT = SNRT – spontaneous cycle length before pacing = <400 ms.

Sinoatrial Conduction Time (SACT)

This is calculated by firing an atrial premature stimulus late in the spontaneous cycle. The atrial premature beat collides with and extinguishes the next sinus impulse. A pause follows as the sinus node is reset. The atrial premature

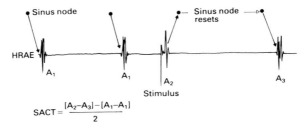

$$SACT = \frac{[A_2-A_3]-[A_1-A_1]}{2}$$

Figure 7.14 Calculation of sinoatrial conduction time.

stimulus has to enter the sinus node and the subsequent reset sinus impulse has to leave it to the atrium. Thus:

$$SACT = [(A_2-A_3) - (A_1-A_1)]/2 = <100\,ms \text{ (Figure 7.14)}$$

where (A_1-A_1) = spontaneous cycle length and (A_2-A_3) = premature atrial stimulus to next spontaneous cycle.

The distance of the catheter from the sinus node is important. The SNRT and SACT are useful only if abnormal. Normal results are unhelpful and cannot be relied upon to predict normal sinus node function.

His Bundle Intervals

Prolongation of the PR interval may result from electrical delay in any part of the AV conducting system. His bundle studies divide the PR interval into A–H interval (AV node conduction) and H–V interval (His–Purkinje conduction) (Figures 7.15 and 7.16).

PA Interval (200 ms)

Lengthening of this is uncommon, usually associated with atrial dilatation or large atrial septal defects. The delay is before the P wave.

A–H Interval (50–120 ms)

This represents AV-node conduction time. The AV node normally shows decremental conduction (increasing delay in conduction with increased frequency of impulses). With graded atrial pacing the A–H time is gradually prolonged to the 'Wenckebach point'. This depends on vagal tone and may be altered by drugs.

Long A–H time is intra-AV-nodal delay. It occurs in:

- first-degree heart block, vagal overactivity, athletes
- Wenckebach second-degree AV block
- inferior infarction
- congenital heart block
- drugs, i.e. digoxin, verapamil, β-blocking agents, amiodarone.

Shortening of the A–H time is usually caused by accessory pathways or sympathetic overactivity. It occurs in:

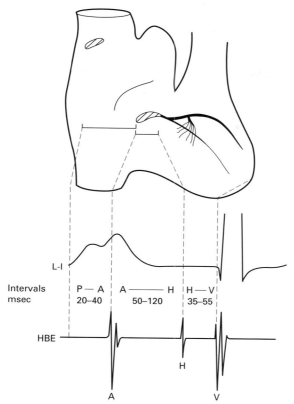

Figure 7.15 Normal HBE intervals: L-I standard lead I of ECG. HBE = His bundle electrogram.

- sympathetic overactivity
- drugs: atropine, catecholamines
- accessory atrionodal or atrio-His pathways (James' pathways)
- junctional ectopics.

In Wolff–Parkinson–White syndrome, the accessory pathway (Kent pathway) is not part of the AV node and does not affect the A–H time.

H–V Interval (35–55 ms)

This represents His–Purkinje system conduction. Rarely, two His spikes may be seen (split His potential), suggesting conduction delay within the His bundle. Lengthening of the H–V time indicates delay in conduction within the His bundle or intraventricular conduction system. It occurs in:

- acquired heart block in elderly people (Lev's, Lenegre's disease)
- Mobitz type II AV block
- anterior infarction
- surgical trauma
- drugs (quinidine, disopyramide, ajmaline, flecainide).

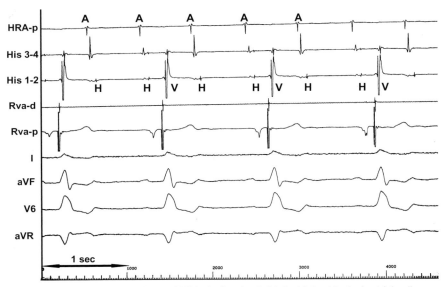

Figure 7.16 His bundle study in 2:1 AV block showing 2:1 infra-Hisian block. A, atrial spike; H, His bundle spike; V, ventricular spike. Permanent pacing needed.

Measurement of the H–V interval in patients with bifascicular block will not predict the small number who will develop complete AV block (approximately 6% patients with RBBB and LAHB). An example of His bundle recordings is shown in Figure 7.16, in a patient with 2:1 AV block caused by a block below the His bundle.

Shortening of the H–V interval usually is a result of accessory pathways arising from the normal AV node or His bundle (Mahaim pathways) or direct AV pathways (Kent pathway). Shortening occurs in:

• sympathetic overactivity
• drugs: catecholamines
• nodoventricular or His-ventricular pathways (Mahaim)
• atrioventricular pathways (Kent)
• idioventricular rhythm arising from one of the fascicles.

Spurious short H–V intervals may be produced by recording RBB activity. Delivery of increasingly premature atrial stimuli until RBBB develops should help differentiate this. If the so-called His spike disappears with the development of RBBB, the spike was not a true His spike but arose from the RBB.

7.8 Advice to the Pacemaker Patient Before Going Home

Pacemaker Interference from Environmental Factors

Before a patient with a permanent pacemaker goes home he or she should be warned that external signals may rarely interfere with the pacemaker and alter its function. The pacemaker wire acts as an aerial for the signal and it is usually only a problem with a unipolar system. The typical response of the pacemaker to an external signal is to switch to fixed-rate pacing (see Magnet Rate, Section 7.3). This increase in heart rate is noticed by the patient, who can then walk away from the source of interference and negate the problem.

Bursts of interference may cause inhibition of the pacemaker and pulsed electromagnetic fields are particular culprits (e.g. airport weapon detectors). The inhibition is quickly noticed by the patient.

As long as the patient is aware of the possibility of pacemaker interference he or she can check his or her own pulse if near a possible signal source. Particular warning should be given about getting too close to the following situations:

• Mains-driven electric motors, especially if sparking or with faulty suppression (e.g. electrical kitchen equipment, vacuum cleaners, electric razors, electric power drills, motor cycles, lawn mowers, outboard motors, old car engines).
• Airport weapon detectors: hand-held detectors are safe.
• Microwave ovens if faulty with inadequate door seal.
• High-power radar stations: hand-held police radar guns are safe.
• CB radio-transmitting systems.
• Some dental drills (e.g. ultrasonic cleaner).
• Some equipment used by physiotherapists (e.g. short-wave heat therapy, faradism).
• Shop anti-theft equipment: the pacemaker may trigger the alarm system as the patient walks out of the shop, and he or she should warn the shopkeeper.
• Public libraries have a system that can inhibit the pacemaker.
• Vibration: hovercraft, helicopters and other sources of vibration may increase the rate of activity-sensing pacemakers. Patients should be warned that this effect may occur.
• Other unexpected magnets such as: magnets in clothing, retention clips in jewellery, fasteners for shoulder bags and back packs, button-hole holders, magnetic storage clips for headphones, sushi bar conveyor belts, audiotape erasure machines, anti-theft security tag release machines.

If a patient is at frequent risk from external interference he or she can use a magnet to switch the pacemaker to fixed-rate mode, during which it is immune to external signals. Generally the risks are very small and are essentially a sudden switch to asynchronous fixed rate pacing, which reverts to normal as soon as the patient walks away from the source of the signal.

Pacemakers and Sport

Vigorous contact sports are best avoided by patients with permanent pacemakers, to avoid injury to the unit (e.g. rugby football, soccer, boxing, judo or karate). Squash should be discouraged if possible. A full golf swing may

'able with a pacemaker in the supramammary pouch, often more
'anted on the left side.

and Radiotherapy

, ...uiation may damage pacemaker circuitry. If possible the pacemaker should be shielded during courses of irradiation. Close monitoring of
pacemaker function is necessary after each dose of irradiation. A typical sign
of pacemaker damage is a noticeable drift in the automatic pacing interval to
a slower rate.

Pacemakers and Surgery

Should a patient with a permanent pacemaker require surgery there is usually
no problem provided that the anaesthetist is aware of the hazards. A common
problem is prostatic surgery with permanent pacemakers *in situ* and a few
precautions are necessary:
- The patient should have ECG monitoring throughout.
- Full DC cardioverting equipment should be available.
- The diathermy plate should be as far from the pacemaker as possible
(i.e. not on the chest or back). Diathermy should not be performed near the
pacemaker box.
- Short bursts of diathermy may inhibit the pacemaker temporarily. This
can be avoided by placing a magnet over the unit, converting it to fixed-rate
mode (VOO). Alternatively the pacemaker can be programmed to VOO
mode at the start of the operation and reprogrammed immediately after the
operation.
- There is a remote risk of VT or VF induced by diathermy with the pacing
electrode acting as an aerial. This will not be prevented by magnet override.

Pacemakers and Driving (see Appendix 6)

Patients should not drive a car for 1 week after the unit's implantation. Provided that they are under regular pacemaker follow-up they may hold a
driving licence and should not have to pay an extra insurance premium.
Patients with permanent pacemakers or ICDs may not hold group 2 licences
(formerly LGV or PCV licences).

Pacemakers and Mobile Telephones

Close proximity of a mobile telephone to a pacemaker may cause pacemaker
inhibition. This is most likely to occur with a high-power output from the
phone, maximum sensitivity of the pacemaker and unipolar pacing. It is much
more likely with digital phones than analogue phones. The most common
interference is inappropriate atrial tracking up to the upper tracking limit of
the pacemaker. Ventricular inhibition may also occur.

Patients wishing to use digital phones must be programmed to bipolar
pacing with sensing thresholds programmed as high as possible and be tested
in the pacing clinic using the phone. Patients should not carry the phone close

to the pacemaker. They should hold the phone away from the body when dialling, and use the ear remote from the pacemaker. If interference from digital phone still occurs in spite of these caveats patients should revert to an analogue system.

7.9 Pacing for Heart Failure: Cardiac Resynchronization Therapy

In heart failure the QRS duration is often prolonged (e.g. LBBB with QRS >150 ms) and delayed activation of the LV results in uncoordinated systolic contraction with paradoxical septal motion, presystolic mitral regurgitation and reduced diastolic filling time. Prolonged QRS duration is associated with a poor prognosis in heart failure.

Changes in Physiology

Atrial synchronized biventricular pacing optimizes AV delay and shortens the QRS duration on the standard 12-lead ECG. Peak systolic pressure (max dP/dt) and stroke volume increase. In patients who respond, reverse remodelling occurs with a reduction in LV and LA dimensions and reduction in presystolic mitral regurgitation. This technique has been labelled cardiac resynchronization therapy (CRT).

Early studies of CRT in heart failure in patients in sinus rhythm have shown an improvement in the 6-minute walk distance, a slight increase in peak Vo_2, a considerable improvement in quality of life, and objective improvement in LVEF assessed by radionuclide studies (MUSTIC trial). Biventricular pacing alone was of some value also in those patients who were in AF. Further studies are under way, but there are no long-term mortality data yet.

Pacing Technique

For the patient in sinus rhythm three pacing leads are used: the conventional atrial J wire in the RA appendage and RV lead in the RV apex, plus a third LV lead advanced through the coronary sinus into a suitable lateral vein overlying the LV (Figures 7.17–7.19). The anatomy of the coronary venous system is first demonstrated by retrograde dye injection through a balloon catheter inflated in the coronary sinus. For patients with additional ventricular tachyarrhythmias, a biventricular ICD system is used. Fortunately thrombosis of the coronary sinus with a long-standing pacing lead in situ does not appear to be a problem.

Problems with the LV lead may be encountered:
• Accessing a suitable vein
• Difficulty in accessing the coronary sinus in patients with a dilated right atrium
• High pacing threshold with what is effectively an epicardial lead

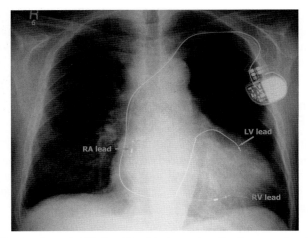

Figure 7.17 Chest radiograph: P/A film. Biventricular pacing. Cardiac resynchronization therapy. CRT.

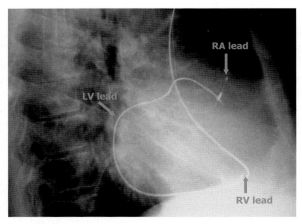

Figure 7.18 Chest radiograph: right lateral view. Biventricular pacing.

• Stability of the miniaturized tined lead; improving lead design is improving lead stability
• Very rarely perforation of the coronary sinus with the guiding catheter
• Three leads in the subclavian vein may rarely cause a subclavian vein thrombosis
• If no satisfactory LV lead position can be found, try a second active fixation RV lead screwed in high up on the RV septum.

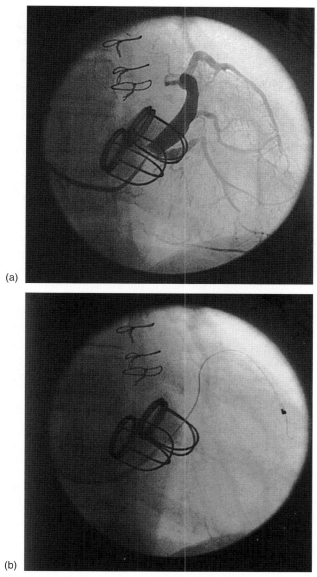

(a)

(b)

Figure 7.19 Permanent pacing in a patient with mitral and tricuspid Starr–Edwards valve replacements: (a) coronary venous anatomy demonstrated by retrograde injection of dye up the coronary sinus with the balloon catheter inflated in the ostium of the coronary sinus. (b) The pacing lead has been advanced down the anterior interventricular vein. Satisfactory LV pacing established.

Patient Selection

The ideal candidate for CRT is theoretically a patient with grade III or IV heart failure (NYHA class), a low LVEF (<35%) in SR with a wide LBBB (QRS >150 ms). Conventional indications for pacing (second- or third-degree heart block, syncope, etc.) are not necessary.

Studies attempting to identify the best criteria for patient selection continue. It is increasingly realized that the QRS duration on the 12-lead ECG is not a reliable guide to patient response to CRT. Increasing reliance is now placed on echocardiography and tissue Doppler imaging to identify inter- and intra-ventricular dyssynchrony. Patients with a narrow QRS or even a wide RBBB may still benefit.

7.10 Pacing for Tachyarrhythmias and the ICD

Implantation of a designated antitachycardia pacing device without defibrillation capacity is now rarely needed. Catheter radiofrequency ablation has replaced antitachycardia pacemakers as treatment for supraventricular arrhythmias. Antitachycardia pacing is still useful in certain situations:
• As part of tiered therapy in the ICD in the management of VT (Figure 7.20; see Section 7.11)
• As an emergency in the catheter laboratory when SVT or VT may occur during cardiac catheterization
• In the CCU or ITU setting where drug therapy has failed or is inappropriate
• Very occasionally in patients with permanent pacemakers by programming the rate up and AV delay down. Permanent overdrive pacing at a higher rate may help prevent VT.

Antitachycardia pacing in the ICD for VT has several advantages:
• Automatic: no patient cooperation required
• Less drug therapy
• No drug effects on LV function
• Less battery requirements than for DC shocks
• Rapid termination prevents deterioration of the rhythm, hypotension or cerebral hypoperfusion
• No drug side effects
• Possible method of arrhythmia control in pregnancy
• No negative inotropic effect on LV function
• May work when drugs fail
• Rapid termination preventing hypotension or cerebral hypoperfusion
• Patient normal between attacks
• Easily reversible (explantation or reprogramming).

Methods of Antitachycardia Pacing

Overdrive Suppression

1 Permanent overdrive pacing: single chamber. Suppression of ectopics by overdrive pacing may prevent SVT or VT. Prevention of bradycardia may

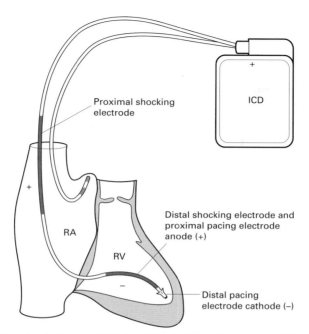

Figure 7.20 Example of a two-lead ICD: the distal shocking electrode is positioned against the RV septum. For shock delivery, the proximal shocking electrode and the ICD unit itself (hot can) act together as the anode (+) and the distal shocking electrode as the cathode (–). For pacing, the distal shocking electrode acts as the anode and the distal pacing electrode as the cathode.

abolish episodes of bradycardia-dependent VT, although this is not very effective in the long term.

2 Permanent overdrive pacing: dual chamber. AV pacing with a short programmed AV delay (e.g. 50–150 ms) can prevent recurrent re-entry tachycardia using the AV node as part of the circuit. It may also help reduce episodes of VT.

Tachycardia Termination/Version
Bursts of tachycardia can be terminated using overdrive or underdrive pacing or bursts of extra-stimuli. Underdrive pacing (VOO mode) is the least effective relying on random competition and rarely effective at faster rates (>160/min).

In VT termination using the ICD careful electrophysiological studies are needed to select the best algorithm. The number and timing of extra-stimuli need to be programmed. Ramp or autodecremental pacing may be needed if standard extra-stimuli at fixed intervals fail (Figure 7.21).

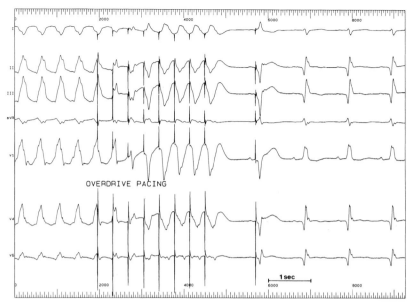

Figure 7.21 Successful overdrive pacing of VT by the ICD. The VT is relatively slow (135/min) and is overdriven by a train-of-eight paced beats at 166/min. The first beat after the pacing train is back-up paced and then SR resumes.

7.11 Implantable Cardioverter Defibrillator

Following the pioneering work of Mirowski implanting a device in a dog in 1969, the first unit was implanted in 1980 in a human. The box was 200 cm³ in volume. Initially the box was implanted in the abdomen with a thoracotomy also required for an epicardial patch plus two intravenous wires. The units have become much smaller now (down to 39 cm³), a thoracotomy is rarely required and one transvenous wire provides shocking, sensing and pacing electrodes. A second (atrial) wire allows dual chamber pacing and sensing. ICDs with biventricular pacing are now available. Advances in technology now provide greater control:

• Tiered pacing therapy for VT with programmed initial antitachycardia pacing followed by a DC shock if attempts at pacing overdrive are unsuccessful. An example of successful overdrive pacing by an ICD is shown in Figure 7.21 and a 15 J shock defibrillating the patient on another occasion Figure 7.22.

• Tiered shock therapy: initial shock is about 15 J with further shocks of 29–34 J if the initial shock is unsuccessful. Biphasic shock waveform (with the polarity of the shock reversing halfway through the shock) allows for a lower defibrillation threshold (DFT). For patients with a high DFT high output ICDs are available (maximum output 42 J), or a subcutaneous array electrode may be used (Figure 7.23).

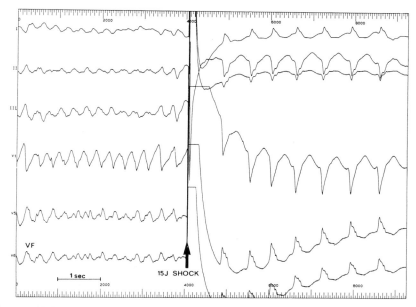

Figure 7.22 Defibrillation of VF by the ICD with a single 15J shock to an LBBB tachycardia.

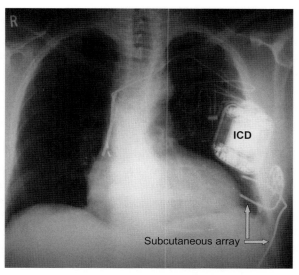

Figure 7.23 ICD with subcutaneous array fitted as high defibrillation threshold. Previous Ross operation for aortic stenosis.

• Back-up VVIR or DDDR pacing for bradycardia.
• Full telemetry and programming facilities: this can store information such as battery status, number of previous shocks, stored electrograms.
• Improved sensitivity with automatic gain control allowing better differentiation of fast AF or atrial flutter from VF.
• The hot can (active can). The ICD itself acts as an anode in conjunction with the proximal shocking electrode (see Figure 7.20). This lowers defibrillation thresholds.

This technology is not cheap: units with wire(s) are up to £20000 each, but bulk purchasing reduces the cost. The UK implant rate for ICDs has risen from 19 to 63 per million population in 2005, but this rate could well double in the next 5 years with the new NICE guidelines (see below). European rates are 85 per million and 400 per million in the USA.

Indications for ICD Therapy

There should be no treatable cause, e.g. drug toxicity, metabolic disturbance or reversible ischaemia. Patients with coronary disease and demonstrable ischaemia on treadmill testing or stress thallium scanning should be revascularized first. These indications are based on NICE guidelines.

Secondary Prevention

• This group have had a previous failed sudden death episode or haemodynamically significant VT.
• Cardiac arrest caused by either VT or VF.
• Recurrent sustained (>30s), preferably monomorphic VT causing syncope or presyncope.
• Sustained VT without syncope or cardiac arrest with an LVEF <35%.
• Three trials in secondary prevention have confirmed the superiority of ICDs over amiodarone or β blockade (Table 7.4). Drugs proved of no value in preventing cardiac death.

Primary Prevention

• Previous MI with non-sustained VT on Holter monitoring, inducible VT on electrophysiological testing and an LVEF <35%.
• Previous MI, LVEF <30% and QRS duration >120ms.
• Familial condition with high sudden death risk: this includes patients with long QT syndrome, Brugada syndrome (see Section 8.6), hypertrophic cardiomyopathy (see Section 4.2), arrythmogenic RV dysplasia (see Section 4.4) and some patients with repaired congenital heart disease.
• Patients who have sustained VT with good LV function (LVEF >35%), or syncope of unknown cause and inducible VT on electrophysiological testing, are not necessarily candidates for ICDs as initial therapy. Table 7.5 details the eight largest primary prevention trials.

Table 7.4 The three ICD randomized controlled secondary prevention trials

Trial	n	Patients	Control arm	Primary endpoint	Results
AVID 1997	1013	Resuscitated VT/VF, VT + syncope or LVEF <40% + haemodynamic compromise	Amiodarone or sotalol	All-cause mortality, mean 2.6-year follow-up	18 months: 15.8% deaths in ICD group, 24% in controls. At 1, 2 and 3 years deaths reduced by 39%, 27% and 31%
CIDS 2000	659	Resuscitated VF or VT + syncope or VT + LVEF <35% or sustained VT	Amiodarone	All-cause mortality, mean 3-year follow-up	Deaths reduced from 10.2 to 8.3%/ year (NS) with ICD
CASH 2000	288	Survivors of cardiac arrest	Amiodarone or metoprolol (propafenone withdrawn)	All-cause mortality, mean 57-month follow-up	At 57 months deaths reduced from 44.4% in drug group to 36.4% in ICD group (NS)

See Appendix 4 for references.

Table 7.5 The larger ICD randomised control primary prevention trials

Trial	n	Patients	Control arm	Primary endpoint	Result
MADIT 1996	196	MI > 3 weeks LVEF <35% Asymptomatic VT or NSVT on EP	Conventional therapy	All-cause mortality	Lower mortality at 5 years with ICD Drugs: no effect
CABG-patch 1997	1055	LVEF <35% awaiting CABG	CABG No ICD	All-cause mortality	No improvement with ICD
MUSST 1999	704	LVEF <40% Ischaemic Inducible VT	Drugs or ICD EP guided vs no drugs	Cardiac arrest Arrhythmic death	2-year deaths 33% in drug group, 10% in ICD group
MADIT II 2002	1232	LVEF <30% Previous MI No documented arrhythmia	Conventional therapy ± ICD	All cause mortality mean 20-month follow-up	Deaths: 19.8% in drug group, and 14.2% in ICD group
COMPANION 2004	1520	LVEF <35% QRS >120ms Ischaemic or DCM patients	Optimal medical therapy ± CRT or ± CRT-D	Death or any cause of hospitalization	CRT-D reduced endpoint 40% CRT reduced endpoint 34%
DEFINITE 2004	458	LVEF <35% DCM only NSVT or PVCs	Standard medical therapy ± ICD	All-cause mortality 29-month follow-up	At 2 years deaths reduced from 14.1% (drug group) to 7.9% with ICD
DINAMIT 2004	674	LVEF <35% 6-40 days post-MI	Optimal medical therapy ± ICD	All-cause mortality	No difference between groups
SCD-HeFT 2005	2521	LVEF <35% Ischaemic or DCM patients NYHA II/III	Conventional therapy ± ICD or amiodarone	All-cause mortality	5years. Deaths with ICD group 28.9% Amiodarone group 34.1% Placebo group 35.8%

See Appendix 4 for references.

Although drug therapy has proved of no benefit in preventing sudden death in secondary prevention trials, drug therapy has been shown to reduce the number of shocks experienced. A combination of amiodarone plus β blocker reduced shocks by 73% in a group of patients receiving an ICD for secondary prevention (the OPTIC trial). These drugs may also work in part by reducing inappropriate shocks by reducing heart rate. This trial cannot be extrapolated to primary prevention although the combination may be equally effective.

Conclusions from ICD Primary Prevention Trials

Although not all these trials are positive for ICDs the overall message is clear. Any patient with poor ventricular function (LVEF <35%) after an MI should have an ICD whether or not they have documented ventricular arrhythmias. Amiodarone or other suppressive drug therapy is of no value in reducing mortality. In addition if the QRS >120ms, a biventricular ICD should be considered with the decision usually based on an echocardiographically proven dyssynchrony study. The evidence is less clear for patients with dilated cardiomyopathy, but based on the SCD HeFT trial these patients should be managed along the same lines as the ischaemic group.

Contraindications to ICD Therapy
• VT secondary to drugs or metabolic disturbance
• VT in acute myocardial ischaemia or infarction
• Acute myocarditis
• Unsustained VT (<30s)
• Incessant or very frequent VT
• The arrhythmia is supraventricular
• There is a unipolar pacing system in situ; it must be removed and converted to a dedicated bipolar system only
• Symptomatic patients with spontaneous episodes suspected of having VT but without ECG evidence.

ICD Implantation

Most ICDs can now be implanted in a similar fashion to permanent pacemakers and general anaesthesia is occasionally required. The device is very little bigger than a DDD pacing unit. The ICD is implanted if possible beneath the pectoralis major with the wires introduced via the cephalic or subclavian veins. The left side is preferable. Newer leads are smaller (French 11). In very thin patients the box can be implanted in the abdomen beneath the rectus sheath.

High Defibrillation Thresholds

The defibrillation threshold is checked at implantation and should be <20J. The wire position is the most crucial factor with the shocking electrode lying up against the septum. The use of the hot can and a subcutaneous array electrode can help if the DFT is high (see Figure 7.23). A high energy box may be needed and changing the polarity of the shock may help. Amiodarone and flecainide tend to increase the DFT, and sotalol reduces it. If an ICD implant has borderline DFTs the patient can be treated with sotalol and the DFT retested. An alternative is an extra-active fixation coronary sinus shocking coil which widens the defibrillation/shocking field and lowers the DFT.

In a very few patients in whom satisfactory DFTs are unobtainable using a single transvenous wire with a subcutaneous array a thoracotomy as a separate procedure is needed to implant an epicardial patch.

Antitachycardia Pacing Facility

The antitachycardia facilities are programmed in at the end of the procedure. The choice of antitachycardia programmes depends partly on the VT rate seen preoperatively and partly on clinical judgement. The antitachycardia pacing facility has greatly improved battery life which should be good for >100 shocks.

The ICD Shock

It takes 5–15 s for the capacitors to charge once antitachycardia pacing has been unsuccessful. Some units incorporate an audible bleeping tone to warn the patient that a shock is imminent (useful if he or she is cooking for instance). The patient, if still conscious, may describe a sensation of being suddenly kicked in the back. Anyone touching the patient at the time of the shock will not be harmed. Initial shocks can be programmed to 15 J. This should be 10 J more than the lowest successful shock strength at the EP study at implantation. Further shocks of 29–34 J are then delivered if the 15 J shock was unsuccessful.

Problems and Complications

Operative mortality rate is now 1%, but the slightly more bulky unit and wire results in a higher morbidity than conventional pacing with problems such as wire or box extrusion, pocket infection and sensing malfunction resulting in inappropriate shocks. Extensive psychological support is also needed both before and after implantation. Regular follow-up is needed in the pacing clinic (more frequently than for routine pacemaker follow-up) and this places an increasing burden on the cardiac scientific officers. In some units an audible bleeping tone indicates end of battery life (ERI – elective replacement indication).

Inappropriate Shocks

These are becoming less frequent with the increasing sophistication of the ICD being able to discriminate between various cardiac rhythms, but up to 20%

of cases may receive them. The most common problems are with sinus tachycardia with a wide QRS or fast paroxysmal AF. Fifty per cent of cases with ICDs probably develop AF during their lifetime. After a shock the patient should attend the ICD clinic for device interrogation.

Follow-up of Patients with ICDs

Driving

Group 1 (car) driving is not allowed for 6 months post-implantation (secondary prevention cases). Subsequently a patient with an ICD must have been free from all forms of therapy (antitachycardia pacing or shock) for 6 months to be allowed a driving licence. The ban is shorter for primary prevention (see Appendix 6).

A group 2 driver (vocational licence) will not be allowed to drive a heavy goods vehicle again whatever the reason for the ICD implant.

Patients should be told to avoid the following:
• Big electrical transformers
• Large loudspeakers with strong magnets
• Digital portable telephones: an analogue phone may be used but should not be put in the breast pocket over the ICD (see earlier)
• MRI
• Electrocautery: if surgery with diathermy is needed the ICD must be deactivated. If no programmer is available, a magnet should be taped over the unit; the magnet will not affect back-up pacing
• Transcutaneous electrical nerve stimulation (TENS) device: this may be possible, but with the ICD on monitor only the sensed electrogram should be recorded with the TENS machine switched on to check there is no oversensing; if there is, the TENS electrodes must be moved
• Additional antiarrhythmic therapy is allowed but drugs such as amiodarone may increase the DFTs and shock impedance, which will have to be checked once the patient is loaded on the drug
• There are no problems with X-rays, microwave ovens, bathing, sex, etc. Anyone touching a patient at the time of a shock will not receive a shock.

Long-term Results

These vary from series to series but a mortality rate of about 10% per year may be expected chiefly dependent on LV function. Although much criticized, the MADIT trial compared ICD therapy with conventional drug therapy in a randomized trial over 5 years in patients with inducible, non-suppressible, VT post-infarction and an LVEF < 35%. Patients receiving an ICD had a better prognosis with no evidence that drug therapy influenced survival. Meta-analysis of three ICD trials showed 27% relative risk reduction for total mortality and 52% for arrhythmic death. One death is prevented for 10 patients treated over 3 years. About 30% patients who have an ICD implanted do not use it in the first year after implantation.

Patients with better prognosis include the following:
- Patients whose arrhythmia is well tolerated
- Patients whose VT cannot be induced at EP study
- Patients with VT inducible and suppressible at EP study by drug therapy
- Patients whose tachycardia is slowed by drug therapy even if not suppressed
- LVEF >0.4.

Analysis of cost-effectiveness in secondary prevention is difficult, but from the AVID trial it has been estimated that the cost per life year gained using a 5-year model was £26000–£31000.

Explanting the Unit

The unit must be deactivated before it is removed. This applies particularly after a patient's death when the battery life may not be depleted. Failure to deactivate the ICD may result in the operator receiving shocks or burns.

7.12 Pacing in Children and Congenital Heart Disease

Permanent pacing in children may be required for congenital complete heart block, after surgical correction of congenital heart disease or for complete heart block developing as the natural progression of disease (e.g. corrected transposition). The choice of pacing route is crucial. Life-long pacing will be needed and venous obstruction can be a major problem. Three options are available.

Pacing via the Transvenous Route

This carries all the advantages of endocardial pacing but there are major long-term problems:
- Venous obstruction: this will prevent further use of the vein, make lead extraction difficult or impossible, and may also result in SVC stenosis (see Figures 7.7 and 7.8) or obstruction.
- Child growth: attempts to use extra coils of wire in the right atrium or ventricle to allow for child growth are not the answer because the coils may cause dysrrhythmias and the wire coils become attached to the endocardium.
- Lead extraction and reoperation.
- Endocardial leads are best avoided if there are residual atrial or ventricular shunts.

Pacing via the Epicardial Route

In children this has many advantages:
- Saves the venous route for later when the child has grown.
- Allows dual chamber pacing with the use of LA and LV epicarc trodes. DDD pacing will improve haemodynamics and reduce atrial dysrhythmias.
- Avoids the risk of paradoxical embolism, e.g. after a Fontan procedure.

However, the disadvantages of epicardial pacing must also be considered (see Section 7.3). Epicardial leads tend to have a bigger electrode surface area and a higher lead impedance.

Pacing via the Transatrial Route

This can be performed via a mini-thoracotomy using a purse string suture in the right atrium or at the time of cardiac surgery. The lead is advanced to the right ventricle via intraoperative fluoroscopy. The generator is buried in the rectus abdominis sheath as with epicardial pacing.

The transatrial route:
- avoids the pitfalls of epicardial pacing
- has the long-term advantages of transvenous pacing with long-term reliability of the electrode
- can be used in patients with SVC obstruction
- leaves venous access free for when the child has grown.

From the above pros and cons it can be seen that the first choice of pacing route in infants and young children is either the epicardial or the transatrial route. A combined procedure with a transatrial endocardial lead and an epicardial lead is possible. Conventional transvenous pacing can then be established once the child has grown.

VVIR vs DDDR Pacing

Theoretically dual chamber pacing (DDDR) has the advantages of improved haemodynamics, and in children with poor ventricular function this may be important. ANP levels should be lower and atrial dysrhythmias less with the addition of atrial pacing.

However, cardiac output in the younger heart is more rate dependent than atrial–kick dependent and VVIR pacing may suffice. Generally if the child <25 kg use a single chamber VVIR system, and if >25 kg consider a DDDR unit.

Biventricular Pacing for Heart Failure in Congenital Heart Disease

A failing systemic ventricle is an increasing problem in congenital heart disease. It may become a problem when the right ventricle is the systemic ventricle as in congenitally corrected transposition (see Section 2.6), or transposition after a Mustard procedure or in a single (primitive) ventricle. The long-term effects and possible benefits of biventricular pacing in these conditions are simply not known.

It can be established with epicardial RV and LV leads in the transposition groups. In the short term a reduction in AV valve regurgitation and increased systemic ventricle ejection fraction have been seen. In the long term it is hoped that reverse remodelling will occur with improved ventricular function and survival.

8 Disturbances of Cardiac Rhythm: Tachycardias and Ablation

8.1 Principles of Paroxysmal Tachycardia Diagnosis

In patients with intermittent (paroxysmal) tachycardias, diagnosis may be difficult. It is useful to know if the arrhythmia starts and stops suddenly, whether it is regular or irregular, and if there are any factors that start it or stop it. 'Catching' the arrhythmia may not always be possible with the limited services of 24-hour ECG monitoring, and the patient may not be able to get to a hospital to have the arrhythmia recorded when it occurs. A patient-activated recorder may help. In cases where the arrhythmia is infrequent and disabling an implantable loop recorder (e.g. Medtronic Reveal device) is useful. Sometimes the 24-hour Holter monitor produces some startling results (Figure 8.1).

Diagnosis of paroxysmal tachycardia involves the following:
• Recognition of likely associated cardiac lesions:
AF: alcohol, mitral valve disease, thyrotoxicosis, coronary artery disease, pericarditis, postcardiac surgery, etc.
VT: LV aneurysm, recent myocardial infarct.
• Recognition of resting 12-lead ECG abnormalities, e.g. pre-excitation with short PR interval:
– without δ wave: Lown–Ganong–Levine syndrome
– with δ wave Wolff–Parkinson–White (WPW) syndrome
– apparent long QT interval caused by prominent 'u' wave: hypokalaemia
– long QT interval: may be caused by metabolic abnormalities, drugs or rare genetic defects; torsades de pointes may result (see Section 8.6).
• Recognition of other cardiotoxic drugs, e.g. sympathomimetic agents – β_2 agonists (SVT or VT), digoxin (paroxysmal SVT with varying block), l-dopa, tricyclic antidepressants (VT), doxorubicin (Adriamycin) (SVT or VT).

Swanton's Cardiology, sixth edition. By R. H. Swanton and S. Banerjee. Published 2008 Blackwell Publishing. ISBN 978-1-4051-7819-8.

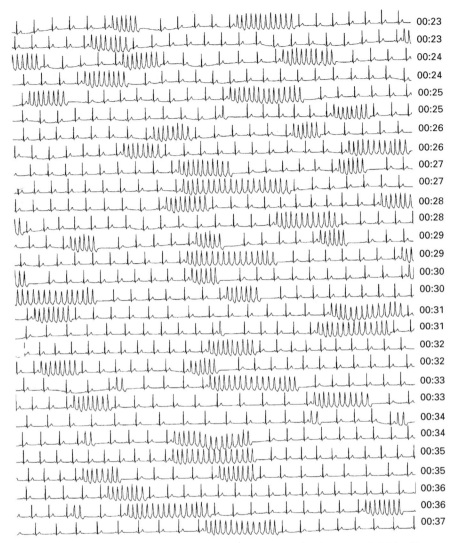

Figure 8.1 Fourteen minutes from a 24-h Holter monitor recording in a man at night, with a main LAD stenosis, who presented with palpitation after one episode of chest pain. Tracing shows bursts of self-terminating monomorphic VT. Treated by coronary stenting.

- Recognition of other precipitating factors: caffeine (tea or coffee excess), smoking, alcohol, emotional stress, fatigue.
- Metabolic upsets: K^+ or Ca^{2+} high or low, hypoxia, hypercapnia, metabolic acidosis, hypomagnesaemia, phaeochromocytoma, febrile illnesses, pneumonia, etc.
- ECG monitoring for 24 hours: several recordings are often needed in a single patient. Telemetry is an alternative, and is useful for ambulant patients

during hospital admission. With infrequent episodes associated with symptoms an implantable Reveal device may be needed.

• Provocation of the arrhythmia: this is sometimes necessary to establish a diagnosis, to assess provocation factors and to assess treatment. The most common provocation test is the exercise test. Unifocal ectopic beats in the normal heart are common and usually decrease in number during exercise, recurring with rest. The abnormal heart may develop multifocal frequent ectopics or even VT on effort. A few patients with WPW syndrome may develop tachycardia on effort, but this is uncommon.

Other provocative tests in patients with paroxysmal tachycardia include the use of the tilt table (orthostatic tachycardia), isoprenaline infusion (WPW syndrome), electrophysiological stimulation or cardiac catheterization with LV and coronary angiography. A more detailed protocol for provocation studies of ventricular tachycardia is discussed in Section 8.5.

Most intermittent tachycardias can usually be diagnosed without provocation tests. Electrophysiological studies may be needed to assess the effect of drug therapy.

8.2 Classification of Antiarrhythmic Drugs

Table 8.1 shows the Vaughan–Williams classification. Some drugs fit into more than one class and some drugs fit into none of them. In spite of its limitations the classification is still commonly used and is included here. Table 8.2 also shows a classification based on the clinical effects of the drugs and their sites of action. It does not contain any electrophysiological data but is probably more useful at the bedside.

8.3 Supraventricular Arrhythmias

These are commonly classified as:
• AF
• Atrial flutter
• Atrial tachycardia
• Junctional tachycardia
• Pre-excitation syndromes
• SVT with aberrant conduction (a wide complex tachycardia).

Atrial Fibrillation
Prevalence increases with increasing age of the population: 0.5% in ages 50–59 years and 8.8% in ages 80–89 years. Incidence is 0.2%/year in ages 30–39 years and 2.3% in ages 80–89 years.

In the USA there were 2.08 million people known to have AF in 1995, with the number expected to reach 5.61 million by 2050.

Table 8.1 Classification of antiarrhythmic drugs (Vaughan–Williams)

	Class 1			Class 2	Class 3	Class 4
Method of action	Block fast sodium channel			β-Sympathetic blockade	Potassium channel blockade	Slow calcium channel blockade
Effect on cardiac action potential	Slow phase 0 rate of rise Depress phase 4 rate of rise Also effect on APD varies: 1a ↑ APD	1b ↓ APD	1c no effect APD	Depress phase 4 rate of rise	Increase APD	Depress phases 2 and 3
Primary site of action	Atrium Ventricle Bypass	Ventricle	His–Purkinje Ventricle Bypass	Sinus and AV nodes	Atrium AV node His–Purkinje Ventricle Accessory pathway	AV node
Examples of drugs	Quinidine Procainamide Disopyramide Ajmaline	Lidocaine Phenytoin Mexiletine Aprindine Tocainide Moricizine	Flecainide Encainide Lorcainide Propafenone	β-Blocking agent Bretylium Guanethidine	Dofetilide Amiodarone Disopyramide Sotalol Several other β-blocking agents Bethanidine Bretylium	Verapamil Diltiazem Adenosine
Effect on AV node and His–Purkinje system	Variable on AV node ↑ His–Purkinje refractory period	Variable on AV node ↑ His–Purkinje refractory period	↑ A–H ↑ H–V time ↑ His–Purkinje refractory period	↑ A–H time ↑ AV node refractory period No effect on His–Purkinje refractory period	↑ A–H time Little effect on H–V time ↑ Refractory periods of both AV node and His–Purkinje system	↑ A–H time ↑ AV node refractory period

Table 8.2 Drugs available for specific tachycardias

Sinus tachycardia	AF, atrial flutter, SVT	Junctional tachycardia	WPW syndrome bypass tachycardia	VT
None initially, look for cause:	*Version to SR:* Disopyramide	(Vagal manoeuvres):	*At AV node:* β Blockade	*Prevention and termination:*
Pain	Amiodarone	Verapamil	*At accessory pathway:*	Lidocaine
Anxiety	Flecainide	β Blockade		Mexiletine
Fever, sepsis	*Rate control at AV node:*	Digoxin	Disopyramide	Tocainide
Hypovolaemia		Flecainide	Quinidine	Procainamide
Low-output state	Adenosine		Amiodarone	Quinidine
Shock	Digoxin		Procainamide	Phenytoin
Thyrotoxicosis	Verapamil		Flecainide	β Blockade
	β Blockade		Sotalol	Amiodarone
	Prevention		Propafenone	Disopyramide
	Disopyramide		Ajmaline	Propafenone
	Amiodarone			*Version only:*
	Flecainide			Bretylium tosylate
	Propafenone			Ajmaline
	Procainamide			
	Quinidine			

A classification by Camm has divided AF into the following:

• *Paroxysmal*: self-terminating at least once. Patients may be unaware of bursts of AF.

• *Persistent*: >48 h with no spontaneous termination. Can be converted to sinus rhythm with drugs or DC cardioversion.

• *Permanent*: established AF. Cannot be terminated by drugs or DC cardioversion. Patients need rate control therapy plus consideration of anticoagulation.

There is a gradual tendency over time for paroxysmal AF to become persistent and finally permanent. Drug and device therapy aims at maintaining sinus rhythm for as long as possible. 'AF begets AF' and it is still important to try to reduce the frequency of paroxysmal bursts of AF.

Aetiology
There are many possible provoking factors.

Common Causes
• Ischaemic heart disease
• Alcohol: binge drinking ('holiday heart') or chronic alcohol consumption
• Thyrotoxicosis
• Mitral valve disease: LA dilatation caused by mitral stenosis and/or regurgitation
• Hypertension: accounts for about 50% cases

- Cardiac surgery: right atrial cannulation; thoracotomy
- Pyrexial illness, chest infection, etc.

Less Common Causes
- General anaesthesia
- Hypoxia: chronic pulmonary disease
- Pulmonary embolism
- After ASD closure
- Chest trauma
- Pregnancy
- Heart muscle disease: dilated cardiomyopathy > hypertrophic
- Obstructive sleep apnoea
- Provocation by pacing wire, catheter in either atrium
- Part of the rhythm spectrum of sinoatrial disease
- Malignant infiltration.

If no cause is apparent and the heart is otherwise normal clinically and on echocardiography, the term 'lone AF' is used.

The Importance of Atrial Volume and Stretch
Many of the aetiological factors above induce LV diastolic dysfunction (age, hypertension, ischaemic heart disease, cardiomyopathies, etc.), which results in higher LA pressures and atrial stretch. LA volume is a predictor of AF, as well as CVA and cardiovascular death. A dilated LA causes stasis, but atrial stretch also directly increases thrombomodulin levels contributing to coagulation. Increased LA volume also occurs in athletes and long-distance runners, which may provoke AF.

Permanent AF

Rate control

In permanent AF, drug therapy is used to control the rate of ventricular response by increasing AV node refractoriness. Vagal manoeuvres will do this temporarily and may be useful in the diagnosis of fast AF.

Digoxin is still the drug of choice in AF (see Inotropes, Section 6.8). Digoxin is unlikely to control ventricular rate adequately if catecholamines are raised (e.g. effort, pyrexia). If the ventricular response is still too fast in a well-digitalized patient, a small dose of a β-blocking agent is added (e.g. metoprolol 25–50 mg three times daily) and the dose gradually increased if necessary. Before adding a β-blocking agent it is important to be sure that LV function is adequate and the patient is not thyrotoxic. If the LV function is poor a calcium antagonist or amiodarone is safer than β blockade. Verapamil is added to digoxin, starting at 40 mg three times daily and increasing the dose if necessary up to 120 mg three times daily (or diltiazem 60 mg three times daily initially). If this fails to control the response, amiodarone can be tried. Digoxin and β blockade combination usually controls the ventricular response.

AF and Accessory Pathway Conduction
Very occasionally in AF the conduction pathway to the ventricles is anomalous (e.g. Kent accessory pathway in WPW syndrome). In this situation digoxin, β blockade and verapamil are not effective. Digoxin and verapamil may even increase anterograde condition in the accessory pathway and are contraindicated (see Figure 8.19). If an ECG in AF shows intermittent or constant δ waves or if the ventricular response in AF is very fast (e.g. RR intervals of 200–250 ms), then WPW syndrome is a strong possibility (see Figure 8.8). Intravenous disopyramide 50–150 mg or flecainide 50–150 mg i.v. is the drug of choice. Other agents that can be effective are quinidine, procainamide and amiodarone. Do not use more than one drug intravenously; if your choice fails then proceed to DC cardioversion.

Paroxysmal AF
In the euthyroid patient, alcohol is the most common precipitating factor. Caffeine, nicotine and emotional stress have been implicated but with little evidence. Attacks are not usually effort related except in the younger patient (see below). Drug therapy is aimed at reducing the number and duration of attacks but is unlikely to suppress them completely. It is likely over the years that in spite of drug treatment attacks will become more frequent and eventually AF becomes permanent unless the patient has an RF ablation.

Upstream Drug Therapy
Drugs that control hypertension are particularly useful at reducing the frequency of recurrent episodes. Trandolapril and irbesartan plus amiodarone have been shown to reduce the recurrence rate.

Rhythm Control: Drug Treatment or Ablation?
With the increasing success of RF ablation for AF more patients are being referred early in the course of their condition for ablation, which is curative in about 80% of cases. Some units claim higher figures but the length of follow-up, the use of amiodarone and the extent of Holter monitoring must be noted because many episodes of AF are silent and not noticed by the patient.

Generally, if the patient's symptoms are mild and infrequent a single drug can be tried using the 'pill in the pocket approach' (see below). With patients who are getting symptomatic attacks, say every week, a single drug taken daily can be tried initially. If a single drug fails to control symptoms adequately, ablation should be considered as an alternative to adding in a second antiarrhythmic agent.

Choice of Drug Therapy
Drugs of value are amiodarone, flecainide, propafenone, disopyramide and β blockade. Quinidine is of proven value but rarely used in the UK because of side effects (see Section 8.9). Class 1b agents should be avoided. Flecainide is the initial drug of choice provided that LV function is good and there is no

known coronary disease. The same cautions hold for propafenone. Amiodarone (probably the most effective drug) is reserved for patients with LV dysfunction, coronary disease or failed treatment with flecainide or propafenone. Side effects (see below) limit its use. β Blockade is useful adjunctive therapy. Possible proarrhythmias, induced particularly by class 1 agents, must be considered. Digoxin is not in this list and merely controls ventricular response at rest if AF occurs. It has no value in AF prevention.

A few younger patients with normal hearts will have episodes of AF induced by autonomic factors. Those where AF is induced by exercise or on waking or with emotional stress should be β blocked. Others where AF occurs, while asleep or after meals (vagal activity), should be tried on disopyramide or flecainide.

It is important to note that there is an embolic risk with paroxysmal AF just as there is with permanent AF. Anticoagulation should be considered.

Pill in the Pocket Regimen

This works well for patients with infrequent episodes of AF (previously confirmed on Holter monitoring). The class 1C agents propafenone and flecainide are used, which have a rapid onset of action compared with amiodarone. Patients should be instructed to take a single dose based on body weight:

	Weight < 70 kg	Weight > 70 kg
Flecainide	200 mg	300 mg
Propafenone	450 mg	600 mg

Success rates as high as 94% have been found using this regimen with the drug working in about 2 h. Inevitably with disease progression some patients will have to be switched to daily prophylactic therapy. Proarrhythmia is rare and the main problem is atrial flutter with high ventricular rates (e.g. 1:1 flutter with a ventricular rate of 300/min). This occurs in about 1% of cases using this regimen.

The pill in the pocket method should be avoided in patients with the following:
• Frequent episodes of AF
• ECG showing pre-excitation, BBB, previously documented second- or third-degree AV block, or long QT interval
• Severe LV dysfunction or history of heart failure
• Severe valve disease
• Known ischaemic heart disease
• Sinoatrial disease
• Pregnancy.

It can be seen that the most suitable cases are those with lone AF and infrequent episodes.

Anticoagulation and AF (Figures 8.2 and 8.3)

This should be considered in patients with frequent episodes of uncontrolled AF, in patients needing DC cardioversion (see below) and in the long-term management of permanent AF. The annual CVA risk for patients in their 60s with lone AF is between 3 and 8%. Approximately 35% of patients in permanent AF who are not anticoagulated will have an embolic event in their lifetime.

There are now seven major trials comparing warfarin with placebo and four comparing warfarin with aspirin in AF. It is now clear that warfarin is superior to aspirin in the prevention of thromboembolic events.

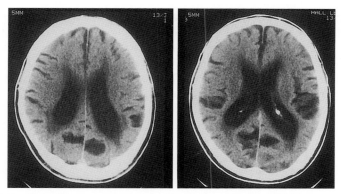

Figure 8.2 Cerebral CT in a man presenting with presenile dementia. Multiple cerebral infarcts caused by emboli from atrial fibrillation.

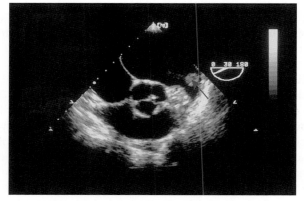

Figure 8.3 Transoesophageal echocardiogram in a man with atrial fibrillation showing thrombus in the left atrial appendage (arrowed).

These trials have identified patients at particular risk of thromboembolism:

- Hypertension: systolic blood pressure > 160 mmHg
- Poor LV function. LVEF < 25%
- Age > 75 years
- Patients with diabetes
- Previous emboli, CVA or transient ischaemic attack.

In these high-risk patients, warfarin is important in controlling the INR between 2.0 and 3.0. There are no equally effective alternative regimens yet. A regimen of low-dose warfarin plus aspirin is not an alternative and is ineffective. Dual antiplatelet therapy with aspirin plus clopidogrel is less effective than warfarin alone (ACTIVE-W study). However, in patients <60 years with lone AF (structurally normal heart on echocardiography), the embolic risk is small and aspirin alone is adequate.

One trial comparing warfarin with the now withdrawn antithrombin ximelagatran (SPORTIF II) showed that only 57% patients in the warfarin arm of the trial were in the correct therapeutic range.

CHADS$_2$ Scoring System

A simple approach is to use the CHADS$_2$ scoring system which scores on these five major risk factors for thromboembolism in AF:

Risk factor	Score
Congestive cardiac failure	1
Hypertension	1
Age > 65	1
Diabetes	1
Stroke	2

A total score of 0–1 should be managed with soluble aspirin. A score of 2 or more should be anticoagulated with warfarin, but the hypertension must be well controlled.

Drug Cardioversion

This is most likely to succeed with recent-onset AF. Flecainide 2 mg/kg i.v. over 10 min is the drug of choice but should be avoided in patients with poor LV function because it has a negative inotropic effect. Disopyramide 50–150 mg i.v. slowly over 5 min is an alternative. Fibrillatory waves may coarsen and the ventricular response increase before sinus rhythm is achieved. Amiodarone given orally (200 mg three times daily up to 400 mg three times daily for 1 week) may also result in version to sinus rhythm. The dose is reduced after 1 week. Amiodarone is also very useful given intravenously: 5 mg/kg over 4 h in 5% dextrose. The maximum intravenous dose over 24 h in an adult is 1200 mg. An immediate result should not be expected: it may take 24–48 h to convert the patient back to sinus rhythm. The patient can be converted to oral amiodarone when practical.

DC Cardioversion

This is not used for permanent or paroxysmal AF. Its role is chiefly in two types of situation:

1 As an elective procedure after a first attack of AF with an identifiable cause, e.g. attack of pneumonia, a thoracotomy, pulmonary embolus, controlled thyrotoxicosis after thyroidectomy, after coronary artery surgery (see Aetiology above). In lone AF with no apparent cause DC cardioversion should also be tried.

2 As an emergency procedure where atrial transport is vital to the maintenance of a reasonable cardiac output. The patient is usually very sick and the chances of success are not great. Examples are in HCM, aortic valve stenosis and acute MI. Generally every effort should be made to get the patient back into sinus rhythm. Age is no barrier.

Cardioversion and the Need for Anticoagulation

If the left atrium is small and AF has only been present for 24–48 h, prior anticoagulation is unnecessary. If the LA is dilated, there is mitral valve disease or AF has been prolonged, the patient is anticoagulated with warfarin for 4 weeks before DC cardioversion. The risk of systemic emboli is about 5–7% without anticoagulation and < 1.6% with it. Recent experience with transoesophageal echocardiography (TOE) has shown that thrombi in the atrial appendage occur in about 13% of patients with AF (Figure 8.3). If no thrombi are seen on TOE DC cardioversion may be performed safely without prior anticoagulation. If bi- or multiplane TOE is not available patients should be anticoagulated beforehand. Patients with spontaneous echocardiographic contrast in the left atrium (thought to be a prelude to thrombi) should also be anticoagulated (see Figure 17.57).

A dilated LA and prolonged AF make it less likely that DC cardioversion will succeed. Anticoagulation should be continued for 1 month after successful cardioversion. Reversion to AF is common and about 30% stay in sinus rhythm. Disopyramide, β blockade or amiodarone helps maintain sinus rhythm.

Suggested Protocol for DC Cardioversion

• Serum potassium between 4.5 and 5.5 mmol/l if possible.
• There is no need to stop digoxin beforehand but DC cardioversion is not performed if there is any suspicion of digoxin toxicity (see Section 6.8).
• Fast for 6 h. Consent should include explanation of remote risk of cerebral emboli.
• General anaesthesia with short-acting intravenous agent (e.g. propofol).

• Start with 200J shock (100J if in atrial flutter). If failure to cardiovert: second shock, 300J. If failure: give disopyramide 100mg i.v or flecainide 50–100mg slowly over 5–10min. Third shock 360J with paddles in anteroposterior position. If still fails: consider treatment with amiodarone for 1 month and a further attempt, or just accept AF as definitive rhythm and treat with digoxin and long-term warfarin.

Left Atrial Appendage Occlusion Devices

It is thought that the vast majority of systemic emboli in AF originate from the left atrial appendage (LAA). Plication of the appendage at mitral valve surgery reduces the postoperative embolic risk. Several devices are now available that can be inserted into the LAA (PLAATO, Watchman devices) occluding it and preventing further emboli. A 12 F sheath is inserted into the LA via a transseptal puncture and guidance with fluoroscopy and TOE is necessary. The orifice diameter of the LAA is measured to size the device. Patients are kept on warfarin for 3 months after device implantation and then switched to aspirin.

Problems with LAA occlusion device implantation (about 5% of cases) include:
• Device embolization into the LA (falling out of the appendage)
• Pericardial effusion or tamponade
• Thromboembolic events
• Erosion of the LA wall by the device.

These devices are still in their infancy and few cardiologists have experience with them. NICE guidance does not sanction their use. However, in patients who have a history of a bad bleed on warfarin, are not suitable for AF ablation (e.g. LA too large) and have had systemic emboli, device closure of the LAA should be considered.

Devices to Suppress or Convert AF

Atrial Pacing

Although atrial pacing has been shown to reduce AF and systemic emboli in patients with sinoatrial disease or sinus bradycardia it has not been shown to be a useful strategy in the long-term prevention of recurrent paroxysmal AF.

Internal Atrial Defibrillator

Although successful at recognizing and defibrillating AF to SR, any shock >1J is uncomfortable for the patient. The use of these devices has largely been superseded by the development of RF ablation.

Atrial Flutter (Figure 8.4 and see Chapter 16, Figure 16.3)
The atrial rate in atrial flutter is 280–320/min and 2:1 ventricular response results in a ventricular rate of 150/min. With a 4:1 response, the ventricular

Atrial flutter with 2:1 AV block. Flutter rate is 270/min. Ventricular rate is 135/min

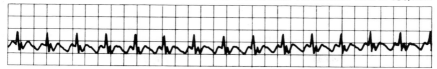

Carotid sinus massage (CSM) in atrial flutter produces transient complete AV block revealing the atrial flutter waves. Lead III

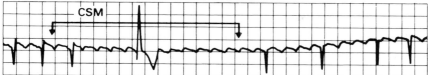

Chronic atrial flutter. Effect of digoxin. Atrial flutter rate 280/min. 4:1 AV block reduces ventricular rate to 70/min

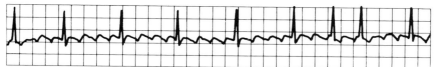

Chronic atrial flutter. Effect of amiodarone. Slows intrinsic flutter rate to 190/min. 3:1 AV block results in ventricular rate of 63/min. Lead II

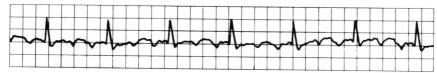

Figure 8.4 Atrial flutter.

rate is 75/min; however, it is unusual to be able to keep the response at a regular 4:1.

Carotid sinus massage will increase the degree of AV block temporarily and this can be useful in diagnosis of the rhythm, as the typical saw-tooth pattern of flutter becomes obvious (especially in leads II and VI in the ECG). An isolated event of atrial flutter is best treated by DC cardioversion. It is the most likely arrhythmia to convert to SR and only small energy shocks are needed (50–100 J in the adult). If AF is produced, the patient is shocked again into SR.

Paroxysmal atrial flutter is controlled initially by drug therapy. Digoxin may produce AF, which tends to be easier to manage. In difficult cases of paroxysmal atrial flutter the atrium can be fibrillated using a right atrial endocardial pacing lead.

Flecainide used to suppress paroxysmal AF may occasionally produce atrial flutter, which very rarely may conduct 1:1 to the ventricles. β Blockade may reduce the number of flutter episodes.

Amiodarone is also useful because it reduces the atrial flutter rate, making even 2:1 ventricular response more acceptable (e.g. down to 130–140/min). It probably also reduces the number of bursts of flutter.

Generally, however, long-term drug treatment is not the answer and the patient should be referred early for flutter ablation (see Section 8.8).

Atrial Tachycardia (Figure 8.5 and see Chapter 16, Figure 16.3)

- Ectopic atrial tachycardia (SVT, primary atrial tachycardia or PAT): atrial rate is 150–250/min. Often atrial rate is about 160–170/min, and ventricular response is 1:1 (P waves may not be visible on the ECG but appear with carotid sinus massage). Figure 8.5 shows an ectopic atrial tachycardia with a faster atrial rate of 260/min and 2:1 AV block.
- Paroxysmal atrial tachycardia with varying block secondary to digoxin toxicity (PATB). Ventricular response is less likely to be a 1:1 response. P waves are usually visible (Figure 8.5).

Adenosine

The purine nucleoside adenosine has taken over from verapamil as the drug of choice in an acute episode of atrial tachycardia. It is given as 3 mg i.v. followed by a saline flush. If necessary a second dose of 6 mg and a third of 12 mg may be given at 2-min intervals (dose for children 0.0375–0.25 mg/kg). The very short half-life of the drug (5–10 s) makes it safe even in wide complex tachycardias, but this means that the SVT may recur. If it does then verapamil is used (see below).

Ectopic atrial tachycardia with 2:1 AV block. Atrial rate 260/min. P waves arrowed. Ventricular rate 130/min

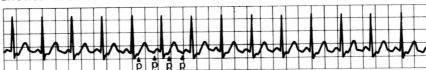

Atrial tachycardia with varying block. P waves arrowed. Atrial rate 214/min. PATB. Could be digoxin toxicity

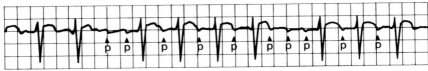

Atrial flutter with 4:1 AV block. Flutter rate 288/min. Ventricular rate 72/min

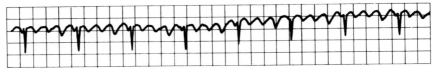

Figure 8.5 Atrial tachycardias.

Side effects of adenosine include transient chest pain, flushing, nausea, headache and dyspnoea. If troublesome, these can be reversed with intravenous aminophylline. Dose reduction needed in patients on dipyridamole (inhibits breakdown). Dose increase is needed in patients on aminophylline (blocks adenosine receptor).

Verapamil

This is almost as effective in SVT as adenosine but has a negative inotropic effect and is contraindicated in wide complex tachycardias, in case these are ventricular in origin. The exception is fascicular tachycardia (see Figure 8.9 and Section 8.5). It can be used in recurrent SVT after initial success with adenosine. It is given as 5–10 mg as a fast intravenous bolus. The dose can be repeated in 20 min if still necessary. It is more hazardous in patients already on β blockade but can still be used with careful monitoring (risk of complete AV block) in an emergency. DC shock may be needed.

Paroxysmal atrial tachycardia in the long term can be managed on oral verapamil, β blockade or even digoxin. Disopyramide, flecainide, propafenone and amiodarone are also very useful. Long-acting quinidine preparations are still used, but gastrointestinal side effects may prove a problem.

In atrial tachycardia with block (digoxin toxicity) the drug is stopped, and the K+ checked. The potassium should be >4.5 mmol/l and oral or intravenous KCl may be necessary. Verapamil or β blockade is used to slow ventricular response if necessary. DC cardioversion is avoided if possible, and if used low-energy shock is given (25–50 J) under lidocaine cover. Rapid atrial pacing can be used to extinguish the atrial focus.

Verapamil and Coronary Angioplasty

Verapamil can be given via the intracoronary route during coronary angioplasty if coronary spasm is a problem (e.g. as a result of the wire) or as a useful agent to prevent spasm during rotablation. It is also used in the no reflow situation. Start with 0.5 mg i.c. but temporary pacing should be available particularly with rotablation.

Disopyramide

The use of disopyramide in atrial tachycardia may slow the atrial rate, but quicken the ventricular response before version to sinus rhythm. Disopyramide prolongs atrial effective refractory period, slowing atrial rate, but its anticholinergic effect on the AV node may increase ventricular response. The net effect depends on vagal tone. It is a more useful drug for long-term prophylaxis than for acute intravenous administration in atrial tachycardia.

Junctional Tachycardias (AV Nodal Tachycardias) (Figures 8.6 and 8.7)

These are commonly divided into:
- AVNRT: atrioventricular nodal re-entry tachycardia
- AVRT: atrioventricular re-entry tachycardia
- His bundle tachycardia.

Atrioventricular re-entry tachycardia (AVRT). Common type. Inverted P waves seen just after QRS complexes. PR > RP, i.e. a short RP tachycardia

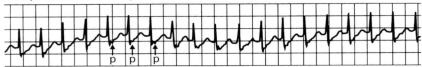

Atrioventricular re-entry tachycardia (AVRT) at 160/min reverting spontaneously to sinus rhythm. Although no P waves can be seen following the QRS complex as in the trace above, this ECG shows QRS alternans. If the narrow complex tachycardia is < 210/min QRS alternans is diagnostic of AVRT

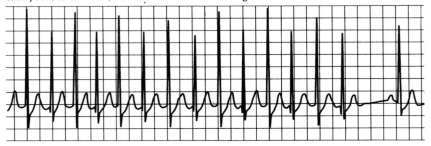

AV nodal re-entry tachycardia (AVNRT). Rate 214/min. Common type. P waves buried in QRS complexes as ventricle and atrium depolarize simultaneously

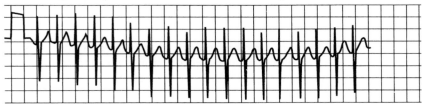

Figure 8.6 Junctional tachycardias.

AVNRT (Common Slow-fast Type) (Figures 8.6 and 8.7)

This involves a re-entry circuit in or very close to the AV node. There is usually a slow anterograde limb and a fast retrograde limb to the circuit. Atrium and ventricle are depolarized simultaneously so that the P wave is typically buried in the QRS complex. If visible it occurs as a positive blip just at the end of the QRS and may be mistaken for incomplete RBBB.

AVNRT (Uncommon Fast-slow Type – a Long RP Tachycardia)

This is as above but the anterograde limb is fast and the retrograde limb slow. Atrial depolarization is thus late and there are inverted P waves in inferior leads halfway between the QRS complexes. PR interval is less than RP'. This is a long RP tachycardia.

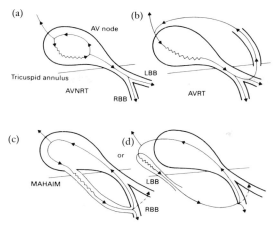

Figure 8.7 Examples of re-entry pathways involving the AV node: junctional tachycardias. Each circuit has a slow pathway (the zigzag line representing decremental conduction) and a fast pathway. (a) AV nodal re-entry tachycardia (AVNRT): the re-entry circuit is entirely within the AV node. Atria and ventricles are depolarized together. The P waves are buried within the QRS complexes (see also Figure 8.6). (b) AV re-entry tachycardia (AVRT): the re-entry fast pathway is remote from the AV node (as in WPW syndrome tachycardia). Atrial depolarization occurs after ventricular and P waves follow QRS complexes. PR is thus greater than RP'. A short RP tachycardia. Common type (see also Figure 8.6 and Figure 16.3). (c) Mahaim nodofascicular pathway. Late depolarization of the left bundle branch (LBB) results in the tachycardia having an LBBB morphology. (d) Mahaim free-wall pathway. The slow limb of the circuit is often in the anterior tricuspid annulus.

AVRT (Common Type: a Short RP' Tachycardia) (Figures 8.6 and 8.7)

These tachycardias involve accessory pathways remote from the AV node such as WPW syndrome. During tachycardia there is slow anterograde conduction through the AV node and fast retrograde conduction through the accessory pathway (see Figure 8.19). The δ waves are lost (no anterograde conduction through the accessory pathway) and the P waves, which may be difficult to see, are between the QRS complexes with PR > RP'. QRS alternans may occur at fast rates (see Figure 8.6). QRS alternans below rates of 210/min is virtually diagnostic of AVRT. At rates higher than this it may occur in AVNRT.

AVRT (Uncommon Type – a Long RP' Tachycardia)

Usually occurring in children, this incessant tachycardia has a fast limb through the AV node and a slow retrograde limb close to the AV node – similar to the uncommon form of AVNRT with the P wave late in the cycle so that PR < RP'. The accessory pathway is usually concealed and the resting ECG normal.

His Bundle Tachycardia (Junctional Ectopic Tachycardia)

This is rare. Again it is seen in children, sometimes after cardiac surgery. The QRS complexes look normal but there is AV dissociation with dissociated (slower) sinus P waves. This is best managed with class 1 antiarrhythmic agents not verapamil.

Management

Where anterograde conduction through the AV node is involved in the tachycardia circuit, vagal manoeuvres are worth trying initially and the patient should be taught these (eyeball massage is dangerous and so is excluded):
• Ice-cold water splashed on the face or ice-cubes in a polythene bag placed on the face – the 'duck-diving' reflex.
• Carotid sinus massage: one side at a time with the patient lying flat.
• Stimulation of the soft palate (gag reflex).
• Valsalva or Müller's manoeuvres.
• Straining, lifting heavy weights, changes in posture.

If the AV node is involved, anterograde conduction will be blocked by adenosine or by β blockade. Verapamil should be avoided (see Section 8.7). In the long term, β blockade and amiodarone are very useful, but RF ablation is playing an increasing role in both AVRT and some cases of AVNRT where the slow pathway is very close to the AV node.

The WPW syndrome is discussed separately (see Section 8.7).

Wide Complex Tachycardia: Differentiation of SVT from VT

QRS complexes > 120 ms are classified as wide. Table 8.3 gives a general guide and see also Figure 8.8 and Chapter 16, Figure 16.4.

It is important to remember that the haemodynamic state of the patient is no guide at all to the source of the tachycardia, because this depends on heart rate and LV function, irrespective of the origin of the tachycardia. It is safer to assume that wide complex tachycardia is ventricular in origin unless the patient has had a firm diagnosis made before. Vagal manoeuvres are worth trying (Valsalva or carotid sinus massage), as is a test dose of intravenous adenosine. If this fails to influence the tachycardia and the patient is in a reasonable haemodynamic state, then amiodarone is the drug of choice (see Section 8.4). It may be impossible to decide on the origin of tachycardia, especially with paroxysmal wide complex tachycardia picked up on a 24-hour ECG. An oesophageal electrode (easily swallowed as a 'pill on a wire') may help in identifying atrial activity from the left atrium. Electrophysiological studies with provocation may be necessary to decide between the two.

8.4 Ventricular Arrhythmias

These are commonly classified as follows:
• Ventricular premature beats (VPBs), premature ventricular complexes (VPCs), ventricular ectopics
• Ventricular tachycardia: sustained or non-sustained
• Ventricular flutter/fibrillation
• Fascicular tachycardia

Ventricular tachycardia.

Wide complex tachycardia with RBBB pattern in a man with an inferior infarct (see first complex in standard leads). Rsr' in V1 and V2. QRS duration > 140 msec. No p wave preceding first bizarre QRS. Extreme left axis > –30 degrees. RS ratio in V6 < 1.

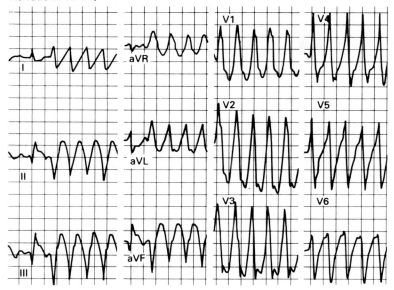

Atrial fibrillation with pre-excitation. WPW Type A.

Bizarre wide QRS with delta waves. Negative delta waves in I aVL and V6 suggest left lateral pathway. Note irregular tachycardia (sustained VT is regular as above).

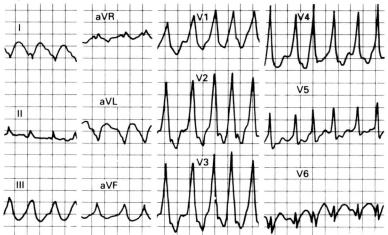

Figure 8.8 Wide complex tachycardias.

Table 8.3 Differentiation of SVT with aberrant conduction from ventricular tachycardia

Sign	SVT with aberrancy	Ventricular tachycardia
Vagal manoeuvres or intravenous adenosine	May slow ventricular response to reveal atrial activity	Ineffective
Signs of AV dissociation		
Cannon waves	Absent	Present
First heart sound	Normal	Variable
Fusion beats	Absent	May be present
Capture beats (narrow QRS)	Absent	May be present
Independent P waves	Absent	May be seen
ECG pattern	Usually RBBB	Bizarre wide QRS, RBBB or LBBB
Onset of tachycardia	P wave preceding first wide QRS	No P wave preceding first bizarre QRS
QRS duration	<140 ms	>140 ms
QRS axis	Normal	More negative than −30°
V leads polarity	Discordant (some positive some negative)	Concordant (all negative or all positive)
If in RBBB		
Features in V1	rSR' in V1	Rsr' in V1
RS ratio in V6	>1	<1
Tip of S wave in V1	Down to or below isoelectric line	Well above isoelectric line
If in LBBB		
Initial R wave in V1	<30 ms	>30 ms
S wave in V1	No notch on S wave	Notch on S wave
Onset r to nadir S in V1	<60 ms	>60 ms
Onset to nadir S in other chest leads	<100 ms	>100 ms
Q in V6	Absent	Present
rS complexes in V leads	Present	May be absent

- Genetic arrhythmia syndromes: long QT syndrome, short QT syndrome, Brugada syndrome
- Torsades de pointes
- Sudden cardiac death.

Ventricular Premature Beats

Ventricular Premature Beats on Routine 24-hour Monitoring

Routine 24-hour ECG monitoring in an apparently healthy population will reveal ectopic beats in more than half, and in about 10% these will be multifocal. They do not necessarily imply underlying heart disease. They probably occur with increasing frequency in the older population. The following are important points in the decision to treat them:

- Are the ectopics producing troublesome symptoms?
- Is there an excessive consumption of alcohol, tea, coffee, cola, tobacco?
- Any recent febrile or influenza-type illness?
- Any associated drug therapy that might be implicated, e.g. digoxin, sympathomimetics, tricyclic antidepressants, diuretics inducing hypokalaemia?
- Is there any underlying cardiac condition, e.g. mitral leaflet prolapse, recent MI, sinoatrial disease, cardiomyopathy, aortic valve disease?

Clearing up these points will require echocardiography and probably exercise testing. Innocent ectopics tend to disappear with increasing heart rate. More pathological ones may increase in frequency with possible short salvos of ventricular tachycardia on effort (see Chapter 16, Figure 16.4).

If full clinical examination is normal, echocardiography is normal and an exercise test is negative (see Section 16.2), the patient should be reassured. Treatment will be necessary only if, in spite of reassurance and avoidance of possible precipitating factors, symptoms are still troublesome. Usually a small dose of a β-blocking agent or disopyramide is effective, but should rarely be necessary.

Excessive zeal in trying to quench ectopic beats may result in drug side effects being worse than the condition itself.

Ventricular Premature Beats after MI

The treatment of ventricular premature beats after MI is still controversial. Lown (1967) proposed certain types of premature beats were more likely to lead to VF and should be suppressed. These warning arrhythmias were:

- frequent VPBs
- multifocal VPBs
- R-on-T phenomenon
- salvos of VPBs (two or more).

Since then it has been established that as many as 50% of cases of VF post-infarction occur with no warning arrhythmias at all. It has also been established that there is no case for routine use of antiarrhythmic drugs in all patients entering a CCU. There is no justification for a single-drug policy for all patients.

Ventricular premature beats are possibly just a marker of the extent of myocardial damage and do not necessarily cause sudden death. In an uncomplicated myocardial infarct, suppression of simple unifocal ectopic beats is not justified.

This has been shown to be dangerous in the cardiac arrhythmia suppression trial (CAST study) in which patients receiving flecainide or encainide had a higher mortality (7.7%) than if just taking a placebo (3%) and the trial was stopped early. The drugs were presumed to have a proarrhythmic effect.

Suppression of ventricular premature beats after MI:

- Check K^+, other drugs (e.g. digoxin), acid–base state and blood bases (hypoxia, hypercapnia), and correct them if possible. K^+ should be 4.5–5.5 mmol/l.

• Consider prophylactic antiarrhythmic drug if: poor haemodynamic state, frequent multifocal VPBs, R-on-T or salvos of VPBs. Lidocaine is given as an infusion, switching to an oral agent after 48 h. If LV function is good, consider β blockade or disopyramide. If LV function is poor, use amiodarone. Two big trials, the European and the Canadian myocardial infarct amiodarone trials (EMIAT and CAMIAT), have shown a reduction in arrhythmic deaths (but not overall mortality) in patients treated with amiodarone after MI. Amiodarone should be particularly considered in patients with >10–20 ventricular premature beats/h on Holter monitoring after infarction plus poor LV function (LVEF <40%).

• Consider temporary pacing if ectopics are related to atropine-resistant bradycardia.

8.5 Ventricular Tachycardia

(Figures 8.8, 8.9 and 8.10; see also Chapter 16, Figure 16.4)

Ventricular Tachycardia Classification

Fascicular Tachycardia

This is an uncommon wide complex tachycardia with characteristic appearances on 12-lead ECG, which shows an RBBB pattern (but not very wide RBBB), usually with left axis deviation and a superior axis – positive in aVR (Figure 8.9). It is the only wide complex tachycardia in which verapamil can be used and the most effective drug.

Non-sustained VT

This is a salvo of three or more ventricular premature beats at a rate of >100 beats/min (cycle length <600 ms), terminating in <30 s.

Sustained VT

This is VT lasting >30 s, or requiring termination resulting form haemodynamic compromise in <30 s.

In both types the VT may be monomorphic with a stable single QRS morphology, or polymorphic with a changing multiform QRS morphology at a cycle lengths between 600 and 180 ms.

RV Outflow Tract Tachycardia

This has a characteristic LBBB pattern with an inferior (vertical) axis (Figure 8.10). It is the tachycardia most suited to VT ablation (see Section 8.8).

Ventricular Flutter

This is a term occasionally used to describe monomorphic VT at a rate of approximately 300/min (cycle length 200 ms). No isoelectric interval between QRS complexes.

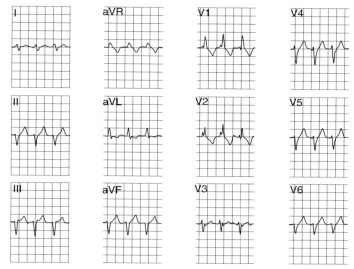

Figure 8.9 Fascicular tachycardia: wide complex tachycardia with RBBB pattern, extreme left axis deviation. Superior axis with aVR positive. Responded to verapamil only. Amiodarone was ineffective.

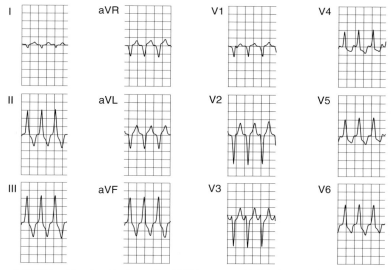

Figure 8.10 RV outflow tract tachycardia. LBBB pattern with inferior axis (most positive in III). Consider VT ablation.

Ventricular Fibrillation

This is a rapid ventricular rate >300/min with marked variability in QRS cycle length and QRS amplitude. Usually starts as coarse VF with good QRS amplitude (most likely to defibrillate) degenerating into fine VF with very low QRS amplitude (least likely to defibrillate) (see Figure 16.4).

Symptoms

These are very variable. Patients may be totally unaware of an arrhythmia that may be found on the CCU, Holter monitoring or pacemaker interrogation. Alternatively patients may experience transient palpitations, or a stronger, fast, regular pounding in the chest, and/or symptoms of haemodynamic compromise: dizziness, light-headedness, feeling faint, a greying out of vision, presyncope or syncope.

Available Drugs

Commonly used drugs in the management of VT are shown in Table 8.4. Many of the class 1 agents (e.g. lidocaine, mexiletine) have similar side effects predominantly affecting the CNS (tremor, dizziness, confusion, cerebellar ataxia, fits) and the gastrointestinal tract (nausea, anorexia, vomiting). The large number of drugs testifies to the failure of a single drug to work in all cases of VT, and sometimes several drugs need to be used in prophylaxis.

Treatment of VT (Figure 8.11)

Treatment of VT depends on the patient's condition. If present right at the onset of VT in a monitored patient, a chest thump or getting the patient to give a vigorous cough may succeed in re-establishing sinus rhythm. In the very sick patient DC cardioversion is necessary (see below).

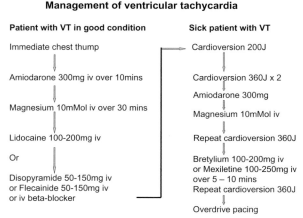

Figure 8.11 Treatment of VT.

Management of VT in a Haemodynamically Stable Patient (see Figure 8.11)

• Establish intravenous access. Check blood for K$^+$, acid–base balance and arterial blood gases and correct if necessary. Aim to get K$^+$ >4.5 mmol/l. Maximum potassium replacement rate is 30 mmol/h.
• High-flow oxygen.
• Start amiodarone 300 mg in 5% dextrose over 10 min then aim to deliver a total of 1200 mg over 24 h.
• Assume hypomagnesaemia. Give 10 mmol magnesium sulphate over 30 min (5 ml 50% solution).
• If VT persists, or haemodynamics deteriorates: for DC shock (see unstable haemodynamics below). It is much safer to shock a patient early for VT than to try several different antiarrhythmic drugs.

Management of VT in a Haemodynamically Unstable Patient

• Establish intravenous access. Check blood for K$^+$, acid–base balance and blood gases in all patients and correct if necessary (including artificial ventilation). Aim to get K$^+$ >4.5 mmol/l. Maximum potassium replacement rate is 30 mmol/h.
• Cardiac massage may help correct the arrhythmia.
• High-flow oxygen.
• Sedate the patient if awake and alert: midazolam 1–2 mg i.v.
• In the sick patient with low-output state consider intubation and general anaesthesia.
• DC synchronized shock 200 J. If fails: DC shock 360 J.
• Give amiodarone 300 mg i.v. in 20 ml 5% dextrose over 5–10 min. If unavailable, give lidocaine 100–200 mg bolus followed by infusion (Table 8.4).
• Assume hypomagnesaemia. Give 10 mmol magnesium sulphate over 30 min (5 ml 50% solution).
• If still in VT: further 360 J shock.
• Consider overdrive pacing.
• Consider alternative antiarrhythmic drug, e.g. intravenous mexiletine.

Long-term Prophylaxis

Once successfully cardioverted, prophylactic therapy is started orally and ICD implantation is considered (see Section 7.11). The effect of the chosen drug is monitored with 24-hour Holter taping and/or VT provocation study (see below). It is important to keep the serum K$^+$ between 4.5 and 5.5 mmol/l. If VT was secondary to MI or acute myocarditis, it is probably wise to continue drug therapy for 3 months in the first instance, and then repeat 24-hour monitoring both on the drug and after its withdrawal. In some cases more than one drug will be necessary and indefinite oral therapy may be required. Cardiac catheterization is indicated to delineate coronary disease or an LV aneurysm if this is a suspected cause of recurrent VT.

Table 8.4 Drugs commonly used in ventricular arrhythmias

Drug (proprietary name)	Oral dose	Intravenous dose	Half-life (approximate) (h)	Therapeutic plasma level (μg/ml)	Side effects
Lidocaine (Xylocard)	—	100–200mg i.v. bolus 4mg/min for 30min 2mg/min for 2h then 1mg/min	30min	1.5–6.0	Drowsiness + confusion, paraesthesiae and numbness, dysarthria, fits
Quinidine (Kinidin, Kiditard, Quinicardine)	200mg test dose 200–400mg three or four times daily Long-acting preparation twice daily	Rarely used 6–10mg/kg over 0.5h (quinidine gluconate)	7	2–5	Visual disturbances, tinnitus, vertigo, thrombocytopenia, agranulocytosis, diarrhoea, paroxysmal VT or VF, half-dose digoxin, warfarin, etc.
Procainamide (Pronestyl)	375mg 4-hourly	100mg over 5min Repeat up to max. 1g over 1h 2–5mg/min infusion	3	5–10	Hypotension, AV block, insomnia, fever, rash, arthralgia, arteritis (lupus syndrome), agranulocytosis
Disopyramide (Rhythmodan, Norpace)	100–200mg (max.) 6-hourly	50mg i.v. over 5 min repeat to max. 150 mg, and to 300 mg in 1 hour	6	2–6	Dry mouth, blurred vision, urinary retention, constipation, hypotension, VT
Propafenone (Arythmol, Rythmonorm)	150mg three times daily up to 300mg three times daily	2mg/kg then 2mg/min	6	0.2–3.0	Dizziness, headache, anticholinergic
Phenytoin (Epanutin)	100mg three times daily to 200mg twice daily	50mg over 5min, repeating to 500 mg	22	10–18	Cerebellar signs, gum hypertrophy, megaloblastic anaemia (folate), lupus syndrome, bradycardia, hypotension

Drug	Oral dose	Intravenous dose	Half-life (h)	Plasma concentration	Side effects
Mexiletine (Mexitil)	Loading dose 400mg then 200mg three times daily	100–250mg over 10min 4mg/min for 1h, 2mg/min for 1h, then 0.5mg/min	16	1–2pg/ml	Anorexia, nausea, vomiting, tremor, cerebellar signs, bradycardia, hypotension
Aprindine (Fiboran, Fibocil)	Loading dose 200mg, then 100–200mg once daily	25mg over 5min repeated to 150mg	12–66 28	1–3	Tremor, giddiness, diplopia, hallucinations, ataxia, agranulocytosis, jaundice (rare)
Tocainide (Tonocard)	400–800mg three times daily	0.5–0.75mg/kg per min over 15min	14	5–10	Nausea, vomiting, CNS disturbance, giddiness, cerebellar signs, blood dyscrasias
Flecainide (Tambocor)	100–200mg twice daily	1.5–2mg/kg over 10min	12–27 Mean 20	200–800ng/ml	Avoid in paced patients. Giddiness, blurred vision
Propranolol (Inderal)	40mg three times daily (range 10–240mg three times daily)	0.1–0.2mg/kg over 5min	3	30–50 ng/ml oral 50–100 i.v.	Hypotension, AV block, depression, LV failure, cold peripheries, bronchospasm
Amiodarone (Cordarone X)	200mg three times daily for 1 week reducing to ≤200mg once daily	5mg/kg over 2–4h 10–20 mg/kg per day infusion	28 days	0.1	Photosensitivity, corneal microdeposits, thyroid dysfunction, sleep disturbance, etc., alveolitis, half-dose digoxin, warfarin
Bretylium tosylate (Bretylate, Bretylol)	Poorly absorbed	5 mg/kg over 10 min then 1–2 mg/min bolus dose if in VF	8	0.5–1	Hypotension, dizziness, avoid in digoxin toxicity
Ajmaline (Cardiorhythmine)	Not suitable as very short half-life	5–10mg over 2min Repeated after 10min	1–2min	1–3	Caution if also on digoxin as may induce AV block

Regimens of choice are one or more of these drugs:
- Disopyramide 100 mg three or four times daily
- Mexiletine 200 mg three times daily
- Amiodarone 200 mg three times daily for 1 week then reducing
- Propafenone 150–300 mg three times daily
- β-Blocking agent flecainide 100–200 mg twice daily.

Drugs of second choice may be added or tried separately:
- Procainamide 375 mg 4-hourly
- Quinidine durules, two twice daily
- Phenytoin 100 mg three times daily to 200 mg twice daily.

The best combinations of the first group are those from different Vaughan–Williams classes (e.g. disopyramide or mexiletine and amiodarone). There is evidence that amiodarone may be more effective than long-term β blockade in prevention of recurrent VT in patients with HCM. The ICD is now important in the long-term management of recurrent VT (see Section 7.11), and additional amiodarone has been shown to reduce the need for shock therapy.

Provocation of VT

It is important to check that the VT is being successfully suppressed by drug treatment. Patients who have VT that is still provokable at catheter studies are at much greater risk than those whose rhythm is successfully suppressed. A provocation study and Holter monitoring are the two equally important methods for identifying those at risk (the ESVEM trial).

Figure 8.12 shows the simple form of a provocation study. An anaesthetist should be available in case DC cardioversion is needed. Ventricular pacing is established at 100/min (R–R interval 600 ms). After at least eight paced beats a ventricular extra-stimulus (E1) is interposed at an interval of 300 ms. If VT is not provoked the extra-stimulus is brought in in 10 ms (R–ectopic interval 290 ms) and the cycle repeated. The cycle is repeated each time with the R–extra-stimulus interval 10 ms less until the extra-stimulus no longer captures – the effective refractory period (ERP). The extra-stimulus is then moved to an interval of ERP + 50 ms. A second extra-stimulus (E2) is then added at 300 ms and E2 moved in each time with an E1–E2 interval 10 ms less than the previous cycle. When E2 fails to capture, E1 is moved in 10 ms until E2 captures. The sequence is then repeated moving in E2.

The protocol is repeated with three extra-stimuli, and then at a ventricular paced rhythm of 120/min (R–R interval 500 ms) and if necessary at 150/min (R–R interval 400 ms). If VT is still not provoked, a different pacing site can be chosen in the RV, and isoprenaline infused if a really rigorous protocol is wanted. An example of a ventricular provocation study is shown in Figure 8.13.

8.6 Long QT Syndromes (LQTSs)

A long QT interval may be congenital (inherited gene defects) or acquired (drug or electrolyte effects), resulting from abnormalities of the ion channels controlling the duration of repolarization.

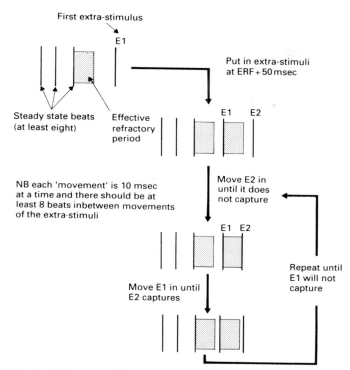

Figure 8.12 A simplified approach to ventricular provocation.

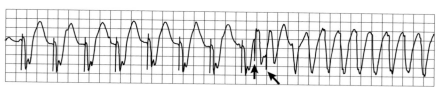

Figure 8.13 Ventricular provocation study using Wellen's protocol: 56-year-old man with dilated cardiomyopathy. A drive train of eight RV paced beats (100/min) is followed by two extra-stimuli (arrowed) at 240 and 220 ms resulting in VT. This patient proceeded to ICD implantation.

The normal QTc is 0.38–0.46 s (see Section 16.1). A long QT interval may predispose to VT often of the polymorphic torsades de pointes type (Figure 8.15 and see Chapter 16, Figure 16.4). Table 8.5 sets out the diagnostic criteria.

QT Dispersion

This is the difference between the maximum and minimum QT interval on the surface 12-lead ECG. In ischaemic patients QT dispersion will be increased by pacing. It is possible that wide QT dispersion may be a marker for

Table 8.5 Diagnostic criteria of long QT syndrome

Major criteria	Minor criteria
Long QT interval	Congenital deafness
Stress-induced symptoms	T-wave alternans
Family history of long QT interval	Low heart rate in children
	Repolarization abnormalities on ECG (e.g. notched T wave)

Criteria set out in 1985 are still valid today. Need two major criteria or one major and two minor.

ventricular arrhythmias and sudden death because it indicates wide differences in repolarization times in the myocardium.

Congenital LQTS Genetic Defects

These are rare syndromes. Only 500 families worldwide were on a registry by 1995. Two clinical syndromes were originally recognized:

1 Jervell and Lange–Nielsen (1957): a family with long QT interval, congenital deaf mutism and sudden death. Autosomal recessive.

2 Romano–Ward (1963–64): QT prolongation and risk of sudden death. Normal hearing. Autosomal dominant transmission. Genetic heterogeneity present as more common in females.

Both syndromes are characterized by the following:

• Genetically prolonged QT interval. ECG may also show T-wave alternans, notched or biphasic T waves, sinus pauses or even AV block.

• Frequent syncopal attacks provoked by emotional or physical stress. Symptoms still may occur during rest or sleep.

• High mortality in untreated cases: 21% dying in 1 year from first syncope; 50% at 10 years.

Dominance of the left sympathetic nerves appears to be pathogenetic and therapy is aimed at this. β Blockade is 80% effective. If this fails left sympathetic nerve denervation is considered (cardiac sympathectomy), or a combination of pacing plus β blockade. Higher rate pacing (e.g. 100/min) keeps the QT interval short. ICDs have been used but these patients are usually children. An ICD shock may induce pain or fear, regenerating the original VT. There are also all the problems of child growth, marriage prospects, etc. Fortunately most children can be managed without an ICD. Particularly bad prognostic features are:

• family history of syncope and sudden death
• QTc >0.5 s
• congenital deafness
• AV block
• documented ventricular arrhythmias
• LQT3 mutation in male patients.

Table 8.6 Summary of the most common long QT syndromes

Syndrome	Gene	Channel	Risk factors	Treatment
LQT1	KVLQT1	I_{ks}	Exercise, emotion, swimming	β Blockade Left cardiac sympathectomy Rarely need ICD
LQT2	HERG	I_{kr}	Sudden arousal Loud noises	Avoid alarm clocks, loud noises and bedroom telephones Keep K^+ > 4.0 mmol/l
LQT3	SCN5A	I_{Na}	Bradycardia, sleep	Mexiletine, pacing, ICD

Schwarz and his colleagues have now identified three principal genetic types with different ion channel defects, and in time this will make therapy more specific. A summary of these types is shown in Table 8.6.

1 *LQT1:* mutation on chromosome 11. The most common type. *KVLQT1* gene. A novel voltage-gated K^+-channel abnormality. High risk with effort/emotion, low risk in sleep. Unlikely to benefit from pacing. Treat with β blockade or left cardiac sympathectomy. β Blockade can be started even with a low resting heart rate.

2 *LQT2:* mutation on chromosome 7 (1995). *HERG* gene. Defect in inward K^+ rectifier. High risk with exercise or arousal. Low risk in sleep. Unlikely to benefit from pacing because it does not shorten the QT interval with increasing heart rate. β Blockade first choice.

3 *LQT3:* mutation on chromosome 3 p21–23. *SCN5A* gene. Na^+-channel dysfunction. Rarest. Highest risk during bradycardia (sleep). Should benefit from pacing but less from β blockade. Mexiletene may be helpful by blocking the persistent current in the defective Na^+ channel. The most difficult of the three to treat.

Mexiletine is most effective in LQT3, shortening the QT interval by blocking the continuing faulty inward sodium current (I_{Na}) although it does also shorten the QT interval in LQT1 and LQT2.

The genotype of the patient can be a useful prognostic guide, helping in the decision for the need for intervention. Patients with the LQT1 or LQT2 mutations tend to be younger at symptom onset and also to have a higher likelihood of cardiac events, but the highest risk of death during a cardiac event appears to be in men with the LQT3 mutation.

LQTS Mutation Carriers

Low penetrance of the gene mutation is now known to occur in the LQTs with silent mutation carriers in families. This carries medicolegal consequences if the patient is not notified of any risk. The hidden risk is of additional drug treatment or hypokalaemia prolonging the QT interval (Table 8.7) and inducing symptoms.

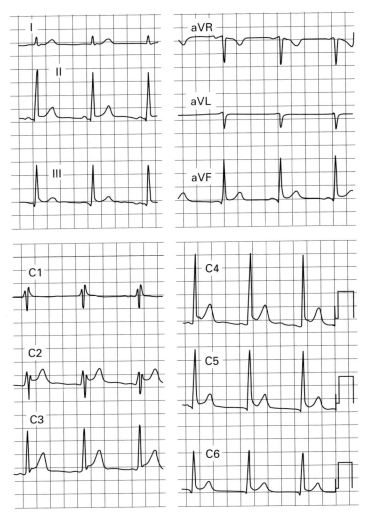

Figure 8.14 Brugada syndrome: 12-lead ECG in a man with a history of three syncopal attacks and a family history of sudden death in his 26-year-old-brother. ECG shows incomplete RBBB and persistent ST elevation in anterior chest leads. Coronary angiography and left ventriculography were normal. VT provocation study induced VT degenerating into VF after two extra-stimuli. An ICD was implanted.

Brugada Syndrome

Described in 1992 by Brugada and Brugada, this rare condition is a cause of sudden death from idiopathic VF in apparently normal hearts. Genetic studies by Chen et al. have found abnormalities in the sodium channel gene *SCN5A* (compare LQT3 above) in some patients. Recently more detailed studies of the RV outflow tract using electron beam CT imaging has shown abnormalities in some of these patients.

Table 8.7 Drugs prolonging the QT interval

Antiarrhythmics	Psychiatric drugs	Antimalarials/ antibiotics	Serotonin antagonists	Others
Quinidine	Thioridazine	Erythromycin	Ketanserin	Probucol
Procainamide	Pimozide	Pentamidine		Vasopressin
Disopyramide	Chlorpromazine	Halofantrine		Terfenadine
Amiodarone	Haloperidol	Amantidine		Astemizole
Sotalol	Tricyclics	Quinine		Tacrolimus
d-Sotalol	Lithium	Chloroquine		Domperidone
Bretylium	Sertindole	Clarithromycin		Ranolazine
Bepridil	Methadone			
Ibutilide				
Dofetilide				

The condition is diagnosed by a characteristic ECG appearance together with a history of syncope or a family history of sudden death. The ECG changes may be quite subtle and show incomplete or complete RBBB, together with persistent ST elevation in precordial leads (see Figure 8.14). Performing the ECG using the chest leads V1–3 two intercostal spaces higher improves the diagnostic sensitivity.

Ajmaline, a class 1a sodium channel-blocking agent, is used as a provocation drug to study changes induced in the anterior chest lead morphology. It causes a scalloped/concave upward ST elevation in anterior chest leads in Brugada syndrome patients with only no change or minimal QT widening in the normal patient. Dose is 1 mg/kg i.v. slowly, up to a maximum of 60 mg.

Ventricular provocation studies should be performed. There is a high incidence of inducing VT/VF with multiple extra-stimuli and the ICD has greatly reduced the mortality in this condition.

Acquired Long QT Interval

This is most commonly drug-induced or secondary to hypocalcaemia or hypomagnesaemia. It may occur in anorexia nervosa. Prolongation of the QT interval is part of the therapeutic benefit of drugs such as amiodarone and sotalol, and the finding of a long QT interval is not necessarily an indication to stop the drug unless the QT interval is >500 ms. Torsades de pointes is unlikely to occur unless the QT interval exceeds this. Patients should not receive two of the drugs from the list in Table 8.7 at the same time with the increased risk of inducing polymorphic VT. Hypokalaemia must be avoided. Two more common examples of along QT interval are shown in Figure 8.15, caused by amiodarone therapy and hypocalcaemia. Although amiodarone commonly prolongs the QT interval polymorphic VT as a result of the drug is rare.

Measurement of the QT interval before and shortly after starting treatment is needed. Several drugs have been withdrawn because of their effect on the

QT interval (prenylamine, terodiline, cisapride) and terfenadine, originally an over-the-counter drug, is now available only on prescription in the UK.

Torsades de Pointes

Polymorphic VT with twisting spirals of QRS complexes around the isoelectric line (see Figures 8.15 and 16.4). It is commonly associated with a long QT interval (congenital or drug-induced), or may complicate an MI, especially if the QT interval is prolonged.

Risk Factors Identified for Drug-induced Torsades

- Female sex
- Hypokalaemia

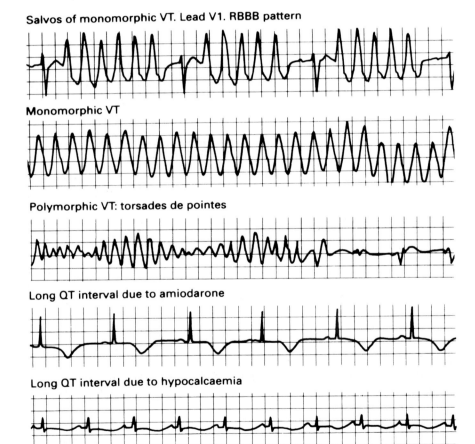

Salvos of monomorphic VT. Lead V1. RBBB pattern

Monomorphic VT

Polymorphic VT: torsades de pointes

Long QT interval due to amiodarone

Long QT interval due to hypocalcaemia

Figure 8.15 Monomorphic and polymorphic ventricular tachycardias. Two common causes of long QT on ECG.

- Hypomagnesaemia
- Bradycardia
- Recent conversion from AF with a QT-prolonging drug
- CCF
- Digoxin therapy
- Rapid intravenous infusion of a QT-prolonging drug or high drug levels
- Pre-existing ion channel polymorphisms (see above).

Management of Torsades de Pointes

Torsades respond poorly to conventional drugs and may be made worse by class Ia agents, e.g. lidocaine, or class III agents. The probable culprit drug is stopped.

Consider the following:

- Pacing: temporary or permanent. Atrial pacing at 90–110/min shortens the QT interval, helping to prevent torsades.
- Magnesium sulphate infusion (even if magnesium level is normal): 1–2 g i.v. over 2–3 min (equivalent to 2–4 ml 50% magnesium sulphate). Then infuse at 2–8 mg/min.
- Isoprenaline infusion 2–10 μg/min, intravenous magnesium (even if magnesium level is normal) or overdrive atrial pacing to rates of 90–110/min.
- Potassium replacement to get K^+ to 4.5–5.0 mmol/l.

8.7 Wolff–Parkinson–White Syndrome

A variety of eponyms has become attached to accessory pathways that cause paroxysmal tachycardia using the pathway as a re-entry circuit. The three most well known are:

1 *Kent bundle* (1893): AV accessory pathway separate from AV node. Short PR interval on ECG and δ wave. WPW syndrome. The great majority of accessory pathway tachycardias (Figure 8.19).

2 *Mahaim pathway*: often young patients with LBBB-pattern tachycardia. Nodoventricular pathway including fasciculoventricular and His-ventricular pathways. Most Mahaim paths seem to be in the anterior tricuspid annulus separate from the AV node. Rare (see Figure 8.7).

3 *James' pathway*: atrionodal or atriofascicular/atrio-His tracts. Short PR interval on ECG but no δ wave. Lown–Ganong–Levine syndrome. Uncommon.

WPW syndrome occurs in 1–3/1000 of the population but less than a quarter have episodes of sustained tachycardia. This may result partly from the fact that the accessory pathway can lose its ability to conduct anterogradely over the years. The δ wave results from premature activation of part of the ventricular myocardium by the accessory pathway. There may in addition be repolarization abnormalities resembling ischaemia and a false-positive exercise test is common. The accessory pathway may be in the anterior or posterior septum or in either the right or the left atrial free wall. Two broad types were originally recognized (Table 8.8). Type A (positive δ wave in V1–LV pathway – Figure 8.16) and Type B (negative δ wave in V1–RV pathway – Figure 8.17). This classification is no longer used because it is now realized that the accessory pathway may be anywhere in the free wall between either atrium or ventricle, or in the interventricular septum. A guide to localization of WPW syndrome accessory pathways is shown in Figure 8.18. More detailed localization is possible, analysing the initial δ wave polarity.

Table 8.8 Original WPW syndrome classification

Original WPW Type	Site of accessory pathway	ECG appearances
Type A	Posterior left atrial wall to left ventricle or paraseptal	Positive δ wave in leads V1–6. Negative δ wave in lead I
Type B	Lateral right atrial wall to right ventricle	Biphasic or negative δ wave in leads V1–3. Positive δ wave in lead I

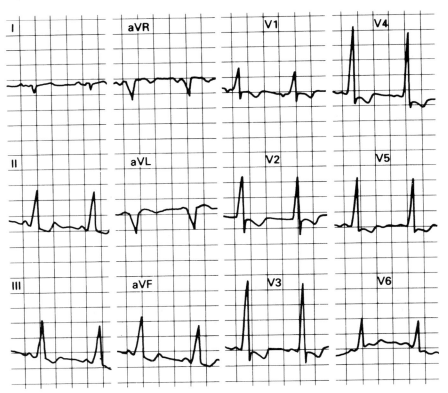

Figure 8.16 Wolff–Parkinson–White syndrome: left-sided pathway. Using the algorithm in Figure 8.18 it is shown to be a left lateral pathway. Originally classified as type A.

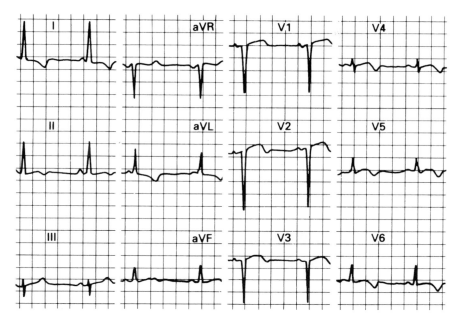

Figure 8.17 Wolff–Parkinson–White syndrome: right-sided anteroseptal pathway. Note repolarization abnormalities mimicking myocardial ischaemia. Originally classified as type B.

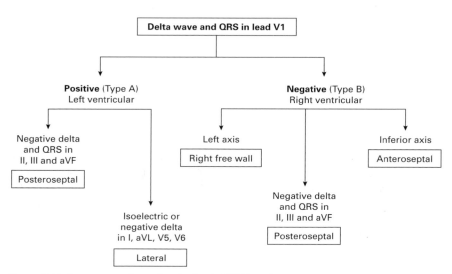

Figure 8.18 Accessory pathway localization in WPW syndrome.

The ECG complex in the WPW syndrome is thus a fusion complex of abnormally activated and normally activated myocardium. The ECG appearances may mimic other conditions:

- LBBB (type B)
- True posterior infarction, RV hypertrophy or RBBB.

Associated Lesions

The WPW syndrome may occur as an isolated condition or in association with other cardiac lesions (e.g. Ebstein's anomaly, hypertrophic obstructive cardiomyopathy, mitral valve prolapse), and paroxysmal tachycardia is a common problem in these conditions. The WPW syndrome may be concealed and not obvious on the surface ECG. In this situation the accessory pathway conducts only retrogradely.

WPW Syndrome Tachycardia

The development of tachycardia results from unidirectional block in the accessory pathway (Figure 8.19). A circus movement is set up with anterograde conduction down the AV node, and retrograde conduction in the Kent bundle (caused by prolonged anterograde refractoriness of the Kent bundle). During tachycardia the δ wave is lost, because ventricular activation occurs only via the AV node, and the ECG and its axis may appear very different from the ECG in normal sinus rhythm. Occasionally, in small children the circuit is established the wrong way round (i.e. anterogradely via the accessory pathway) and the QRS complexes are wide. This antidromic tachycardia may be confused with VT, or SVT with bundle-branch block. Frequently there is more than one accessory pathway (e.g. in Ebstein's anomaly – see Section 3.7), and antidromic tachycardia is more common in patients with multiple pathways.

Sudden Death

Most patients with WPW syndrome are asymptomatic, and the sudden death risk is rare (incidence <0.6%). This is thought to result from the development of AF with rapid conduction down the accessory pathway, leading to VF. In atrial flutter with 1:1 conduction the ventricular rate can reach 300/min before converting to VF.

Drug Treatment

Drugs can act at three sites in WPW tachycardia (see Figure 8.19). Vagal manoeuvres may help in some cases.

WPW syndrome tachycardia can be treated by disopyramide 50–150 mg i.v., flecainide 50–150 mg i.v., propranolol 1–10 mg i.v. or ajmaline 10–50 mg i.v. Intravenous amiodarone is dangerous unless given very slowly (over 1–4 h). Long-term prophylaxis may require a combination of drugs (e.g. disopyramide + β blockade, amiodarone + β blockade). DC cardioversion should be used early if the tachycardia is poorly tolerated.

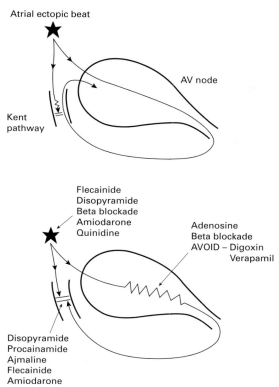

Atrial ectopic beat

AV node

Kent pathway

Flecainide
Disopyramide
Beta blockade
Amiodarone
Quinidine

Adenosine
Beta blockade
AVOID – Digoxin
Verapamil

Disopyramide
Procainamide
Ajmaline
Flecainide
Amiodarone

Figure 8.19 Mechanisms and drug treatment of re-entry tachycardia in WPW syndrome. The upper panel shows the re-entry circuit. A premature atrial beat (star) is blocked at the Kent bundle anterogradely and conducted normally through the AV node. The Kent bundle is not refractory to retrograde conduction and the circus movement is set up. The lower panel shows the sites of drug action. The atrial premature beat can be abolished by disopyramide, β blockade, amiodarone, flecainide or quinidine. Anterograde conduction down the AV node is delayed by adenosine or β blockade. Retrograde conduction up the Kent pathway is blocked by disopyramide, amiodarone, flecainide, ajmaline, procainamide, sotalol and propafenone. Verapamil and digoxin are contraindicated.

Digoxin and verapamil should be avoided in WPW syndrome tachycardia, because the drugs may accelerate anterograde conduction down the Kent bundle.

RF Ablation

This procedure is curative in the vast majority of patients with WPW syndrome and drug treatment is now used only for the acute attack. There is an argument for RF ablation even in the asymptomatic patient with WPW syndrome to prevent longer-term sequelae (see below). The need for permanent pacing with septal pathway ablation is very low (<2%).

8.8 Catheter Ablation

DC Ablation

In 1982 Gallagher described the use of high-energy DC shocks delivered to the His bundle by a standard tripolar recording catheter in the catheter laboratory in eight patients with refractory SVT. It was described as a 'tactic of last resort'. Shocks of up to 300 J were used, and a general anaesthetic was required. Although the shocks were subsequently modified, it became clear that high-energy catheter ablation produced explosive barotrauma in the heart sometimes resulting in:

• hypotension requiring volume loading
• coronary spasm
• cardiac perforation
• transient pulseless electrical activity
• permanent RV dysfunction
• ventricular arrhythmias at follow-up.

AV nodal ablation with the development of complete AV block was possible with the implantation of a permanent pacemaker. It proved very valuable for patients with fast intractable AF or SVT. However, complete AV block was sometimes induced inadvertently in an attempt to ablate accessory pathways near the AV node, and the technique was imprecise.

RF Ablation

Radiofrequency current uses energy similar to surgical diathermy. First reported in 1987, the use of this form of energy is a huge advance and at last has brought a permanent non-surgical cure to many patients with disabling tachycardias, whose lives were a misery on drug treatment. Particular advantages of the technique are:

• only low voltages required (40–60 V), no cardiac barotrauma
• no neuromuscular stimulation so no general anaesthetic required; sedation only
• discrete precise lesions with minimal cardiac damage
• possibility of performing electrophysiological study and ablation in one procedure
• high success rate and low recurrence rate with very few complications.

The disadvantage with the technique is that it is time-consuming, with a long learning curve and often a long screening time. Average length of the procedure is 1–3 h, but occasionally >6 h with screening times of 2 h. Two to five catheters are introduced via the femoral vein. A femoral artery catheter to the left heart is needed for left-sided accessory pathways, and possibly a subclavian puncture or arm vein catheter for coronary sinus catheterization. A TOE is performed at the start of the procedure to exclude LA thrombus if LA access is needed (e.g. all AF ablation procedures). The ablating catheter tip must be negotiated gradually to within <1 mm of the accessory pathway. The use of orthogonal and steerable catheters has helped. The technique can be used for WPW syndrome tachycardias of any type even if the pathway is close to the AV node.

Sometimes multiple accessory pathways have to be dealt with. Ablation can, if necessary, be performed in the coronary sinus but there is a small risk of pericarditis or perforation here. Shocks lasting for a few seconds are delivered once the accessory pathway action potential has been recorded and the device switches off automatically if the impedance rises as a result of blood coagulum. Recurrence rate is small (5%) and complications few. Patients are sedated and heparinized throughout the procedure. After RF ablation the patient is kept in overnight and echocardiography is sometimes performed before discharge to exclude a possible pericardial collection.

RF Ablation of Accessory Pathways

Patients who are unresponsive to medical treatment, dislike their treatment or have frequent or disabling attacks are candidates for RF ablation, which is curative and avoids the need for any further drug treatment. The electrophysiological (EP) study and the RF ablation can be done as one procedure. Recurrence rate is <5%.

An electrophysiological study is used as risk stratification by measuring the anterograde effective refractory period (ERP) of the bypass tract(s). Attempts are made to initiate the tachycardia and this may include atrial burst pacing to induce AF. Higher-risk features include:

- bypass tract ERP <270 ms
- multiple accessory pathways
- septal accessory pathway
- easily inducible SVT
- male sex.

So successful is RF ablation now that patients rarely require surgical ablation of the bypass. Epicardial mapping is necessary before surgical ablation because the pathway is usually invisible. Septal tracts are difficult with a risk of complete AV block, and posteroseptal pathways are difficult with the proximity of the coronary sinus.

Asymptomatic WPW Syndrome

Earlier advice was that patients who were absolutely asymptomatic and found to have WPW on a routine ECG did not need an EP study unless they planned high-rise activities, such as rock-climbing, were pilots or athletes. However, a recent randomized study from Pappone's group of asymptomatic patients at high risk of arrhythmias (inducibility at EP study) showed a highly significant reduction in arrhythmias over a 5-year period in patients who had had an RF ablation.

AF Ablation

The discovery that potentials from muscle sleeves round the ostia of the pulmonary veins were largely responsible for the generation of AF has led to a huge demand for this procedure, which is still being developed and refined. It has since been realized that these potentials may arise from sites other than the pulmonary veins (e.g. coronary sinus, interatrial septum, posterior LA wall).

Initial enthusiasm for ablation of the ostia of the pulmonary veins waned with the complication of ostial pulmonary vein stenosis in a few patients. Wide area circumferential ablation (WACA), developed by Pappone, is now used, ablating a complete circle around, but well clear of, the pulmonary vein ostia. Additional ablation lines are drawn across the left atrium, joining the upper PV's ablation circuits and one line down to the mitral annulus. If these lines are complete, this effectively locks out any fibrillation wave from propagating into the left atrium and causing a recurrence of AF. Finally complex atrial fractionated electrograms (CAFEs) are targeted.

Recurrence of AF in the first 2 months is not uncommon and does not necessarily mean long-term failure. Anticoagulation and antiarrhythmic drugs are usually continued for several months after the procedure.

Who Should be Considered for AF Ablation?
• The young patient with frequent paroxysmal AF, and an otherwise normal heart
• Paroxysmal AF refractory to one or more antiarrhythmic drugs
• Paroxysmal AF with rapidly developing symptoms (e.g. hypertrophic cardiomyopathy)
• Persistent AF with warfarin intolerance or bleeding complications

Who is Unsuitable for AF Ablation?
• Very large left atrium
• Severe mitral valve disease
• Recent embolic event or LA thrombus on TOE

There are no large randomized trials yet comparing AF ablation with long-term anticoagulation and antiarrhythmic drug treatment (medical group). A large non-randomized trial from Pappone's team in Milan suggested that event-free survival, and freedom from AF recurrences, were higher in the ablation group.

Complications
Major complications occur in about 6% of procedures and include:
• Pulmonary vein stenosis: incidence reduced by the WACA approach (see above)
• Systemic embolism: incidence reduced by TOE before the procedure, heparinization during the procedure and subsequent anticoagulation
• Pericardial effusion or tamponade: echocardiography and pericardiocentesis equipment should be available in the lab
• Atrio-oesophageal fistula: fortunately rare. Occurs with multiple ablations on the posterior LA wall. Usually fatal

- LA flutter: treated with further ablation
- Left phrenic nerve paralysis: may be transient.

AVNRT Ablation

AV nodal re-entrant tachycardia has also been successfully cured by RF ablation. The slow component of the pathway in the posterior septum can be safely ablated without damaging the AV node. There is a 2% risk of complete AV block requiring permanent pacing, and this must be discussed with the patient before the procedure, especially the younger patient with infrequent attacks.

Flutter Ablation

Most cases of atrial flutter can be managed by delivering several shocks to the triangle of Koch between the His bundle and the ostium of the coronary sinus. This destroys the area of slow conduction and the need for permanent pacing is rare. Patients with congenital heart disease may have multiple flutter circuits and recurrence of atrial flutter after an initial successful flutter ablation is a possibility (e.g. after a Fontan procedure).

VT Ablation

RF ablation is possible for VT in either ventricle but the success rate is lower than for accessory pathway ablation. VT arising from the RV outflow tract (LBBB pattern with inferior axis – see Figure 8.10, p. 387) is the VT that is most likely to be successfully ablated. It may also be useful in idiopathic VT in otherwise normal hearts, and in very frequent or incessant VT after MI (where an ICD is inappropriate). It may also be possible to ablate VT in patients with an ICD who are experiencing a 'VT storm', getting frequent shocks from the device and refractory to additional drug therapy (e.g. with amiodarone and mexiletine).

AV Node Ablation

This is still sometimes used in patients with fast AF whose ventricular rate cannot be controlled on rate-limiting drugs, and whose AF cannot be ablated successfully. Permanent VVIR pacing is needed as part of the procedure.

Surgical Techniques for the Management of Arrhythmias

The management of arrhythmias that are refractory to drug treatment may include:
- antitachycardia pacing (temporary or permanent) (see Section 7.10)
- catheter ablation of AV node, bypass tract or arrhythmogenic focus (see above)
- implantation of automatic cardioverter defibrillator (see Section 7.11)
- other surgical procedures.

RF ablation for WPW syndrome tachycardia has largely removed this condition from the sphere of the surgeon. Frequent VT refractory to drug treatment may still need surgery. The best surgical case is that of the patient with well-tolerated, inducible, monomorphic VT with a localized infarct or aneurysm and good residual LV function. Results for polymorphic VT are not so good and patients with additional poor LV function are probably best managed with an ICD.

Direct division or ablation of an accessory pathway or arrhythmogenic focus can be performed during open-heart surgery. Careful epicardial and occasionally endocardial electrographic mapping are required to detect the activation sequence over the atrial and ventricular myocardium. Detection of the earliest activation site on the myocardium helps establish the site of the accessory pathway (e.g. in WPW syndrome) or the arrhythmogenic focus (e.g. in VT).

Surgical techniques may involve the following approaches:
• Cryotherapy: a cryoprobe can produce temporary ablation at −10°C, or permanent at −65°C, e.g. of accessory pathway or His bundle.
• Ventriculotomy: encircling ventriculotomy is performed during VT.
• Endocardial resection: performed during cardiopulmonary bypass.
• Endocardial ablation: ablation lines drawn in the LA at the time of mitral valve surgery.
• Ventricular aneurysmectomy: performed alone may miss the site of origin of the VT, because this is often at the junction of scar tissue and more normal myocardium.
• Mitral valve replacement (for arrhythmias with mitral valve prolapse).
• Cardiac transplantation: for the extreme case where drugs and other ablative techniques have failed.

Combinations of these techniques may be necessary, e.g. mapping directed endocardial resection plus the implantation of an ICD.

8.9 Problems with Individual Antiarrhythmic Drugs

Amiodarone

This iodine-containing compound has a very long half-life and is strongly bound to plasma proteins. It is highly fat soluble and probably binds with phospholipids on the cell membrane and modifies adenyl cyclase activity.

Given orally it takes 5–10 days to saturate the tissues. It is of great value in both atrial and ventricular arrhythmias, as well as WPW syndrome, where it acts by increasing the bypass anterograde ERP.

Electrophysiological Effects

It increases action potential duration (APD) in both sinus and AV nodes, but more so in the His–Purkinje system and ventricular muscle. It increases the A–H interval without changing the H–V time. It slightly reduces the sinus node discharge rate and sinus node recovery time. It reduces conduction in the WPW syndrome accessory pathway, and reduces the anterograde ERP more than the retrograde ERP. It reduces excitability of all cardiac tissues, and the automaticity of SA and AV nodes is reduced. There is probably no chronic effect on contractility, although acute intravenous administration produces vasodilatation with afterload reduction, which affects acute contractility measurements.

Drug Interactions

The doses of digoxin and warfarin should be halved in patients starting amiodarone (displacement of digoxin from myocardial receptors increases plasma digoxin, but reduces the direct cardiac effect). Amiodarone can be used with verapamil or β blockers, but care is needed (effects on AV node).

Side Effects (Table 8.9)

These are common and sometimes require the drug to be stopped. Patients should be warned about possible photosensitivity. They should shield themselves from the sun and use barrier creams (factor 30 +) if necessary.

Thyroid function is checked before starting the drug, especially in patients with AF. It is best avoided in patients with known thyroid dysfunction.

Thyroid dysfunction (hypothyroidism) is caused by inhibition of T_3 production and enhancement of reversed T_3 production (inactive). Thyrotoxicosis (less common) is treated with carbimazole. Corneal microdeposits are very common, but only visible on the slit-lamp. They are reversible if the drug is stopped and regular eye checks are no longer needed. Only about 6% of patients on the drug develop visual disturbance.

The drug is safe in moderate renal dysfunction. Amiodarone does increase serum creatinine probably by reducing renal tubular excretion. Sinistrin clearance is not affected and the drug does not reduce the glomerular filtration rate. The rise in serum creatinine gradually reverses when the amiodarone is stopped.

Pulmonary fibrosis occurs in about 5% of patients taking amiodarone. It is more common in patients aged over 70, in those with low pretreatment pulmonary diffusion capacity (D_{LCO}), with high maintenance doses of

Table 8.9 Amiodarone side effects

Common side effects	Rarer side effects
Photosensitivity (>50% patients)	Peripheral neuropathy
Skin rash	Pulmonary fibrosis (fibrosing alveolitis)
Headache	Thyroid dysfunction (hypothyroidism more than
Tremor	hyperthyroidism)
Sleep disturbance, insomnia and	Slate-grey skin and melanosis (Figure 8.20)
nightmares	
Gut effects: nausea, constipation	Hepatic dysfunction (raised enzymes)
Corneal microdeposits	Visual symptoms
Increased prothrombin time	Epididymitis
Elevation of serum creatinine	

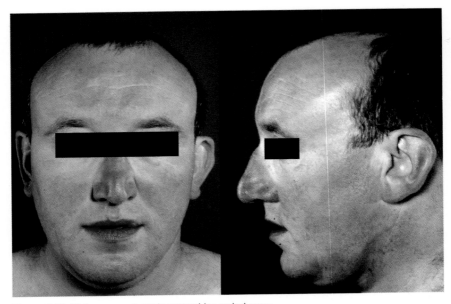

Figure 8.20 Slate-grey melanosis caused by amiodarone

amiodarone, and with therapy for longer than 2 months. It is rare with a maintenance dose <300 mg/day. There is no test that predicts lung fibrosis so patients must be told to report increasing dyspnoea, cough or weight loss. Symptoms and signs may easily be confused with early pulmonary oedema, especially in patients with known poor LV function. Fibrosis may be reversible if the drug is stopped soon enough. Steroid therapy needed for 6 months.

Cardioversion on Amiodarone
If the patient has sinoatrial disease care is needed (effect on reducing sinus node automaticity), but it is usually safe.

Dosage
• Oral therapy: 200 mg three times daily for 1 week, reducing to 200 mg daily or less. It is very important to follow up patients taking amiodarone closely and to ensure that they are taking the smallest possible maintenance dose.
• Intravenous administration can be dangerous if given quickly (α-blocking effect). It is avoided if possible in elderly people and patients with large hearts. In AF or VT it may restore sinus rhythm without the need for DC cardioversion in about 50% of patients. Infusion dose is 5 mg/kg in 100 ml 5% dextrose (not 0.9% saline) over 1–4 h. Maximum dose is 1200 mg in 24 h.

Abnormal rhythm may not be abolished immediately, sometimes reverting several hours after the infusion has stopped. The infusion should, if possible, be given through a central line. It can be given through a peripheral line for the first 24h but the vein must be flushed at the end of the infusion.

Drug Levels
In chronic therapy it may be helpful to assay plasma amiodarone levels, and the level of its principal metabolite, desethyl amiodarone. Normal range for both is 0.6–2.5 mg/l; both are antiarrhythmic.

Disopyramide
A drug with both class 1a and class 3 actions, disopyramide also has an anticholinergic effect. The anticholinergic effect on the heart depends on the vagal tone present (in the normal heart, disopyramide may occasionally increase heart rate slightly by this 'vagolytic' action). About 90% is bioavailable taken orally, and with normal serum levels (2–6 µg/ml) about 30–50% is free in serum. Half is excreted unchanged in urine.

Electrophysiological Effects
It prolongs atrial effective refractory period, has a variable effect on AV node refractory period and prolongs ventricular refractory period. Conduction times in AV node and His–Purkinje system are little affected (unless there is pronounced vagal tone). It slows the accessory pathway conduction. It is a useful drug: in atrial ectopics, prevention of AF or paroxysmal SVT because it causes a rise in atrial ERP; in WPW syndrome tachycardia because it causes a rise in accessory pathway conduction time; and in ventricular ectopics or tachycardia because it causes a rise in ventricular ERP. It is a useful drug in hypertrophic obstructive cardiomyopathy (Section 4.2).

Dosage

Oral
Loading dose is 300 mg in the adult (200 mg if <50 kg) followed by 150 mg 6-hourly (100 mg if <50 kg). Increase dose interval if renal dysfunction (e.g. once daily for creatinine clearance ≤15 ml/min).

Intravenous
Dose of 50 mg is given slowly over 5 min, and may be carefully repeated up to 150 mg if necessary and contraindications have not appeared (see below).

Relative Contraindications to Disopyramide (Where the Drug has to be Used with Great Care)
• CCF with a large heart, poor LV function or cardiogenic shock
• Sinoatrial disease (prolongs atrial ERP)
• Second- or third-degree AV block

Table 8.10 Disopyramide side effects

Common (anticholinergic) side effects	Less common side effects
Dry mouth, eyes, nose	Urinary retention
Blurred vision	Acute psychosis
Hesitancy in men with prostatic hypertrophy	Cholestatic jaundice
Constipation	Hypoglycaemia
Nausea	Agranulocytosis

- Prostatic hypertrophy
- Glaucoma
- Hypokalaemia: rarely it may precipitate VT (torsades de pointes) as with quinidine.

The side effects are detailed in Table 8.10.

Other Points to Note
- A dry mouth is an expected side effect and is a guide to neither plasma level nor drug toxicity.
- Occasionally the drug may potentiate warfarin.
- It does not interact with lidocaine and can be used where lidocaine fails. It has only a weak negative inotropic effect.
- Disopyramide toxicity on ECG: watch for lengthening QT interval, widening of QRS complex, bradycardia or conduction defects.
- Also watch for hypotension. More likely with too rapid intravenous administration, especially if the patient is also on β blockade or other antihypertensive medication.

Procainamide
A class 1a antiarrhythmic with electrophysiological properties similar to quinidine. Up to 90% is absorbed orally and 15% only is protein bound. The drug is acetylated in the liver (first-pass metabolism) and acetylator status is important in determining plasma levels and toxic side effects. About 50% of the drug is excreted in the urine. The acetyl metabolite is also antiarrhythmic and has a longer half-life.

Dosage
- In the adult the drug is given 4-hourly; in some difficult cases this means waking the patient at night to maintain plasma levels (5–10 µg/ml).
- Average adult dose is 375 mg, 4-hourly (250–500 mg 4-hourly).
- Slow-release preparation: procainamide durules can be taken 8-hourly (dose 1–1.5 g, 8-hourly).
- Acetylator status
  - fast acetylators: may not reach necessary plasma levels of procainamide, but acetyl metabolite is antiarrhythmic and less toxic
  - slow acetylators: may have high plasma levels and risk toxicity.

- Intravenous dose is 100 mg slowly over 5 min up to a maximum of 1 g in 1 h.

Electrophysiological Effects of Procainamide

Little effect on AV node conduction (A–H time) and dose-dependent increase in His–Purkinje conduction (H–V time). Increase in refractory period of Kent pathway making it useful in WPW syndrome tachycardia.

Side Effects

These make it a more useful drug in acute management of ventricular arrhythmias than in chronic suppression.

Intravenously it is a little safer than quinidine and can be tried if lidocaine fails. The following are side effects after intravenous administration:

- Hypotension caused by vasodilatation (reversed by phenylephrine)
- Complete AV block: the drug should not be given in complete AV block because it may slow or extinguish the idioventricular rhythm
- In atrial flutter or AF a vagolytic effect on the AV node may increase ventricular response (as with disopyramide). Procainamide is not usually used for atrial dysrhythmias, although it may extinguish atrial ectopics.

Long-term Side Effects

- The lupus syndrome: rash, arthralgia, fever, arteritis, pleurisy and pericarditis, but no renal involvement. The effects resolve on stopping the drug. Antinuclear antibodies occur in half the patients receiving the drug.
- Agranulocytosis.

Unless absolutely essential, procainamide should be restricted to 3–6 months of oral therapy.

Quinidine

This is the original antiarrhythmic drug with class 1a activity. The drug is completely absorbed orally; intravenous administration can be dangerous and so is rarely used.

Unlike procainamide, 80% is protein bound, causing drug interactions. The drug is hydroxylated in the liver and CCF; liver congestion results in high plasma quinidine levels. Alkaline urine may result in toxic metabolic accumulation.

Quinidine may be tried in paroxysmal AF or other atrial arrhythmias, and may help keep a patient in SR after cardioversion. Atrial arrhythmias are the main indication for its use; it is rarely used for ventricular arrhythmias now because less toxic drugs are available. It is contraindicated in sinoatrial disease, digoxin toxicity and complete AV block.

Dosage

A test dose of quinidine sulphate of 200 mg is given to check for drug idiosyncrasy (anaphylaxis).

Quinidine durules are then started, initially two twice daily (= 500 mg quinidine bisulphate twice daily) to three times daily maximum. When starting treatment, quinidine displacement of other drugs from plasma proteins necessitates reducing the doses of other drugs, so the dose of concomitant warfarin or digoxin should be halved.

Electrophysiological Effects
As in procainamide, no change in A–H time (or even slight shortening as a result of vagolytic effect), plus lengthening of H–V time. Surface ECG shows:
- widening QRS
- prolonged QT interval
- T-wave changes.

These are useful guides to toxicity.

QRS widening >120 ms is an indication to stop the drug. With increasing toxicity the following may occur:
- atrial standstill
- VT (torsades de pointes) (see Figure 8.15 and Chapter 16, Figure 16.4)
- VF.

Side Effects
These are commonly gastrointestinal. Any others are indications to stop the drug:
- Gastrointestinal: diarrhoea is expected, with nausea and vomiting.
- Cinchonism: tinnitus, vertigo, deafness, visual disturbances, blindness.
- Haematological: thrombocytopenia, purpura, agranulocytosis.
- Neuromuscular blocking effect: this may potentiate muscle relaxants. Its vagolytic action inhibits anticholinesterase activity in myasthenia.
- Quinidine syncope: this may be caused by AV block, VT or VF.

A prolonged QT interval plus an early ectopic (R on T) may be the cause.

Lidocaine
A class 1b antiarrhythmic that shortens the action potential duration. It differs from procainamide and quinidine in several respects (Table 8.11).

It is used for ventricular arrhythmias in the CCU. It is rapidly metabolized in the liver, allowing flexible control, and has to be given intravenously. Liver dysfunction or congestion (as in heart failure) requires dose reduction. It is not protein bound.

Lidocaine metabolites are excreted in the urine and contribute to CNS toxicity. It is safer than intravenous procainamide in low-output states or in patients with degrees of AV block.

Dosage
There are numerous suggested schedules. One of the easiest is: 200 mg i.v. bolus over 5 min, followed by infusion of 4 mg/min for 30 min, then 2 mg/min for 2 h, then 1 mg/min.

Table 8.11 Differences between class 1a and class 1b antiarrhythmic agents

	Class 1a: procainamide quinidine	Class 1b: lidocaine
Action potential duration	Lengthened	Shortened
Peripheral vessels	Vasodilator	Vasoconstrictor
Oral preparation	Yes	No
Useful in atrial arrhythmias	Yes	No
Conduction of His–Purkinje system	Prolongs H–V time	Little effect
CNS toxicity	Uncommon	Common
Myocardial depression	In toxic doses	Minimal
Use in sinoatrial disease	No	Safe

In low-output states the initial 4 mg/min infusion period is omitted and the infusion is started at 2 mg/min. Plasma levels should be 1.5–6 µg/ml. Significant plasma levels can be obtained after intramuscular lidocaine (300 mg in the adult) after about 15 min. Lidocaine infiltration used for minor surgery, pacemaker insertion, etc. can also produce significant plasma levels.

Side Effects
These are primarily neurological, especially in elderly people, and include: numbness, drowsiness, confusion, nausea, vomiting, dizziness, dysarthria and eventually convulsions. Convulsions are managed with intravenous diazepam.

Lidocaine is safer in cardiac failure or cardiogenic shock than procainamide, provided that lower infusion rates are used. What to do if lidocaine fails:
• Check adequate infusion rate and that drip is still functional
• Check plasma K$^+$: lidocaine is less effective in hypokalaemia
• Check for additional drug therapy, possibly causing arrhythmias: digitalis, other inotropes, etc.
• Gradually increase lidocaine infusion rate until early toxic signs appear
• If still ineffective switch to alternative drug, e.g. disopyramide, flecainide, amiodarone or bretylium tosylate.

Mexiletine
This is a class 1b agent similar to lidocaine, but available for oral administration. Hepatic metabolism is slower than with lidocaine, and renal excretion is reduced if the urine is alkaline.

Electrophysiological effects are variable; the H–V time has been reported to increase or decrease. Generally it has little effect on AV conduction. Its effect on blocking the inward sodium current makes it the drug of choice in the LQT3 syndrome (see Section 8.6).

Dosage
Orally: 400 mg loading dose, then 200 mg 8-hourly in the adult. Intravenous dosage is complicated as with lidocaine, because there is a small margin

between therapeutic effect and side effects. Suggested intravenous regimen: 100–250 mg i.v. over 10 min, 4 mg/min for 1 h, 2 mg/min for 1 h, then 0.5 mg/min.

Close attention is needed with intravenous mexiletine because the long half-life (16 h) compared with lidocaine means that fine-tuning of the regimen is much more difficult. Neurological side effects are common with intravenous therapy. Chronic oral therapy is much easier, and side effects are less likely.

Side Effects

These are as with lidocaine: dizziness, numbness, paraesthesiae, tremor, dysarthria, tinnitus, myoclonus, convulsions, nausea and vomiting, hiccoughs, bradycardia and hypotension. The bradycardia usually responds to atropine.

On oral therapy common complaints are nausea, anorexia and a continuous unpleasant taste in the mouth.

Tocainide

Also similar to lidocaine in structure and antiarrhythmic effect but available orally and has a longer half-life (11–14 h). Fifty per cent is protein bound. About 40% is excreted unchanged in the urine. Electrophysiological effects are similar to those of lidocaine.

As with lidocaine, it is safe in low-output states, but dosage should be reduced in patients with heart failure, renal disease or after MI because the half-life is prolonged (e.g. 17–19 h) and twice-daily dosage is sufficient in these patients.

Dosage

- Oral: 400–800 mg 8-hourly, 400–600 mg 12-hourly in hepatic, disease or CCF.
- Intravenous: 0.5–0.75 mg/kg per min over 15–30 min, followed by oral therapy.

Side effects are similar to those of lidocaine and mexiletine and, unfortunately, as common. The main adverse effects are nausea, vomiting, dizziness and light-headedness, tremors and paraesthesiae.

Recently, neutropenia, agranulocytosis, thrombocytopenia and aplastic anaemia have been reported. The drug should only be used for life-threatening arrhythmias and weekly blood counts are necessary while patients are on the drug.

Flecainide

This is a class 1c antiarrhythmic agent that received bad coverage in the CAST study. This study showed that patients taking flecainide or encainide for ectopic beats after an MI had a higher mortality than those taking a placebo. This was thought to result from a proarrhythmic effect of these drugs. The CAST trial results led to the drug being largely abandoned for a wide

variety of arrhythmias unrelated to MI. Flecainide is still of great value in refractory arrhythmias not responding to other drugs:
- life-threatening VT
- paroxysmal atrial arrhythmias, AF or atrial flutter (see Section 8.3)
- reciprocating tachycardias involving accessory pathways (either intra- or extranodal).

Similar to tocainide it has a long half-life (approximately 20 h) and twice-daily dosage is adequate. In common with other class 1c drugs, it does not prolong the action potential duration, but prolongs the refractory period in His–Purkinje and accessory bypass tracts.

Dosage
- Oral: 100–200 mg 12-hourly. Maximum daily dose 400 mg. The long-term dose should be reduced if possible, especially in elderly people.
- Intravenous: 0.5–2.0 mg/kg i.v. slowly up to a maximum of 150 mg.

Careful ECG monitoring is needed if the patient is in VT. In patients with poor LV function it is safer to give the drug as a mini-infusion over 30 min. Side effects are not common and generally the drug is well tolerated. Giddiness, light-headedness and blurred vision are the most common complaints. The proarrhythmic effect occurs in a small number of patients (probably <10%). It has a mild negative inotropic effect. Flecainide should be avoided in:
- patients in cardiac failure
- patients with permanent pacing who do not have a programmable unit; the pacing threshold may rise and the pacemaker may need programming to a higher output voltage or pulse width; a similar increase in pacing voltage may be needed with temporary wires
- second- or third-degree AV block
- sinoatrial disease
- ectopic beats after MI.

Propafenone
This is another class 1c agent recently available in the UK. It is valuable in the management of both supraventricular and ventricular arrhythmias, as well as those re-entrant arrhythmias involving accessory pathway conduction. It blocks retrograde conduction in the accessory pathway. Bioavailability is 50% and protein binding 90%. Half-life is approximately 6 h. The drug is given 8-hourly. Dose: 150–300 mg three times daily. Side effects are dizziness, unusual taste and headache. It is mildly negatively inotropic. It has anticholinergic effects. Care is needed in patients with airway obstruction because it has mild β-blocking activity. It should be avoided in patients with myasthenia gravis.

Bretylium Tosylate
A drug that tends to be used as a last resort in patients with VT or VF resistant to other antiarrhythmic therapy. It is only available intravenously or intramuscularly.

Its mode of action is not well understood, but it has both class 2 and 3 effects. Eighty per cent is excreted unchanged in the urine. The half-life is about 8 h.

Dosage
- Intramuscularly: 5 mg/kg 8-hourly or 200 mg 2-hourly until the drug works (up to a maximum of 2 g).
- Intravenously: single bolus of 5 mg/kg for VF.

Side Effects
Hypotension, nausea, nasal stuffiness (sympathetic blockade); parotid pain with prolonged use; patients receiving bretylium should be lying flat, and hypotension (the most common side effect) can be reversed by volume loading and a pressor agent if necessary (e.g. phenylephrine).

9 Infective Endocarditis

Sir William Osler first described the condition in 1885, although Riviere described postmortem findings of vegetations in 1723. Mahler died from endocarditis in 1911 and had massive vegetations 'like seaweed' on his valve.

It is no longer termed 'subacute bacterial endocarditis', because non-bacterial organisms are becoming an increasing cause of the condition. The incidence is 1.7–6.2/100000 patient-years. In the UK there are about 1500–2000 cases annually. The male:female ratio is 2:1.

The overall mortality rate still runs at about 20%, but is a great deal less for penicillin-sensitive *Streptococcus viridans* (approximately 5–10%) and tricuspid valve endocarditis in drug abusers (about 10% mortality) and a great deal more for staphylococci and enterococci (25–50%). Prosthetic valve endocarditis is also at higher risk (approximately 40%) where further surgery is usually required as part of the management. The fungal endocarditis mortality rate is at least 60%. Prognostic factors are shown in Table 9.3.

A Changing Disease

Infective endocarditis is a changing disease, but the advent of newer antibiotics has had little effect on mortality figures. The changes in the type of disease are the result of several factors:

- Decline in rheumatic fever and rheumatic valve disease
- Increasing incidence in older patients
- Increased survival of patients operated upon for congenital heart disease
- Prosthetic valve endocarditis
- Different organisms: increasing number of staphylococcal and fungal infections
- Antibiotic resistance
- Drug addicts with tricuspid valve endocarditis

Swanton's Cardiology, sixth edition. By R. H. Swanton and S. Banerjee. Published 2008 Blackwell Publishing. ISBN 978-1-4051-7819-8.

- Multi-drug-resistant organisms
- Increase in immunosuppressed population, e.g. HIV-positive individuals, patients on haemodialysis with chronic renal failure, people with alcohol problems and patients on steroids.

9.1 Predisposing Cardiac Lesions

These are shown in Table 9.1. The haemodynamic situation that predisposes to infection is a high-pressure jet into a lower-pressure system through a narrow orifice, resulting in endothelial wear and tear (Rodbard's factors). Bacteria then settle on this damaged endothelial surface, and platelet, fibrin and inflammatory cellular accumulation follows, surrounding bacteria in a 'protective cocoon'. Thus infective endocarditis is much more likely on a VSD than an ASD (Table 9.1).

There seems little doubt now that infective endocarditis can occur on a previously normal valve. In spite of this the logistics of antibiotic cover for dental procedures, etc. are such that it is at present advised only for those patients with known predisposing lesions listed in Table 9.1.

Other predisposing factors should also be remembered: patients at higher risk of infection from general medical conditions (e.g. diabetes, renal failure, haemodialysis and alcoholism). Immunosuppressed patients and intravenous drug abusers are also at high risk. Overall about 5% of the total population is at risk.

Table 9.1 Infective endocarditis: predisposing cardiac lesions

Commonly in	Less commonly in	Virtually never in
Aortic valve disease (bicuspid or rheumatic)	HCM and subaortic stenosis	Secundum ASD
Mitral valve disease:	Previously normal valve	Pulmonary valve stenosis
Regurgitation > stenosis	Jet lesion	Mitral prolapse without
Floppy valve	AV fistula	regurgitation
Coarctation	Mural thrombus, e.g. post-infarct	Innocent cardiac murmurs
Cyanotic congenital heart disease, e.g. TGA, Fallot's tetralogy		
Patent ductus arteriosus		Divided PDA
VSD		Surgically repaired ASD or VSD with no residual defect
Prosthetic valves: tissue or mechanical	Permanent pacemaker wire	Coronary stent implantation
Tricuspid valve in drug abusers		

9.2 Portals of Entry

These are often unknown, but careful history taking may reveal one of the following in the previous few months:

• *Dental work* of any type: extraction, fillings or even scaling. Patients with poor dental hygiene are at risk and these are often elderly people, immuno-suppressed individuals, patients with polycythaemia (congenital heart disease) or gingivitis associated with gum hypertrophy (e.g. phenytoin or nifedipine). Badly fitting dentures or dental braces may also be dangerous. Retained dental roots are a particularly common source of infection and the teeth are still the most common portal of entry. Overall a confirmed dental source occurs in only about 20% cases. All patients with infective endocarditis should have an orthopantomograph (OPG) to identify any dental pathology or root abscess (Figure 9.1).

• *Urinary tract infection*: cystoscopy, catheterization, lithotripsy.

• *Respiratory infection*.

• *Enterococci* may gain access to the circulation via carcinoma of the colon, and present with infective endocarditis (e.g. *Streptococcus bovis*). Endoscopy is still contentious. It is unlikely after standard gastroduodenoscopy, sigmoid-oscopy or barium examinations.

• *Skin disease*: purulent lesions, wound infections, burns, leg ulcers (Figure 9.2).

• *Intravenous cannulation*: this is particularly a problem with CVP lines and may be a cause of infective endocarditis soon after valve replacement. It is especially likely in patients requiring CVP lines for more than 48 h and in those with additional medical problems (e.g. jaundice, uraemia, additional steroid treatment). Strict aseptic procedures necessary for all CVP line insertions.

• *Intravenous drug abuse* (Figure 9.3).

• *Chronic haemodialysis*.

• *Gallbladder disease*.

Orthopantomogram (OPG)

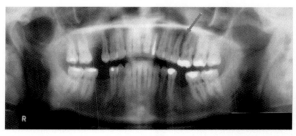

Figure 9.1 Orthopantomogram in a man with infective endocarditis. There is dental root abscess (arrowed).

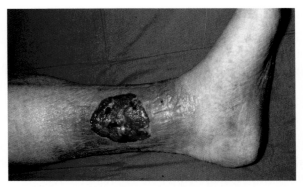

Figure 9.2 Chronic leg ulcer: source of *Staphylococcus epidermidis* endocarditis. Biopsy showed squamous cell carcinoma.

- *Surgery.*
- *Abortion*: operative > spontaneous.
- *Parturition*: although a theoretically likely portal of entry, this is probably less of a risk factor than once thought.
- *Fractures, osteomyelitis* (Figure 9.4).

The fact that the portal of entry is often unknown has led to virtually every invasive procedure being incriminated as a possible cause. As a result many probably 'innocent' procedures (e.g. gastroscopy) have been included in the past. Basically all endoscopy procedures should be covered by antibiotics in

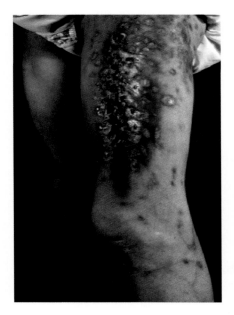

Figure 9.3 Chronic infected ulcers in the thigh of a drug abuser. Source of *Staphylococcus aureus* endocarditis.

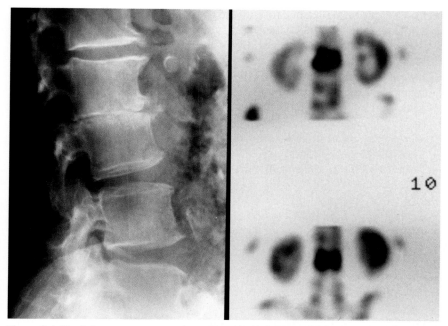

Figure 9.4 *Staphylococcus aureus* endocarditis with discitis and osteomyelitis in lumbar vertebrae (left). Bone scan (right) showing corresponding hot spot.

patients with known predisposing lesions if any biopsy procedure is likely to be performed. Body piercing may also be a culprit.

9.3 Organisms Responsible

Bacteria

- *Streptococcus viridans* group: still the most common cause although less so than in the past. Probably accounts for 40% of cases now. This is a heterogeneous group including *S. milleri, S. oralis, S. mitis, S. mitior, S. mutans, S. salivarius* and other oral streptococci. *S. milleri* is present in the mouth, gut and vagina. It tends to form abscesses more frequently than other types.
- *Streptococcus bovis*: a normal inhabitant of the gut. Similar to the viridans group in its sensitivity to penicillin. May be associated with malignant or inflammatory bowel disease.
- *Enterococcus faecalis* and *E. faecium*: approximately 10% cases, usually in elderly people.
- *Staphylococcus aureus*
- *Staphylococcus epidermidis* } approximately 25% cases
- Diphtheroid bacilli
- Microaerophilic streptococci } especially postcardiac surgery

- Much rarer bacteria can cause infective endocarditis, often with an insidious course and a long period of mild symptoms, e.g.
  - HACEK group of Gram-negative bacilli (*Haemophilus aphrophilus, Actinobacillus actinomycetecomitans, Cardiobacterium hominis, Eikenella corrodens, Kingella kingae*). Also called HB group of bacilli. Fastidious organisms requiring prolonged culture in 10% CO_2
  - anaerobic Gram-negative bacilli: *Fusobacterium* sp., *Bacteroides* sp., *Streptobacillus moniliformis, Propionibacterium acnes, Listeria monocytogenes, Brucella abortus, Legionella* sp. and many others
- *Coxiella burnetii* (Q-fever)
- *Chlamydia psittaci, Chlamydia trachomatis.*

Fungi
- *Candida* sp.
- *Aspergillus* sp.
- *Histoplasma* sp.

Other Organisms
? Viral infection (as yet unproven).

9.4 Diagnosis and Physical Signs

An awareness of the possibility of infective endocarditis is vital, because the condition may occur in the absence of a fever or a murmur initially, especially if the patient is elderly or has received recent antibiotic therapy. Infective endocarditis is also the great mimic, because the wide variety of physical signs may be mistaken for conditions as diverse as a collagen vascular disease, rheumatic fever, a non-specific viral infection, a primary neurological condition, mild haemolytic anaemia, left atrial myxoma or brucellosis.

Duke Criteria for Diagnosis (Durack 1994)
These clinical criteria have now replaced the Von Reyn criteria and are accepted as the most sensitive and specific. They have recently been modified to take into account increasing prevalence of staphylococcal endocarditis, the availability of polymerase chain reaction (PCR) in diagnosis and the latest serological techniques. These modified criteria are now in the European Society of Cardiology Guidelines on Endocarditis.

Diagnosis requires: pathological criteria, or two major criteria, or one major plus three minor, or five minor.

Pathological Criteria
- Positive histology or microbiology of pathological material obtained post mortem or at cardiac surgery (valve tissue vegetations, embolic fragments or abscess contents).

Major Criteria
- Positive blood cultures: two or more with the same organism consistent with endocarditis such as *Streptococcus viridans*.
- Persistent bacteraemia from two blood cultures 12 h apart, or three or more positive cultures with less specific organisms such as *S. aureus* or *S. epidermidis*.
- Evidence of endocardial involvement, i.e. visible vegetations or oscillating structures on echocardiography, or abscess formation, or new paraprosthetic valve leak/partial dehiscence.
- Positive serology for *Coxiella burnettii*, *Bartonella* sp. or *Chlamydia psittaci*.
- Positive molecular assays for specific bacterial DNA on PCR.

Minor Criteria
- Predisposition to infective endocarditis, e.g. known previous valve disease, prosthetic valve, central line within the last 6 months, previous rheumatic fever, previous infective endocarditis, intravenous drug abuser, congenital heart disease, permanent pacemaker *in situ*.
- Fever >38°C.
- Vascular phenomena, e.g. arterial emboli, mycotic aneurysm rupture, septic pulmonary infarcts, splenomegaly, clubbing, splinter haemorrhages, petechiae or purpura.
- Immunological phenomena, e.g. glomerulonephritis, Roth's spots, Osler's nodes.
- Elevated ESR or CRP.
- Further microbiological evidence, e.g. one positive blood culture.

Limitations of Duke Criteria
These criteria have not been evaluated in large numbers of cases of prosthetic valve endocarditis (PVE), and the system is more sensitive for native valve endocarditis than PVE. Patients who have received prior antibiotic therapy with negative blood cultures will be classified only as possible cases. Peripheral venous lines are not included in the minor criteria section, but they are an important cause of bacteraemia.

Presentation
Typically the condition presents with the following:
- *Signs of infection*: fever, night sweats, rigors. Weight loss and general malaise. Anaemia is expected. With chronic untreated infection there is additional clubbing and splenomegaly. Fever may be absent in patients with CCF, chronic renal or liver disease, if antibiotics have been taken previously and in elderly or immunocompromised patients.
- *Signs and symptoms of immune complex deposition*: microscopic haematuria is common and there may be frank glomerulonephritis. A generalized vasculitis can affect any vessel (e.g. brain, skin, kidneys). A toxic encephalopathy

may occur with presentation varying from confusion to stupor, to meningitis. Retinal haemorrhages are common (flame-or boat-shaped). Roth's spots (boat-shaped haemorrhages with a pale centre) on the retina occur in more fulminating or untreated cases (Figure 9.5). Splinter haemorrhages on finger- or toenails (see Figure 1.1). Arthralgia. Osler's nodes – painful pulp infarcts on fingers or toes, or on palms or soles. Janeway's lesions – less common than Osler's nodes: painless flat erythema on palms or soles.

• *Signs of the cardiac lesion*: a new murmur is very significant, as is a change in the nature of an existing murmur. Auscultation daily is necessary in patients with infective endocarditis. Mild aortic or mitral regurgitation may not be audible.

• *Emboli*: these may be followed by abscess formation in the relevant organ. They occur in about 30% cases. Common sites are: cerebral (Figure 9.6), retinal, coronary, splenic, mesenteric, renal or femoropopliteal arteries. Cere-

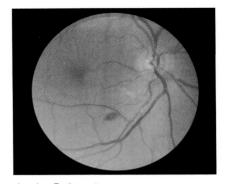

Figure 9.5 Right fundus showing Roth spot.

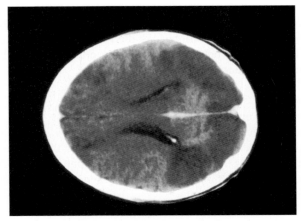

Figure 9.6 Cerebral CT scan: multiple cerebral septic emboli, particularly affecting occipital lobes.

bral abscess may present with seizures, stupor or focal signs. In patients with right-sided endocarditis, pulmonary infarcts are often followed by lung abscesses. A mycotic aneurysm may follow a cerebral embolus and present with subarachnoid and/or intracerebral haemorrhage (Figure 9.7). Possibly Osler's nodes have an embolic element also. Large friable and obstructive emboli are common in fungal endocarditis (Figure 9.8). Embolic events may occur during or after antibiotic treatment, even in an apparently 'cured' case. Secondary abscess formation prevents bacteriological cure.

• *Complications of valve destruction or abscess formation*: this may result in increasingly severe valve regurgitation. Abscess formation can result in the dehiscence of the prosthetic valve-sewing ring (see Figure 3.34). A septal abscess (e.g. aortic valve endocarditis) produces a long PR interval, leading

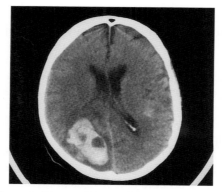

Figure 9.7 Cerebral CT scan in 59-year-old man with aortic valve endocarditis presenting with a sudden collapse secondary to a ruptured mycotic aneurysm in the right occipital cortex.

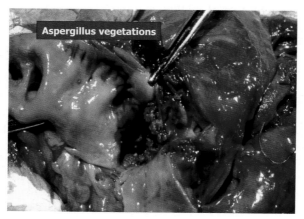

Figure 9.8 Postmortem specimen of a case of aspergillus endocarditis on the aortic valve, with fleshy vegetations obstructing the LV outflow tract.

to complete AV block. Aortic root abscesses may produce a sinus of Valsalva aneurysm, or involve the coronary ostia. Large fleshy vegetations may cause valve obstruction (see Figure 3.35).

- *Left ventricular failure*: this is one of the most common causes of death in infective endocarditis. Primary involvement of the myocardium occurs with reduction in contractility and non-specific ST–T-wave changes on the ECG. There may be an associated pericardial effusion or even pyopericardium. LVF is exacerbated by additional valve dysfunction.
- *Intravenous drug abuser*: tricuspid valve involvement may result in occult pulmonary emboli, and subsequently lung abscesses. Immune complex phenomena may still occur (e.g. glomerulonephritis).
- *Cyanotic congenital heart disease*: as well as the above cerebral abscess is a well-recognized complication (right-to-left shunting).

Investigations
- Three blood cultures from different venous sites 1 h apart. Bacteraemia is constant so it is no longer necessary to wait for peak fever; 85–90% of cases will be cultured in this way.

There is little point in performing arterial or marrow cultures if venous blood cultures are negative. Approximately 10% of cases are culture negative. Blood should also be cultured through a CVP line if there is one in situ, but multi-organism contamination may be a problem here. The CVP line is then removed and the tip cultured.

- Routine FBC and ESR: normally the condition is associated with an anaemia, neutrophil leukocytosis and high ESR. None of these is absolute. A rising haemoglobin and falling ESR are useful signs of therapeutic success. Routine biochemistry, LFTs, creatinine.
- CRP: an acute-phase protein released by the liver in response to cytokines from activated macrophages. Rises acutely with bacterial infection (much less with viral). A falling CRP is a good sign of infection coming under control (Figure 9.9).
- Microscopy of fresh urine for red cells: microscopic haematuria is common early in the disease and should regress during treatment. Midstream urine analysis if indicated.
- Swabs of any skin lesion, drip site; nasal swab.
- Dental radiographs: orthopantomogram + special views as indicated (Figure 9.1).
- ECG and chest radiograph at regular intervals (at least weekly). Beware long PR interval (see below).
- Bacterial or fungal DNA analysis using the PCR on blood, valve or tissue samples. Should be considered where blood cultures are negative (e.g. previous antibiotics). May reveal infection by a fastidious organism.
- Weekly transthoracic echocardiography (TTE): vegetations are not visualized until >2 mm in size. Colour Doppler with TTE is best for the identification of aortic regurgitation, a septal abscess or an acquired VSD.

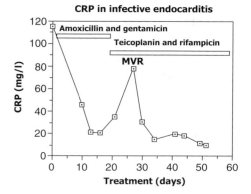

CRP in infective endocarditis

Figure 9.9 Serial measurements of CRP in infective endocarditis on the mitral valve. After initial successful treatment amoxicillin resistance develops with rapid rise in CRP. Switching antibiotics and replacing the mitral valve (MVR) results in a cure.

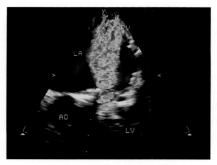

Figure 9.10 Mitral prosthetic valve endocarditis. Transoesophageal echocardiography shows a severe paraprosthetic jet of mitral regurgitation reaching the back of a dilated left atrium.

- Transoesophageal echocardiography (TOE) should be performed (see Section 17.5):
  - if TTE is negative but there is a high suspicion of infective endocarditis
  - for all cases of prosthetic valve endocarditis (possible or definite endocarditis) see Figure 9.10
  - for lengthening PR interval on ECG – suspicion of aortic root abscess which may develop into a mycotic aneurysm
  - for persisting fever or deteriorating medical condition in spite of antibiotic treatment.

TOE is very useful for visualizing mitral valve vegetations, or leaflet perforation. A subaortic LVOTO aneurysm will be picked up only by TOE, and with colour Doppler TOE will identify an LVOTO-to-RA fistula.

An example of vegetations on a native mitral and tricuspid valve is seen in Figures 9.11 and 17.44.

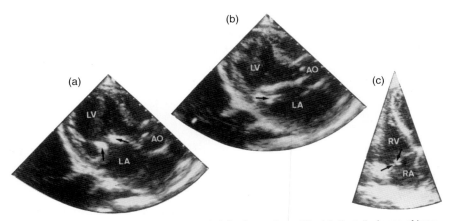

Figure 9.11 Transthoracic echocardiogram in infective endocarditis: (a) diastolic frame of long axis view showing large vegetations on the mitral leaflets (arrowed). (b) Systolic frame of same patient showing prolapse of the posterior mitral leaflet (arrowed). There was severe mitral regurgitation. (c) Apical four-chamber view of right heart showing small vegetations on tricuspid valve (arrowed).

• Other investigations that may occasionally help are assays of immune complex titres and anti-staphylococcal antibodies.

Culture-negative Endocarditis

About 10% of infective endocarditis may be culture negative. Five reasons in order of probability are:

1 *Previous antibiotic therapy*: the longer the course of antibiotics before blood cultures the more likely the chance of cultures being negative. If the condition remains untreated, re-seeding of the blood may occur after several weeks from organisms still alive in the centre of the vegetations. Even a single dose of an antibiotic may result initially in negative cultures.

2 *Wrong diagnosis*: in culture-negative patients it is important to think of alternative diagnoses and re-examine the patient. Many conditions mimic infective endocarditis: particularly collagen vascular disease, polymyalgia rheumatica, malignant disease, atrial myxoma, sarcoid, drug reaction, etc. There may be a non-cardiac infection in a patient who has a heart murmur, or there may be non-infective endocarditis (see Section 9.8).

3 *Fastidious organisms* that require special culture media and conditions, e.g. organisms from the HACEK group (CO_2 incubation), nutritionally-dependent streptococci (*S. defectivus* and *S. adjacens* needing cysteine- or pyridoxine-enriched medium), *Brucella*, *Legionella* or *Neisseria* spp., L-forms or anaerobes.

4 *Cell-dependent organisms*, e.g. *Coxiella burnetii* (Q-fever), *Chlamydia psittaci* or *C. trachomatis*: check Q-fever and chlamydial complement-fixing antibodies.

5 *Fungi*: consider especially in chronically sick patients who are immunosuppressed or who have been on prolonged intravenous feeding, and those with prosthetic heart valves. Check aspergillus precipitins and candida antibodies. Most cases of endocarditis will have a raised titre to candida antibodies (anamnestic response). A rising titre is more important.

9.5 Treatment Management

There is nothing to be gained by waiting to see if cultures are positive. If the condition is suspected and investigations have been performed, treatment should start immediately.

If dental extractions are required, these are ideally performed at the start of the course of antibiotics. This is not always practical and additional antibiotic cover is usually required in the middle of an established course. Culturing teeth is rarely useful as a large spectrum of oral flora results.

If a systemic embolus occurs, it should be cultured and examined for hyphae.

Route

Intravenous therapy is essential initially. The choice rests between central and peripheral lines. Both have their advantages and must be inserted with strict aseptic techniques.

The central line (subclavian or internal jugular) should be changed weekly. The best central line is a tunnelled subclavian inserted via the infraclavicular route (e.g. using a Nutricath or Picc line). The tunnel helps prevent spread of infection from the skin entry site. A tunnelled subclavian line does not require changing weekly if the entry site looks clean and should last the whole antibiotic course with careful management (Figure 9.12). The catheter should be soft, pliable and not reach as far as the right atrium. The catheter in the right atrium or SVC may cause infected mural thrombus. A stiff central line in the right atrium may perforate the wall. The central line skin entry site should be covered by Steri-Drape (e.g. Opsite). Covering with other dressings is not advised and povidone–iodine on the entry site does not prevent infection.

Peripheral lines are less dangerous but more inconvenient and painful. The peripheral line should be changed every 72 h if possible even if the vein has not thrombosed. This helps preserve the life of peripheral veins. The arm is immobilized, dilute antibiotic solution is used and a heparin flush (500 U in 5 ml 5% dextrose) given after each infusion helps preserve the vein.

The giving set should be changed daily with either system. For a patient on warfarin (e.g. mechanical prosthetic valves) a central line should not be inserted until the INR <2.0. Start with a peripheral line and intravenous heparin. Stop the warfarin temporarily. When the INR falls to <2.0, insert a central line and restart warfarin, stopping the heparin when the INR >2.5.

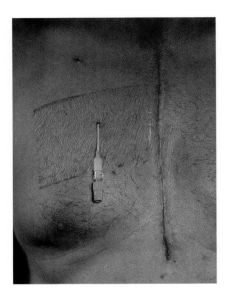

Figure 9.12 Tunnelled subclavian central line (Nutricath) after 6 weeks iv antibiotic therapy in a man with prosthetic valve endocarditis.

Length of Course

There are no fixed rules. This depends on the patient's response to treatment, the sensitivity and nature of the organism, vegetation size on the echocardiogram, patient tolerance and drug access. There is a definite trend to shorter courses in sensitive 'friendly' organisms. The following are suggestions only.

• *Streptococcus viridans* group: if sensitive (MIC <0.1 mg/l) 2 weeks of intravenous therapy followed by 2 weeks of oral amoxicillin. If insensitive, 4 weeks of intravenous therapy.
• *Staphylococcus epidermidis*: 4–8 weeks intravenously.
• *Staphylococcus aureus*: 4–8 weeks intravenously.
• *Q-fever*: indefinite oral therapy.
• *Fungal endocarditis*: 3 months of intravenous treatment followed by oral therapy.
• *Prosthetic valve endocarditis*: a minimum of 2 months' intravenous therapy should cure some cases. Most will need redo valve surgery, followed by a further month's intravenous treatment.

Choice of Antibiotic Regimen

Once the diagnosis is considered probable, treatment should be started before the blood culture results are known. Start with intravenous benzylpenicillin and gentamicin as detailed in the section on penicillin-sensitive streptococci. If staphylococcal infection is likely (e.g. intravenous drug abusers or patients on haemodialysis) use vancomycin instead of penicillin. Always use at least two antibiotics for staphylococcal infection.

Plasma antibiotic levels are measured at trough (pre-dose) and peak (15-min post-intravenous dose). If the peak level is too high, the dose is reduced; if the trough level is too high, the interval between doses is increased.

Antibiotic/Organism Sensitivity Testing

With a positive blood culture, guidance from a bacteriologist is essential, the choice depending on the organism's antibiotic sensitivity. Antibiotic levels are necessary to check both the dose and the risk of toxicity (especially with the aminoglycosides and antifungal agents).

Minimum inhibitory concentration (MIC) is estimated and provides a guide to dosage and drug choice. Therapy should aim to reach trough levels of at least 10 × MIC. In *Streptococcus viridans* infection if MIC >0.1 mg/l, the addition of an aminoglycoside to penicillin should be considered. Disc sensitivity is probably as valuable as MIC testing and much easier to assess.

Minimal bactericidal concentration (MBC) is more difficult to measure and less frequently used now. It may be useful when drug therapy is failing. It is the highest dilution of a patient's serum that kills a standard innoculum of the patient's organism in vitro. A peak bactericidal titre of 1:64 and trough of 1:32 is the therapeutic range required.

Do not stop treatment if the temperature fails to settle within a few days. This may take 2 weeks even with drug-sensitive organisms, but is more likely with large vegetations or abscess formation.

If fever persists:
- Check sensitivity of organism and drug levels
- Echocardiography to check possible change in size of vegetations, aortic root or septal abscess
- Consider other possible sources of fever
- Consider adding another synergistic antibiotic
- Surgery should be considered early for cases with persisting fever resistant to medical therapy.

A bactericidal antibiotic is used except in rare circumstances: tetracycline therapy in Q-fever endocarditis and high-dose erythromycin if there is penicillin and cephalosporin allergy. Probenecid is sometimes used to maintain high plasma amoxicillin levels when a patient is converted to oral therapy from intravenous penicillin.

The clinical response is a most useful guide to therapy. The regimens set out below are the doses suggested in a 70-kg adult with normal renal function. Doses must be reduced in smaller patients, elderly patients and those with renal failure.

All the antibiotic regimens listed below are by intravenous bolus injection unless otherwise specified, and are the shortest possible courses for the organisms discussed. Some patients may require longer courses depending on response to treatment. Gentamicin levels must be taken twice weekly with an

80 mg 12-hourly regimen, and more often with an 8-hourly regimen or if the serum creatinine is raised.

Antibiotics for Patients not Allergic to Penicillin

Streptococcus viridans Group and *S. bovis* (Approximately 40% of cases)
1 Fully sensitive to penicillin (MIC <0.1 mg/l), with favourable conditions (see below):

Benzylpenicillin 1.2 g (2 MU) i.v. 4-hourly plus gentamicin 80 mg i.v. 12-hourly for 2 weeks. Followed by 2 weeks of oral amoxicillin.

If this 2-week i.v. regimen is to be considered there must be:
– no heart failure or conduction abnormalities
– no embolic phenomena
– native valve infection, not prosthetic
– small vegetations only
– response within 7 days of treatment with the temperature returning to normal.

2 Reduced sensitivity to penicillin (MIC >0.1 mg/l) or less favourable conditions. Regimen as in (1) above but continued for 4 weeks of intravenous therapy.

Enterococci (Approximately 10% of cases)
Usually more resistant to penicillin than the viridans group (median MIC 2 mg/l). About 25% are gentamicin resistant:
1 Gentamicin sensitive (MIC <100 mg/l): ampicillin or amoxicillin 2 g i.v. 4-hourly plus gentamicin 80 mg i.v. 12-hourly for 4 weeks.
2 Gentamicin highly resistant (MIC > 2000 mg/l): ampicillin or amoxicillin 2 g i.v. 4-hourly for at least 6 weeks. Streptomycin may be added if the strain is sensitive to it. (Dose: 75 mg/kg i.m. 12-hourly. Dose not to exceed 500 mg.)

Patients infected with enterococci resistant to both gentamicin and streptomycin have a high mortality and are best managed with early surgery and high-dose amoxicillin for 8–12 weeks.

Staphylococci
1 Penicillin sensitive (non-β-lactamase producers): benzylpenicillin 1.2 g (2 MU) i.v. for 4 weeks. Plus fusidic acid 500 mg orally 8-hourly for 4 weeks. Or plus gentamicin 80–120 mg 8-hourly for 1 week.
2 Methicillin sensitive (β-lactamase producers): flucloxacillin 2 g i.v. 4-hourly for 4 weeks. Plus fusidic acid 500 mg orally 8-hourly for 4 weeks, or plus gentamicin 80–120 mg 8-hourly for 1 week.
3 Methicillin resistant (β-lactamase producers and methicillin resistant): vancomycin initially 1 g by slow intravenous infusion over 100 min once or twice daily for 4 weeks. Blood levels determine dose. Aim for trough levels 5–10 mg/l and peak levels taken 1 h post-dose up to 30 mg/l. Plus fusidic acid

500 mg-hourly orally for 4 weeks, or plus gentamicin 80–120 mg 8-hourly for 1 week.

Antibiotics for Other Organisms

Gram-negative Organisms

Ampicillin 2–4 g i.v. 6-hourly. Gentamicin 80 mg i.v. 8-hourly initially. Metronidazole 500 mg i.v. 8-hourly is added for uncontrolled anaerobic organisms (e.g. fusobacterium or bacteroides endocarditis).

HACEK Organisms

Infection caused by one of these organisms can be treated with 4–6 week course of ceftriaxone (1 g i.v. once daily) or cefotaxime (1 g i.v. 8-hourly). Patients who are allergic to penicillin: consider using trimethoprim or aztreonam.

Q-fever (Coxiella burnetii)

There are no rickettsiacidal drugs. Treatment should be regarded as indefinite if the drug regimen is tolerated, because *Coxiella* may survive for years in the liver. Early surgery is advisable. Start drug treatment with doxycycline 100 mg twice daily orally plus either co-trimoxazole, rifampicin or a quinolone (e.g. ciprofloxacin). Monitoring successful therapy is difficult. Complement levels are unhelpful: the serum IgM levels may stay up with successful treatment, but the phase 1 antibody titre should gradually fall.

Candida albicans or Other Yeast Organisms

Large fleshy vegetations occur and tend to embolize, causing metastatic infection. Myocardial invasion occurs. Again early surgery is advised. Start treatment with 5-fluorocytosine (flucytosine) 3 g i.v. 6-hourly (50 mg/kg 6-hourly). Marrow depression and hepatic necrosis are the most dangerous side effects. If flucytosine resistance develops add amphotericin B 250 μg/kg per day initially, increasing if renal function is satisfactory. Miconazole 600 mg i.v. 8-hourly is an alternative if renal function is poor. Oral fluconazole 50 mg daily is substituted after a successful course of intravenous treatment and surgery and continued for some months as late relapse may occur.

Aspergillus spp. or Other Non-yeast Fungi (Figure 9.8)

This is rarely diagnosed in time and medical treatment alone is never successful. Early surgery is the only hope. Amphotericin B 250 μg/kg per day or miconazole 600 mg i.v. 8-hourly if poor renal function. Oral itraconazole 100 mg once daily for a month may be used after an intravenous course of amphotericin. It may in time prove more effective than amphotericin B. Where possible, fungal endocarditis should be treated with two drugs.

Antibiotics for Patients Allergic to Penicillin

Streptococcus viridans group, *S. bovis* and enterococci
The choice is from two:
1 Teicoplanin 400 mg i.v. 12-hourly for three injections, followed by 400 mg i.v. daily for 4 weeks, plus gentamicin 80 mg i.v. twice daily for 2 weeks (*S. viridans* group and *S. bovis*) or 4 weeks (enterococci).
2 Vancomycin 1 g by intravenous infusion over 100 min once or twice daily for 4 weeks. Adjust dose to achieve trough levels of 5–10 mg/l and peak levels 1 h post-infusion of about 30 mg/l, plus gentamicin regimen as detailed for teicoplanin. Strains of enterococci resistant to vancomycin have been reported.

Staphylococci
Vancomycin 1 g by intravenous infusion over 100 min once or twice daily for 4 weeks. Blood levels as detailed above for streptococci. Plus fusidic acid 500 mg 8-hourly orally for 4 weeks and/or gentamicin 80–120 mg 8-hourly for 1 week.

Recurrent Fever During Treatment

Fever recurrence after an initial successful period of medical therapy can pose a diagnostic problem. The following are four common reasons:
1 *Development of the patient's sensitivity to an antibiotic*: most commonly with penicillin, but may occur with any antibiotic. Check for proteinuria and eosinophilia. Neutropenia is common. An interstitial nephritis may develop. The fever, nephritis and eosinophilia usually disappear rapidly if the antibiotic is stopped.
2 *Development of antibiotic resistance*: rapid rise in CRP with recurrent fever. Possible if the MIC is high and inadequate doses of the antibiotic are used initially. Change of antibiotic regimen needed (Figure 9.9).
3 *Additional or uncontrolled infection*: remove central line if present and culture tip. Check chest, urine, etc. Consider occult pulmonary emboli (especially with tricuspid endocarditis), enlarging vegetations (on echocardio-graphy) or hidden abscess formation (e.g. around aortic root, septum or haematogenous spread to abdomen). Check abdominal ultrasound. (e.g. ? hepatic or renal abscess).
4 *Diagnosis still wrong*: consider other possibilities, e.g. malignant disease or collagen vascular disease.

Antimicrobial Side Effects and Other Problems

Penicillin

These are: allergy (fever, urticaria, arthralgia, rash); angioneurotic oedema; interstitial nephritis; sodium loading; encephalopathy; hypokalaemic alkalosis; neutropenia.

The last four are dose-dependent side effects, usually quickly reversible on stopping the drug. They are rare, and are possible if >24 g/day penicillin is used. With a history of penicillin allergy there is roughly a 10% chance of cross-sensitivity to cephalosporins.

Fusidic Acid

These are nausea and vomiting, jaundice and hepatotoxicity, microbial resistance.

Nausea and vomiting are very common, even with intravenous therapy, and may make it impossible to use the drug. Liver damage is reversible if the drug is stopped early. Microbial resistance develops quickly if the drug is used alone. The drug is well absorbed orally.

Aminoglycosides

These are ototoxicity and nephrotoxicity.

About 10% of patients on these drugs develop VIII nerve damage. If long-term treatment is required, weekly audiometry is essential with calorics to detect early damage. Either the vestibular or auditory component may be damaged first or in isolation. High-frequency deafness may occur early without the patient noticing any side effects. Beware the patient using the drip pole as a support, concealing ataxia. The suggested dose schedule is shown below. Doses are reduced in renal impairment.

Nephrotoxicity is exacerbated by concomitant use of furosemide, ethacrynic acid, and possibly some cephalosporins. Frequent tests of renal function are necessary (serum creatinine three times a week). The urine is tested daily for protein, and urine microscopy performed to look for casts at regular intervals.

Antibiotics for other organisms

Guide to Gentamicin Dosage

There is a move to use lower doses of gentamicin. This helps avoid ototoxicity and expensive litigation. The drug is synergistic with penicillin and still very valuable at low serum levels.

- Adults with normal renal function: 80 mg i.v. 12-hourly initially. Adults <60 kg in weight use 60 mg i.v. 12-hourly.
- Children with normal renal function: 3 mg/kg i.v. initially followed by 2 mg/kg i.v. 12-hourly.
- With renal impairment dose is reduced. Until drug levels are known dose is regulated corresponding to blood urea levels:
    - 7–17 mmol/l: 80 mg 12-hourly
    - 18–33 mmol/l: 80 mg daily
    - >33 mmol/l: 80 mg alternate days or less.
- Drug levels: blood for these is taken from the opposite arm if a peripheral line is used. They are performed initially on the third day of treatment.

Trough level: taken just before gentamicin dose. The trough level is the most important measurement of all and must always be < 2 μg/ml.

Levels of 2–5 µg/ml mean drug accumulation and the dose interval should be increased.

Peak level: taken 15 min after intravenous dose. The level should be <10 µg/ml. Preferably 6–10 µg/ml. The dose is reduced if the level exceeds this.

It is safest to restrict gentamicin therapy to just the first 2 weeks of treatment if possible.

Other Drugs of Great Value in Bacterial Cases (Table 9.2)

• Amikacin: in gentamicin-resistant cases. Dose 15 mg/kg per day in two doses 12-hourly.

• Tobramycin: in mild renal impairment, because it is less nephrotoxic than gentamicin. Up to 5 mg/kg per day 8–12-hourly (similar to gentamicin).

• Vancomycin: caution in any degree of uraemia. May be used as a single antibiotic. Maximum adult dose 2 g/day. Start with 500 mg i.v. 6-hourly. May be reduced to as little as 1 g/week in uraemia associated with endocarditis. Infusion may cause histamine release and the 'red man' syndrome. A recent report has shown the production of vancomycin-dependent anti-platelet antibodies, causing thrombocytopenia and bleeding in some patients, which is reversible on stopping the drug.

• Rifampicin: not just an antituberculous drug, but toxicity in 20% of cases. Shock, renal failure, thrombocytopenia, hepatotoxicity, influenza and respiratory symptoms. Oral therapy 450–600 mg daily before breakfast. Never use as a single agent as resistant strains emerge rapidly.

• Netilmicin: this drug is less ototoxic than gentamicin or tobramycin and may supersede both. Dose for average size adult with normal renal function: 150 mg i.v. 12-hourly (total 4–6 mg/kg per day).

• Teicoplanin: can be given as a once-daily dose either intramuscularly or preferably intravenously as 400 mg. It is much less ototoxic and nephrotoxic than aminoglycosides. Useful in streptococci, staphylococci and enterococci. It is particularly useful for *Staphylococcus epidermidis* and in combination with rifampicin for penicillin-resistant or hypersensitive cases. May also cause histamine release (similar to vancomycin). Toxic epidermal necrolysis is a rare complication.

Second-line Drugs

• Lincomycin and clindamycin: very effective in staphylococcal (and some anaerobic) infections. Pseudomembranous colitis limits their use. If it develops, vancomycin is effective given orally.

• Cephalosporin group: may be useful in penicillin hypersensitivity. Nephrotoxicity was a problem with first-generation cephalopsorins but more recent agents such as cefotaxime and ceftriaxone are safe in renal failure and dose reduction is needed only when GFR falls <10 ml/min. Care with additional use with aminoglycosides and diuretics.

Table 9.2 Antibiotic properties

Antibiotic	Renal excretion	Site of damage	? Use in renal disease
Benzylpenicillin (penicillin G)	90% proximal tubular secretion	Rare hypokalaemic alkalosis Hypersensitivity Interstitial nephritis	Yes, with dose reduction 1–2 g 6-hourly
Gentamicin	All glomerular filtration	Tubular necrosis 2–10% Binds to renal tissue	Yes, with great care taking drug levels Cephalosporins probably best avoided
Tobramycin	All glomerular filtration	Tubular necrosis in 1–2% Less than gentamicin	Safer than gentamicin in renal damage
Vancomycin	80% renal excretion	None	Yes, with dose reduction levels, from 1 g/day to 1 g/week
Amikacin	95% renal excretion	Probably similar to gentamicin	As with gentamicin levels
Cephalothin	70–80% renal excretion	Tubular necrosis	Aminoglycosides probably best avoided Care in renal disease
Ceftriaxone	60% renal, 40% hepatic and GI tract	GI tract. Rarely pseudomembranous colitis	Yes. Dose reduced if GFR <10ml/min
Tetracyclines	Principally renal excretion	'Anti-anabolic effect' increases uraemia Old tetracyclines: Fanconi's anaemia	Avoid (except doxycycline)
Fusidic acid	Principally biliary excretion	None in kidney	Yes, no dose adjustment necessary
Amphotericin B	Slow renal excretion	Reduces renal blood flow (arteriolar constriction) Nephrocalcinosis, tubular damage: renal tubular acidosis, potassium wasting	Reduce dose (e.g. 0.25 mg/kg on alternate days)

Table 9.3 Prognosis in infective endocarditis

Good prognosis	Worse prognosis
Young patient	Elderly patient
Native valve endocarditis	Prosthetic valve endocarditis
Normal LV function	Poor LV function
Streptococcus viridans infection	Staphylococcal, enterococcal or fungal infection
Dental organism	Nosocomial organism
Mild valve damage	Severe valve damage
Small vegetations	Large vegetations (>5 mm)
Uncomplicated endocarditis	Complicated endocarditis
Normal renal function	Abnormal renal function
Normal weight, well nourished	Underweight, poorly nourished
	Serum albumin <30 g/l

- Erythromycin: bacteriostatic in low doses. May be useful in penicillin hypersensitivity. Clarithromycin is an alternative. Dose is 500 mg i.v. twice daily. Less toxic to veins than erythromycin.
- Chloramphenicol: best avoided in long courses unless desperate. Causes leukopenia, thrombocytopenia, irreversible aplastic anaemia, peripheral and optic neuritis, gut side effects, erythema multiforme.

Monitoring Therapy Effects
- Daily patient examination: the most important of all to detect new signs.
- Daily weighing.
- Six-hourly temperature chart.
- Daily urine testing: microscopy for RBCs and casts.
- FBC, U&Es and LFTs twice weekly as minimum. A steady or rising haemoglobin and falling CRP and ESR are good signs. The ESR is often the last variable to return to normal after a long antibiotic course in infective endocarditis. It may return to normal only a month or so after the course has finished. The CRP falls more quickly (see Figure 9.9).
- Antibiotic drug levels.
- Weekly echocardiogram: although vegetations are frequently not seen on the echocardiogram, a gradual change in valve configuration may be detected.

Management of the Infected Tricuspid Valve in Intravenous Drug Users
The tricuspid valve is the most frequently affected in intravenous drug users. The pulmonary valve is rarely involved, but the mitral and aortic valves may

be affected in addition in severe cases. Although the lungs act as a barrier to systemic emboli with isolated tricuspid valve involvement, systemic immunological phenomena (e.g. glomerulonephritis) can still occur.

Pulmonary Complications
The lungs bear the brunt of damage from infected embolic material. Pulmonary infarcts may present as chest pain, dyspnoea, cough and haemoptysis. The chest radiograph may show pulmonary infiltrates, pleural effusions, pneumothorax, lung abscesses or an empyema.

Cardiac Complications
Destruction of the tricuspid valve leads to increasing tricuspid regurgitation, dilatation of both the right ventricle and atrium and right heart failure with resultant pulsatile hepatomegaly, peripheral oedema and ascites. AF from the dilated right atrium exacerbates the problem. Involvement of the mitral and aortic valve leads to additional left heart problems and the risk of systemic emboli. Pericardial effusion and pyopericardium may occur and require drainage.

Culprit Organisms
Staphylococcus aureus is the culprit organism in about 70% of these cases with Pseudomonas aeruginosa, streptococci, Gram-negative organisms, diphtheroids and fungi accounting for the rest. In one recent series 58% cases were also HIV positive. Advanced HIV infection is a risk factor for endocarditis (see Section 11.2).

Management
Intravenous antibiotic therapy is on the usual lines, but *Staphylococcus aureus* must be the assumed organism until the result of blood cultures is available. Start with flucloxacillin and gentamicin (see above). Compliance with a hospital regimen is difficult in these cases. Self-discharge or additional self-medication through the intravenous line is not unusual. Ideally aim for at least 4 weeks of intravenous therapy (2 weeks of gentamicin only) followed by a switch to oral therapy such as rifampicin and ciprofloxacin under supervision as an outpatient. Severe valve destruction, recurrent pulmonary complications, and additional aortic or mitral valve endocarditis are likely to need surgery.

Surgery in these cases aims to remove as much infected material as possible from the tricuspid valve (vegetectomy) while preserving its structure if possible. It may be necessary to remove a valve leaflet, or repair a leaflet with a pericardial patch. Tricuspid valve replacement with a xenograft is sometimes necessary, but reinfection may be a problem. Removal of the tricuspid valve without replacing it is no longer considered useful. Pacing will be needed in 25% of patients who need a valve replacement.

Prevention of Recurrence
This is a major problem. Counselling will involve education regarding services available to intravenous drug users in the community, clean injection strategies and needle exchange information.

Prognosis in tricuspid valve endocarditis
Mortality is much lower than for left-sided endocarditis, even when S. aureus is the infecting organism (about 5% mortality rate with medical management alone, and 15–25% in patients needing surgery). The following are bad prognostic features:
- Additional left-sided endocarditis
- Presence of a prosthetic valve
- Methicillin-resistant S. aureus (MRSA)
- Metastatic infection: lung abscesses or empyema
- HIV-positive cases with a CD4 count $<200/mm^3$
- Large vegetations >10 mm
- Failure of medical treatment alone
- Fungal endocarditis.

9.6 Other Interventions and Infective Endocarditis

Anticoagulants and Endocarditis
This is controversial with the risk of haemorrhage at the site of embolus impaction (e.g. mycotic embolus and subarachnoid or intracerebral haemorrhage). Anticoagulation does not prevent the development of vegetations.

It is best reserved for: patients with prosthetic (non-tissue) valves, pelvic vein thrombosis or gross deep vein thrombosis or pulmonary embolism. Patients with mixed mitral valve disease and endocarditis already on anticoagulants should be continued on anticoagulants with a control INR of 2:1 approximately.

Cardiac Catheterization
This is usually not necessary and was once thought to be absolutely contraindicated, with the risk of dislodging friable vegetations. However, it may be useful in patients with aortic valve endocarditis with suspected abscess formation, to obtain more information about the anatomy of the root by an aortogram with the catheter well above the valve. Also the significance of mitral regurgitation in the course of infective endocarditis may rarely require cardiac catheterization with LV angiography. Intravenous digital subtraction angiography (Figure 9.13), CT or MR angiography of the aortic root can provide information about possible aortic root abscesses. TOE is invaluable and obviates the need for cardiac catheterization (see Section 17.5) in most cases.

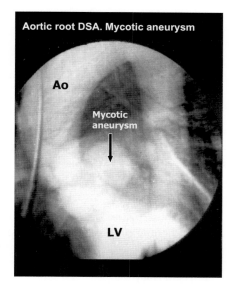

Aortic root DSA. Mycotic aneurysm

Ao

Mycotic
aneurysm

LV

Figure 9.13 Intravenous digital subtraction aortogram in a patient with aortic valve endocarditis showing a posterior aortic root mycotic aneurysm.

Pacemaker Endocarditis

This is a rare complication of permanent pacing and in about 50% cases is caused by erosion of the pacemaker box through the skin. *S. epidermidis* is a common causative organism. TOE is useful diagnostically to identify vegetations on the pacing wire, but the condition is easily missed. Pulmonary infiltrates may occur.

The condition is rarely cured by antibiotics alone and the infection usually recurs in a few months after an initial antibiotic course. Removal of the entire pacing system (box and wire) is necessary. This may involve a thoractomy to ensure complete pacing system removal. Temporary pacing may be needed, or preferably a new pacing system on the other side. Epicardial wires are an alternative but not usually a long-term solution. In the frail patient, or one in whom there is no alternative pacing solution, indefinite oral antibiotics will be required to keep any residual infection at bay.

Indications for Surgical Intervention (Table 9.4)

Approximately 50% of cases referred to a cardiothoracic unit will need surgery. A surgeon can remove at operation a mass of infected material that would never be cured with antibiotics alone:
• Failure of antibiotics to control infection: persisting fever after 1 week's appropriate antibiotic therapy with evidence of valve dysfunction, and no other cause for fever
• Increasing valve regurgitation or destruction
• Large fleshy or mobile vegetations (>10 mm), or increasing vegetation size on echocardiography

---

Table 9.4 Surgery in endocarditis

Needed in 50% cases in tertiary centres
Operate early
Use a homograft or stentless xenograft if possible for aortic valve endocarditis
Redo surgery may be needed for paraprosthetic valve regurgitation several months after the
  initial operation (after the patient has been bacteriologically cured)
Permanent pacing commonly needed for aortic valve cases
Full course of intravenous antibiotics needed after surgery (e.g. 4 weeks)
Get a dental opinion while the patient is still in hospital on treatment
Follow up any patient with a sternal wound infection very carefully (especially those with
  diabetes)

- Valve obstruction resulting from vegetations
- Lengthening of the PR interval: septal abscess formation
- Paravalve abscess on echocardiography
- Development of an aneurysm of the sinus of Valsalva, or paravalve mycotic aneurysm (Figure 9.13)
- Endocarditis caused by *S. aureus*, Q-fever and most fungal cases
- Systemic emboli: in case of cerebral embolism exclude intracranial haemorrhage using CT. If no evidence of an intracranial bleed, operate early (within 3 days) or wait 3–4 weeks
- Almost all cases of prosthetic valve endocarditis
- Relapse of infection after a full course of medical treatment.

If possible, a few days' antibiotics are given before surgery, but in very severe cases this may be only a few doses. When in doubt, operate early before renal and cardiac failure develop.

After valve replacement for infective endocarditis a full course of medical therapy should be given, of a length detailed earlier.

9.7 Prevention of Infective Endocarditis

Much of the evidence on which recommendations are made is based on animal work. The American Heart Association's recommendations of 1977 have been modified to allow a simpler regimen, which is more likely to be followed. This prophylaxis is necessary for:
- any dental work
- any surgical procedure
- cystoscopy and urinary tract instrumentation
- prostatic biopsy (transrectal)
- insertion of permanent pacemakers.

Prophylaxis is not necessary before cardiac catheterization. There is no hard evidence that it is necessary before gastroscopy or sigmoidoscopy, but it is advisable if performing biopsies. Normally used before rectal or colonic biopsy and also before delivery.

It is safer to advise patients to have antibiotic prophylaxis before every dental appointment. If several visits to the dentist are required, the same antibiotic regimen should not be used within a month. Patients should be urged to visit the dentist regularly. The use of chlorhexidinegel (1%) applied to the gingival margin or chlorhexidine mouthwash (0.2%) 5 min before the dental work should reduce the severity of the bacteraemia. Intraligamental injections of local anaesthetics should be avoided.

Controversy

The regimen shown in Table 9.5 is based on the recommendations of the endocarditis working party of the British Society for Antimicrobial Chemotherapy (BSAC). Recently this group have downgraded their recommendations to giving antibiotic cover only to those patients who have had previous endocarditis or have prosthetic heart valves, surgical conduits or complex congenital heart disease. Patients previously deemed to be at moderate risk (e.g. acquired valve disease) were not thought to merit antibiotic prophylaxis These recommendations were based on the lack of evidence for successful prophylaxis and the dangers of antibiotic allergy.

Table 9.5 Antibiotic cover for patients with congenital heart disease or acquired valve disease receiving dental treatment or any operative procedure

---

1. Without anaesthetic or under local anaesthesia

Amoxicillin 3 g orally 1 h before procedure. For patients allergic to penicillin or who have had amoxicillin in the last month: either clindamycin 600 mg as a single dose 1 h before procedure or erythromycin stearate 1.5 g orally before procedure + 0.5 g 6 h later. The 1.5 g dose may cause nausea and the single dose of clindamycin is better tolerated.

For children: age 5–10 years half adult dose for all three drugs above; age <5 years: quarter of the adult dose.

2. Under general anaesthetic

Ampicillin 1 g i.v. with premedication (or amoxicillin 1 g in 2.5 ml 1% lidocaine i.m.) + 0.5 g orally 6 h later. For patients allergic to penicillin or who have had amoxicillin or ampicillin in the last month: either vancomycin 1 g i.v. slowly over 100 min + gentamicin 120 mg i.v. just before induction, or teicoplanin 400 mg i.v. + gentamicin 120 mg i.v. just before induction. This is the easiest regimen. Or clindamycin 300 mg in 50 ml 0.9% saline i.v. over 10 min just before induction followed by clindamycin 150 mg orally or by intravenous injection over 10 min 6 h later. This is not suitable for patients undergoing pelvic instrumentation, or genitourinary or gastrointestinal procedures.

For children: either vancomycin 20 mg/kg + gentamicin 2 mg/kg i.v. or clindamycin 150 mg i.v. (age 5–10 years) or 75 mg i.v. (age under 5 years) diluted as above.

3. Special risk patients under general anaesthetic

Patients with prosthetic heart valves or history of previous infective endocarditis: ampicillin 1 g + gentamicin 120 mg i.v. with premeditation + amoxicillin 0.5 g orally at 6 h. For penicillin allergy use regimen under (2) above.

These guidelines differ from those published by the British Cardiac Society, The European Society of Cardiology and the American Heart Association/ American College of Cardiology. They have proved controversial among cardiologists who have to treat infective endocarditis, a disease with a persistently high mortality, and the regimen in Section 9.5 remains the current recommendation among cardiologists. NICE is expected to report on this topic in April 2008.

Summary of Infective Endocarditis
- A changing disease, new organisms, older patients, more prosthetic valves
- No reduction in hospital mortality
- New revised Duke criteria for diagnosis
- Multidisciplinary team needed for management
- Always use more than one antibiotic for staphylococcal infection if possible
- TOE for prosthetic valve endocarditis
- If there are indications for surgery: operate early and follow with long antibiotic course
- Close follow-up needed after hospital discharge.

9.8 Non-infective Endocarditis

Non-infective Thrombotic Endocarditis (Marantic Endocarditis)
Non-infective vegetations may occur on heart valves. This is sometimes called marantic endocarditis. They may, if large, be identified on echocardiography (>5 mm in size) and may embolize. They occur in:
- mucinous adenocarcinomas of the pancreas, lung and upper gastrointestinal tract
- other malignant disease, e.g. bladder, lung and lymphomas
- associated with a thrombotic tendency and peripheral microthrombi in small vessels in adult respiratory distress syndrome.

In cases of malignant disease there may be an associated migratory thrombophlebitis, disseminated intravascular coagulation and microangiopathic haemolytic anaemia. Often the condition is only discovered post mortem.

Libman–Sacks Endocarditis
This was first described in 1924 as an active verrucous endocarditis with verrucae or vegetations commonly affecting the aortic or mitral valves, chordae, papillary muscles and ventricular endocardium. Occasionally the tricuspid valve may be involved. It occurs as part of the spectrum of organ involvement of systemic lupus erythematosus (SLE) and, rarely, scleroderma. As with non-infective endocarditis, valve regurgitation is uncommon and the condition may only be diagnosed post mortem (in <50% of cases of SLE). The vegetations are small and may be missed on echocardiography. They are much more

likely in patients who have anti-phospholipid antibodies in their serum. Valve cusps contain a large amount of mucopolysaccharide and it has been suggested that steroid therapy may be implicated.

Although valve involvement is common, severe valve regurgitation is not. Occasionally valve replacement is required.

10 Pericardial Disease

10.1 Acute Pericarditis

Inflammation of the parietal and visceral layers of the pericardium may be a primary condition or secondary to systemic disease.

Causes
- Acute rheumatic fever
- Other bacterial infections
- Viruses, e.g. Coxsackie group, Epstein–Barr virus
- Fungal infections: patients on immunosuppressive agents
- Uraemia
- Trauma, e.g. road traffic accident with steering wheel injury
- Collagen vascular disease, particularly systemic lupus erythematosus (SLE), rheumatoid arthritis
- After an acute MI (see Section 5.10)
- Post-cardiotomy syndrome, Dressler (see Section 5.10)
- Malignant disease
- Radiotherapy
- Hypothyroidism
- Many cases are idiopathic and recurrent idiopathic pericarditis is common.

Pericardial Pain and Other Symptoms
Pain is variable in intensity and site. It is usually retrosternal, radiating to the neck, left shoulder, back and around the left scapula. It may be epigastric only. It is often quite sharp in quality, unlike the heavy sensation of angina, but like angina is made worse by effort. Its most important characteristics are the following:
- Its relationship to position: it is relieved by sitting forward and made worse by lying flat, twisting the thorax or lying on the left side.
- Its relationship to respiration: it is frequently worsened by deep inspiration, coughing, etc.

Swanton's Cardiology, sixth edition. By R. H. Swanton and S. Banerjee. Published 2008 Blackwell Publishing. ISBN 978-1-4051-7819-8.

The pain does not necessarily improve as a pericardial effusion develops. Dyspnoea is a common symptom. The patient frequently takes small rapid breaths, because any major respiratory movement causes pain.

An enlarging effusion increases dyspnoea. Other symptoms include and depend on associated conditions, e.g. fever, dry cough, sweating, arthralgia, rash, pruritus.

Physical Signs

Venous pressure may be normal initially, rising as and if an effusion develops. Prominent 'x' descent suggests that tamponade (see Section 10.2) may be developing.

The pericardial rub is best heard at the left sternal edge with the patient leaning forward. It is variable with respiration and often transient, coming and going over a few hours. It may be confused with and sound very similar to true cardiac murmurs (e.g. the to-and-fro murmur of aortic regurgitation). The heart sounds are soft with a pericardial effusion.

There may be bronchial breathing at the left base with large effusions compressing the left lower lobe (Ewart's sign).

The signs also include those of tamponade (see Section 10.2).

Investigations

These obviously depend on the suspected aetiology but the list below is an example of the possible difficulties in making a diagnosis:
- FBC and ESR, CRP, U&Es, creatinine
- ASO titre, anti-DNAse B titre, etc., throat swabs
- Blood cultures × 3
- Viral titres: acutely and, 2 weeks later, urine + faecal samples
- Paul Bunnell screen
- Cold agglutinins: *mycoplasma*
- LE cells, ANF, anti-DNA antibodies, immune complex titres, complement levels
- T_4, T_3, TSH
- Sputum culture and cytology
- Mantoux test
- Fungal precipitins
- Chest radiograph, heart shape and size, lung pathology
- ECG
- Echocardiogram
- Pericardial fluid for culture, Ziehl–Neelsen staining, guinea-pig inoculation, cytology and fungal culture.

ECG Changes (Figure 10.1 and see Chapter 16, Figure 16.10)
These are often non-specific showing T-wave inversion only. 'Saddle-shaped' ST-segment elevation may occur and be confused with MI, but in pericarditis the ST segment is concave upwards (convex upwards in infarction).

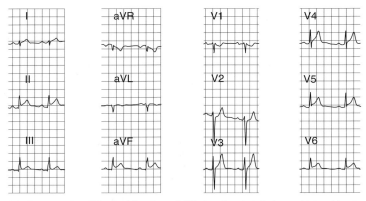

Figure 10.1 Acute pericarditis. Saddle-shaped ST elevation in inferior and lateral leads.

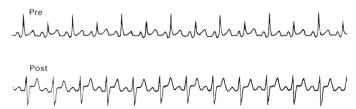

Figure 10.2 ECG lead II in tamponade pre- and post-pericardiocentesis: the ECG before aspiration shows electrical alternans. After pericardiocentesis, this disappears, the voltage has increased and the axis has changed.

With the development of a pericardial effusion the voltage falls, and with very large effusions electrical alternans may occur (Figure 10.2).

Echocardiography (see Chapter 17, Figures 17.39 and 17.40)
This is most valuable in confirming the presence of an effusion, its site and size. LV function is assessed regularly for possible deterioration, e.g. associated myocarditis.

Cardiac Imaging
Cardiac catheterization is rarely necessary now. RA cineangiography before pericardial aspiration will confirm the diagnosis with an obviously thickened pericardium. CT or MRI will also show the thickened pericardium clearly. When calcified the thickened pericardium is clearly visible on the chest radiograph (Figure 10.3).

Management
Analgesia and bed rest are the main forms of therapy. Soluble aspirin or nonsteroidal anti-inflammatory agents are very successful in relieving pain in

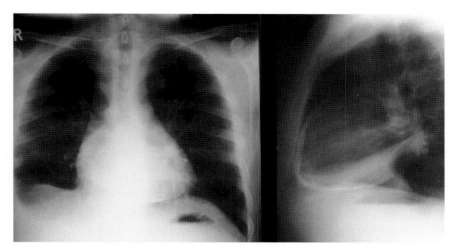

Figure 10.3 Chest radiograph: P/A and left lateral. Tuberculous calcific constrictive pericarditis.

most cases. A course of steroids (e.g. starting with prednisolone 45–60 mg daily, reducing over several weeks) will also work, but care must be taken to follow the patient carefully after cessation of treatment, because the symptoms may recur. Idiopathic benign recurrent pericarditis is treated symptomatically. It is probably of autoimmune origin, although specific autoantibodies have not been identified. Colchicine can be very helpful in preventing relapses and may avoid the need for long-term steroids. A dose of 500 μg twice daily usually avoids the main side effect: diarrhoea. If tolerated the drug may have to be continued for at least a year to avoid a relapse.

Aspiration of the effusion is indicated for diagnosis and/or the relief of symptoms or tamponade. Patients with recurrent effusions not settling on medical treatment should have surgical drainage with a pericardial window and direct histology may be helpful. Occasionally a patient continues to relapse with chest pain and dyspnoea in spite of this regimen. A pericardiectomy is then the only answer. Specific therapy is necessary for the possible associated condition.

Molecular analysis of the pericardial fluid involves the search for bacterial or fungal DNA using PCR, or of viral DNA or RNA. This will increase the identification of the cause, particularly in patients who have had previous antibiotics in bacterial cases.

Recurrent loculated effusions may require extensive pericardectomy.

10.2 Tamponade

This is an acute situation that requires quick diagnosis and pericardial aspiration. Patients, if conscious, complain of dyspnoea, a dull central chest pain, facial engorgement, abdominal and ankle swelling. A chronic form of tamponade does occur.

Acute Causes

- MI with rupture of ventricular wall
- Aortic dissection into the pericardial space
- After cardiac surgery
- Chest trauma
- After trans-septal puncture at cardiac catheter
- Uraemic patients undergoing haemodialysis (and heparinization)
- Malignant disease and/or radiotherapy
- Patients on anticoagulants
- Associated with acute pericarditis
- Perforation of a coronary artery during PCI (see Section 5.9)

Chronic pericardial effusion may, in addition, occur with collagen diseases, Dressler, viral, bacterial or tuberculous pericarditis. Chylous effusions can occur with lymphatic obstruction.

Diagnosis of tamponade should be considered in any patient with a low-output state, high venous pressure, oliguria or anuria who is not responding to inotropes.

Physical Signs

- *JVP*: raised, prominent 'x' descent (systolic). Forward flow from cavae only occurs during ventricular systole. No 'y' descent (see Figure 1.8). Inspiratory filling of the neck veins is not common.
- *BP*: low. May be undetectable on inspiration.
- *Pulse*: low volume. Pulsus paradoxus. An abnormally excessive reduction in pulse volume on inspiration. The exact mechanism is still debated, but increased venous return on inspiration fills the right heart, and left heart filling is less possible with increased RV volume occupying more space in the 'rigid box'. Other factors also contribute (e.g. the normal inspiratory reduction of intrathoracic pressure transmitted to the aorta, and a relative failure of intrapericardial pressure to fall much on inspiration). Diaphragmatic traction on the pericardium is now thought to be irrelevant.

Normally there is a slight reduction of systolic pressure on inspiration (e.g. about 5 mmHg). Reduction of systolic pressure of >10 mmHg is suggestive of pulsus paradoxus (Figure 10.4). Other causes of pulsus paradoxus are:

- constrictive pericarditis (less commonly)
- status asthmaticus (exaggerated pressure swings within the thorax transmitted to the aorta).

Heart sounds are soft. There may be a pericardial rub in tamponade.

Oliguria or anuria rapidly develops with tamponade, and a brisk diuresis occurs when tamponade is relieved.

Other Help in Diagnosis

The ECG shows progressive reduction in voltage, and sometimes electrical alternans (see Figure 10.2). This may be a result of the heart moving around

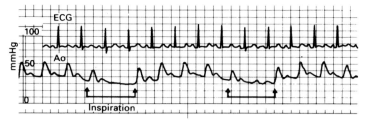

Figure 10.4 Pulsus paradoxus in tamponade: simultaneous arterial pressure (Ao) and ECG in a man with subacute cardiac rupture. The patient was in shock and hypotensive. On inspiration the pulse pressure disappears, and returns immediately on the onset of expiration.

within the fluid-filled pericardium. The chest radiograph shows a symmetrical globular enlargement of the heart. Echocardiography confirms a large pericardial fluid collection with RA and/or RV diastolic collapse. The size of the collection is a better predictor of tamponade than right heart collapse (see Figure 10.4). RA cineangiography confirms diagnosis but is not necessary now with two-dimensional echocardiography.

Management

Pericardial needle aspiration may be life-saving, but usually is only of temporary benefit. Insertion of a surgical drain or creation of a pericardial window is frequently necessary. Needle aspiration is best performed via the xiphisternal route with the patient supine, using ECG control if screening is not available. The V lead of a standard ECG is attached to the aspiration needle with a crocodile clip. The needle is inserted 1–1.5 cm (0.5 inch) below the xiphisternum and, keeping it horizontal, the tip is rotated 45° to the left (towards the left shoulder tip). The cardiac pulsation can usually be felt at the end of the needle, but, if the needle penetrates the myocardium itself, ST-segment elevation occurs ('injury potential'). Pericardial fluid should be sent for cytology if no obvious diagnosis is apparent. Creation of a pericardial window allows a pericardial biopsy to be taken. Removal of even a small amount of fluid from the pericardial sac (e.g. only 50–100 ml) can produce a considerable improvement in haemodynamics as the intrapericardial pressure falls sharply. Instillation of chemotherapeutic agents is possible in confirmed malignant disease with reaccumulation of fluid (e.g. 5-fluorouracil, nitrogen mustard or ^{32}P). Instilling tetracycline in patients with recurrent malignant pericardial effusions may help obliterate the pericardial space.

10.3 Chronic Constrictive Pericarditis

Constrictive pericarditis and restrictive cardiomyopathy usually present in a similar way with signs and symptoms of both right- and left-sided heart failure. However, there is no history of hypertension, angina is rare and the heart is not grossly enlarged (as in dilated cardiomyopathy). Clinically,

Table 10.1 Similarities and differences between tamponade and pericardial constriction

	Tamponade	Constrictive pericarditis
JVP/RA pressure	Prominent 'x' descent	Prominent 'x' and 'y' descents
Kussmaul's sign	Usually absent	May be present
Pulsus paradoxus	Invariable	Not common
Atrial pressures	Equal	Equal
LVEDP/RVEDP	Equal	Equal
Diastolic dip-and-plateau waveform	Absent	Present

right-sided signs are prominent with marked elevation of venous pressure, hepatomegaly, and often ankle oedema or ascites. The right-sided signs in constriction may appear quite suddenly over a matter of days. Table 10.1 details differences between constrictive pericarditis and tamponade.

The cause is often not identified. It is probably the result of haemorrhagic pericarditis producing fibrosis with organization of the exudate. The three most common causes are previous pericarditis (infective), cardiac surgery and mediastinal irradiation.

Possible Causes
- Viral, e.g. Coxsackie virus
- Fungal, e.g. *Histoplasma* sp.
- Tuberculosis
- Other bacterial infections
- Mediastinal radiotherapy
- Malignant disease: lymphoma, breast or lung carcinoma, mesothelioma, melanoma
- Connective tissue disease, e.g. SLE, scleroderma, rheumatoid arthritis
- Uraemia (rare)
- Drugs, e.g. procainamide, hydralazine, isoniazid, minoxidil, methysergide, phenylbutazone
- Sarcoidosis
- Amyloidosis
- Asbestosis
- Trauma
- Post-cardiac surgery
- Post-pacemaker or ICD implantation
- Carcinoid.

Physical Signs
The most important sign is in the JVP with the appearance of prominent 'x' and 'y' descents (Figure 10.5) in the venous pressure. This is an important differential diagnostic point from tamponade. These two prominent descents

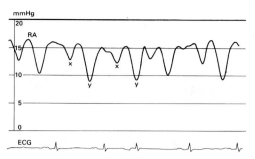

Figure 10.5 Right atrial pressure in pericardial constriction: the mean RA pressure is high and the 'x' and 'y' descents are prominent.

can be seen even if the patient is in AF. Forward flow occurs during ventricular systole and on tricuspid valve opening. Inspiratory filling of the neck veins may occur (Kussmaul's sign) but it is not a particularly reliable sign. Pulsus paradoxus is uncommon in constrictive pericarditis. Ankle oedema and ascites are common, as is hepatosplenomegaly. Heart sounds are soft. There may be an early third sound associated with rapid early ventricular filling (pericardial knock).

AF is common. Although the condition is chronic, the development of oedema and ascites may be acute and sudden. In chronic cases cardiac cachexia may occur leading to a mistaken diagnosis of intra-abdominal malignancy.

Differential Diagnosis of Pericardial Constriction
- Chronic pericardial effusion (Table 10.11)
- Restrictive cardiomyopathy: amyloidosis, endomyocardial fibrosis, Loeffler's eosinophilic endocarditis
- Dilated cardiomyopathy (DCM)
- Mitral stenosis with pulmonary hypertension and tricuspid regurgitation
- HCM involving RV and LV
- Thromboembolic pulmonary hypertension
- Ischaemic CCF
- SVC obstruction
- RA myxoma
- Nephrotic syndrome
- Liver disease
- Intra-abdominal malignancy
- Pregnancy.

The heart is large in DCM and ischaemic CCF but tends to be smaller or normal in constrictive pericarditis and restrictive cardiomyopathy.

LV systolic function is usually normal in restrictive cardiomyopathy and often normal in constrictive pericarditis. It is grossly reduced in DCM and ischaemic CCF.

Table 10.2 Differences between pericardial constriction and restrictive cardiomyopathy

	Constrictive pericarditis	Restrictive cardiomyopathy
Physical signs	Kussmaul's sign +ve	Kussmaul's sign –ve
	No murmurs	Possible MR or TR
	Pericardial knock	Early S3, or S4 if still in SR
ECG	Possible low voltage	Low voltage and may show pathological Q waves
Echocardiography	No LVH	Normal or small LV chamber
	Pericardial thickening/Ca^{2+}	Normal pericardium
	Interventricular septal bounce in early diastole and septal shift to left on inspiration	Granular sparkle (amyloid) Possible LVH Normal septal motion
Colour M-mode	LV flow propagation velocity is fast >100 cm/s	Slow LV flow propagation velocity <100 cm/s
Mitral Doppler	Respiratory variation >25% in transmitral inflow E velocity	Respiratory variation <25% in transmitral inflow E velocity
	Respiratory variation >18% in pulmonary vein D velocity	Respiratory variation <18% in pulmonary vein D velocity
Mitral annulus	High early filling Ea velocity >8.0 cm/s	Low early filling Ea velocity <8.0 cm/s
Hepatic veins	Diastolic flow reversal on expiration	Not seen
Cardiac cathetarization	LVEDP = RVEDP	LVEDP 7 mmHg > RVEDP

Severe pulmonary hypertension is not a feature of constriction or restriction, but is frequently found in the other conditions listed above.

Cardiac catheterization, plus CT/MRI may be the only way to reach a definitive diagnosis.

In restrictive cardiomyopathy measurements of muscle movement and relaxation are abnormal (e.g. flow propagation velocity) whereas these measurements are normal in pericardial constriction. However, in spite of all the differences in Table 10.2 there are still grey areas, such as a patient with constriction who has myocardial scarring and fibrosis from an old infarct.

Investigations

These are usually unrewarding. There is little point in viral titres in such a chronic disease. The important feature is a vigorous search for tuberculosis, e.g.
• Mantoux, early morning sputum and urine
• ANF, DNA antibodies, rheumatoid factor
• Chest radiograph: calcification of the pericardium strongly suggests a tuberculous aetiology (see Figure 10.3); pleural effusions are more common than pulmonary oedema
• Echocardiography shows normal LV size with rapid early filling and diastasis (best seen on posterior wall movement); RA, IVC and hepatic veins are

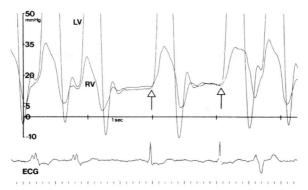

Figure 10.6 Simultaneous recording of left and right ventricular pressures in chronic constrictive pericarditis. On longer R–R intervals there is a dip-and-plateau waveform in diastole. The end-diastolic pressures of both ventricles are high and virtually equal (arrowed). This helps to distinguish the condition from restrictive cardiomyopathy.

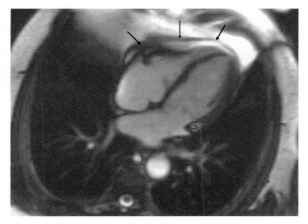

Figure 10.7 Cardiac MRI showing pericardial thickening anteriorly (arrowed).

dilated. Doppler studies should show an increased E:A ratio and diastolic flow reversal in the hepatic veins on expiration

• Cardiac catheterization is necessary to differentiate the condition from restrictive cardiomyopathy. Atrial pressures are high and equal, with prominent 'x' and 'y' descents in constriction. LVEDP = RVEDP (or virtually so) at any phase of respiration and both are high. Systolic function is usually normal in constriction, but may be impaired in severe cases (the constricted pericardium may involve the epicardium). There is a typical diastolic plateau waveform in both ventricles (rapid early filling then diastasis) (Figure 10.6). In constriction the difference between the LVEDP and RVEDP should be <5mm.

• CT/MRI (Figures 10.7 and 10.8): both can be used to demonstrate the thickened pericardium and pericardial thickness >4mm helps to distinguish

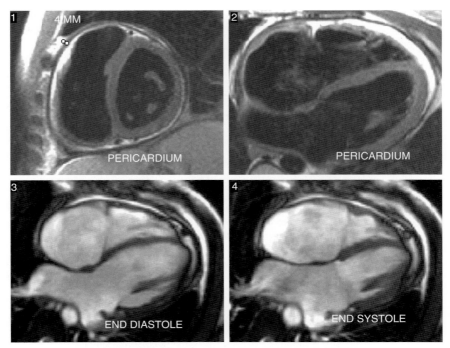

Figure 10.8 Constrictive pericarditis on cardiac MRI.

constriction from restrictive cardiomyopathy. In addition the ventricles are small and tubular-shaped, and the RA and IVC dilated.

Management
Balloon dilatation of the pericardium has been tried in a few cases with some success, avoiding the need for a limited thoracotomy, and this may be useful as a palliative measure in patients with malignant disease.

Pericardial Window
This can be of temporary benefit and also useful diagnostically. This can be performed either through small left submammary thoracotomy or using video-assisted thoracoscopy (VATS). The latter is less invasive and can still yield useful pericardial tissue for histology as well as draining any left pleural effusion.

Pericardiectomy
Although diuretic therapy and salt restriction may also be of temporary benefit, pericardiectomy is usually necessary. As much of the anterior wall of both ventricles as possible is freed. It is a procedure not without difficulties because the pericardium may be strongly adherent to the epicardial muscle.

Freeing the AV groove is important if at all possible. The phrenic nerves are preserved. It is a haemorrhagic business. The pericardium should be sent for histology and culture.

In cases of tuberculous pericarditis, antituberculous therapy is combined with steroids to try to prevent progression to constriction. Total pericardiectomy for patients with established constriction is not delayed and combined with drug treatment: a year's course of antituberculous therapy may be necessary.

Patients who have constriction secondary to malignant disease or as a result of radiotherapy fare worst after pericardiectomy. Every effort should be made to manage these patients medically or with the limited procedures of balloon dilatation or a pericardial window.

10.4 Effusive–Constrictive Pericarditis

This is a rare condition combining features of pericardial tamponade and constriction of the visceral pericardium. It is probably a half-way stage on the pathway from acute pericarditis with effusion, through to classic pericardial constriction without fluid. Patients present with signs and symptoms of tamponade but their RA pressure does not fall after pericardiocentesis even though the intrapericardial pressure falls. Removal of the pericardial fluid has dealt with only half the problem.

Causes are those of classic constriction and are chiefly infective, radiation-induced, neoplastic, after surgery or idiopathic. Radiation is probably the most common cause overall, but tuberculosis the most common in developing countries.

Measurement of intrapericardial pressure is not routinely necessary. The condition should be suspected if the patient's neck veins remain raised after pericardiocentesis, where more than one drainage procedure is required or where the pericardium looks thickened on echocardiography or MRI.

Pericardiectomy
After pericardiocentesis some patients improve clinically. Occasionally the condition resolves spontaneously, but eventually a pericardiectomy is usually required. In these patients the parietal pericardium may be unimpressive at the time of surgery and it is important to remove as much of the visceral pericardium as possible (attached to the ventricular wall).

11 The Heart in Systemic Disease

11.1 Acromegaly

Increased growth hormone (GH) from a pituitary tumour results in increased synthesis of insulin-like growth factors (IGF-I and -II) from the liver. Diabetes occurs in about 50% of cases. The following are the cardiovascular changes:
• Systemic hypertension in 30%. Total exchangeable sodium increased. Some have increased aldosterone levels. All have increased sensitivity to angiotensin II. The hypertension is usually mild and controllable medically.
• LV hypertrophy present in more than half the cases.
• HCM: this is independent of hypertension or coronary disease. It may be massive, with interstitial fibrosis and changes very similar to hypertrophic obstructive cardiomyopathy. Patients will need managing exactly on the same lines (see Section 4.2). Subaortic myotomy/myomectomy may be needed for severe cases.
• Diabetes mellitus may result in small vessel disease.
• Coronary disease is more frequent as a result of hypertension, diabetes and raised plasma free fatty acid levels.

11.2 AIDS (Acquired Immune Deficiency Syndrome)

Clinical evidence of cardiac involvement occurs only in about 10% of cases, although post mortem 25% of cases may have cardiac disease. The following are typical problems:
• Dilated cardiomyopathy (DCM) pictures in about 8% cases of HIV infection. The incidence is higher with a CD4 count <400 cells/mm^3. In situ hybridization studies of myocardial biopsy specimens show HIV nucleic acid sequences in the myocyte in most cases. Inflammatory lymphocytic infiltrates with CD3 and CD8 cells are seen. Myocarditis may occasionally result from a wide variety of opportunistic infections (e.g. toxoplasmosis, histoplasmosis, CMV, Coxsackie virus) but is usually caused by the HIV itself. An autoimmune component induced by the HIV or other viruses is possible. Thirty per

Swanton's Cardiology, sixth edition. By R. H. Swanton and S. Banerjee. Published 2008 Blackwell Publishing. ISBN 978-1-4051-7819-8.

cent of patients have antibodies to α-myosin. Symptoms from CCF may be incorrectly attributed to pre-existing lung disease.

- Drug treatment (e.g. zidovudine) and malnutrition (e.g. selenium deficiency) have been implicated in contributing to the cardiomyopathy picture.
- Pericardial effusion: may lead to tamponade and require aspiration.
- Ventricular arrhythmias.
- Non-bacterial thrombotic endocarditis (marantic endocarditis).
- Infective endocarditis, e.g. *Aspergillus* sp.
- Metastatic involvement from Kaposi's sarcoma.
- RV failure (recurrent chest infections causing pulmonary hypertension).
- Diffuse coronary disease (see below).

Treatment is only palliative. Pericardial aspiration, standard treatment for cardiac failure or drug therapy for specific opportunistic infection may be needed. The incidence of cardiac problems is related to the viral load and inversely to the CD4 count. Highly aggressive anti-retroviral treatment (HAART) has reduced this.

Protease Inhibitors and the Dyslipidaemia Syndrome

Used as part of HAART, protease inhibitors can induce a metabolic disturbance with dyslipidaemia, a lipodystrophy syndrome, impaired glucose tolerance, insulin resistance and diabetes. β Cell function is impaired and free fatty acid turnover increases. The dyslipidaemia can be startling with a 30–40% increase in triglycerides and a 200% increase in serum cholesterol. There is an increased hepatic production of triglyceride-rich lipoproteins (VLDLs) as a result of activation of lipogenic genes under control of *SREBP*-1c. This is reversible on stopping the drug(s). Endothelial dysfunction has been shown in patients on protease inhibitors with an increase in carotid intima–media thickness, coronary disease and coronary calcification. There is now a recognized increased risk of MI in patients taking protease inhibitors (not seen with reverse-transcriptase inhibitors).

Treatment

Rosuvastatin is the statin of choice because it not metabolized through cytochrome P450 3A4 (which is inhibited by protease inhibitors). Use Omacor for the hypertriglceridaemia, and conventional treatment for insulin resistance (diet, exercise, weight loss, metformin and thiazolidinediones).

Diffuse coronary disease can often be dealt with by angioplasty, but CABG is very occasionally necessary.

11.3 Amyloidosis

Amyloid fibrils are derived from a monoclonal immunoglobulin light chain (κ or λ) or its N-terminal fragment. They circulate in the blood as Bence Jones protein and are deposited in the tissues as β-pleated sheet fibrils. They may be deposited in any tissue.

It is histologically identifiable by staining orange/pink with Congo red, exhibiting green/yellow birefringence in polarized light and a characteristic fibrillary structure under electron microscopy.

Immune Origin Amyloid (Formerly Primary Amyloid): AL-type Protein

A plasma cell dyscrasia produces monoclonal immunoglobulin light chains that become pleated together to form amyloid fibrils. About 20% of patients with AL amyloidosis have myeloma and about 50% patients with AL amyloid have cardiac involvement.

Restrictive Cardiomyopathy (see Sections 4.3 and 10.3)

Amyloid deposits in the myocardium give the muscle a 'rubbery rigidity' but the diagnosis is easily missed in the early stages because it presents with just diastolic dysfunction.

Infiltration between myocardial cells results in a small stiff heart with high LVEDP and RVEDP, whereas systolic function remains normal until late in the disease. Small pericardial effusions may occur, but the typical picture is of CCF with a normal sized heart on the chest radiograph. Coronary artery occlusion may occur with amyloid deposits in the arterial wall. Tachyarrhythmias are common, AF producing a rapid deterioration with a stiff ventricular muscle. Sinus arrest and AV block may require pacing. Mild AV valve regurgitation occurs but valve replacement is rarely indicated. Pulmonary infiltration is common.

Clinical findings show a raised JVP with prominent 'x' and 'y' descents and a possible Kussmaul sign (inspiratory filling of the neck veins). The apex is usually impalpable but an S4 and/or early S3 may be heard. The picture is very similar to constrictive pericarditis, which is the chief differential diagnosis (see Section 10.3).

Other non-cardiac features include the following: macroglossia, peripheral neuropathy, postural hypotension (autonomic neuropathy), large joint arthritis, renal involvement, waxy skin deposits, spontaneous purpura (often periorbital) and ecchymoses.

Cardiac Investigations and Diagnosis

ECG shows low voltage with Q waves in anterior or inferior leads simulating old infarction. There may be sinus arrest, AF or degrees of AV block.

Echocardiography shows a concentrically thickened myocardium with a speckled appearance, 'granular sparkle', on two-dimensional imaging. There may be an insignificant pericardial effusion. Initially early diastolic filling is impaired with EA reversal (see Section 17.3), but later in the course of the disease this 'pseudo-normalizes' as diastolic filling becomes more restrictive. There is rapid early diastolic filling then diastasis.

Think of cardiac amyloid with the combination of low voltage on the ECG with apparent LVH on the echocardiogram.

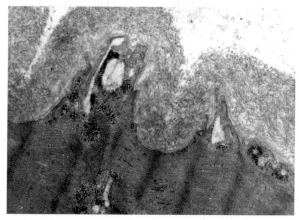

Figure 11.1 Cardiac amyloid: electron micrograph of endomyocardial biopsy specimen. Amyloid fibril deposition on myocardial fibre basement membrane. Reproduced from Swanton *et al.*, Am J Cardiol 1977; 39:7, with permission of Elsevier Ltd.

Cardiac magnetic resonance imaging (CMRI) will confirm the apparent LV hypertrophy, plus a possible small pericardial effusion. There is late gadolinium enhancement.

Cardiac catheterization shows a typical diastolic dip-and-plateau waveform in both ventricles. However, RVEDP and LVEDP differ, usually by >7 mmHg, in all phases of respiration in contrast to constrictive pericarditis where they are the same. Diagnosis is confirmed by endomyocardial biopsy (Figure 11.1).

Rectal biopsy will be positive in more than half the cases.

Serum amyloid protein scanning is useful for diagnosing amyloid in abdominal viscera, but is not helpful in picking up cardiac amyloid.

About 10% of patients with AL amyloidosis turn out to have hereditary amyloid (see below). In this group chemotherapy is of no value and liver transplantation must be considered.

Treatment

There is no specific treatment for a depressingly relentless condition, with most patients dying within 15 months of diagnosis. Low-dose chemotherapy for the plasma cell dyscrasia (e.g. with melphalan and prednisone) may produce some regression in cardiac amyloid if continued for >1 year. This combination is superior to colchicine. Unfortunately chemotherapy seems to clear amyloid from the heart slower than from other organs and improvement in cardiac function is unlikely for several years.

Patients with cardiac amyloid may be very sensitive to digoxin. Amiodarone is used for paroxysmal tachyarrhythmias, pacing for sinus arrest and AV block plus diuretics for systemic or pulmonary oedema. Vasodilators and calcium antagonists are best avoided, with the main management being titration of diuretics.

Free light chains can now be assayed in the serum and monitoring the light chain level over time is a useful guide to prognosis.

Cardiac transplantation is not contraindicated in cardiac amyloid and about 20 patients with cardiac amyloid have been transplanted in the UK. This should be considered only if the patient is likely to survive >5 years with regard to visceral infiltration. Attempts should then be made to reduce the fibril precursors with chemotherapy. As with multiple myeloma autologous peripheral blood stem cell transplantation has been successful in a few cases.

Future Research
This is needed to prevent the development of amyloid fibrils by stabilizing precursor proteins, and inhibiting glycosoaminoglycan binding. We need β-sheet breakers to breakdown the β-pleated sheets once formed.

Senile Cardiac Amyloid: ATTR Amyloid Protein
Amyloid deposits derived from wild-type transthyretin (TTR) are very common in the atria of elderly people and may be the cause of atrial arrhythmias in this age group. Senile cardiac amyloid is found in 25% of postmortem examinations in patients >80 years. It is more common in black patients than in white, and in men more than in women. Wild-type TTR amyloidosis is almost always confined to the myocardium, with a better prognosis than other types. Smaller deposits may be found in the ventricles and aorta of patients post mortem but these are rarely of pathological significance. Rectal biopsy and biopsy of other organs will be negative.

The condition is rarely diagnosed in life and treatment is rarely necessary, usually involving management of atrial dysrhythmias.

Reactive Amyloid (Formerly Secondary Amyloid): AA-type Amyloid Protein
Amyloid deposition secondary to chronic inflammatory disease: TB, leprosy, chronic rheumatoid arthritis, Crohn's disease, bronchiectasis, paraplegia (urinary infections), etc. Infiltration in liver, spleen and kidney occurs but the heart is much less commonly involved (only about 2% of cases). Patients usually present with renal dysfunction and hence systemic oedema is much more likely to result from nephrotic syndrome than from heart failure.

Hereditary Familial Amyloid (Mutant TTR) or ATTR
TTR is produced in the liver. An autosomal dominant condition of familial amyloid is caused by a mutant/variant γ-TTR causing a familial polyneuropathy. Liver transplantation is the mainstay of treatment (removing the source of the variant TTR), and has improved the peripheral neuropathy, but unfortunately cardiac involvement is common and may progress in spite of liver

transplantation. Ten patients in the Mayo Clinic have had combined heart and liver transplants for familial amyloidosis with a 83% 5-year survival rate.

Cardiac amyloid has the following features:
- Usually caused by AL amyloid (plasma cell dyscrasia)
- Typically presents as restrictive cardiomyopathy
- Low-voltage ECG with LVH on echocardiography
- Cardiac biopsy usually diagnostic, rectal biopsy less reliable
- Diuretics the main cardiac treatment
- Poor prognosis almost invariable
- Cardiac transplantation followed by chemotherapy a rare possibility.

11.4 Anderson–Fabry Disease

Described in 1898 this is a lysosomal storage disease resulting from an X-linked defect of glycosphingolipid metabolism which causes a relative deficiency of α-galactosidase. The failure of biodegradation of glycosphingolipids causes an accumulation of globotriosoceramide (GB3) in the tissues. Over 300 mutations have been identified on chromosome Xq22. Unlike other X-linked recessive disorders females may be affected. It occurs in approximately 1 in 40 000 population and, although it commonly presents in childhood, the disease may not present until adult life with cardiac, neurological or renal involvement. The diagnosis is easily missed at this stage with such a wide spectrum of organ involvement. Diagnosis is important because enzyme replacement therapy is now available from the specialized units dealing with the condition.

Clinical Features
- Skin: angiokeratomas – tiny raised dark red spots in the bathing trunk area, on the back and around the mouth. Similar in appearance to purpura, but the spots are raised and have a different distribution.
- Hypohidrosis: loss of sweating causing heat intolerance
- Eyes: cornea verticillata – diagnostic whorls radiating from the centre of the cornea. Posterior subcapsular cataract and retinal vascular lesions also cause loss of vision.
- Gastrointestinal involvement: recurrent bouts of abdominal pain, diarrhoea or constipation, nausea and vomiting. May be mistaken for an irritable bowel syndrome.
- Cardiac involvement: small vessel disease resulting from endothelial cell swelling causes angina and MI. Large epicardial coronary arteries may be normal. Coronary flow reserve is reduced as a result of this small vessel disease. Valve regurgitation and conduction disturbances occur. A HCM picture may present in adults aged over 30 years. About 6.3% of late-onset HCM have Fabry's disease. This is concentric hypertrophy and LVOT obstruction is not usually a feature. Systolic function is usually normal. AF occurs in >10% cases and anticoagulation may be needed.

• Renal involvement: proteinuria, haematuria and nephritic syndrome occur. Chronic renal failure may require dialysis.
• CNS involvement: transient ischaemic attack or CVA may occur in young adults. Acroparaesthesiae may be the presenting symptom: burning neuropathic pain in hands and feet. Usually a problem in childhood, improving with age. Often provoked by fever, alcohol, exercise or temperature change.

Treatment

Recently developed enzyme replacement therapy has at last offered patients some symptom relief. Intravenous infusions are given in alternate weeks. Two forms of recombinant enzyme replacement are available: agalsidase α produced in human fibroblasts (0.2 mg/kg alternate weeks) and agalsidase β from Chinese hamster ovary cells (1 mg/kg alternate weeks).

Treatment reduces deposits of GB3 and has been shown to reduce pain and improve quality of life. It stabilizes renal function, reduces LV mass and improves diastolic dysfunction. As yet improvements in coronary flow reserve have not been shown, and fibroblast and myofibrillar inclusions persist.

11.5 Ankylosing Spondylitis

A progressive inflammatory disease of the vertebral column, sacroiliac, hip, shoulder and manubriosternal joints, with chronic back pain and eventual fusion and calcification of the intervertebral discs and anterior spinal ligament. It occurs 90% in men. High incidence of the human leukocyte antigen histocompatibility antigen HLA-B27. There is cardiac involvement in 10% of cases and secondary amyloidosis in about 6%:
• Conduction disturbance leading to AV block
• Aortic regurgitation less common, as a result of aortic root dilatation (medial necrosis).

Permanent pacing and aortic valve replacement may sometimes be needed in the same patient.

Arteritis and valve granulomas do not occur, unlike rheumatoid cardiac disease.

11.6 Cardiac Myxoma

This may occur in any cardiac chamber but occurs most commonly in the left atrium. It is typically a gelatinous friable tumour attached to the atrial septum by a short pedicle. It is three times more common in the left atrium than in the right. Middle-aged women are most commonly affected. Untreated, it is usually fatal, although disease progression may be very slow over a period of years. The tumour often prolapses through the mitral or tricuspid valve and can cause sudden obstruction to blood flow. Fragments of the tumour easily break off and cause systemic emboli. Multiple tumours occur very rarely.

There is also a rare familial form (autosomal dominant) associated with lentiginosis (multiple freckles) or HCM. This condition – the Carney complex – is also associated with multiple myxomas, some of which may be extracardiac, and endocrine adenomas.

Symptoms

The atrial myxoma commonly presents in one of four ways in order of frequency:

1 *Dyspnoea*: this may be of gradual onset or sudden severe pulmonary oedema.

2 *Systemic emboli*: any organ may be involved, e.g. brain (fits, hemiplegia, etc.), MI, acute ischaemia of a limb.

3 *Constitutional upset*: weight loss, fever, myalgia (low albumin and raised globulin with a high ESR are often associated).

4 *Sudden death*: the atrial myxoma is found post mortem occluding the mitral valve orifice.

Physical Signs

The left atrial myxoma most closely mimics mitral stenosis but there are one or two pointers suggesting a myxoma:

• The patient is in sinus rhythm. Atrial dysrhythmias are rare.

• Signs of mitral stenosis may be transient and occur only if the tumour approaches the mitral valve orifice. Sometimes postural changes will influence the murmur.

• There is no opening snap.

• There may be an early diastolic plop as the tumour prolapses through the valve.

Right atrial myxomas are more difficult to pick up clinically. There may be signs suggesting RV dysfunction (raised JVP, oedema, etc.) or pulmonary infarction from emboli. A tricuspid diastolic flow murmur is often difficult to hear.

Investigations

Chest radiograph shows a small heart with enlargement of the LA appendage and possible pulmonary oedema. There is no mitral valve calcification. In long-standing cases, calcification may occur in the tumour itself.

Echocardiography is diagnostic. Two-dimensional echocardiography (see Figure 11.2) will be diagnostic in almost all cases of prolapsing myxoma. Transoesophageal echocardiography will give more accurate information of the size and site of the myxoma.

Cardiac catheterization is now virtually never required. In cases of left-sided myxomas where there is diagnostic doubt after echocardiography, pulmonary angiography with follow through to the left heart may help. Direct left heart catheterization should be avoided because this may dislodge friable material from the myxoma. With right-sided myxomas, if there is doubt after

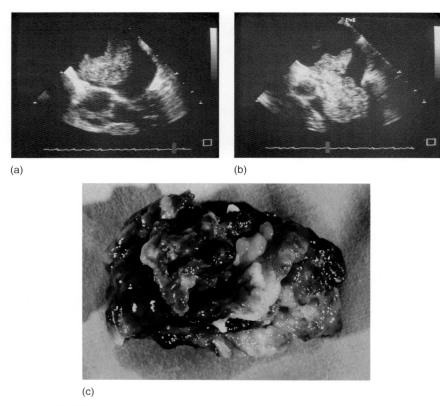

(a)

(b)

(c)

Figure 11.2 Atrial myxoma: transoesophageal echocardiogram. (a) A large myxoma is seen in the left atrium, which (b) prolapses through the mitral valve in diastole. (c) The removed specimen.

echocardiography, digital subtraction angiography from a peripheral venous injection is helpful.

Histology
This may be obtained from analysis of peripheral embolic material. Although the tumour embolizes frequently, it does not grow in its peripheral site.

Differential Diagnosis
The following conditions should also be considered in a patient with a mitral murmur, mild pyrexia, weight loss, abnormal plasma proteins and high ESR:
- rheumatic mitral stenosis
- infective endocarditis
- SLE
- reticulosis

- cor triatriatum
- LA thrombus.

Treatment

'Never let the sun set on a myxoma.' Goodwin's advice remains true today. The friable nature of the tumour is unpredictable. After echocardiographic diagnosis, surgical removal of the myxoma should be performed as soon as possible using cardiopulmonary bypass (Figure 11.2). Occasionally atrial septectomy and an interatrial patch are required. Recurrence of the myxoma is extremely rare but patients should be followed up for the first 5 years.

11.7 Cytotoxic Chemotherapy and the Heart

Acute Toxicity

Vincristine and 5-Fluorouracil

High doses of vincristine or 5-fluorouracil given intravenously may cause an acute coronary syndrome in about 4% of patients. This is caused by endothelium-independent coronary constriction associated with platelet adhesion. An infusion of 5-fluorouracil seems more likely to provoke this than a bolus injection. The infusion should be stopped and the patient treated with coronary vasodilators (nitrates and calcium antagonists). Stents should be avoided if possible.

Cyclophosphamide

An acute myocarditis/pericarditis picture may occur rarely with cyclophosphamide in the first 10 days of administration. This may be associated with multiple ectopic beats, repolarization changes on the ECG and ventricular arrhythmias. There may be a pericardial effusion with falling voltage on the ECG, and even tamponade. In one study this reaction occurred in 0.9% patients, but is becoming less of a problem now with lower dose schedules.

Anthracyclines

Three phases of cardiac damage have been described with anthracycline use. The first is the immediate pericarditis/myocarditis syndrome similar to cyclophosphamide above. This acute injury is proportional to peak plasma levels (too high an infusion rate). The second is CCF developing during or soon after anthracycline treatment, and the third is heart failure developing many years after treatment. Peak incidence of damage is a few months after treatment.

Chronic Toxicity with Anthracyclines
The mechanism of cardiac damage is poorly understood because these antimitotic agents damage non-dividing myocardial cells. Lipid peroxidation with the generation of free radicals by the anthracycline–iron complex has been implicated with subsequent mitochondrial damage, impairment of the electron transport chain and resulting calcium overload. However, this may also be the mechanism whereby the drugs have their therapeutic effect.

Recognised Risk Factors
- Children (especially age <4 years)
- Old age
- Cumulative life-time dose of daunorubicin or doxorubicin >500 mg/m^2
- Mediastinal radiotherapy
- Female sex
- Time from treatment
- Pre-existing cardiac disease or hypertension.

Assessment of LV Function during Treatment
Early detection of myocardial injury is vital. Mild elevations of troponin T (>0.01 ng/ml) have been shown to be associated with early damage. Approximately 10% of patients are troponin positive after a first course of anthracyclines, and 15% after a second course.

Measurements of natriuretic peptide ANP and BNP levels show a sharp rise once the LVEF falls below 50%. It is likely that biochemical variables will be a more sensitive marker of early damage than echocardiographic measurements but no study has yet confirmed this. Regular echocardiography should detect diastolic dysfunction before systolic dysfunction and a fall in LVEF. Any drop in LVEF means that LV damage has already occurred.

MUGA scanning is an alternative, if available. Generally this is likely to be impractical and reproducibility of the measurement is ±5%. Myocardial biopsy is theoretically useful but also impractical.

Prevention of Cardiotoxicity
- Avoiding the use of anthracyclines: is there an alternative chemotherapeutic regimen or a less toxic anthracycline? Epirubicin is probably less cardiotoxic than daunorubicin or doxorubicin, with maximum dose being 900–1000 mg/m^2. Idarubicin is also less cardiotoxic, but a maximum dose has not yet been defined.
- Keep the total cumulative dose of doxorubicin to <300 mg/m^2, particularly in children.
- Weekly administration schedule rather than larger doses every 3 weeks.
- Use of liposomal doxorubin.
- Dexrazoxane: this binds free and bound iron and reduces the formation of anthracycline–iron complexes. One trial has shown a reduction in cardiac injury using dexrazoxane in children. However, there are concerns that it may reduce the effectiveness of the anthracycline, or contribute to marrow suppression.
- ACE inhibitors: recovery of ventricular function with the use of ACE inhibitors has been documented. It is not known whether pre-treatment with ACE inhibitors is protective.
- Reactive oxygen species scavengers: these might theoretically be of value.

Table 11.1 Cardiotoxicity of trastuzumab

Drug regimen	Cardiotoxicity (%)
Trastuzumab monotherapy	1–2
Previous anthracyclines	7
Concomitant paclitaxel	12
Concomitant anthracyclines	29

Imatinib Mesylate (Gleevec)

This drug is used to treat chronic myeloid leukaemia and gastrointestinal stromal tumours. It is known to cause fluid retention, but a recent study has shown that it may cause severe systolic LV dysfunction. This has been documented in a few patients developing LVF a mean of 7 months after starting therapy with imatinib. Their pre-treatment systolic function was normal. Regular echocardiography is needed in patients receiving imatinib.

Trastuzumab (Herceptin)

This is a monoclonal antibody to epidermal growth factor receptor-2 (ErbB2 receptor) which is overexpressed in 25% patients with breast carcinoma. Trastuzumab reduces the 2-year mortality rate in patients who are HER2 positive from 5.3% to 3.5%. Overall, 2% of patients develop heart failure but concomitant chemotherapy can increase the incidence of cardiotoxicity as shown in a study of 700 patients with metastatic breast cancer treated with trastuzumab (Table 11.2).

ErbB2 signalling is necessary to keep myocardial cells alive and ErbB2 is essential in the prevention of DCM. Loss or inhibition of ErbB2 renders the cell more susceptible to anthracycline damage and ErbB2 knock-out mice do worse when treated with anthracyclines than wild-type mice.

Trastuzumab should not be given to patients receiving anthracyclines, or to patients recently treated with anthracyclines.

11.8 Diabetes Mellitus

There are an estimated 2 million people with diabetes in the UK (95% type 2), of whom 75% will die from coronary disease. Aggressive management of diabetes has been more effective at controlling the microvascular (e.g. retinal) complications than the macrovascular ones (e.g. coronary). Conventional risk factors account for only about 25% of the excess risk of coronary disease in diabetics. Other mechanisms responsible for these vascular complications include the following:

• Hypertriglyceridaemia, raised levels of VLDL and small atherogenic LDL particles.

- Reduced levels of HDL: low HDL levels are an independent risk factor for cardiac events.
- Procoagulable state: raised levels of factors VII and X, thromboxane (TxA2), lipoprotein(a) and plasminogen activator inhibitor (PAI-1), leading to reduced fibrinolysis. Platelet aggregability is increased. Antithrombin III levels are reduced.
- Insulin resistance, hyperinsulinaemia, metabolic syndrome X (see Section 11.10).

Endothelial dysfunction is common in people with diabetes and results partly from hyperglycaemia and insulin resistance. Hyperglycaemia has a toxic effect on endothelium through the formation of superoxide and other reactive oxygen species. Advanced glycation end-products (AGEs) are formed in plasma and blood vessel walls. Once these are bound to a receptor for these glycation end-products (RAGEs) there is increased expression of vascular adhesion molecule (VCAM), increased monocyte adherence, plus an increase in tissue factor and endothelin release. This increases the procoagulable state, and promotes vasoconstriction and oxidation of LDLs in the vascular wall.

Autonomic impairment in people with diabetes results in reduced heart rate variability and silent ischaemia. This may deprive people with diabetes of a signal to stop exercising during ischaemia. Cardiac autonomic neuropathy can be demonstrated in one in six individuals with diabetes. Sudden death may occur (often at night) and is associated with a long QT interval exacerbated by hypoglycaemia.

Diabetic cardiomyopathy: the existence of this condition is hotly debated. In many patients the diastolic dysfunction seen is a result of diffuse coronary disease or LV hypertrophy secondary to uncontrolled hypertension. Nevertheless there are claims that a specific restrictive cardiomyopathy exists secondary to a metabolic disturbance.

Management of Angina in People with Diabetes

This should be on similar lines to angina management for those who do not have diabetes. β Blockade is important and should not be withheld on the basis of masking hypoglycaemic attacks. Use a cardioselective agent (see Section 5.3). Aspirin is used in all patients with known coronary disease. Hypertension control is vital and the single most important manageable risk factor. ACE inhibitors are very useful with their additional renal protective effects and reduction in microalbuminuria.

Coronary disease tends to be diffuse in people with diabetes and angioplasty is best in short lesions. Abciximab should be used just before the procedure. In the EPISTENT trial abciximab reduced the 1-year mortality in patients with diabetes who are undergoing coronary stenting (4.1% vs 1.2%) and the target vessel revascularization rate at 6 months (16.6% vs 8.1%). There is a higher restenosis rate even with stents and abciximab in people with diabetes compared with those who do not have it. In the BARI trial published in 1996, conducted in the era before the use of stents or abciximab, CAB surgery in multivessel disease improved the long-term survival over balloon angioplasty alone (80.6% vs 65.5% 5-year survival rate). Analysis of this trial showed that the sole determining factor for better survival in the surgical group was the use of the left internal mammary artery graft (LIMA) as an arterial conduit. Even with surgery long-term results are not as good as in patients who do not have diabetes.

Drug-eluting stents have improved the restenosis rates. In the SIRIUS trial the bare metal stent restenosis rate in patients with diabetes was 50.5%, reduced to 17.6% with drug-eluting stents. (In those who do not have diabetes the figures were 36.3% vs 8.9% respectively.) The outcome of the CARDia trial comparing the long-term outcome of patients with diabetes treated with surgery vs drug-eluting stents and abciximab is eagerly awaited.

MI in Patients with Diabetes

This is silent in 12% and unrecognized in 39% of patients with diabetes (Framingham data). There is a higher rate in female and Asian patients. There is no diurnal variation in the timing of the infarct. Patients with diabetes are known to have a higher complication rate with a higher incidence of LVF and stroke.

Thrombolysis is important and should be given to patients with diabetic eye disease unless they have had a recent symptomatic retinal or vitreous haemorrhage. β Blockade should be started acutely. Oral hypoglycaemic agents should be stopped. There are theoretical concerns that sulphonylureas may inhibit ischaemic pre-conditioning by blocking the K^+ ATP channel, but this does not seem to be a clinical problem.

All infarcts in patients with diabetes should be managed with a regimen of intravenous insulin and glucose (DIGAMI trial).

11.9 Haemochromatosis

This should be considered in any young man with a DCM. It occasionally presents as a restrictive type of cardiomyopathy. Increased iron absorption with iron overload results in iron deposition in the myocyte sarcoplasm, with subsequent cell death and fibrosis. HLA-A3 and HLA-B14 are common. Additional features are liver disease, diabetes, skin pigmentation, hypopituitarism with hypogonadism, arthritis similar to rheumatoid and pseudogout. A similar illness may occur after repeated blood transfusions (e.g. for sickle cell anaemia, aplastic anaemia or thalassaemia major) with cardiac haemosiderosis.

There is a clinical picture of CCF, usually with a large heart. AF is common, ventricular arrhythmias and heart block less so. Iron does not deposit in the conducting system.

Diagnosis is usually made by liver biopsy or sternal marrow. Endomyocardial biopsy will show up iron stores on Prussian blue staining. Raised serum iron, low iron-binding capacity and high serum ferritin levels (often >1 g/ml with normal range 18–300 ng/ml or μg/l).

Treatment for haemochromatosis heart disease is venesection to remove iron over 1–2 years. Documented improvement in LV function has occurred with both venesection and desferrioxamine mesilate infusions to chelate the iron.

Desferrioxamine dose: 30–50 mg/kg per day infused intravenously over 8–10 h on at least 4 days a week. This is performed through a tunnelled central line. Patients with deteriorating LV function need constant infusions over 24 h 7 days a week. The social and psychological difficulties with this regimen are considerable. Long-term warfarin is needed to avoid thrombus formation at the tip of the central line.

Deferiprone: this is an oral iron chelator with a licence for use in thalassaemia. It could be considered an alternative to patients with haemochromatosis unable to tolerate venesection or desferrioxamine or their regimen.

Imaging the Iron-overloaded Heart

Conventional echocardiography can show early changes in diastolic dysfunction followed by ventricular dilatation and features of a dilated cardiomyopathy (see Section 4.1). Tissue Doppler imaging can pick up early subtle changes in diastolic function.

CMRI will show up iron-overloaded myocardium darker than normal. Early changes resulting from iron deposition can also be detected by MRI $T2^*$ imaging. This is a measure of the decay of the image with time. Normal $T2^*$ is >20 ms. Patients with a $T2^*$ of <8 ms have highly significant iron overload.

11.10 Metabolic Syndrome (Reaven 1988)

Unlike cardiac syndrome X with which, unfortunately, it is easily confused, patients with this condition are at risk of developing cardiovascular disease and progressing towards type 2 diabetes. It consists of patients with the following:
- Central (abdominal) obesity: BMI >30. Waist circumference in men >102 cm, and in women 88 cm. Waist:hip ratio >0.9 in men, >0.85 in women.
- Hypertriglyceridaemia: triglycerides >1.7 mmol/l.
- Low HDL-cholesterol <1.0 mmol/l (male) and 1.3 mmol/l (female)
- Systemic hypertension (>135/85)
- Fasting blood glucose >5.6 mmol/l (100 mg/dl).

Although these variables are generally accepted there are still substantial differences in definition of this syndrome in Europe. Of all of these variables the BP is the most important and a simple BP and waist measurement in the clinic is all that is really necessary initially.

The abdominal obesity resulting from an excessive accumulation of visceral fat seems to be particularly dangerous. These adipocytes not only store fat but are a biochemical factory producing a variety of hormones and cytokines (Figure 11.3).

Visceral adipocyte activity

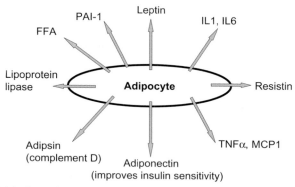

Figure 11.3 Metabolic syndrome section: visceral adipocyte activity. FFA, free fatty acids; PAI-1, plasminogen activator inhibitor 1. IL-1 and IL-6, interleukin-1 and -6; TNF, tumour necrosis factor; MCP1, macrophage chemoattractant protein 1.

The dyslipidaemia is similar to that in type 2 diabetes with a relative increase in small dense (atherogenic) LDL particles and increased levels of apolipoprotein B. Adiponectin levels are low. Insulin resistance occurs and hyperinsulinaemia is an independent cardiovascular risk factor. There is an interesting overlap, however, because insulin resistance has been found in some patients with cardiac syndrome X. Patients also have raised levels of plasminogen activator inhibitor (PAI-1) and hence reduced intrinsic fibrinolysis.

Risks of the Metabolic Syndrome
Approximately 4% of men and 2% of women will develop type 2 diabetes within 5 years of diagnosis. By the time symptomatic diabetes is diagnosed, 50% of pancreatic islet cells are lost and it is important to intervene early in diabetes before symptoms develop. Patients with the metabolic syndrome have a fourfold increased risk of cardiovascular death in 10 years.

Lifestyle Intervention
Workers in Finland have found that vigorous lifestyle intervention can prevent the onset of new diabetes:
• Weight reduction by >5%
• Reduce fat intake to <30% total calories and in particular reduce saturated fat intake by 10%
• Exercise >4 h/week
• Increase fibre and fresh vegetable intake.
   Patients achieving these aims did not develop diabetes and lifestyle intervention is probably more effective and certainly cheaper than multiple drug therapy.

Rimonabant in the Metabolic Syndrome

This drug inhibits the type 1 cannabinoid receptor (CB1 receptors both central in the hypothalamus and nucleus accumbens, and peripheral in adipocytes, liver, skeletal muscle, gastrointestinal tract and pancreas). It thus reduces appetite and is of benefit in quitting smoking. When 20 mg daily was given to patients with the metabolic syndrome (mean BMI 34) in the RIO trials it:

- reduced body weight by >5% in 50% of patients (vs 28% in controls), and 10% weight loss in 27%
- increased HDL 25% (8% greater than placebo)
- reduced triglycerides 15%
- normalized the glucose tolerance test; reduces fasting insulin without much change in fasting glucose, i.e. reduced insulin resistance
- showed no change in total LDL-cholesterol but rimonabant shifted the balance to larger, less atherogenic LDL particles
- increased adiponectin levels 46% (the protective cytokine).

In addition it reduced HbA1c in patients with diabetes and reduced progression of patients with the metabolic syndrome to type 2 diabetes. In hypertensive patients it reduces blood pressure (but not in non-hypertensive patients).

This is a new (but expensive) drug for the metabolic syndrome that does seem to reduce abdominal/visceral fat. It has no cardiovascular side effects but can cause some nausea and dizziness. The main problem is that on discontinuation of the drug all the biochemical variables above revert to their pre-treatment state. It is contraindicated in patients with a history of depression.

11.11 Myxoedema

This is most common in elderly people as a result of Hashimoto's thyroiditis. It affects women more than men. It may result from surgery, radio-iodine or drugs (amiodarone, lithium). Typical findings are the exact opposite to thyrotoxicosis: a low metabolic rate, raised SVR, hypodynamic circulation with low cardiac output. Patients may have:

- weight gain, cold intolerance, dry skin and hair, lethargy, menorrhagia, constipation, memory loss leading to frank dementia, myotonic jerks
- typical facial appearance: puffy eyes, eyebrow thinning, dull expression (Figure 11.4)
- sinus bradycardia, low pulse pressure
- pericardial, pleural, peritoneal and synovial effusions with high protein content; pericardial effusions accumulate slowly and tamponade is rare
- coronary disease: LDL-cholesterol is raised; ischaemia may often be silent
- ECG low voltage: long QT interval, conduction defects, bradycardia; permanent pacing may be needed.

Again it is an easily missed diagnosis in elderly people. Check free T_4 (low) and TSH (must be elevated for the diagnosis).

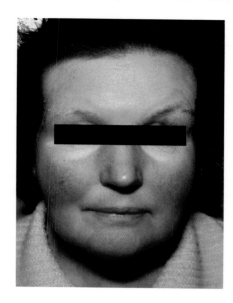

Figure 11.4 Hypothyroidism.

Management

Dose of L-thyroxine 50 μg daily up to 200 μg daily if indicated. Thyroid replacement requires great care in patients with coronary disease. Start at thyroxine 25 μg daily and increase very slowly (monthly or less). Patients with severe coronary disease should have CABG before replacement therapy.

Postcoronary bypass management can be difficult. Epicardial pacing wires are useful. Patients are sensitive to hypnotics and analgesics, and they do not respond to fluid challenge by increasing cardiac output. Pulmonary oedema may develop at relatively low LA pressures as capillary permeability is increased. Fluid input must be tightly controlled because there is a tendency to dilutional hyponatraemia.

11.12 Rheumatoid Arthritis

This causes symmetrical synovial thickening and inflammation leading to an erosive arthritis. It affects women more than men. Loss of articular cartilage leads to joint subluxation and destruction, coupled with weakening of ligaments and tendons. There is generalized illness with fever, normochromic/normocytic anaemia, possibly with splenomegaly (Felty syndrome), Sjögren syndrome and later secondary amyloidosis.

The heart is one of many organs involved in the extra-articular complications of rheumatoid arthritis. Cardiac involvement is not common and may be asymptomatic:

- *Pericarditis*: the most common form of cardiac involvement. Usually benign fibrinous pericarditis, often an asymptomatic pericardial rub associated with pleural involvement. Pericardial effusions may need aspiration. Occasionally leads to constriction.

• *Myocardial involvement*: rheumatoid nodules within the myocardium can rarely cause LV dysfunction. Conduction system involvement, leading to complete AV block.

• *Valve lesions*: small nodules on valves (aortic > mitral) can cause aortic regurgitation.

• *Coronary arteritis* is rare.

Other Organ Involvement

• Lung: pleural effusion, multiple pulmonary nodules, progressive interstitial fibrosis leading to honeycomb lung and pulmonary hypertension. Rheumatoid plus pneumoconiosis (Caplan syndrome).

• Vasculitis: Raynaud's phenomenon. Digital arteritis with focal pulp infarcts. Chronic leg ulcers. Gastrointestinal haemorrhage. Mesenteric or renal arteritis. Mononeuritis multiplex.

• Nervous system: peripheral neuropathy. Nerve compression, e.g. carpal tunnel syndrome.

• Eye: iridocyclitis (juvenile arthritis). Scleritis leading to scleromalacia perforans.

Management

This is the conventional treatment for cardiac complications if symptomatic. Most patients will already be on specific anti-inflammatory agents. It is not known whether steroid therapy in acute fibrinous pericarditis helps prevent later constriction.

11.13 Sarcoidosis

This is a multisystem granulomatous disease with a prevalence of about 20 per 100 000 in the UK. There is equal sex distribution. It is more common in Irish and African–Caribbean individuals. About 5% of cases of generalized sarcoid have overt cardiac involvement, but cardiac involvement occurs in about 25% of cases of widespread sarcoid post mortem.

Any part of the heart may be involved. Common sites are LV or RV free wall, interventricular septum, papillary muscles, AV node and the His–Purkinje system. Uncommonly, atrial muscle, pericardium, valve tissue or great vessels may be infiltrated. In order of frequency patients present with:

• complete AV block (20–30% of cases): Stokes–Adams attacks; often in young age group

• ventricular tachycardia or extrasystoles

• supraventricular arrhythmias

• chest pain simulating ischaemia

• sudden death in about 15%

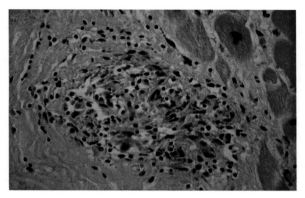

Figure 11.5 Cardiac sarcoid granuloma.

* acute myocarditis-like picture
* CCF with extensive infiltration.

Complete heart block may be transient. It is often rapidly reversible on steroid therapy but is an absolute indication for permanent pacing whatever the results of steroids. Myocardial infiltration may produce Q waves on an ECG, simulating old infarction. Mural thrombus can occur over infiltration sites. AV valve regurgitation occurs in 8% of patients but papillary muscle infiltration is a more common cause than granulomas on the valve. Old, healed, ventricular scars may cause small aneurysms. Diffuse myocardial involvement can cause a restrictive cardiomyopathy.

There is no single imaging technique that reliably picks up cardiac sarcoid, and granulomatous deposits (Figure 11.5) may be microscopic and missed on endomyocardial biopsy. Treatment may involve permanent pacing, steroid therapy for acute attacks (not curative) and antiarrhythmic therapy. Known ventricular aneurysms are not a contraindication for steroids. Digoxin is safe if AF develops.

11.14 Scleroderma/Systemic Sclerosis

This is a progressive systemic sclerosis, affecting women more than men. Fibrous thickening and degeneration of skin develop with changes also in the heart, lung, gastrointestinal (GI) tract and kidneys. Focal necrosis and subsequent fibrosis result from recurrent spasm of the small arterioles and intimal proliferation:

* Thickening and tightening of the skin, particularly in the fingers and face (mask-like). Loss of skin creases. Necrosis, scarring and tapering of the fingertips (sclerodactyly) with acrocyanosis. Restriction of finger movement and claw hand. Skeletal muscle atrophy.
* Raynaud's phenomenon.
* Lung involvement: pulmonary fibrosis and pulmonary hypertension. Stiff lungs. Reduced transfer factor (Kco) (see Section 13.5).

• Renal involvement with progressive renal failure and systemic hypertension. GI tract involvement with atrophy and fibrosis: dysphagia, hypomotility of small bowel, bacterial overgrowth, malabsorption.
• CREST syndrome: calcinosis, Raynaud's phenomenon, oesophageal involvement, sclerodactyly and telangiectasia.
• Pericarditis in 20%: may develop large effusions or later pericardial constriction.
• Myocardial involvement: focal fibrosis is the end-result of myofibrillar degeneration and contraction band necrosis. Large epicardial coronaries are usually normal. Microvascular intimal proliferation contributes to spasm-induced ischaemia. The end-result may be a DCM- or HCM-type picture.
• Primary valve disease is very rare (unlike other collagen vascular diseases).
• Conduction defects: pacing with a DDD unit may be necessary (dilated or stiff LV).

Management
The condition is relentless, with symptomatic control all that can be offered. Large doses of calcium antagonists such as nifedipine help the symptoms of Raynaud's phenomenon as well as controlling hypertension and possibly delaying progression of pulmonary hypertension. Conventional treatment for cardiac failure plus pacing may be needed.

11.15 Systemic Lupus Erythematosus

This is a multi-organ chronic inflammatory disease typically with fever, poly-arthralgia and arthritis, erythematous rash, including facial 'butterfly' rash, pleurisy, pericarditis, anaemia, thrombocytopenia, splenomegaly, renal failure and CNS involvement. It is much more common in young women. Drug-induced lupus (e.g. from procainamide) rarely causes CNS or renal disease.
  Cardiac involvement is common:
• Premature atherosclerotic coronary disease: patients with lupus who develop coronary disease are more likely to have raised LDL-cholesterol, tri-glycerides and lipoprotein(a) and reduced HDL. They are also more likely to have lupus anticoagulant and anti-phospholipid antibodies. Hypertension secondary to renal disease or exacerbated by steroids is an additional risk factor.
• Coronary arteritis is rare. Fibrinoid necrosis in small intramural vessels, with secondary thrombotic occlusion.
• Pericarditis: the most frequent form of cardiac involvement. As with rheumatoid arthritis, often silent. May be recurrent or need pericardial aspiration. Tamponade or later constriction can occur.
• Valve disease: Libman–Sacks endocarditis (see Section 9.8). TOE studies have shown valve involvement in 60% of patients with SLE, usually on the aortic and mitral valves. Therapy for SLE does not prevent valve vegetations,

and they cannot be used as a marker for successful therapy. Valve involvement is usually silent. Patients with definite vegetations in SLE should be advised to have antibiotic cover for dental procedures, etc. because the Libman–Sacks endocarditis may become secondarily infected.
• Myocarditis is rare. LV failure is more likely to result from hypertension or anaemia.

Other organ involvement:
• Skin: symmetrical rash on face, hands, fingertips; malar butterfly rash not all that common; periungual telangiectasia; discoid lupus lesions; reversible alopecia; hyperpigmentation or vitiligo; purpura; urticaria.
• Joints: similar distribution but less destructive than rheumatoid.
• Lung: pleurisy with or without effusion; basal atelectasis.
• Raynaud's phenomenon.
• Lupus nephritis: hypertension and progressive renal failure are common.
• CNS: CVAs are common and may result from vasculitis, emboli or intracerebral haemorrhage. If the CT shows an infarct and there is no evidence of vasculitis elsewhere, anticoagulation should be considered. Other CNS involvement includes depression, fits, cranial nerve palsy and peripheral neuropathy. Retinal lesions include white cytoid bodies.
• Sjögren syndrome.

Management
• Steroids for acute exacerbation of the illness with possible additional azathioprine or cyclophosphamide.
• Non-steroidal anti-inflammatory agents where possible for recurrent pericarditis.
• Valve replacement rarely necessary for Libman–Sacks non-infective endocarditis.
• Renal failure most common cause of death.

11.16 Thyrotoxicosis

Thyroxine increases cardiac β-receptors (effects similar to catecholamine excess) but also acts separately.

Results in an increased total blood volume, metabolic rate, heart rate, stroke volume, cardiac output, coronary and skeletal muscle blood flow, contractility, LVEDV, rate of diastolic relaxation and atrial excitability. Results in a decreased SVR, diastolic filling time and contractility reserve (no increase in LVEF on exercise). Patients may have:
• weight loss, heat intolerance, eye signs with proptosis, ophthalmoplegia, chemosis, amenorrhoea
• tachycardia: high sleeping pulse rate; wide pulse pressure
• loud heart sounds: S3; exertional dyspnoea
• ejection systolic flow murmur: high stroke volume
• hyperdynamic apex

- pleuropericardial rub with hyperkinetic heart
- AF in 9–22% (normal population 0.4%)
- systemic embolic risk
- angina even with normal coronaries; rarely, MI
- high-output failure: large heart may resemble DCM; similar to chronic anaemia.

In elderly people thyrotoxicosis is easily overlooked. There may be no eye signs or obvious goitre. Total T_4 and T_3 levels may be normal even in the thyrotoxic patient in cardiac failure because peripheral conversion of T_4 to T_3 is reduced, and thyroxine-binding globulin (TBG) levels are low, reducing total T_4. Therefore measure free T_4 (high) and TSH (low) in any patient with AF of unknown cause.

Management
- Rate control: digoxin alone is rarely enough. Additional β blockade or verapamil needed. Avoid β blockers with intrinsic sympathomimetic activity. Large doses may be needed (increased clearance). If large heart on chest radiograph, avoid β blockade and calcium antagonists, and just use digoxin, diuretics and antithyroid drugs. For the rare thyroid storm propranolol is given intravenously 0.1 mg/kg slowly over 10 min.
- Start carbimazole 10–15 mg or propylthiouracil 100 mg three times daily.
- Avoid cardioversion until the patient is definitely euthyroid.
- Anticoagulate until back in SR: LV function should improve with successful treatment and the heart becomes smaller on the chest radiograph but it may never return completely to normal.

12 Systemic Hypertension

Definition

Blood pressure rises with age (Table 12.1), with cold environment or anxiety, with effort, and varies with the time of day (lowest at 4.00 am, rising rapidly by 9.00 am). With mild hypertension the blood pressure is taken twice or more before calling a patient 'hypertensive'. With more severe hypertension this is not necessary. Elevation of systolic or diastolic pressure is of equal importance.

Table 12.1 Blood pressure and age

Age (years)	Normal (mmHg)	Borderline (mmHg)	Definite (mmHg)
17–40	<140/80	150/90	>160/100
41–50	<140/80	150/90	>160/100
≥60	<150/90	160/90	>170/100

12.1 Pitfalls in Measurement

A long cuff is needed to encircle the arm. Too small a cuff or too fat an arm results in spuriously high readings. The patient should be calm having had 5-min rest and having abstained from drinking coffee and smoking. The blood pressure should be measured to the nearest 2 mmHg in the seated position. It is preferable to use Korotkow's phase 5 (disappearance of the sounds) for the diastolic reading rather than phase 4 (muffling of the sounds).

The initial BP should be measured in both arms and the higher reading taken (sometimes BP is a little higher in the right arm). If the patient has symptoms of postural hypotension measure the BP standing.

Swanton's Cardiology, sixth edition. By R. H. Swanton and S. Banerjee. Published 2008 Blackwell Publishing. ISBN 978-1-4051-7819-8.

Ambulatory 24-hour BP recording may occasionally be necessary in patients whose BP recordings are wildly different at subsequent visits, or to check the effectiveness of drug treatment (Figure 12.1).

Self-testing with home monitoring devices should not be encouraged but in the enthusiastic or anxious patient their use may be unavoidable. Their value has not been established.

12.2 Significance of Hypertension and Who to Treat

Hypertension is associated with an increased risk of cerebrovascular disease, retinopathy, cardiac failure, MI, occlusive peripheral arterial disease and renal failure. Each increment of 10 mmHg systolic pressure reduces life expectancy. Successful blood pressure control reduces mortality from CVA and renal failure (but not definitely myocardial infarct deaths). Each reduction in systolic pressure of 6 mmHg reduces the CVA risk by 40%. Start treatment if:
- BP >160/100 mmHg
- Isolated systolic hypertension with systolic pressure >160 mmHg
- BP >140/90 plus a calculated 10-year CVD risk >20%, or evidence of existing target organ damage (e.g. coronary, renal or cerebrovascular disease).
- Diabetics: Treat if BP >130/85

The aim is to achieve a BP of 140/90 or less. In elderly people with isolated systolic hypertension this may be a very difficult target and any reduction in BP is worthwhile.

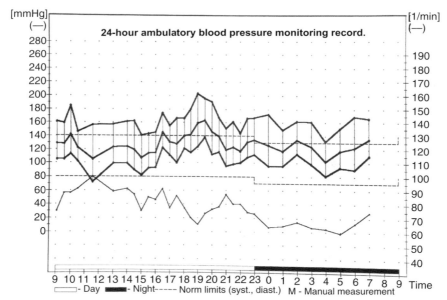

Figure 12.1 Ambulatory 24-hour BP monitoring: hypertensive patient showing both systolic and diastolic pressures above the 140/80 target lines and no nocturnal drop in BP.

12.3 Typical Symptoms and Signs

Symptoms
There are usually none. An elevated BP is most frequently just found on a routine examination.
- Headache: frontal or occipital headaches are typically worse in the morning
- May have migraine
- Dizziness or light-headedness
- Dyspnoea on effort progressing to orthopnoea or PND
- Angina (increased muscle mass + coronary disease) and/or claudication
- Nocturia even if off diuretics
- Possibly haematuria and/or dysuria in history
- History of transient ischaemic attacks
- Mild visual disturbance
- Epistaxes.

Signs to Note
- Blood pressure in both arms
- Synchrony of radial and femoral pulses
- Check all peripheral pulses
- Arterial bruits: carotid, aortic, renal
- LV hypertrophy
- ? S_3 present
- Fundal examination: AV nipping, haemorrhages, exudates, papilloedema
- Check for proteinuria.

Causes
- Essential: 95% of cases
- Renal disease, glomerulonephritis, pyelonephritis, polycystic disease, hydronephrosis
- Renal artery stenosis (atheromatous plaques or fibromuscular hyperplasia)
- Coarctation of the aorta
- Phaeochromocytoma
- Primary hyperaldosteronism (Conn syndrome)
- Cushing syndrome
- Iatrogenic drug therapy: glucocorticoids, carbenoxolone, MAOIs, sympathomimetics, oestrogens
- Acromegaly
- Hypercalcaemia
- CNS disturbances: raised intracranial pressure, familial dysautonomia
- Postoperative: especially cardiopulmonary bypass
- Pre-eclampsia
- Pseudohyperaldosteronism (Liddle syndrome).

12.4 Investigations

Almost all patients will have essential hypertension (? family history) and the necessary investigations are: FBC, U&Es, creatinine (preferably U&Es off diuretics). Urine testing: protein, blood, sugar (if positive, urine culture); chest radiograph; ECG.

A routine intravenous urogram (IVU) is not necessary. It should be considered in patients with a history of renal disease and in those who are most likely to have renovascular hypertension:
• Onset of hypertension under the age of 30 years
• Accelerated hypertension or deteriorating renal function
• Hypertension after renal trauma, or an episode of renal pain
• Presence of a renal bruit.

The estimation of 24-hour urine catecholamines is expensive but the test should be done in all cases of hypertension + glycosuria, patients with a history of paroxysmal hypertension, sweating, palpitations, episodes of hypotension or the young patient. Three 24-hour urine vanillylmandelic acid (VMA) levels were required with the patient on a vanilla-free diet and preferably off all drugs (normal range up to 35 µmol/24 h). A test with a single 24-h urine collection for catecholamines is now diagnostic (see Section 12.6). Urine saves must be done before the IVU.

Echocardiography is much more useful in establishing LV hypertrophy than the ECG. It also provides useful information on LV function and quantifies any associated aortic regurgitation (root dilatation).

12.5 Renovascular Hypertension (Renal Artery Stenosis)

This is an easily missed diagnosis. There are two types of pathological lesion: fibromuscular hyperplasia and atheromatous/arteriosclerotic disease. Disease presentation differs (Table 12.2).

The following are clinical features that suggest renal artery stenosis is contributing to or causing hypertension:
• Young patient with no family history of hypertension
• Peripheral vascular disease

Table 12.2 Pathology of renal artery stenosis

Fibromuscular hyperplasia	Atheromatous stenosis
Mainly effects females	More common in males
Younger age group	Older age group
Renal function often normal	Renal function impaired
Normal peripheral vessels	Peripheral vascular disease
Not smoking related	Heavy smokers

- Resistant hypertension or deteriorating BP in a compliant patient
- Rising serum creatinine on an ACE inhibitor or an AIIRA
- Renal impairment with minimal proteinuria
- Secondary hyperaldosteronism
- Sudden pulmonary oedema.

Investigations

- Abdominal ultrasonography with renal artery Doppler studies. This is not possible in obese patients.
- Magnetic resonance angiography (MRA): the investigation of choice. Both radiation and femoral artery catheterization can be avoided.
- Abdominal aortogram (Figure 12.2) if MRA unavailable.
- Digital subtraction arteriography (DSA) of the renal vessels: this is preferable to direct intubation of the renal arteries themselves and a flush descending aortogram with DSA is usually all that is needed. Rarely necessary now with good MRA.
- IVU: features suggesting renal artery stenosis on an IVU are a disparity of renal size by >1.5 cm, delayed appearance of dye on the affected side with increased density of dye later on that side. With a positive IVU, the following investigations may be considered necessary to demonstrate that the abnormal kidney is the cause of the hypertension:
  - captopril-enhanced renal scintigraphy is a reliable and safe investigation
  - technetium-labelled DTPA renogram is performed before and after a 12.5 mg dose of captopril; renal function drops sharply on the affected side; less helpful if bilateral stenoses

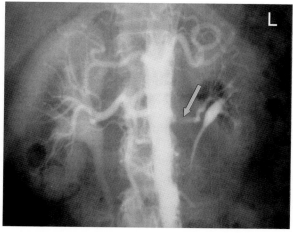

Figure 12.2 Systemic hypertension: left renal artery stenosis. Note smaller left kidney with denser urogram.

– plasma renin activity (peripheral blood) lying and after 1 hour standing

– renal vein:renin ratio: simultaneous sampling with the patient off β blockade. A ratio >1.5:1 (abnormal to normal) is significant. Differential ureteric sampling is now rarely needed in most patients.

Angioplasty or Surgery for Renal Artery Stenosis

Renal angioplasty is more successful in fibromuscular hyperplasia than in arteriosclerotic vessels. There is a risk of renal artery dissection or acute occlusion. Before stenting the cure rate for dilatation of fibromuscular hyperplasia was about 50%, but only about 20% for successful dilatation in arteriosclerotic vessels. Proximal and ostial renal artery stenoses have until recently been managed surgically. Stenting all these lesions is now increasingly popular and successful, but as with coronary stenting in-stent restenosis may occur.

There is no point in renal artery intervention if there is no evidence of renal function on the affected side, the kidney is <8 cm in size or the renal artery is totally occluded.

Surgery is now rarely required. It involves renal endarterectomy, autotransplantation, aortorenal saphenous vein bypass or nephrectomy. The splenic artery can be used to replace the renal artery because it is usually free of atheroma. Removal of a small kidney does not necessarily result in improvement in blood pressure.

12.6 Phaeochromocytoma

Most of these tumours occur in the adrenal medulla arising from neurochromaffin cells. Extramedullary tumours (paragangliomas or ganglioneuromas) can occur anywhere along the sympathetic chain, posterior mediastinum or heart. About 5% are associated with the multiple endocrine neoplasia syndrome (MEN) type II, or with the von Hippel–Lindau syndrome (retinal and cerebellar haemangiomas) or in neurofibromatosis (von Recklinghausen's disease). These neuroendocrine tumours can secrete a variety of polypeptides, e.g. calcitonin, parathyroid hormone, calcitonin gene-related peptide (CGRP), vasoactive intestinal peptide (VIP, causing watery diarrhoea and hypokalaemia) or neuropeptide Y.

Symptoms are often paroxysmal with episodes of palpitation, angina, headaches, dizziness, sweating and visual disturbance. There may be intense peripheral vasoconstriction producing a pale, mottled, cold skin. Postural hypotension may occur with volume depletion. Acute pulmonary oedema may occur as a result of a catecholamine-induced myocarditis plus hypertensive LVF.

ECG is usually abnormal, with variable T-wave inversion in chest leads and signs of LV hypertrophy.

Urine testing: may have catecholamine-driven glycosuria.

Diagnosis

• Urinary catecholamines. The estimation of urinary adrenaline, noradrenaline and dopamine has superseded the old estimation of urinary VMA, which is less sensitive. Until recently diagnosis rested on three 24-hour urine collections because hormone release is pulsatile. However, it is possible to screen for a phaeochromocytoma by comparing the catecholamine concentration in a single 24-hour urine sample with the urine creatinine, avoiding the problem of multiple or incomplete urine collections (Table 12.3). Urine collection is in acid bottles.

Adrenal venous blood contains adrenaline:noradrenaline in a 4:1 ratio. High adrenaline levels suggest an adrenal tumour. Very high noradrenaline levels compared with adrenaline suggest an extramedullary tumour:

• Abdominal ultrasonography: if adrenal tumour is not visualized consider:

  – CT and/or MRI of adrenals, 5% of the tumours are multiple (may be bilateral) and approximately 5% are malignant.

  – IVU with tomography of the adrenals. Urine collections should precede the IVU.

  – pentolinium suppression test: plasma catecholamines should be suppressed by 2.5 mg pentolinium. Failure of suppression is a positive test, but false-positive results can occur in renal failure.

  – clonidine suppression test: after 0.3 mg clonidine orally, plasma catecholamines should fall to <500 pmol/ml in 3 h.

  – MIBG scan: iodine[123]-labelled *meta*-iodobenzylguanidine ([123I]MIBG) is a guanethidine analogue, and is taken up by presynaptic adrenergic neurons. Dense uptake occurs in phaeochromocytoma tissue. It is a very valuable imaging method for extramedullary tumours.

• With modern imaging techniques, further investigations are rarely necessary. More dangerous investigations such as arteriography or adrenal venous and IVC sampling are performed only after adequate α and β blockade with intra-arterial pressure monitoring.

Table 12.3 Catecholamines: normal ranges

Normal ranges	Adrenaline	Noradrenaline	Dopamine
24-hour urine total	8–150 nmol	50–570 nmol	0–3240 nmol
Catecholamine/	≤15 nmol/mmol	≤53 nmol/mmol	≤338 nmol/mmol
urine creatinine	urine creatinine	urine creatinine	urine creatinine
Plasma	0.1–1.2 pmol/ml	0.5–3.5 pmol/ml	
Platelet	0.03–0.7 pmol/mg	0.33–3.2 pmol/mg	
	platelet protein	platelet protein	

Therapy before Invasive Investigation or Surgery

A minimum of oral phenoxybenzamine 10 mg three times daily and pro-pranolol 80 mg three times daily is needed for 2 weeks, starting the phenoxy-benzamine first. Diuretics should be avoided because there is already volume depletion. Long-acting calcium antagonists may be used. Gradual control of blood pressure is important. Sudden falls could provoke retinal or cerebral infarction. Persistent hypertension in spite of adequate α and β blockade may be a result of other peptides (e.g. endothelin, neuropetide Y) secreted by the tumour. Further control of hypertension is managed during investigation or surgery by intravenous phentolamine, hydralazine or trimetaphan (see Section 12.7).

Immediately after tumour removal, intense vasodilatation may occur requiring close attention to volume replacement. Central venous and intra-arterial pressure monitoring are essential.

Malignant phaeochromocytoma will require long-term α and β blockade, additional chemotherapy, and attempts to block further catecholamine secretion with α-methyltyrosine or [^{131}I]MIBG.

12.7 Treatment of Systemic Hypertension

General Measures

Weight reduction, reducing alcohol intake, increasing exercise and even medi-tation have all independently been shown to reduce blood pressure in hyper-tensive patients. Discourage the addition of salt to food (but patients may use it in cooking). Women on the pill should be advised to switch to a different form of contraception if treatment is not quickly successful. Patients with severe hypertension (>230/130) should be admitted for bed rest and carefully monitored treatment.

Drug Treatment

Patients should be advised that almost all antihypertensive therapy has some side effects. Treatment will be necessary for life in most cases. Stopping therapy usually results in the blood pressure climbing again. Drug treatment should be tailored to the individual patient and there is no single ideal regimen. Multiple drug therapy is often necessary. As well as being more effective, this may reduce drug side effects by avoiding large doses of indi-vidual drugs. Aim if possible for a once-daily drug regimen.

It used to be thought that it did not matter which drug regimen was chosen as long as it brought the blood pressure down to target levels. After the LIFE and ASCOT trials this philosophy no longer holds. In the LIFE trial losartan was superior to atenolol in stroke prevention in spite of equal blood pressure reduction. This was particularly so in patients >75 years. In the ASCOT trial amlodipine (with added perindopril if necessary) was found to be superior to a regimen of atenolol (adding a thiazide if necessary) in terms of reducing cardiovascular events and inducing less diabetes. Again blood pressure reduction in the two groups was very similar (2.7 mmHg better in the amlodipine arm) but the outcomes were different. In addition the amlodipine/perindopril regime helped prevent the development of type 2 diabetes.

Diuretics

Thiazides increase salt and water excretion but can cause hyperuricaemia, hypercalcaemia, hypokalaemia, hypertrigyceridaemia and lower HDL-cholesterol. They may cause impotence. Furosemide is not a good drug for hypertension unless used with captopril, or there is a degree of renal failure. Spironolactone is most useful for primary hyperaldosteronism, but is of great value in resistant hypertension even in small doses (12.5–25 mg daily). Vasodilators and β-blocking agents are discussed in Chapter 5.

There has been a gradual shift away from diuretics and β blockade as initial treatment (even before the ASCOT trial results) to drugs with fewer long-term side effects: calcium antagonists, ACE inhibitors or α_1 blockers. Table 12.4 summarizes the effects of these five groups of drugs on metabolic and other variables.

It can be seen that β blockade and thiazides have deleterious effects on lipid metabolism. HDL levels are lowered, and triglycerides and fasting glucose levels are raised by the β blockade/thiazide combination.

Angiotensin Receptor Antagonists AIIRA (see also Section 6.6)

These drugs are tolerated well by patients who find the cough induced by ACE inhibitors intolerable. As they are specific for the angiotensin receptor, bradykinin levels are not increased, and there is no first-dose effect (gradual onset of action). They reduce but do not completely inhibit aldosterone release, so hyperkalaemia is less likely than with ACE inhibitors. They have a mild uricosuric action.

It can be seen that, although all classes of drugs reduce blood pressure, diuretics and β blockers have the worst metabolic profile. Most patients can

Table 12.4 Metabolic effects of antihypertensive drugs

Parameter	Diuretic	β Blocker	Calcium antagonist	ACE inhibitor	α_1 Blocker
LDL-cholesterol	–	–/0	0	0	+
HDL-cholesterol	0	–	0	0	+/0
Triglycerides	–	–	0	0	+
Glucose intolerance	–	–	0	+	+
Activity	0	–	0	0	0
LV hypertrophy	0	+	+	+	+
Blood pressure	+	+	+	+	+

0, no effect; –, deleterious effect; +, beneficial effect.

be managed on an ACE inhibitor, or an AIIRA or a long-acting calcium antagonist as a single agent.

Summary of Classes of Drugs Available for Hypertension

• Calcium antagonist: amlodipine 5–10 mg once daily, or nifedipine LA 30–60 mg once daily or verapamil slow release 120–240 mg once daily. Main side effects are ankle oedema (dose dependent), constipation, flushing and gingival hyperplasia.

• ACE inhibitor: enalapril 2.5–5.0 mg once or twice daily (maximum dose 20 mg twice daily), or lisinopril 2.5–5.0 mg once daily (maximum dose 40 mg once daily) or ramipril 1.25 mg once daily (maximum dose 10 mg once daily), or perindopril 2–4 mg (maximum dose 8 mg once daily). Diuretic needed with bigger doses (see Section 6.6). Spironolactone can be added (watching for hyperkalaemia) as 40% patients on long-term ACE inhibitors have raised levels of aldosterone (ACE escape).

• Angiotensin II receptor antagonist (AIIRA), e.g. losartan 50–100 mg or valsartan 80–160 mg or irbesartan 150–300 mg or candesartan 4–16 mg, all once daily. Similar in effect to ACE inhibitors, but do not cause a cough because they have no effect on bradykinin levels. Useful in ACE-intolerant patients, or as additional therapy to ACE inhibitors in resistant hypertension (watching for possible hyperkalaemia). AIIRAs or ARBs also reduce microalbuminuria in patients with diabetes.

ACE inhibitors and AIIRAs are contraindicated in renal artery stenosis. Interglomerular filtration pressure is maintained in renal artery stenosis by increased tone in the efferent arteriole (mediated by angiotensin II). ACE inhibitors and ARAs may prevent this autoregulatory mechanism and glomerular filtration may fall sharply, precipitating renal failure.

• α_1-Blocking agent: doxazosin slow release 4 mg once daily (maximum dose 16 mg once daily). This has a longer half-life than prazosin and tachyphylaxis is not a problem. Ankle swelling and nasal stuffiness are common side effects. Doxazosin received bad press in the ALLHAT trial, but the trial itself has been much criticized. Probably best avoided as monotherapy but useful as an additional drug in more resistant cases.

• β-Blocking agent, e.g. atenolol 50–100 mg once daily, or the longer-acting bisoprolol 2.5–10 mg once daily, or labetolol 50–100 mg three times daily (which has additional α-blocking activity). These drugs are no longer the routine initial drug of choice. Their metabolic profile is inferior to ACE inhibitors (table). However, β-blocking agents are indicated for:

  – the hyperactive or anxious patient with sympathetic overdrive
  – the patient with additional angina or a previous history of MI
  – women of child-bearing years (ACE inhibitors and ARBs contraindicated in pregnancy)
  – intolerance of ACE inhibitors or AIIRAs.

If the β-blocking agent is being withdrawn, do so gradually. If additional treatment is needed add in a dihydropyridine calcium antagonist (amlodipine or nifedipine) rather than a thiazide.

- Methyldopa: rarely used now except in the hypertensive pregnant patient where it can be a drug of first choice (see Section 15.2). Start at 250 mg three times daily. Side effects: drowsiness, nasal stuffiness and rarely haemolytic anaemia.
- Imidazoline (I_1)-receptor agonist: moxonidine 200–400 µg daily. Centrally acting. Reduces sympathetic outflow lowering peripheral resistance. Similar to clonidine but does not activate α_2-receptors. Avoid in severe renal or cardiac failure. With more resistant hypertension different classes of drugs are used in combination. Always consider patient compliance with failing treatment.
- Renin inhibition: aliskiren is a new oral agent that specifically inhibits renin. It is synergistic when used with angiotensin II receptor blockers. Hyperkalemia must be watched for. Dose 150 mg o.d.
- Rimonabant: a centrally acting cannabinoid receptor antagonist. Primarily of value in obese patients, causing very effective weight reduction and diabetes control; it also lowered blood pressure in the RIO trials in the hypertensive, but not the normotensive, patient. Dose 20 mg o.d.

Joint NICE–BHS Treatment Algorithm (2006) (Table 12.5)
This is also known as the ACD algorithm. It emphasises that ACE inhibitors are not first-choice drugs in black patients (less effective), several drugs are often needed and β-blocking agents are now relegated to fourth-choice agent.

Failure to Control BP: Resistant Hypertension (Table 12.6)
There are many reasons for this; in order of probability:
- Inadequate treatment regimen: some patients will require several different drugs together using doses low enough to avoid side effects as much as possible.
- Compliance: failure to take the drugs because of side effects. This is common particularly in men who may become impotent on therapy.

Table 12.5 ACD algorithm

Patient age	Age < 55 years	Age > 55 years or black patient of any age
Step 1	A (ARB)	C or D
Then for both		
Step 2	A (ARB) + C or A (ARB) + D	
Step 3	A (ARB) + C + D	
Step 4	A (ARB) + C + D + B	
or	A (ARB) + C + D + AB	
or	A (ARB) + C + D + 2nd D	

A (ARB), ACE inhibitor or angiotensin receptor blocker if ACE intolerant; B, β blocker; C, calcium antagonist; D, diuretic; AB: α blocker; 2nd D, additional second diuretic.

Table 12.6 Causes of resistant hypertension

Wrong drug regimen
Poor compliance (side effects)
Severe arteriosclerosis
Excess salt intake
Sodium-retaining drugs
ACE escape
Renovascular hypertension
Surgical hypertension

- The elderly arteriosclerotic patient: old rigid arteries do not dilate well. Care must be taken not to be too enthusiastic about BP control in this age group. Acute reduction in pressure will reduce cerebral perfusion and may cause syncope or a CVA.
- Excessive salt intake: patients must be told to avoid all added salt, and to avoid salty foods.
- Additional drug therapy causing sodium retention: steroids and non-steroidal anti-inflammatory drugs (NSAIDs). Can the steroid therapy be reduced? Can the NSAID be switched to a different analgesic?
- ACE escape: 40% patients on long-term ACE inhibitors have raised levels of aldosterone and additional low-dose spironolactone (or dual blockade with an angiotensin II receptor blocker) may be useful.
- Renovascular hypertension.
- Rarely 'surgical' lesions, e.g. phaeochromocytoma.

Malignant (Accelerated) Hypertension and Pre-eclampsia (see also Section 15.2)

With severe malignant hypertension, complete bed rest and parenteral therapy are needed with intra-arterial pressure monitoring:

- nitroprusside intravenous dose regimen mentioned earlier
- labetalol 200 mg in 200 ml 0.9% saline infused at 1–2 mg (1–2 ml)/min.

CHAPTER 13

Pulmonary Hypertension and Pulmonary Embolism

13.1 Pulmonary Hypertension (PHT)

There is a considerable fall in PVR in the first 24 hours of life when the ductus closes. The PVR continues to fall for the first few months.

PHT exists when peak systolic PA pressure exceeds 25 mmHg at rest or 30 mmHg on exercise.

Histologically there is a reduction in calibre of pulmonary arterioles. This is a result of a combination of intimal hyperplasia 'onion skinning', medial hypertrophy in larger arterioles, and occlusion of pulmonary arterioles from intimal and endothelial proliferation with secondary thrombosis and plexi-form lesions.

The most common causes are the result of left heart problems, thromboembolic disease, lung disease or left-to-right shunts, with high pulmonary blood flow causing reactive changes in the pulmonary vasculature in the first year of life. The WHO classification below has recently been revised.

World Health Organization Classification of PHT

Group I: Pulmonary Arterial Hypertension
- Idiopathic primary PHT
- Familial
- Associated with other conditions: collagen vascular disease (scleroderma), congenital left-to-right shunts (e.g. ASD, VSD, PDA), portal hypertension, HIV infection, drugs (e.g. anorexigens, l-tryptophan, methamphetamine, cocaine), bush tea (crotalaria fulva) rapeseed oil, glycogen storage disease, Gaucher's disease, hereditary haemorrhagic telangiectasia, haemoglobinopathies (e.g. sickle cell disease, β-thalassaemia), myeloproliferative disorders with thrombocythaemia.
- Associated with significant venous or capillary involvement: pulmonary veno-occlusive disease, pulmonary capillary haemangiomatosis
- Persistent PHT of the newborn.

Swanton's Cardiology, sixth edition. By R. H. Swanton and S. Banerjee. Published 2008 Blackwell Publishing. ISBN 978-1-4051-7819-8.

Group II: Pulmonary Venous Hypertension
- Left-sided atrial or ventricular heart disease: includes ischaemic heart disease, cardiomyopathies, atrial myxoma, cor triatriatum, pericardial constriction
- Left-sided valvular heart disease: aortic and mitral valve disease.

Group III: PHT Associated with Hypoxaemia
- Chronic obstructive pulmonary disease
- Interstitial lung disease (pulmonary fibrosis)
- Obstructive sleep apnoea, Pickwickian syndrome
- Chronic exposure to high altitude
- Developmental disorders
- Alveolar hypoventilation disorders
- Neuromuscular disorders: polio, myasthenia.

Group IV: PHT Caused by Chronic Thromboembolic Disease
- Thrombotic obstruction of major proximal or distal pulmonary arteries
- Non-thrombotic pulmonary embolism: tumour, parasites, foreign material.

Group V: Miscellaneous Causes
- Sarcoidosis
- Histiocytosis
- Lymphangiomatosis
- Compression of pulmonary vessels by tumour, lymphadenopathy, mediastinal fibrosis.

Variability of PHT
Various factors (Table 13.1) may alter pulmonary artery pressure and these are relevant to treatment. The most important is the role of oxygen in regulating pulmonary vascular tone.

Table 13.1 Variability of pulmonary hypertension

Increasing PHT	Decreasing PHT
Hypoxia, high altitude	Oxygen
Acidosis	Acetylcholine
Hypercapnia	Hydralazine
High haematocrit	α-Blocking agents
Prostaglandin $F_{2\alpha}$ and A_2	Prostaglandin E and I_2
? Histamine	Pirbuterol
α Agonists	Calcium antagonists
	Nitrates, nitric oxide
	PDE5 inhibitors
	Endotheline antagonists

Elevated haematocrit is important in patients with cyanotic congenital heart disease and Eisenmenger syndrome.

13.2 Pulmonary Embolism

Symptoms
- Dyspnoea: acute-onset dyspnoea is typical. In retrospect mild dyspnoea may precede the acute attack by a day or two. In a few cases dyspnoea presents as acute bronchospasm.
- Pain: sudden-onset pleuritic chest pain probably occurs with smaller emboli. Involvement of the diaphragmatic pleura causes shoulder-tip pain. Pain may be primarily abdominal.
- Cough: persistent dry cough is common.
- Haemoptysis: streaky or frank. Haemoptysis may persist with resolution of the infarcted segment.
- Sweating, fear and apprehension.
- Syncope occurs with massive pulmonary embolism. Pre-syncope and transient episodes of hypotension may occur with smaller ones. Overall mortality rate is approximately 8–10%.
- There may be none if the embolus is small.

Signs
- A restless, centrally cyanosed, sweaty, distressed and dyspnoeic patient
- JVP raised with prominent 'a' wave if in SR
- Tachycardia, low-volume pulse, transient rhythm disturbance
- RV: S_3/S_4 gallop
- Accentuated delayed P_2
- Fever
- Chest signs: rates, later a pleural rub
- Leg signs: only about a third of patients have evidence of deep vein thrombosis (DVT with phlebitis, oedema, etc.)
- Cardiac arrest and sudden death.

Many of the signs above are non-specific and a high index of suspicion should be maintained for patients at risk (Table 13.2). In addition smaller pulmonary emboli may be missed clinically, presenting as a flick in the temperature chart, mild dyspnoea and transient AF, SVT or just ventricular ectopic beats.

Not all these factors are of equal risk. Table 13.3 details odds ratios of increased risk for venous thromboembolism from the common secondary risk factors.

ECG Changes (Not Specific for Pulmonary Embolism)
Typical acute RV strain shows as: $S_1\ Q_3\ T_3$ pattern in standard leads, incomplete or complete RBBB, T-wave inversion in anterior chest leads (see Chapter 16, Figure 16.9).

Table 13.2 Patients at risk for venous thromboembolism

Secondary factors	Procoagulant factors
History of previous DVTs	Polycythaemia/hyperviscosity
Patients on prolonged bed rest	Anticardiolipin antibodies
Stroke	Protein C deficiency
Prolonged use of central venous lines	Protein S deficiency
After MI (see Section 5.10)	Lupus anticoagulant
Patients on diuretics – haemoconcentration	Factor V Leiden (activated protein C
Patients with CCF – low flows	resistance: APC-R)
Surgery: especially pelvic and prostatic surgery	Thrombocythaemia
Leg trauma: especially recent hip or knee	Antithrombin III deficiency
replacement	Raised levels of PAI-1 (plasminogen
Pelvic inflammatory disease	activator inhibitor)
Malignant disease ± chemotherapy	Factor XII deficiency
Prolonged travel: lengthy flight or train journey	Hyperhomocysteinaemia
Pregnancy/puerperium	Dysfibrinogenaemia
Smokers	Prothrombin G20210A mutation
Oral contraceptive pill	
Obesity	

Table 13.3 Relative risk of various secondary factors

Odds ratio >10	Odds ratio 2–9	Odds ratio <2
Hip or leg fracture	Arthroscopy	Bed rest > 5 days
Hip or knee replacement	CVP lines	Age > 40
General surgery	Chemotherapy	
Major trauma	Malignancy	
Spinal cord surgery	CCF	
	CVA	

Other possibilities to note: right axis shift. Rhythm changes: ectopic atrial or ventricular, AF or SVT; ST–T changes with ST depression over inferior leads. All these may be transient.

Chest Radiograph Changes

There may be very little to see on the chest radiograph of patients with small pulmonary emboli.

Features to look for include in the acute stage: elevated hemidiaphragm, pulmonary oligaemia in one or more segments, large pulmonary artery conus or enlargement of a single hilar artery with rapid pruning or tapering.

Later on (from 24 hours to 1 week), if pulmonary infarction occurs, the chest radiograph may show: pulmonary infiltrates, plate atelectasis, small pleural effusions or pleural thickening.

Super-added infection in an infarcted segment may cause cavitation.

Table 13.4 Pulmonary emboli

May be silent
5% of all hospital deaths
Mimics acute inferior myocardial infarction clinically and on ECG (see Figure 16.9)
Very unlikely if arterial Po_2 is normal
Spiral CT scanning the best diagnostic test
Volume load: the acute case (500 ml)
Intravenous unfractionated heparin for all, and thrombolysis if haemodynamically unwell
Pulmonary embolectomy for the shocked moribund case

Table 13.5 Wells scoring system for prediction of pulmonary embolism

Variable	Score
Previous DVT or pulmonary embolism	1.5
Immobilization	1.5
Malignancy	1.0
Haemoptysis	1.0
Heart rate >100/min	1.0
Signs of a DVT	3.0

Low likelihood score <2, intermediate 2–6, highly likely >7.

Echocardiography

The echocardiograph is used to detect RV dysfunction and dilatation and to estimate PA pressure from Doppler analysis of the tricuspid regurgitant jet (see Section 17.3). It is not a useful diagnostic tool, but moderate or severe RV dysfunction is an indication for thrombolysis or embolectomy (see below).

Making the Diagnosis

This may be difficult. Small emboli may be easily missed (Table 13.4). Being aware of the possibility is half the battle. Diagnosis is based on the following factors.

• *Patient at risk*: numerous factors are recognized to put the patient at risk (see above).
• *Clinical predictors*: the Wells (Canadian) scoring system adds up points for a few simple variables (Table 13.5).
• *ECG and chest radiograph*.
• *Blood gases*: the Po_2 should be <10.6 kPa (<80 mmHg) as a result of ventilation/perfusion mismatch. Large pulmonary emboli result in severe hypoxia, hypocapnia and metabolic acidosis – a 'mixed' picture.
• *D-dimer (DD) assay*: D-dimer is a degradation product of cross-linked fibrin.

This assay is a useful test where there is low or intermediate probability of a diagnosis of pulmonary embolism. There are several different assays. The highly sensitive assay is ELISA-DD (Vidas). A level <500 μg/l (a negative DD assay) makes a pulmonary embolus very unlikely. The assay can be repeated after stopping a course of warfarin if there is a suspicion of a recurrence.

• *Spiral (helical) CT with contrast*: this is now the investigation of choice. The CT can also be used to image the pelvic veins, which may be the source of the embolus. See Figure 13.1

• *Ventilation/perfusion scan*: this is a useful test for recurrent small emboli that may be missed by pulmonary angiography or CT. It is useful in high probability cases where CT is negative. It is also useful in those for whom CT with contrast is inadvisable (e.g. contrast allergy or chronic renal failure). The ventilation scan must be normal. The diagnosis is difficult in the presence of chronic obstructive airway disease, severe emphysema or bronchopneumonia. Segmental perfusion defects in the presence of normal ventilation scan are strongly suggestive of pulmonary emboli. Tomography of the perfusion study in various planes is useful. The chest radiograph should be available to the interpreter of the scan. Follow-up scans may show rapid resolution of the perfusion defects as a result of lysis of the thrombus.

• *Pulmonary angiography*: no longer the gold standard, this is occasionally performed in the sicker patient in whom the diagnosis is still uncertain. The angiography catheter can be used for thrombolysis delivery and left in the PA for 48–72 h after angiography if necessary (see Figure 13.2).

The PA pressure is elevated for 10–21 days after a first substantial pulmonary embolus and then usually returns to normal as a result of endogenous

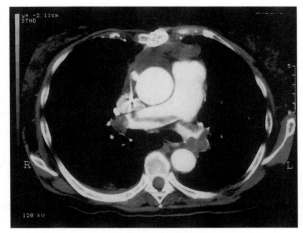

Figure 13.1 CT scan of thorax in massive plumonary embolism showing a long thrombus extending into both right and left pulmonary arteries.

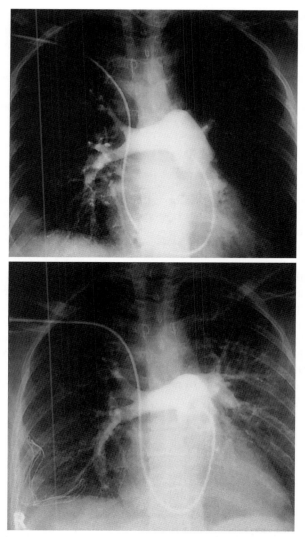

Figure 13.2 Pulmonary angiography in massive pulmonary embolism before (above) and after (below) streptokinase infusion via the PA catheter. Prestreptokinase there is virtually no flow to the left lung, and after streptokinase, a considerable improvement.

fibrinolysis. It remains elevated and causes chronic thromboembolic pulmonary hypertension after a first PE in only 3.8% cases.

Angiograms should show vessel 'cut-offs' or obvious filling defects in the artery. There should be segmental filling defects in addition. Patients with chronic thromboembolic pulmonary hypertension will have large proximal arteries with tortuous distal vessels with peripheral pruning.

Investigations of Less Value
• *Cardiac enzymes*: pulmonary infarction causes elevation of troponin, BNP, LDH and sometimes AST and bilirubin. BNP is released from RV myocardium when under stress.
• *Leg venograms*, ^{125}I-labelled fibrinogen scanning, Doppler ultrasonography: tests to document peripheral leg vein thrombus merely prove an association. They cannot make a diagnosis of pulmonary emboli. An example of DVT on leg venography is shown (Figure 13.3).

Diagnosis in Pregnancy
The concern is the risk of radiation versus the risk of failing to make a diagnosis in a potentially lethal condition. If analysis of D-dimer is positive then spiral CT with contrast is the next step. Radiation is less than with ventilation/perfusion scanning.

Differential Diagnosis
The most common condition to be confused with acute PE is inferior MI. Both cause chest pain, elevated neck veins and similar ECG changes. Transmural inferior infarction causes ST-segment elevation, and PE more commonly causes ST-segment depression in inferior leads. Patients with inferior infarcts are generally not dyspnoeic unless there is additional mitral regurgitation from papillary muscle dysfunction.

Other causes of pulmonary hypertension should be considered.

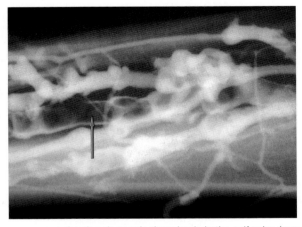

Figure 13.3 Leg venogram showing deep vein thrombosis in the calf veins (arrowed).

13.3 Management of PE

The acute attack is managed with anticoagulation, and thrombolytic therapy in more severe cases. Pulmonary embolectomy is rarely necessary. Attention is then focused on preventive measures.

General Measures

Oxygen and analgesia are usually required. The severe apprehension associated with large pulmonary emboli will require opiate analgesia.

Volume loading: in more severe cases plasma or colloid substitutes should be given even with a raised venous pressure. This may help increase RV stroke volume in severely compromised patients. Start with 500 ml colloid and repeat if necessary.

Anticoagulation

This is all that is required with mild-to-moderate embolization because natural lysis occurs in the lung spontaneously. Heparin is not directly thrombolytic.
• *Unfractionated heparin (UFH)* 10 000 U i.v. stat followed by 5000 U i.v. 2- to 4-hourly. A continuous infusion of heparin probably reduces bleeding complications (dose = 1000 U/h). After 1 week, if no further emboli have occurred, oral anticoagulants are started and the heparin stopped 2 days later. Heparin dose is monitored by APTT estimations.
• *Oral anticoagulants* are continued for 3 months only in the first instance unless there are recurrent emboli; these are rare in patients treated with anticoagulation alone.
• *Low-molecular-weight heparins (LMWHs)*: studies with enoxaparin and tinzaparin have shown that these are as safe and as effective as UFH. No APTT monitoring is required.
• *Fondaparinux*: this oral factor Xa inhibitor has also been shown to be safe and effective and is now the treatment of choice for stable, non-massive or life-threatening pulmonary emboli. Bleeding complications are less than with heparins. Dose: 7.5 mg once daily.

Thrombolytic Therapy

This is reserved for more seriously ill patients who appear unlikely to survive 24–48 h, have demonstrable RV strain on echocardiography or have two or more lobar arteries occluded on angiography (see Figure 13.2).

Thrombolytic therapy has been shown to resolve emboli faster than heparin, to lower the pulmonary artery pressure more than heparin, and appearances on repeat pulmonary angiography and lung scanning show greater improvement with thrombolytic therapy than with heparin.

The improvement is greatest with massive pulmonary emboli. No trial has shown a greater reduction is mortality of thrombolytic therapy over heparin.

The drugs tPA, TNK and reteplase are all more expensive than streptokinase, but may be necessary if streptokinase reactions occur (fever, rashes and allergic reactions are more common with streptokinase).

Before streptokinase therapy, blood is taken for the following tests: FBC, haematocrit, platelet count, INR, APTT, fibrinogen titre and FDPs. Tests are repeated during therapy (every 4 h if possible).

For more details of thrombolytic agents and their action, see Section 5.8.

Streptokinase Dose (Kabikinase, Streptase)

Hydrocortisone 100 mg i.v. stat, streptokinase 250 000 U in 100 ml 0.9% saline infused into PA or peripheral vein over 30 min. Then streptokinase 100 000 U hourly up to 72 h maximum. Heparin is then gradually restarted over the next 12 h.

The streptokinase dose is controlled by the fibrinogen titre. A titre falling below 1:4 in saline may require a decrease in streptokinase dose (e.g. by 50 000 U/h). The thrombin time should be prolonged by two- to fourfold normal value.

The main control, however, is the clinical state. Prolonged thrombin times do not predict bleeding complications.

Complications of Streptokinase

• Allergic reactions are common. Rise in temperature is expected; rashes and pruritus are common. Nausea, vomiting, flushing and headaches may occur. Acute hypotension may occur with the first dose. Hydrocortisone and volume replacement are necessary.

• Bleeding complications: local bleeding at catheter entry sites is expected, and a fall in haemoglobin is common on treatment. Heparin increases the bleeding risk. Pressure on a local bleeding site is all that is generally necessary. A pledget soaked in ε-aminocaproic acid may help.

Streptokinase is stopped with major bleeding complications and fibrinogen replacement started (FFP, cryoprecipitate or fresh blood).

The effects on stopping are usually reversed after 1–2 h when emergency surgery could be contemplated if absolutely necessary. In a desperate situation with continued bleeding, fibrinolytic inhibitors (ε-aminocaproic acid) or kallikrein inactivator (Trasylol) can be tried.

Contraindications to Streptokinase

See Section 5.8.

Fibrin-specific Thrombolytic Agents (see Section 5.8)

The agents rtPA, reteplase and tenecteplase are three fibrin-specific thrombolytic agents with bleeding complications similar to streptokinase. They are used primarily for coronary thrombolysis, but they should also be considered for patients with large pulmonary emboli who have had streptokinase in the past with the persistence of neutralizing antibodies.

Failed Thrombolysis
This occurs in approximately 8% of patients with acute PE. If the patient remains shocked or hypoxic, then pulmonary embolectomy must be considered. Just as in acute MI repeat thrombolysis is not advisable. Repeat thrombolysis carries a 38% mortality rate in non-randomized studies.

Pulmonary Embolectomy
This is rarely necessary. It carries a high mortality (23–57%) in various series, especially if the operation is performed very early. (Two-thirds of patients who die from pulmonary embolism do so in the first 2 h anyway.) Surgical mortality is lower if no cardiac arrest has occurred.

It should be considered in patients with cardiogenic shock who have had 1 h maximum medical therapy, in whom streptokinase is contraindicated or who are unlikely to survive the next hour.

Cardiac massage should be prolonged in an arrest caused by massive PE because it may help to fragment the thrombus. Pulmonary embolectomy can only remove large proximal thrombus, whereas streptokinase may in addition deal with smaller peripheral thrombi.

Pulmonary Thromboendarterectomy
First pioneered by Jamieson in San Diego in 1993 this operation is indicated in patients with grade III or IV NYHA class symptoms with lesions in the main, lobar and segmental arteries. It is not suitable for peripheral thrombi. Operative mortality rate is about 10%. Acute reperfusion pulmonary oedema may be a problem postoperatively and is managed on conventional lines (see Section 6.5). Long-term symptomatic improvement occurs with better gas exchange and pulmonary haemodynamics.

Prognostic Factors in Acute PE
The most critical factor is RV function and preceding cardiac status, but the following are recognized adverse prognostic factors:
- Age >70
- Clinical condition: shock, syncope, hypotension (systolic pressure <90 mmHg)
- Co-morbidities, e.g. chronic renal failure
- RV dysfunction and strain: peak RV pressure >30 mmHg, RV/LV size ratio >0.9, peak tricuspid jet velocity >2.6 m/s
- PA pressure > 50 mmHg
- Patent foramen ovale
- Raised troponin and BNP (RV wall stress).

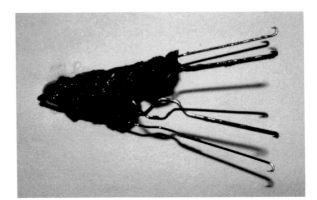

Figure 13.4 Greenfield filter showing trapped thrombus.

Prevention of Pulmonary Emboli

Low-dose subcutaneous heparin has been shown in several trials to prevent pulmonary emboli after surgery (e.g. 5000 U s.c. 2 h preoperatively, then 5000 U s.c. 8-hourly for 7 days). A combination of Dextran 70 given at the end of surgery plus the use of pneumatic leggings has also been shown to reduce postoperative pulmonary emboli. Early mobilization is vital.

Most cases of recurrences of pulmonary emboli will be prevented by oral anticoagulants. Studies for a procoagulant condition do not usually reveal a problem, but about 10% of patients will have a lupus anticoagulant, anticardiolipin antibodies and raised factor VIII levels or factor V Leiden (activated protein C resistance).

IVC Filters (Figure 13.4)

Various operations on the IVC below the renal veins have attempted to prevent PE (plication, ligation, filters, umbrellas, etc.). This is only of temporary benefit because large collateral channels rapidly develop. It may be life-saving in rare instances. The IVC filter is not a substitute for anticoagulation, but may be considered when anticoagulation is contraindicated. If possible patients with an IVC filter should be on long-term anticoagulation. Once anticoagulation is stopped there is an increased incidence of deep vein thrombosis in patients with an IVC filter. One study showed no improvement in mortality with the use of the IVC filter over 2 years.

13.4 Sickle Cell Disease

Of patients with sickle cell disease 30% have PHT, which is often undiagnosed. Other chronic haemolytic anaemias also cause PHT. The mechanism is thought to be free haemoglobin scavenging nitric oxide with the resultant increase in free radicals. Nitric oxide synthase is reduced by red cells releasing arginase, limiting the availability of arginine – the substrate for nitric oxide. Endothelin-1 levels are increased. Asplenia may increase platelet counts and contribute to microemboli. Hypoxic episodes cause pulmonary vasoconstriction and an obliterative vasculopathy develops.

Diagnosis

Symptoms and physical signs are unreliable for the diagnosis of mild PHT. Dyspnoea may be ascribed to anaemia, there may be no wheeze and pulse oximetry may still be normal in the early stages.

Echocardiography is used to estimate the PA pressure from continuous wave Doppler studies of the tricuspid regurgitant jet. PA pressure is $4V^2 + RA$ pressure where V is the peak velocity of the tricuspid regurgitant jet in metres per second, and RA pressure is estimated clinically from the height of the JVP (see Section 17.3). Alternatively the RA pressure can be estimated from the degree of inspiratory collapse of the IVC (5 mmHg for collapse of >50%, 15 mmHg for collapse of <50%). Peak velocities of 2.5–3.0 m/s should be regarded as a diagnostic threshold. Patients with sickle cell disease tolerate even mild pulmonary hypertension badly and a peak velocity of >2.5 m/s has been shown to be a strong predictor of death.

Treatment

Prevention is based on avoiding hypoxic situations (high altitude, air travel), the use of domiciliary oxygen and immediate treatment of concomitant chest infections. In addition:

- Systemic hypertension: associated with PHT, this is a risk factor for stroke in sickle cell disease and should be treated early.
- Pulmonary artery vasodilators: see below.
- Nitric oxide donors: inhaled NO in the short-term emergency. L-Arginine improves NO synthesis lowering PHT 15%. Hydroxyurea also increases NO levels as well as fetal haemoglobin.
- Transfusion therapy: may help prevent stroke.
- Anticoagulation should be considered if systemic pressures are normal.

13.5 Primary Pulmonary Hypertension

Described in 1950 by Paul Wood, this is a rare disease: annual incidence approximately 1 per 200 000 to 1 000 000 population. It is more common in young women. Endothelial dysfunction has been identified in primary PHT, as either a cause or an effect. The condition is a combination of vasoconstriction, intimal hyperplasia, medial hypertrophy and secondary thrombosis. Numerous lung biopsy, platelet, plasma and urine studies have demonstrated an imbalance between levels of vasoconstrictors and vasodilators in this condition (Table 13.6).

Table 13.6 Vasoactivity in primary pulmonary hypertension

Increased: vasoconstrictors	Decreased: vasodilators
Thromboxane A2	Prostacyclin synthase
Endothelin-1	Nitric oxide synthase
Serotonin (5-HT)	Vasoactive intestinal peptide (VIP)
VEGF + receptors	

Production of vascular endothelial growth factor (VEGF) is increased in the lung in chronic hypoxia and contributes to the endothelial proliferation.

Genetic Factors

Two genes in the transforming growth factor β (TGF-β) receptor family have been linked to familial primary PHT.

Angiopoietin-1 and its receptor TIE2 are strongly upregulated in various types of PHT. This protein is involved in the recruitment of smooth muscle cells.

Bone morphogenetic protein and its receptors: BMPR1A and BMPR2. These are downregulated (in response to angiopoietin-1 upregulation) and result in unrestrained signalling of growth-promoting Smads, (intracellular effector proteins) which stimulate the proliferation of vascular smooth muscle cells. Mutations of this gene occur in familial PHT.

Clinical Factors

Clinical factors implicated include: chronic small pulmonary emboli; collagen vascular disease (association with Raynaud's phenomenon); allergic vasculitis (polyarteritis nodosa; drugs (aminorex fumarate and dexfenfluramine – anorexic agents); bush tea – *Crotalaria fulva*, alkaloid ingestion by African–Caribbean individuals; hormonal influences (female sex predominance, association with the pill, presentation during or after pregnancy, etc.); association with cirrhosis.

Symptoms are similar to patients with pulmonary emboli: increasing dyspnoea fatigue and syncope.

Signs to note are: mild central cyanosis, prominent 'a' wave in JVP especially after mild effort. RV heave (left parasternal); RV S_4 and S_3 in later stages; palpable pulmonary artery pulsation in second left interspace; pulmonary ejection click (best with patient holding breath in expiration); loud and often palpable P_2. Listen for a diastolic murmur of pulmonary regurgitation (Graham Steell) and a systolic murmur of tricuspid regurgitation.

ECG shows severe RV strain (T-wave inversion in V1–3), right-axis deviation and incomplete or complete RBBB. Usually in sinus rhythm.

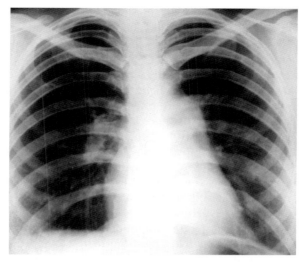

Figure 13.5 Chest radiograph: P/A. Primary pulmonary hypertension. Enlarged PA conus. Oligaemic lung fields.

Chest radiograph shows a normal size heart with enlarged pulmonary artery conus and central pulmonary arteries, but pruned peripheral arteries. Lung peripheries look dark and oligaemic (Figure 13.5).

Echocardiography confirms pulmonary hypertension (see Section 17.3 for calculation), RV hypertrophy and pulmonary and tricuspid regurgitation. Exclude occult left heart problems as a possible cause of PHT: mitral or aortic valve disease, atrial myxoma, cor triatriatum, etc.

Cardiac catheterization is necessary only to check the effect of drug treatment on pulmonary and systemic vascular resistance (see Section 16.3), or as a possible work-up to transplantation.

Management

Mean survival is 5 years from diagnosis: a depressing condition to manage, with no definite aetiology, and much of the therapy palliative. Therapy is aimed at trying to inhibit the contraction and proliferation of smooth muscle cells in the PA wall and the prevention of secondary thrombosis:

• *Anticoagulation*: routine. Shown to improve survival in Mayo Clinic series of 1984.

• *Diuretics*: will improve right heart failure symptoms.

• *Calcium antagonists*: high doses of long-acting drugs are needed but only about a quarter or less of patients will respond with a fall in PVR. Gradual increase in dose advisable unless monitored with Swan–Ganz catheter *in situ*. Typical doses needed are: nifedipine 180–240 mg daily or diltiazem 720 mg daily. Systemic hypotension may be a problem. Responders have improved prognosis. Some centres attempt to target responders by assessing the PVR before and after NO inhalation or intravenous adenosine, and a reduction of 20% in the PVR has been suggested as a target for successful long-term calcium channel blockade.

- *Domiciliary oxygen* may help patients who can still be managed at home.
- *Bosentan*: a dual inhibitor of endothelin A and B (ET_A and ET_B). ET_B receptors are upregulated in PHT and are constrictive. Bosentan has been shown to improve the 6-minute walk distance at 62.5 mg twice daily for 4 weeks, increasing to a maintenance dose of 125 mg twice daily. Measure LFTs before starting and after 2 weeks' therapy. Wean off if ALT > 3 x normal (do not stop suddenly). Avoid concomitant treatment with glibenclamide, fluconazole and ciclosporin. Bosentan has also been shown to be valuable in the Eisenmenger syndrome. It reduces PVR and improves exercise capacity without causing any deterioration in oxygen saturation.
- *Sildenafil*: this phosphodiesterase-5 inhibitor, more commonly used for erectile dysfunction, has been shown in a multicentre trial to improve the exercise capacity (6-minute walk distance) and lower PA pressure when given (20–80 mg three times daily) to patients with pulmonary hypertension. Sildenafil increases intracellular cGMP and enhances NO-mediated vasodilatation. It is not known yet whether sildenafil might delay progression of the disease and reduce longer-term mortality.

Prostacyclin Therapy

- *Prostacyclin* (PGI_2, epoprostenol) infusion via a tunnelled central line: shown to improve symptoms, haemodynamics and survival. Generally reserved for the more severe or deteriorating case when it may be used as a bridge to transplantation. Infusion dosing is performed with right heart catheterization. Start at 2 ng/kg per min increasing by 2 ng/kg per min every 15 min. Increments are stopped when arterial pressure falls by 40%, or heart rate increases by 40%, or patient develops intolerant symptoms: nausea, vomiting, headache, jaw pain, leg pain, diarrhoea, etc. Reduce maximum dose by 2 ng/kg per min to achieve maximum tolerable dose.
- *Inhaled iloprost*: more recently an analogue of prostacyclin can be administered via a nebulizer (aerosolized iloprost 100–150 µg daily in divided doses every 3 h). This avoids the potential infection risk of long-term intravenous therapy and can safely be managed at home. Side effects: headache, cough and jaw pain in some patients.
- *Oral beraprost*: approved in Japan. The first orally active prostacyclin analogue; 80 µg four times daily improved the 3-month 6-minute walk test distance but the benefit was not maintained at 9 or 12 months.
- *Subcutaneous trepostinil*: approved in the USA. A continuous subcutaneous infusion is a useful alternative in patients who are getting into trouble with central lines. Improves signs, symptoms and 6-minute walk test. Pain at the infusion site is common and its limiting factor.

• Future pharmacological directions include the use of endothelin-receptor antagonists or NO precursors.

Surgery

• *Atrial septostomy*: creating a right-to-left shunt. This may help by decompressing the right heart and improve LV filling and cardiac output.

• *Transplantation*: offers the only real hope of long-term survival. Heart and lung, double-lung or single-lung transplantations are possible and severe RV dysfunction may recover once the afterload has been reduced with a new lung. One-year survival rate after lung transplantation is about 70% and recurrence in the transplanted lung has not been seen. Surgical mortality is higher than for other conditions and obliterative bronchiolitis more common. Spontaneous improvement does occur but is very rare.

14 Diseases of the Aorta

14.1 Aortic Root Dilatation/Aneurysm

The aortic root is the initial part of the aorta from the aortic leaflets up to the sinotubular junction). Part of the base of the aortic root consists of ventricular muscle. The aortic root is readily seen on transthoracic echocardiography and measurements of root diameter are made at four levels (Figure 14.1):

1 Leaflet base
2 Maximum diameter at the sinuses
3 Sinotubular junction: dilatation of the aortic root results in effacement (smoothing out or loss) of the sinotubular junction
4 Ascending aorta: the aortic root incorporates the sinuses of Valsalva the vortices of which (responsible for aortic valve closure) were made famous by Leonardo da Vinci in his drawings.

Causes of Aortic Root Dilatation:
- Idiopathic dilatation: annuloaortic ectasia
- Cystic medial necrosis
- Systemic hypertension
- Post-stenotic dilatation in aortic stenosis
- Intramural haematoma and aortic dissection
- Atherosclerosis (Figures 14.2–14.4)
- Sinus of Valsalva aneurysm
- Trauma (Figure 14.5)
- Syphilis: associated with calcification of the aortic root (Figure 14.6).

Several imaging techniques are now available for obtaining the aortic root dimensions (see aortic dissection section). Three-dimensional reconstruction of 64-slice CT scans produces remarkable images. Figures 14.2 and 14.3 show an aortic root aneurysm in a patient with two patent vein grafts, one of which

Swanton's Cardiology, sixth edition. By R. H. Swanton and S. Banerjee. Published 2008 Blackwell Publishing. ISBN 978-1-4051-7819-8.

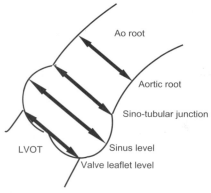

Figure 14.1 Diagrammatic representation of aortic root as seen on transthoracic echocardiography long axis view. Measurement of maximum aortic root diameter should be specified at four levels. The maximum diameter in the normal root will be at sinus level. In aortic root dilatation the sinotubular junction disappears.

has been stented. Measurement of the maximum diameter of the aortic root is important because it is of prognostic value (Table 14.1).

Surgical intervention is indicated once the aneurysm exceeds 5.0 cm, but patients with Marfan syndrome must be considered for surgery once the diameter exceeds 4.0 cm if they have a family history of aortic dissection.

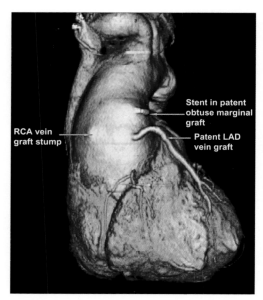

Figure 14.2 64-slice CT of heart in P/A view. Atherosclerotic aortic root aneurysm (6.4 cm), with patent vein grafts to LAD and lateral circumflex. Stent in ostium of circumflex vein graft. RCA graft stump visible.

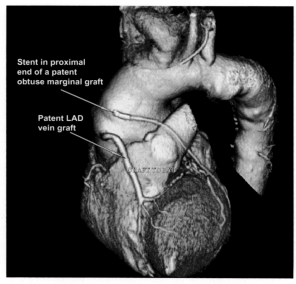

Figure 14.3 64-slice CT of heart in left anterior oblique view (same patient as Figure 14.2). Patent vein grafts to LAD and obtuse marginal.

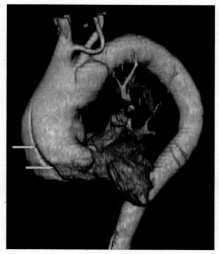

Figure 14.4 64-slice CT with three-dimensional reconstruction showing a dilated aortic root with a type A aortic dissection (arrowed). Left anterior oblique view.

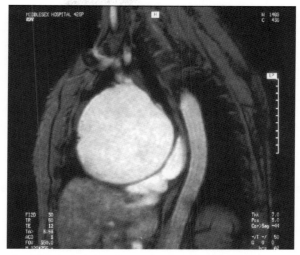

Figure 14.5 Cardiac MRA: lateral view. Traumatic ascending aortic root aneurysm.

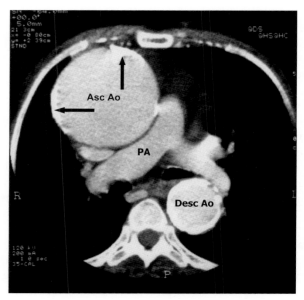

Figure 14.6 CT of thorax with contrast syphilitic aortitis with aneurysmal dilatation of aortic root. Note calcification in aortic root wall (arrowed).

Table 14.1 Aneurysm diameter and annual risk

Maximum aneurysm diameter (cm)	Annual risk of rupture, dissection or death (%)
≥4.0	4
≥5.0	9.3
≥6.0	14.7

With a family history of aortic dissection. Figures from the International Registry of Aortic Dissection (IRAD).

14.2 Dissecting Aneurysm of the Thoracic Aorta

This commonly occurs in men aged 40–70 years and is frequently fatal if untreated. Incidence is 10–20/million per year. Fifty per cent die within 48 h, 70% in 1 week and 90% in 3 months. It is three times as common in men, more so in African–Caribbean than white men, and rare in Oriental races. It is usually a spontaneous event and a history of trauma is unusual. Predisposing factors include:
• hypertension (distal > proximal)
• bicuspid or unicommissural aortic valve (see Section 3.4)
• coarctation of the aorta (see Section 2.4)
• pregnancy (see Section 15.8)
• Turner or Noonan syndrome
• Marfan syndrome (see Section 14.3)
• other connective tissue disorders, e.g. Ehlers–Danlos syndrome, SLE, relapsing polychondritis, giant cell aortitis
• surgical aortotomy sites.

Pathophysiology
A combination of high intraluminal pressure and medial damage seems to be the prime factor (e.g. cystic medial necrosis in Marfan syndrome). Syphilis causes saccular aortic aneurysms not dissections, and atheroma is usually associated with saccular aneurysms. Cause of medial damage is unknown (a genetic mucopolysaccharide deficiency in Marfan syndrome, possibly ischaemic necrosis as a result of occlusion of vasa vasorum in other cases).

Presentation
• *Pain*: the most common form of presentation. A sudden-onset, literally tearing sensation felt in the chest. Usually retrosternal, radiating through to the back, neck and left chest. The pain may be similar to ischaemic cardiac pain. It is very severe. Leaking dissections will produce pleuritic pain in addition. Dissection round a coronary ostium may produce an additional myocardial infarct.

- *Symptoms from arterial involvement*:
  CNS: monoplegia, paraplegia (spinal artery occlusion), hemiplegia, stupor to loss of consciousness, visual disturbances, speech disturbance
  Gastrointestinal: abdominal pain (mesenteric artery dissection), haemorrhage (bowel infarction or aortointestinal fistula), dysphagia (oesophageal compression)
  Renal: renal pain, haematuria (renal artery dissection) or anuria
  Limb: pain and pallor in any limb.
- *Pleuritic pain*: aneurysm leaking may also cause haemoptysis.
- *Giddiness or syncope*: either cerebral effect or secondary to effective volume loss, e.g. retroperitoneal haematoma.
- *Dyspnoea* (LVF, massive haemothorax, pleural effusions, pulmonary haemorrhage).

Aortic dissection may thus mimic clinically a wide variety of conditions from a CVA, acute appendicitis, acute pancreatitis, perforated peptic ulcer, saddle embolism to MI or pulmonary embolism. A patient may present with one ischaemic and one paralysed limb simultaneously.

Physical Signs and Examination

The patient may be in great pain, shocked, cyanosed and sweating profusely. The blood pressure may be high, normal or low. The most important things to check are:

- *Blood pressure* in both arms; all peripheral pulses, their presence and equality (a change in the nature of the pulses may be a valuable clue); there may be arterial bruits, arterial tenderness or palpable aneurysms.
- *Presence of aortic regurgitation*.
- *Sign of tamponade* (see Section 10.2): pericardial rub itself is unusual. SVC obstruction rarely confuses the issue, because it is more common with saccular aneurysms.
- *Signs of LVF*: pleural effusions; staining of chest or abdomen (haemorrhage from leaking aneurysm is an ominous sign).
- *Abdominal signs*: rigidity, palpable mass: ? pulsatile, abdominal tenderness is common.
- *CNS signs*: fundal examination, hypertensive changes; Horner syndrome; urinary retention; limb movement and sensation; general state of consciousness; ? Marfan syndrome habitus.

Chest Radiograph

Widening of the upper mediastinum is strongly suggestive of a dissection, but not diagnostic. An unfolded aorta with a tortuous descending aorta may resemble a dissection.

Fluid in the left costophrenic angle associated with a wide mediastinum is a particularly ominous sign.

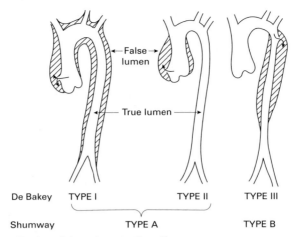

De Bakey   TYPE I   TYPE II   TYPE III

Shumway   TYPE A   TYPE B

Figure 14.7 Classification of thoracic aorta dissection.

Classification

The original De Bakey classification is shown in Figure 14.7.
- *Type I*: the ascending and descending aorta are involved usually into the abdomen. The 'walking stick' distribution.
- *Type II*: involvement of ascending aorta only. The least common. May occur in Marfan syndrome.
- *Type III*: involvement of descending aorta only distal to the left subclavian downwards. The most favourable type prognostically.

This classification was proposed in 1965 and is less used now. More recently Shumway has proposed a more simple classification into two types only. The Shumway classification has largely taken over from the De Bakey one:
- *Type A* (proximal): ascending aorta involved.
- *Type B* (distal): ascending aorta not involved.

Management

Stage 1
Pain relief, intravenous diamorphine as required. ECG monitoring, chest radiograph. Establish two CVP lines and radial artery pressure if possible. Crossmatch 10 units blood, because volume replacement may be necessary if aneurysm leakage has occurred. Plasma should be given initially, followed by whole blood. Dextran 70 or colloid may have to be used. Echocardiography is employed to visualize the aortic root and to check for pericardial fluid. Transoesophageal echocardiography is diagnostic. (Figure 14.8)

Stage 2
Correction of hypertension if present. Wheat, in 1965, realized the importance of lowering both mean systolic pressure and dP/dt. This he accomplished by

trimetaphan 1–2 mg/ml i.v., guanethidine 50 mg twice daily and reserpine 1–2 mg i.m. A variety of other drugs has been used since, e.g. methyldopa, β-blocking agents and diuretics.

The simplest regimen is intravenous nitroprusside (see Section 6.5). It is easier to control, having a very short half-life. Frequent checks on acid–base balance are necessary to check for a metabolic acidosis.

Peak systolic pressure should be <120 mmHg and mean aortic pressure <90 mmHg.

Stage 3: Definitive Diagnosis
Diagnostic method depends on the technology available.

Transoesophageal Echocardiography
This is proving very useful in the diagnosis of dissection and is particularly good at visualizing the dissection flap in the descending aorta. Even with TOE there is a 5% false-negative diagnosis (Figure 14.8).

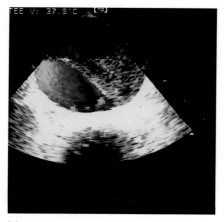

(a)

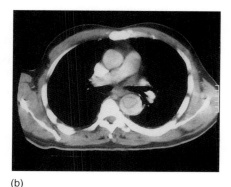

Figure 14.8 (a) Transoesophageal echocardiogram: transverse plane. Aortic dissection. Double-barrelled aorta is shown with flow in compressed true lumen. (b) CT of type B aortic dissection showing false lumen in descending aorta.

(b)

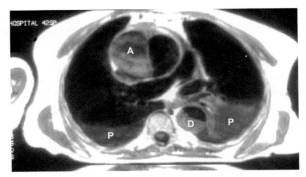

Figure 14.9 CT of thorax: type A aortic dissection. Note double lumen in both ascending (A) and descending (D) thoracic aorta. False lumen containing thrombus. Bilateral pleural effusions (P).

Spiral CT

This is the investigation of choice in aortic dissection but is not always available on an emergency basis. A double lumen can be visualized and the dissection flap (Figure 14.9). It may not, however, be quite as good as aortography for visualizing the origin/point of entry of the dissection, but is very helpful in making the diagnosis and determining the extent of the dissection. It is obviously safer than aortography.

64-slice CT with Three-dimensional Reconstruction

This is not generally available but produces remarkable images of the extent of dissection and size of the aortic root (see Figure 14.4).

Emergency Aortography

This is rarely necessary now with the advent of CT and TOE. It should be performed under heavy sedation or general anaesthesia. A pigtail catheter from the femoral route is preferable and usually this catheter stays in the true lumen. Separate aortic root and aortic arch injections with follow-through to descending aorta are necessary. The patient should be on intravenous nitroprusside or similar drugs before the injections: the force of the injection of large volumes of contrast media into a dissected root has occasionally proved fatal. Renal film should be taken at the end of the procedure.

MRI

When available, this is a safe, quick and most reliable method of diagnosis. The danger of an aortic injection is avoided and no X-irradiation needed (Figures 14.10 and 14.11).

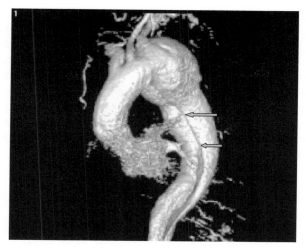

Figure 14.10 MRI three-dimensional reconstruction of thoracic aorta showing a type B dissection with the flap (arrowed) in the descending thoracic aorta.

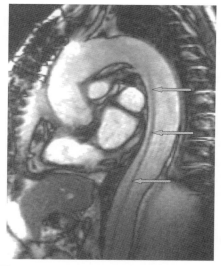

Figure 14.11 Cardiac MR angiogram of type B aortic dissection. Left anterior oblique view. The dissection flap (arrowed) is visible in the descending thoracic and abdominal aorta.

Stage 4

Type A

Surgery is the treatment of choice for type A dissections and medical treatment alone carries a bad prognosis. CPB with coronary perfusion is necessary. The ascending aorta is transected, the two cuffs of true and false walls are sutured together at both sides of the transection and then an end-to-end anastomosis performed, sometimes with a Dacron interposition graft. The aortic valve often becomes competent again once it has been resuspended, making aortic valve replacement unnecessary. Occasionally a root replacement is necessary using a tube valve conduit with re-implantation of the coronaries in the graft (modified Bentall's operation).

If the great vessels are involved, surgery becomes difficult with a greater risk of postoperative stroke. CPB is set up and the patient profoundly cooled to 18 °C. Circulatory arrest is performed and the great vessels joined to an arch graft on a single pedicle flap.

Type B
This has medical management initially, unless complications develop such as an infarcting organ or limb, leaking aneurysm or extension with unremitting pain. If the dissection re-enters above the diaphragm it is possible to replace the descending thoracic aorta with a Dacron graft (using a temporary proximal-to-distal aorta bypass). Difficulties with this operation are the distal anastomosis and the possibility of paraplegia as a result of damage to the anterior spinal artery branches.

Involvement of the abdominal aorta in a type B dissection is much more of a problem, and medical treatment is advocated initially. However, local surgery at the aortic bifurcation may be necessary to save ischaemic legs.

14.3 Marfan Syndrome

Genetics
An autosomal dominant condition with a prevalence of 1 in 10000. It is the results of mutations in the gene coding for fibrillin synthesis on chromosome 15 (*FBN1*). Over 600 different mutations have been found in this gene, and mutations can be identified in >80% cases with a Marfan syndrome phenotype. This wide diversity of mutations accounts for the different phenotypes in Marfan syndrome, but as yet it is not possible to predict the phenotype from the specific mutation. The mutations result in reduced fibrillin synthesis or early fibrillin degradation. In 25% of cases neither parent appears to be affected and careful screening of the parents is needed. The condition affects either sex and 87% die from cardiovascular abnormalities.

Marfan syndrome may be caused by upregulation of transforming growth factor β (TGF-β) caused by a low level or absence of fibrillin-1 protein. Increased TGF-β signalling has been found in the aortic aneurysm of a mouse model of Marfan syndrome. Losartan, an inhibitor of TGF-β, has been shown to prevent aneurysm development in this mouse model and may be a future, important, long-term treatment in humans.

Diagnosis
Diagnosis is still based on finding two or more of the classic clinical signs in the musculoskeletal system, the CVS and the eyes. Possible findings are:

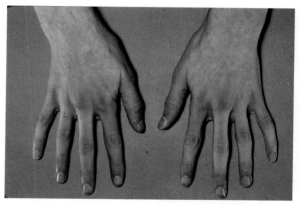

Figure 14.12 Marfan syndrome: arachnodactyly.

- Tall thin patient: dolichostenomelia. Arm span greater than height.
- Long narrow face and skull (dolicocephaly) often with prognathism of the mandible, prominent supraorbital ridges and frontal bossing.
- Arachnodactyly: long tapered fingers (Figure 14.12).
- High-arched palate and dental problems: in some cases this results in collapse of the upper dental arch, malocclusion, crowding with supernumerary teeth, crown dysplasia, enamel hypoplasia and other dental problems.
- Musculoskeletal problems (Figure 14.13), e.g. scoliosis, pectus excavatum, protrusio acetabulae, causing early hip joint osteoarthritis. Dilatation of the lumbar dural sac occurs in 75% of cases.
- Hypermobility of joints and skin laxity: history of joint recurrent dislocation (e.g. temporomandibular joint).
- Possible history of pneumothorax: apical bullae occur.
- Eye problems: ectopia lentis – lens dislocates upwards. Iridodonesis. Usually manageable with corrective spectacles. Lens may need extraction. Increased incidence of myopia, retinal detachment, strabismus (squint), glaucoma.
- Floppy mitral valve. Mild-to-severe mitral regurgitation. Chordal rupture (see Section 3.3).
- Dilatation of aortic root with consequent aortic regurgitation.
- Aortic dissection: see above.

One of the most used signs has been the metacarpal index: the lengths of the second to fifth metacarpals are added and divided by the sum of their minimum widths. In Marfan syndrome this index is >8.5.

In childhood, the more common problems are the development of a progressive scoliosis, which may need surgical correction possibly with a Harrington rod, and the correction of visual difficulties.

Later problems include progressive mitral regurgitation and/or dilatation of the aortic root.

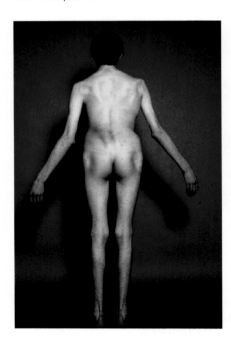

Figure 14.13 Marfan syndrome: note scoliosis.

The Aorta in Marfan Syndrome

The whole aorta may demonstrate cystic medial necrosis. The weakened media allows the aorta to stretch even in the normotensive patient. The typical site for the Marfan syndrome aortic aneurysm is just above the aortic valve, with the aorta returning to more normal dimensions at the origin of the innominate artery, forming a sort of 'onion' shape. However, any part of the aorta may become aneurysmal in time (Figure 14.14). Stretching of the aortic annulus (annuloaortic ectasia) causes aortic regurgitation. Aortic dissection may occur.

Regular echocardiography is essential at least annually to check aortic root dimensions. TOE is useful if available.

Surgery

A composite aortic root and valve replacement (modified Bentall's operation) is indicated once the aortic root dimension is >4.0 cm on echocardiography, whether or not the patient has symptoms. All patients with Marfan syndrome should be on β blockade, reducing aortic dP/dt and hopefully the rate of progression of the aortic aneurysm. Losartan should also be considered (see above).

A new approach is to wrap an Exostent around the ascending aorta, which acts as an external support preventing further aortic dilatation. Long-term results with this technique are awaited.

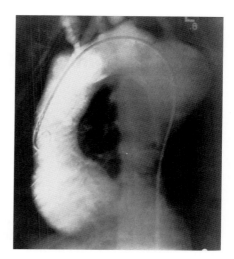

Figure 14.14 Aortogram in Marfan syndrome. There is a typical onion-shaped aneurysmal dilatation of the aortic root and a further aneurysm of the descending thoracic aorta just distal to the origin of the left subclavian artery.

Pregnancy (see Section 15.8)

Parents must be aware that 50% of their progeny will be affected in an autosomal dominant condition. Monthly echocardiography should be performed during pregnancy. The mother should continue β blockade throughout. There is a small (<10%) but definite risk that pregnancy will result in rapid dilatation of the aortic root with the effect of oestrogens on the aortic wall.

Psychosocial Problems

Children will frequently be absent from school and patients with Marfan syndrome may spend many hours in outpatient clinics (cardiac, orthopaedic, dental, eye, etc.). Their overall management is best organized by a specialist in the condition.

Motor and intellectual development is normal. However, absences, poor eyesight and physical restrictions mean that children may get behind and need special help in the classroom. It is hardly surprising that children may develop behavioural problems, or become withdrawn with anxiety and depression. They may have low self-esteem and concerns with their body image, and are targets for bullies.

Forme Fruste Marfan

This term has been used to describe patients with one feature of the syndrome, e.g. annuloaortic ectasia. The genetic defect of this alone has not been identified but it may progress in the same way as a true Marfan syndrome aorta.

15 Pregnancy and Heart Disease

Pregnancy places a normal heart under immense physical strain. If the heart is already compromised by an existing anomaly, this can result in a poor outcome for both fetus and mother. Hence pregnancy in a patient with existing heart disease should be a carefully planned and considered event.

The data for maternal mortality in 2000–2002 show that cardiac disease is now the most common cause of maternal mortality in the UK (Figure 15.1). The cardiac causes of maternal death include those shown in Figure 15.2.

All patients with heart disease should be assessed before conception. The assessment should include a full history (including exercise capacity, history of heart failure or arrhythmia), an exercise test and echocardiography (looking at pulmonary pressures, valve dysfunction and LV dimensions and function).

The patient should be assessed during each of the trimesters and at any time a change of symptoms occurs.

15.1 Physiological Changes Associated with Pregnancy

These changes occur to meet the increased demands of the mother and fetus. The heart itself is displaced to the left and upwards, by the enlarging uterus. This results in apparent cardiomegaly on the chest radiograph. There is a true increase in LV cavity size in that the LVEDD increases, causing a degree of functional valvular regurgitation.

Cardiac Output

Stroke volume and heart rate contribute to cardiac output; both increase in pregnancy. As a result, cardiac output increases rapidly by about 30–40% in the first 12–16 weeks. Cardiac output remains elevated until 30 weeks, but then may decrease slightly as a result of the effect of the enlarging uterus on

Swanton's Cardiology, sixth edition. By R. H. Swanton and S. Banerjee. Published 2008
Blackwell Publishing. ISBN 978-1-4051-7819-8.

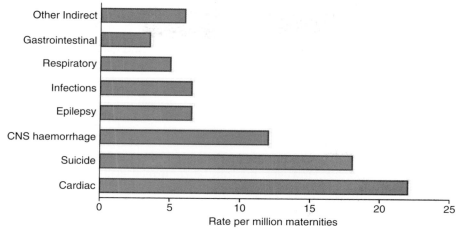

Figure 15.1 Maternal mortality rate from leading causes of deaths per million maternities as reported to the RCOG: Confidential Enquiry into Maternal Deaths: United Kingdom 2000–2.

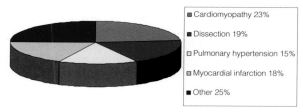

Figure 15.2 Breakdown of cardiac causes of maternal deaths.

the vena cava. During labour, cardiac output increases by a further 30%. After delivery, the cardiac output falls to about 15–25% above normal levels and gradually declines until normal levels are reached at about 6 weeks post partum.

Heart Rate

The rise in cardiac output is mirrored by the rise in heart rate. The rate rises from about 70 beats/min to 90 beats/min. in addition, there is a steady reduction in systemic vascular resistance of about 10–20%, which contributes to the hyperdynamic circulation.

Blood Pressure

Both systolic and diastolic blood pressures drop by about 10 mmHg, reaching trough levels at about 20 weeks. However, by term, BP levels return to pre-pregnancy levels.

15.2 Hypertension in Pregnancy

There are three recognized varieties of hypertension in pregnancy:
1 Pre-existing hypertension
2 Pregnancy-induced hypertension
3 Pre-eclampsia.

The end-effects of each type of hypertension are similar in that they contribute significantly to maternal and fetal mortality and morbidity.

Pre-existing Hypertension

If hypertension is diagnosed in the first trimester, it is likely to have been a pre-existing disorder. However, this can be confirmed at 3–6 months post partum if the baseline BP fails to return to normal.

As with all new diagnoses of hypertension, no assumption of primary or essential hypertension should be made without the exclusion of important causes of secondary hypertension, such as renal or cardiac disease, coarctation, Cushing syndrome, Conn syndrome or phaeochromocytoma (see Section 12.4).

Examination findings to look for include radiofemoral delay (coarctation) and renal bruits (renal artery stenosis). Investigations should include urine dipstick, urea and electrolytes, renal ultrasonography and urinary catecholamines.

Pregnancy-induced Hypertension

This usually appears in the second half of pregnancy and resolves within 6 weeks of delivery. It can persist for up to 3 months post partum. It is a complication seen in about 5–10% of pregnancies.

Pregnancy-induced hypertension is defined as hypertension *without* proteinuria or other features of pre-eclampsia. The main difference between the two conditions is that the outcome is much worse with pre-eclampsia. The later the presentation in the pregnancy, the less likely the progression to pre-eclampsia. (Magee showed that 40% developed pregnancy-induced hypertension before 30 weeks vs 7% after 38 weeks.)

Pre-eclampsia

Pre-eclampsia is defined as pregnancy-induced hypertension in association with proteinuria or oedema. It is a multi-system disorder, caused by diffuse vascular endothelial dysfunction.

Women can present with headache, visual disturbance, epigastric or right upper quadrant pain, nausea, vomiting or rapidly progressive oedema. The most common cause of death is cerebral haemorrhage and adult respiratory distress syndrome. Fetal effects are intrauterine growth retardation, placental abruption and intrauterine death.

Management

BP control has to find a balance of reduction of maternal BP, while protecting the uteroplacental circulation and maintaining fetal blood flow.

Any BP levels >140/90 mmHg should provoke consideration of treatment. It is mandatory for BPs >170/110 mmHg to be treated.

First-line Therapy – Methyldopa

This is a superb drug for BP control and is known to be safe for the fetus. It can cause depression, so should be changed immediately post partum. Other effects include sedation (to which patients eventually become tolerant) and postural hypotension, liver function abnormalities and haemolytic anaemia.

Second-line Therapy

Used in conjunction with methyldopa, calcium antagonists (e.g. slow-release nifedipine) and oral hydralazine are often helpful in those in whom mono-therapy with methyldopa has failed. α-Receptor blockers (doxazosin) are also useful in conjunction with methyldopa.

Third-line Therapy – β Blockers

These are generally well tolerated by pregnant women in addition to being effective antihypertensive agents. However, β blockers are known to cause intrauterine growth retardation and hence patients need regular scans to assess for fetal growth. It is advisable to avoid atenolol in pregnancy. Labetalol in both tablet and parenteral form is a favoured formulation, preferably given in the second or third trimester.

Other Antihypertensives

Diuretics are not the drugs of choice in this physiological state, unless there is evidence of fluid overload: in conditions such as heart failure, pulmonary oedema or idiopathic intracranial hypertension.

ACE Inhibitors

These can cause significant fetal abnormalities including oligohydramnios, renal failure and hypotension. If a patient on ACE inhibitors becomes pregnant this is NOT an indication for termination, because the structural malformations caused are not related to the first trimester. The patient should be promptly converted to methyldopa. Post partum, ACE inhibitors can be restarted as their use in breast-feeding mothers is safe.

Angiotensin Receptor Blockers

These are similar to ACE inhibitors, and it is suggest that they are avoided in pregnancy.

Acute Severe Hypertension

Management includes the use of:
- hydralazine (intermittent intravenous bolus)
- labetalol (continuous intravenous infusion)
- nifedipine tablets (never used sublingually).

If using hydralazine or nifedipine as second-line agents, the concomitant use of methyldopa reduces the side effects of headache and tachycardia.

Magnesium sulphate is the drug of choice in eclampsia. However, when used with nifedipine, profound hypotension may ensue.

15.3 Palpitations and Arrhythmia

The physical and hormonal changes associated with pregnancy may produce a proarrhythmic state. Increasing cardiac output results in myocardial stretch and increases LVED volumes. These changes can promote arrhythmogenesis.

Palpitations can occur in up to 50–60% of pregnant women. Holter data for pregnant women were analysed in one study, which showed that 76% of those experiencing palpitations were found to be in sinus tachycardia alone. Ostrezega demonstrated that only 24% of the Holter tests demonstrated any arrhythmia, most of which was benign.

Most palpitations experienced will be a result of isolated atrial and ventricular ectopic beats. Treatment includes reassurance and avoidance of precipitants.

Sinus Tachycardia
This is common in normal pregnancy. However, if the tachycardia is more than 15% greater than the normal heart rate, consider hyperthyroidism, or other causes such as hypovolaemia, sepsis or respiratory or cardiac pathology.

Supraventricular Tachycardia
Paroxysmal SVT is the most common arrhythmia encountered in pregnancy. Tawan demonstrated that a pregnant patient has a 35% greater risk of developing new SVT than at other times in her life. Episodes of tachycardia are more symptomatic in pregnancy and can occur in any of the trimesters. In patients with pre-existing tachycardia, a catheter ablation should be planned before conception if possible.

Management of an AVNRT is similar in pregnant and non-pregnant women. Vagal manoeuvres should be the first choice. If successful in terminating the arrhythmia, no further treatment is necessary. Intravenous adenosine, propranolol or metoprolol is also safe to use in pregnancy. Some suggest that adenosine use in late pregnancy should be used with fetal heart rate monitoring. Flecainide and amiodarone are best avoided. Both carry the risks of teratogenesis.

If the arrhythmia is resistant to all therapies suggested, DC cardioversion is safe, especially if performed within 48 hours of onset, obviating the need for anticoagulation.

Curative catheter ablation is also possible in pregnancy, preferably in the second trimester with radiation shields placed over the abdomen. Pulsed fluoroscopy should help to limit radiation exposure.

Atrial Fibrillation and Flutter

AF and atrial flutter are rarely seen in isolation in pregnancy. These rhythms are often seen together with congenital heart disease (Ebstein's anomaly), rheumatic heart disease or hyperthyroidism.

In patients with permanent AF, addition of β blockers (*not* atenolol) and digoxin can optimize rate control. Anticoagulation should be considered in those at high risk of stroke, such as women with structural heart disease, rheumatic mitral valve disease and previous emboli. Heparin is safe in early pregnancy (before 12 weeks) and this can be replaced with warfarin in the second and third trimesters.

Long QT Syndrome (see Section 8.6)

Inherited long QT syndrome is seen more commonly in women. However, Rashba found that women who are pregnant experience most cardiac events in the immediate postpartum period (9%), as opposed to during the pregnancy (1.8–4.5%). The recommendation for this group is therefore to continue β-blocker therapy throughout the pregnancy and postpartum period. There is a small risk of β blocker entering breast milk and causing neonatal bradyarrhythmia. However, the maternal risk is greater and takes precedence.

Ventricular Tachycardia

RV outflow tract tachycardia (Figure 8.10) is the most likely source of VT seen in pregnancy. RVOT tachycardia is known to occur in patients without recognized structural heart disease. Most episodes are related to stress and are probably catecholamine driven, given that they respond to β-blocker therapy. Nakagawa's study showed that, in 11 women with VT in pregnancy, 73% had monomorphic VT originating from the right ventricle (i.e. LBBB morphology), with an inferior axis. The tachycardia resolves after delivery and the prognosis for mother and baby is good.

An echocardiogram and ECG are necessary to determine if there is any evidence of structural heart disease. The antiarrhythmic of choice for VT in pregnancy is lidocaine and electrical cardioversion should be performed if haemodynamic compromise occurs.

DC Cardioversion

This procedure is safe in pregnancy and is a quick and useful tool for rapidly terminating potentially troublesome tachyarrhythmias.

Implantable Cardioverter Defibrillators (see Section 7.11)

Women with ICDs implanted should not be discouraged from becoming pregnant. The data are favourable for both maternal and fetal outcomes in the presence of cardiac conditions necessitating ICDs. A study of 44 pregnant women with structural heart disease and ICDs found that none received inappropriate shocks during pregnancy. Indeed, Natale found that 75% received no shocks at all. Fetal outcomes were: 89% born healthy, 4% small for dates and 2% stillborn.

Bradyarrhythmias

Patients with symptomatic bradycardia or congenital complete heart block should have a permanent pacemaker implanted before conception. The placing of temporary wires should not be encouraged peri-delivery.

15.4 Ischaemic Heart Disease

Acute MI is a rare occurrence in women of reproductive age, but pregnancy itself increases the risk of an acute myocardial infarct 3–4 times. The incidence is 1 in 10000 but is increasing, probably in the current climate of increased maternal age, smoking and obesity.

Factors such as maternal age over 30 years, diabetes, hypertension, thrombophilia, transfusion, smoking and peripartum infection are significant risk factors for acute MI in pregnancy. Indeed the odds of acute MI in one study were 30-fold increased for a maternal age ≥40 years, when compared with those for maternal age <20 years. Mortality rate from MI in pregnancy is in the range 37–50%.

The management is difficult because thrombolysis is contraindicated pre-delivery and for 10 days post-delivery. Hence, the treatment of choice is primary angioplasty, although there is no evidence base to support this choice.

15.5 Cardiomyopathy (see also Chapter 4)

Dilated Cardiomyopathy (DCM)

The haemodynamic changes of pregnancy, specifically the increase in cardiac work, may provoke ventricular failure, pulmonary oedema and fetal loss in women with DCM. Those with symptoms NYHA class III and above should be counselled against pregnancy because there is an associated maternal mortality of 7%.

Hypertrophic Cardiomyopathy (HCM)

Pregnancy in patients with HCM is considered to be lower risk than in those with severe DCM. Only those with end-stage hypertrophy that has progressed to dilatation and thinning of the LV wall are classed as high risk for sudden death. Maternal mortality is increased by factors including family history of sudden death, extreme hypertrophy, unexplained syncope, non-sustained ventricular tachycardia and an abnormal BP response to exercise.

β Blockers and diuretics are advised for those who develop dyspnoea and exertional limitations. Normal delivery is advised as the risk of haemorrhage and hence excessive fluid loss is reduced.

Peripartum Cardiomyopathy (PPCM)

This occurs between the last month of pregnancy and 5 months post partum. The aetiology is unknown. The LV systolic dysfunction that occurs can be reversible.

Cardiomyopathy presenting earlier in pregnancy is defined as pregnancy-associated cardiomyopathy. Worldwide, Fett found that there is a huge variation in the incidence of PPCM with high rates in Haiti (1 in 299 livebirths) compared with only 1 per 4000 livebirths in the USA. The following are risk factors for the development of PPCM:

- Increasing gravidity
- Primiparous
- Hypertension/pre-eclampsia
- African race
- Twin pregnancy.

There are many hypotheses as to the aetiology of PPCM, including causes such as selenium deficiency, immune-mediated mechanism, myocarditis and viral triggers (such as enteroviruses – Coxsackie virus, parvovirus B19, adenovirus and herpes virus). The role of fetal microchimaerism (fetal cells enter the maternal circulation apparently to enhance maternal tolerance of the fetus) is still under discussion. It is probable that no one factor is directly contributory and that PPCM is multifactorial. Further research is awaited.

Management

The management is similar to the management of other forms of heart failure and includes ACE inhibitors, or hydralazine if PPCM occurs during pregnancy, β blockers, digoxin and diuretics. Anticoagulation should be considered in those with significantly impaired LVEF (<35%)

15.6 Valvular Heart Disease (see also Chapter 3)

Valvular heart disease is the main acquired cardiac defect likely to cause problems in women during childbirth, across the world. Most commonly, disease is rheumatic in origin but can also be the result of congenital abnormalities or previous endocarditis. The main lesion to cause difficulties is mitral stenosis (>90% of cases). Rheumatic heart disease is rare in the UK and, if seen, is primarily in the immigrant population.

Mitral Stenosis

The natural history of mitral stenosis typically starts with a 20- to 25-year asymptomatic period. As a result, many patients may first present in pregnancy when the haemodynamic demands on the heart make the valve stenosis more apparent. Classically, pregnant women with mitral stenosis present with pulmonary congestion, pulmonary oedema and atrial arrhythmias. The pregnancy-related rise in cardiac output makes the pressure gradient across the valve more critical and leads to an increase in LA volume and pressure and elevated pulmonary filling pressures, and results in increasing symptoms of dyspnoea and diminishing exercise capacity. Pregnancy-induced tachycardia further increases LA pressure by decreasing diastolic filling time. The development of secondary pulmonary hypertension may result in RV failure presenting with peripheral oedema, ascites and hepatic engorgement.

Predictors of maternal mortality include a valve area <1.5 cm^2 and NYHA functional class II, III or IV. Fetal mortality increases with increasing NYHA class.

Medical Management

This should be directed at reducing volume overload. Diuretic therapy, reduced salt intake and reduced physical activity are the mainstay of this approach.

β Blockers reduce tachycardia, improving diastolic filling time and hence help to reduce LA pressure. If AF occurs, this requires prompt correction with cardioversion. Prevention of recurrence of AF is best performed using procainamide and quinidine. Digoxin in combination with β blockers is used for rate control in permanent AF. Anticoagulation is essential in the prothrombotic pregnant state with AF and mitral stenosis.

Percutaneous Balloon Mitral Valvuloplasty (see also Section 3.2)

Ideally performed before conception on patients with valve areas <1 cm^2, this procedure can improve complication rates of pregnancy in women with mitral stenosis, compared with medically treated women.

If necessary, the procedure can be performed during pregnancy, ideally in the second trimester, and has a proven track record of normal subsequent deliveries and excellent fetal outcomes. However, it is contraindicated in women with moderate-to-severe mitral regurgitation, calcification of the mitral valve or clot in the left atrium. Risks of radiation exposure can be avoided by performing the procedure purely under TOE (transoesophgeal echocardiography) control but x-ray guidance is needed to cross the septum.

If a woman with mitral valve disease who is pregnant becomes significantly symptomatic, valve replacement is an option and is best performed in the second trimester. However, this is not without increased risk. Maternal outcomes are virtually the same as in the non-pregnant patient but fetal loss can be anything between 10 and 30%.

Delivery

Vaginal delivery is recommended but with epidural anaesthesia and a short second stage of labour, with assisted delivery devices. Oxygen will reduce pulmonary pressures, and fluid restriction and use of diuretics will help to reduce peripartum rises in LA and pulmonary pressure caused by fluid shifts.

Mitral Regurgitation (see also Section 3.3)

This is most commonly a result of mitral valve prolapse, which is usually well tolerated in pregnancy because the left ventricle is offloaded as a result of the reduced systemic vascular resistance. This results in a diminution of mitral regurgitation.

Symptoms may include exertional dyspnoea, orthopnoea and paroxysmal nocturnal dyspnoea. Some patients will present with AF-associated heart failure.

Medical Management

In the presence of impaired systolic function, treatment with hydralazine, and diuretics can help to further offload the left ventricle. In addition, digoxin is well tolerated in pregnancy and can be a helpful and well-tolerated positive inotrope.

Surgical Management

If symptoms are very limiting and the MR severe, surgical repair of the mitral valve is a good option and obviates the need for ongoing anticoagulant therapy. Mitral valve replacement is possible, with good maternal and fetal outcomes, although any LV dysfunction present before surgery is unlikely to recover after surgery.

Aortic Stenosis (see also Section 3.4)

Symptomatic aortic stenosis is less common than mitral valve disease in the pregnant population. The most common cause for aortic valve disease is congenital valvular abnormalities, usually a bicuspid aortic valve with stenosis secondary to a membrane. Surgical correction before conception is advised for all symptomatic patients and those with a peak gradient >80 mmHg. Termination is advised for patients already symptomatic in the first trimester.

It is important to remember that, in women with congenital aortic stenosis, there is a 15% risk of a similar anomaly in the fetus.

During pregnancy, patients with bicuspid aortic valves are at increased risk of aortic dissection as a result of pregnancy-related hormonal effects on the connective tissue of the aorta.

In aortic stenosis, the need to maintain the pressure gradient across the obstructed LVOT puts an increased stress on the LV wall. As a result, LVH and diastolic dysfunction develop, which can progress to fibrosis, resulting in diminished coronary flow reserve and finally systolic heart failure.

Women with aortic valve areas >1 cm^2 should tolerate pregnancy without any symptoms. The main symptoms of those with more severe aortic stenosis are predominantly caused by left-sided heart failure (exertional dyspnoea) rather than syncope or presyncope. Pulmonary oedema is very rare.

Medical Management
Those with mild-to-moderate stenosis and asymptomatic are best managed medically. It is important to protect LV output by avoiding strenuous exercise, vasodilators and diuretics.

Percutaneous Balloon Valvuloplasty
This procedure can be used as a bridge to aortic valve replacement in patients too unwell to undergo the procedure. The current quoted mortality rate in non-pregnant patients is 5%. There is obviously considerable risk to the fetus during the procedure because the fetal circulation is transiently occluded.

Surgical Management
Patients with calcific aortic valves or with significant AR are best treated with an aortic valve replacement. In women of child-bearing age, a bioprosthetic valve would be advisable as the need for anticoagulation is obviated.

Delivery
Vaginal delivery is suggested. Careful fluid balance and protection against vasodilatation are advised in order to avoid perilous BP drops that may compromise cardiac output.

Aortic Regurgitation (see also Section 3.5)
Acute AR may be seen in aortic dissection, infective endocarditis or prosthetic valve malfunction. Marfan syndrome, bicuspid aortic valve and hypertension are conditions that predispose to aortic dissection. Acute AR is a surgical emergency. Patients present with pulmonary oedema and cardiogenic shock because the ventricle has no time to adapt to the sudden increase in LV volume overload.

Chronic AR is, similar to MR, well tolerated in pregnancy. It is usually seen in the presence of a bicuspid aortic valve or rheumatic heart disease. The peripheral vasodilatation of pregnancy helps to offload the overloaded left ventricle by reducing the volume of regurgitant blood.

Patients with AR present with dyspnoea, exertional fatigue and chest pain. If there is any significant degree of systolic dysfunction (NYHA I or II), the pregnancy may not be so well tolerated.

Management
ACE inhibitors are contraindicated throughout pregnancy so alternative vasodilating agents including nifedipine, nitrates, diuretics and hydralazine should be used. Careful echocardiographic monitoring during pregnancy is recommended.

Pulmonary Valve Disease
The most common problem is pulmonary stenosis and is often associated with Noonan syndrome or Fallot's tetralogy. Patients become symptomatic with

moderate or severe stenosis. Pregnancy is generally well tolerated in those with mild pulmonary stenosis.

It should be remembered that, as with congenital aortic stenosis, there is a considerable risk of the fetus being affected (20%).

Tricuspid Valve Disease

Tricuspid regurgitation is usually a result of endocarditis-related damage or related to Ebstein's anomaly. Tricuspid stenosis is usually congenital.

Patients with Ebstein's anomaly (low-seated tricuspid valve, ASD and TR) should be assessed before conception and treated for the presence of abnormal conduction pathways causing tachyarrhythmias.

15.7 Prosthetic Valves (see also Section 3.8)

Bioprostheses are most probably the best solution in women of child-bearing age. Although they do not have the longevity of mechanical prostheses, the elimination of the need for anticoagulation reduces both maternal and fetal risk. The deterioration of bioprostheses is mildly exacerbated by pregnancy (15 years vs 13.5 years).

Pregnancy is a prothrombotic state. The risk of venous thromboembolism is five times higher in pregnancy than in non-pregnant women. The least thrombotic mechanical valve is the bileaflet tilting disc valve in the aortic position. The following are risk factors for thromboembolism of prosthetic valves in pregnancy:

- Valve type – Björk–Shiley
- Valve position – mitral valve
- LA dilatation
- Additional arrhythmias – AF
- Previous thromboembolism
- Inadequate anticoagulation.

For patients with mechanical valves, the safest option is to maintain warfarin therapy throughout pregnancy, with an elective caesarean section to reduce time off warfarin. There is still some discussion as to when to restart warfarin post partum. Some suggest that it should be restarted immediately post partum, and others at day 10, when the risk of postpartum haemorrhage is significantly lowered. Warfarin is safe in breast-feeding.

The risk of fetal anomalies with this strategy would be about 6%. The anomalies include nasal and musculoskeletal hypoplasia, learning disabilities, chondrodysplasia punctata, epithelial and central nervous system abnormalities. There is also an increased risk of fetal haemorrhage because warfarin crosses the placenta. The critical time for warfarin embryopathy is between 6 and 12 weeks' gestation. With this strategy, the maternal thromboembolism risk is estimated to be 3.9%, with a risk of death of 1.8% (Table 15.1). Interestingly, warfarin embryopathy seems to be dose related, the critical level being 5 mg.

Table 15.1 Rates of maternal thromboembolism and death with differing anticoagulant strategies in prosthetic heart valve pregnancy (Chan et al 2000)

Anticoagulant strategy during pregnancy	Rate of thromboembolism (%)	Rate of death (%)
Warfarin throughout	3.9	1.8
Heparin for first trimester, subsequent warfarin	9.2	4.2
Dose-adjusted heparin throughout	25	7

Table 15.2 Guidelines for antenatal prophylactic and therapeutic doses of low-molecular-weight heparin (RCOG: Confidential Enquity into Why Mothers Die 2000–2002)

Prophylaxis	Enoxaparin (100 units/mg)	Dalteparin	Tinzaparin
Normal body weight	40 mg daily	5000 units daily	4500 units daily
Body weight <50 kg	20 mg daily	2500 units daily	3500 units daily
Body weight >90 kg*	40 mg 12-hourly	5000 units 12-hourly	4500 units 12-hourly
Therapeutic dose	1 mg/kg 12-hourly	90 units/kg 12-hourly	90 units/kg 12-hourly**

*These doses also apply to a woman who has a BMI of >30 kg/m^2 in early pregnancy.
**The manufacturer recommends 175 units/kg once a day.

Other alternatives include heparin (LMWH – twice daily) plus aspirin between 6 and 12 weeks' gestation, converting to warfarin from the second trimester. With this strategy, the maternal thromboembolism risk increased to 9.2%, with a risk of death of 4.2%.

The use of dose-adjusted heparin alone for the duration of the pregnancy was linked to a maternal thromboembolism risk of 25%, with a risk of death of 7% but lower foetopathy.

There are insufficient data on the use of LMWH in this situation (Table 15.2), although it is known that there is a lower risk of maternal heparin-induced thrombocytopenia and osteopenia. In addition, LMWH is associated with low neonatal mortality, and low rates of spontaneous abortion and intrauterine death.

15.8 Congenital Heart Disease (see also Chapter 2)

About 1% of all live births will have some form of congenital heart disease. With improving and focused health care, 85% of infants with congenital heart disease will survive into adulthood.

For women with congenital heart disease, there is a risk varying between 3–12% of the fetus having a similar structural cardiac defect. Therefore specialist fetal ultrasonography should be mandatory at 14–16 weeks and may need to be repeated at 18–22 weeks. If the nuchal fold thickness is normal on a scan, it suggests a significantly lower incidence of CHD (1 in 1000).

As with patients with valvular heart disease, all patients with congenital heart disease should be counselled pre-pregnancy. Effective discussions about contraception should take place in those in whom pregnancy is classed as high risk. The following are predictors of poor outcome in pregnancy:

- Pulmonary hypertension
- Systemic ventricular impairment (EF <20%)
- Severe left-sided outflow tract obstruction
- Marfan syndrome with a dilated root.

Aortopathy

Marfan Syndrome (see also Section 14.3)

There are over 2000 women in the UK with Marfan syndrome. The main risk during pregnancy is type A dissection, which is associated with a maternal mortality rate of 22%. It classically occurs in the third trimester or immediately post partum, when wall stress of the aorta is maximal.

The Marfan syndrome patient with no high-risk features still has a 1% risk of pregnancy-related complications. A healthy UK woman has a 1 in 10 000 risk. The features of high-risk pregnancy in Marfan syndrome are:

- FH of sudden death
- aorta >40 mm diameter
- rapid rate of aortic dilatation.

Management

All patients with Marfan syndrome should be treated with β blockers with regular fetal scanning to assess for intrauterine growth retardation. Elective transthoracic echocardiography should be performed between 6 and 10 weeks' gestation, followed by 4- to 6-weekly scans if the aorta is ≥40 mm. MRI can be used if further imaging is required.

Delivery

Elective caesarean sections are suggested for high-risk Marfan syndrome patients, especially those with an aorta >45 mm diameter (European Society of Cardiology) (Table 15.3). However, the American Societies suggest a natural delivery advocating a short second stage of labour.

Aortic Dissection

Dissection can occur in pregnancy without pre-existing disease caused by the hormonal effects of pregnancy on the connective tissue of the aorta wall.

Table 15.3 Aorta size vs maternal risk of dissection

Aorta size (mm)	Maternal risk of dissection (%)
<40	1
>40	10

Patients with bicuspid aortic valves also have an increased risk of aortic dissection in pregnancy.

Coarctation

Most women with coarctation will have had a repair fashioned. MRI can be used to assess the site of repair accurately and to check for re-coarctation or aneurysm formation safely during pregnancy. Pregnancy is classed as low risk as long as there is no aneurysm at the repair site.

Management

β Blockers can control blood pressure well. The target BP should be ≤130/80. Stenting of the coarctation is not recommended during pregnancy because there is a high risk of dissection at this time.

Delivery

Normal delivery is fine, as long as the second stage is assisted and not prolonged. In the presence of an aneurysm, an elective caesarean section should be performed.

If a patient presents with a newly diagnosed coarctation, BP should be aggressively lowered with β blockers and delivery organized at 35 weeks, by elective section.

Septal Defects

ASD/PFO

In the presence of a small shunt with normal pulmonary pressures, pregnancy is usually well tolerated.

Problems can occur as a result of paradoxical emboli because pregnancy itself is a procoagulant state (fivefold increased risk) and the presence of an arteriovenous connection facilitates the passage of thrombus.

Management

As a result, compression stockings and prophylactic heparin should be used in late pregnancy. Device closure of the ASD should be considered before conception. Antibiotic prophylaxis is not necessary for delivery.

VSD/PDA

A small defect is generally better tolerated than ASDs as the pressure gradient across the VSD does not allow the passage of paradoxical emboli. However, there is a risk of infective endocarditis, so prophylactic antibiotics are required for instrumented or complicated deliveries.

15.9 Complex Congenital Heart Disease (see also Chapter 2)

Repaired Tetralogy of Fallot

In the presence of good LV function and no significant RV outflow tract obstruction, pregnancy is well tolerated. Even with significant pulmonary regurgitation, pregnancy is generally trouble free apart from an increase in complaints of fatigue and breathlessness.

Congenitally Corrected Transposition of the Great Arteries (CCTGA) (see also Section 2.6)

In CCTGA, the AV node is absent and hence complete heart block can occur at any time. All patients with complete heart block should have a pacemaker implanted before conception.

Generally, pregnancy is well tolerated if the patient is symptom free before pregnancy. The systemic tricuspid valve may become more regurgitant during pregnancy as a result of the dilatation of the systemic ventricle (morphologically right ventricle). Furthermore, the systemic ventricle can easily fail with the significant haemodynamic demands of pregnancy.

Transposition of the Great Arteries (see also Section 2.5)

The Mustard or Senning repair comprises an atrial rerouting, so that the tricuspid valve and right ventricle support the systemic circulation. Pregnancy is tolerated similarly to those with CCTGA, although the risk of CHB is less because the AV node is intact. However, the extensive scar tissue can lead to sinus node disease with its resultant atrial arrhythmias.

Pulmonary venous pathways should be imaged pre-pregnancy by TOE or MRI. It is important to demonstrate no obstruction because any obstruction produces a clinical presentation similar to severe mitral stenosis in the pregnant patient.

In the presence of good systemic ventricular function (EF>40%), symptoms of NYHA class II or less, and unobstructed pulmonary venous pathways, pregnancy is classed as low risk.

Fontan

For patients with a functional single ventricle, the Fontan procedure creates two separate circulations in series. The patients are therefore oxygenated and no longer cyanotic. The ventricle supports only the systemic circulation, so there is a propensity to low output states. The pulmonary circulation is not facilitated by a ventricular pump, resulting in free drainage of venous blood into the pulmonary artery without pulsatile flow. However, certain problems ensue as a result of this novel circulation:

- Limited ability to increase cardiac output
- Atrial arrhythmias
- Prothrombotic circulation.

As a result, patients are anticoagulated with warfarin long term. If ventricular function is good and patients are in NYHA class I–II, pregnancy is not contraindicated. However, there is still a 30% risk of fetal loss in the first trimester.

Table 15.4 The safety of drugs in pregnancy and breast-feeding

Drug type	Safe	No adverse data in humans	Use with caution	Contraindicated	Possible effects	Safe in breast-feeding
Antiarrhythmics						
Lidocaine		✓			CNS effects (both mother and fetus) Cardiac effects (both mother and fetus) Uterine artery spasm	
Procainamide		✓			Long-term usage associated with lupus-like syndrome	✓
Flecanide			✓		Teratogenic in animal studies Embryotoxic in animal studies Associated with birth defects and fetal deaths Drug of last resort	
Disopyramide			✓		Associated with premature labour if used in third trimester Embryotoxic in animal studies	
Bretylium		✓			Small-for-date babies	
Amiodarone			✓		Learning difficulties in children of treated mothers Fetal hypothyroidism Fetal death in animal studies	
Mexiletine		✓			Can reduce uterine blood flow by 25%	✓
Verapamil		✓			Can treat fetal tachycardia transplacentally but may result in cardiac depression and arrest	✓
Propranolol		✓			IUGR reported in one study Fetal apnoea Fetal bradycardias Neonatal hypoglycaemia	✓
Quinidine		✓			Used to treat fetal tachyarrhythmias	
Adenosine	✓✓				Significant fetal effects in overdose	
Digoxin	✓✓				Used to treat fetal tachyarrhythmias	✓
Warfarin			✓		Skeletal effects on fetus Brain effects on fetus	
Heparin			✓		Inferior anticoagulation of prosthetic valves (see	

					Comments
Antihypertensives					
Methyldopa	✓				
Hydralazine	✓	✓			Transient neonatal thrombocytopenia
Labetalol	✓	✓	✓	✓	IUGR
Metoprolol	✓	✓	✓		
Acebutalol	✓	✓	✓		
Pindolol	✓	✓	✓	✓	
Clonidine	✓				
Nitroprusside					IUGR; IUGR and cleft palate in animal studies; Cyanide toxicity from accumulation in the fetal liver; Teratogenic in high doses in animal studies
Nifedipine					
Nicardipine	✓				
ACE inhibitors				✓	Anuria; Renal failure; Hypocalvaria; Perinatal death
Angiotensin II receptor blockers				✓	Anuria; Renal failure; Hypocalvaria; Perinatal death; Oligohydramnios; Decreased cranial calcification
Diuretics					
Bumetanide	✓				Adverse effect on plasma volume
Furosemide				✓	Fetal hyperbilirubinaemia
Amiloride				✓	Increased fetal loss and skeletal anomalies in animal studies
Spironolactone	✓			✓	Feminization of the genitalia in animal studies
Triamterene	✓	✓			
Bendrofluazide	✓	✓		✓	
Chlorthiazide/hydrochlorthiazide					Neonatal thrombocytopenia

15.10 Cyanotic Heart Disease without Pulmonary Hypertension

The fetal circulation is dependent on maternal oxygen saturation. Maternal saturations of 85% are associated with a 12% chance of fetal survival. Maternal saturations over 90% are associated with a 92% chance of fetal survival. Problems in the cyanotic patient include the following:

• Haemorrhage: caused by impaired clotting factors and reduced platelet function
• Paradoxical embolism: because of right-to-left shunt
• Heart failure: as a result of pregnancy volume loading on an already overloaded ventricle
• Increased cyanosis: because of the vasodilatation of pregnancy.

Management
This should include prolonged bed rest, which will result in increased maternal oxygenation and subsequent increased fetal survival.

Delivery
Normal delivery should be attempted if possible, but there are often fetal problems that necessitate a caesarean section.

15.11 Eisenmenger Syndrome

Over the last 40 years, the maternal mortality rate from Eisenmenger syndrome has remained at 40%. No single medical or obstetric intervention has changed the excessively high level of mortality associated with this condition. Currently the only treatment possible is heart transplantation. Patients with Eisenmenger syndrome need to be fully informed of the increased risk of death both ante and post partum, and also the risk of severe morbidity. Sterilization (using an irreversible method such as tubal ligation) or termination should be advised with this level of risk. If pregnancy is chosen, strict bed rest for the third trimester is essential. In addition, patients should be monitored for 2 weeks post partum because of the ongoing risk of sudden death.

Fetal Outcomes
The fetal and perinatal mortality rates associated with mothers with significant pulmonary hypertension are approximately 30%. One third of infants born suffer from IUGR and only 25% of pregnancies reach term.

15.12 Cardiac Drugs in Pregnancy

For details of this, see Table 15.4.

16 Cardiac Investigations

16.1 Electrocardiography

The Electrical Axis

The normal mean QRS axis in the frontal plane is −30° to +90°. The normal T-wave axis in the frontal plane should be within 45° of the mean frontal QRS axis, i.e. the QRS-T angle should be <45°.

The following gives a quick calculation of the mean frontal QRS axis: find the isoelectric lead; the QRS axis is at right angles to this. Find the lead at right angles to the isoelectric lead from the hexaxial reference system (Figure 16.1). If the QRS is positive this lead is the electrical axis; if it is negative the axis is 180° away.

Left axis deviation = −30° to −90°

Right axis deviation = +90° to +180°

The quadrant −90° to +180° = extreme right or extreme left axis deviation.

Common causes of axis deviation are shown in Table 16.1.

Intervals

Normal PR interval: 0.2 s

Normal QRS duration: 0.1 s.

Normal Q wave is <0.04 s wide and <25% of the total QRS complex.

The QT interval must be corrected for heart rate (QTc):

$$\text{Normal QTc} = \frac{QT}{\sqrt{R}\text{-R interval}} = 0.38 - 0.42\,s$$

Heart rate calculation from R–R interval: at standard paper speed of 25 mm/s, each big square = 0.2 s. Count the number of 'large squares' between each R wave (Table 16.2).

For intracardiac electrophysiological measurements see Section 7.7.

Swanton's Cardiology, sixth edition. By R. H. Swanton and S. Banerjee. Published 2008 Blackwell Publishing. ISBN 978-1-4051-7819-8.

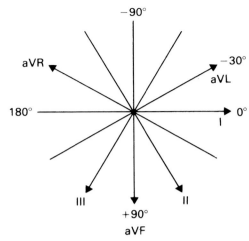

Figure 16.1 Hexaxial reference system.

Table 16.1 The ECG and axis deviation

Right-axis deviation	Left-axis deviation
Infancy	
RV hypertrophy	LV hypertrophy
RBBB	LBBB
Cor pulmonale	Left anterior hemiblock
Acute RV strain: pulmonary embolism	Cardiomyopathies
Secundum ASD	Primum ASD
Fallot's tetralogy, severe PS	Tricuspid atresia
TAPVD	

Table 16.2 Calculation of heart rate from the ECG

R–R interval (s)	Number of large squares	Heart rate (beats/min)
0.2	1	300
0.4	2	150
0.6	3	100
0.8	4	75
1.0	5	60
1.2	6	50
1.4	7	43
1.6	8	37

Hypertrophy

Atrial Hypertrophy and the P Wave

The normal P-wave axis is +30° to +80° in the frontal plane. It is normally <2.5 mm in height. Right atrial depolarization occurs first and causes the initial P-wave deflection. Left atrial depolarization causes the terminal deflection (see Figure 16.2).

Ventricular Hypertrophy

There is no single marker of ventricular hypertrophy on the ECG (Table 16.3).

Several factors are taken into consideration (electrical axis, voltage, delay in the intrinsicoid deflection and ST–T-wave changes) and then the ECG is correlated with the patient's condition. Relying on a single marker of ventricular hypertrophy, e.g. ventricular voltage, may not be reliable. A thin chest wall in young men results in a large voltage; a thick chest wall may mask it.

Factors Influencing Chest Lead Voltage
- LV cavity size
- LV muscle mass
- Presence of pericardial fluid

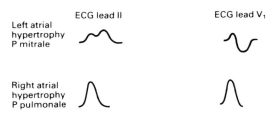

Figure 16.2 The P wave and atrial hypertrophy.

Table 16.3 Diagnosis of ventricular hypertrophy from the ECG

Right ventricular hypertrophy	Left ventricular hypertrophy
Right-axis deviation > 90°	Left-axis deviation > –30°
RV1 + SV6 > 11 mm	SV1 or V2 + RV5 or V5 or V6 > 40 mm
RV1 or SV6 > 7 mm	SV1 or V1 or RV5 or V6 > 25 mm
R/SV1 > 1	RI + SIII > 25 mm
R/SV6 < 1	R in I or aVL > 14 mm
T-wave inversion V1–V3 or V4, ST depression	T-wave inversion in I, aVL ST depression V4–V6
Low voltage V1	
Delay in intrinsicoid deflection in V1 > 0.05 s	Delay in intrinsicoid deflection in V6 > 0.04 s
P pulmonale	P mitrale

- Lung volume in front of heart
- Chest wall thickness.

Examples of acute RV strain are shown in Figure 16.10 and of LV hypertrophy in Figure 16.3.

RV Hypertrophy in Children

The neonate has RV predominance on the ECG with dominant R waves in V1 and aVR, and deep S waves in V6. The pattern gradually swings leftwards through childhood and has reached adult configuration by the age of 15 years. By the end of the first week T waves are negative in V1 and V2 and positive in V5 and V6. By 1 month, the positive R wave in aVR has disappeared. The dominance of the RV in the first 3 months makes the diagnosis of pathological RV hypertrophy difficult and serial ECGs may be needed.

- Presence of a Q wave in V1
- Delay in intrinsicoid deflection in V1 > 0.04 s in the absence of RBBB
- R/S or R/Q in aVR > 1
- QRS axis > 120°
- P pulmonale with P wave > 3 mm in II
- R/S in V1 7 (at 3 months); R/S in V6 0.5 (at 3 months).

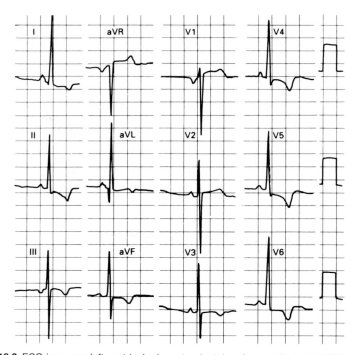

Figure 16.3 ECG in severe left ventricular hypertrophy taken from patient with HCM.

Combined Ventricular Hypertrophy

The effects of both RV and LV hypertrophy on the ECG may cancel each other out and the QRS complexes appear normal. Suspect it if:

- LV hypertrophy + right axis
- RV hypertrophy + left axis
- LV hypertrophy + dominant R in V1 and aVR and deep S in VS
- RV hypertrophy + large Q and R waves in V5 and V6.

Common rhythm problems

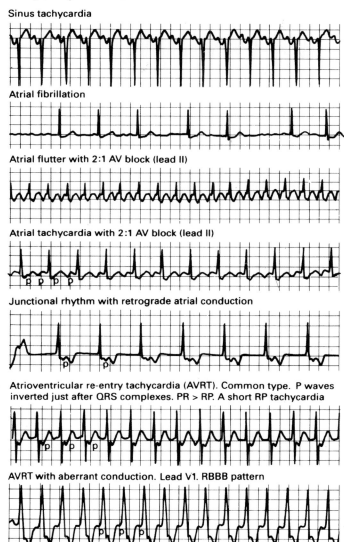

Figure 16.4 Common atrial rhythms.

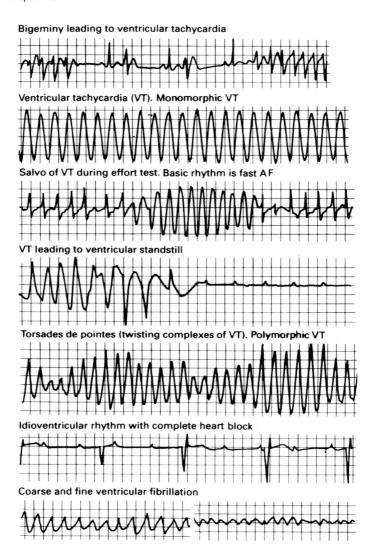

Figure 16.5 Common ventricular rhythms.

Conduction Disturbances

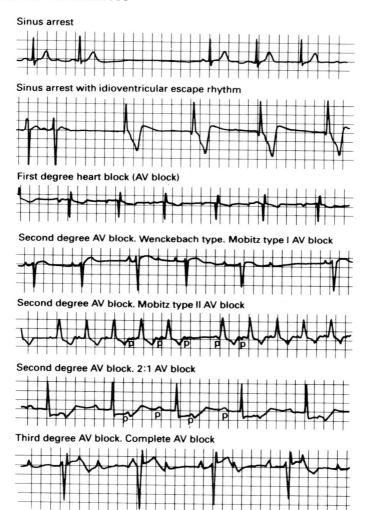

Sinus arrest

Sinus arrest with idioventricular escape rhythm

First degree heart block (AV block)

Second degree AV block. Wenckebach type. Mobitz type I AV block

Second degree AV block. Mobitz type II AV block

Second degree AV block. 2:1 AV block

Third degree AV block. Complete AV block

Figure 16.6 Examples of conduction disturbances.

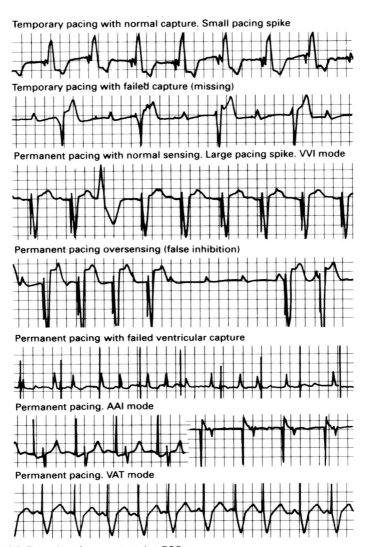

Figure 16.7 Examples of common pacing ECGs.

Bundle Branch Blocks

(a)

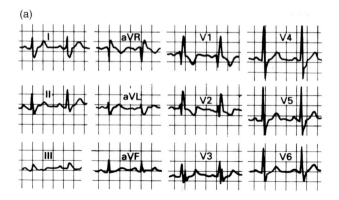

(b)

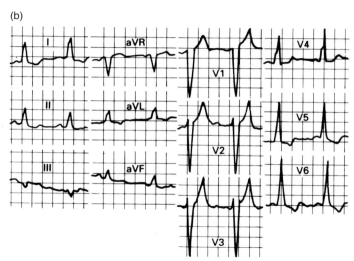

Figure 16.8 (a) Right bundle-branch block, (b) left bundle-branch block.

Bifascicular blocks

(a)

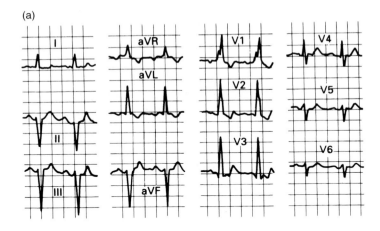

(b)

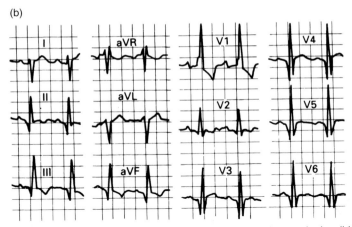

Figure 16.9 (a) RBBB and left anterior hemiblock, (b) RBBB and left posterior hemiblock.

Myocardial infarction and its mimicks

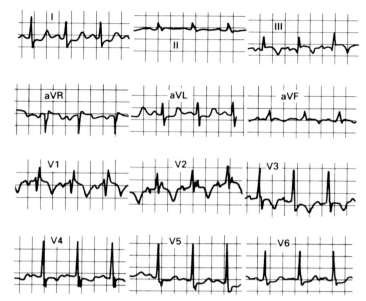

Figure 16.10 ECG in acute pulmonary embolism: this shows typical S_1, Q_3, T_3 pattern, incomplete RBBB and RV strain.

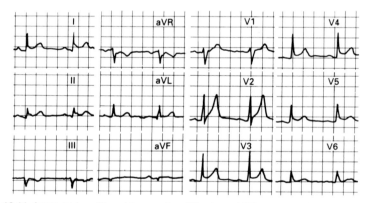

Figure 16.11 Acute pericarditis: widespread saddle-shaped ST segment elevation.

Acute	Recent	Old
2–5 days	2–6 months	6 months
ST segment	T wave inverted	Just Q
elevation		waves

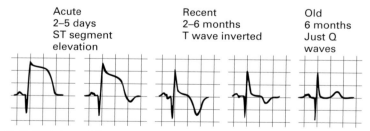

Figure 16.12 Evolution of ST segments after an MI. Persistent ST segment elevation after 3 months suggests an LV aneurysm.

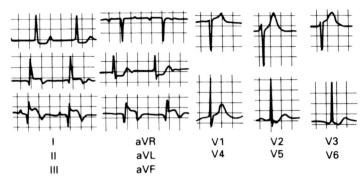

I	aVR	V1	V2	V3
II	aVL	V4	V5	V6
III	aVF			

Figure 16.13 Acute transmural inferior MI: this shows typical Q waves and raised ST segments in inferior leads. There is variable sinus and nodal rhythm. Reciprocal or mirror image ST depression in I and aVL.

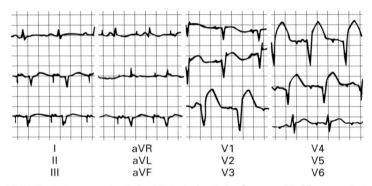

I	aVR	V1	V4
II	aVL	V2	V5
III	aVF	V3	V6

Figure 16.14 Acute transmural anterior MI: typical anterior Q wave with ST-segment elevation; atrial pacing.

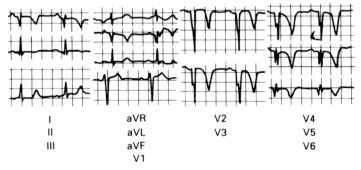

I	aVR	V2	V4
II	aVL	V3	V5
III	aVF		V6
	V1		

Figure 16.15 Recent transmural anterior MI.

Electrolyte Disturbances and the ECG

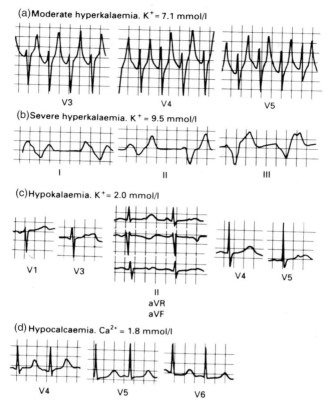

Figure 16.16 Electrolytes and the ECG: (a) moderate hyperkalaemia produces tall, peaked T waves. (b) Severe hyperkalaemia produces gross widening of the QRS also, with a resulting 'sine wave' appearance. P waves disappear. (c) Hypokalaemia produces prominent U waves with small T waves resulting in an apparently long QT interval. The T wave is often lost in the U wave. (d) Hypocalcaemia produces a long QT interval with small T waves, whereas hypercalcaemia produces a short QT interval with normal T waves.

16.2 Exercise Testing

The reliability, limitations and uses of exercise testing have been carefully established in recent years. Although the sensitivity and specificity of treadmill exercise testing have been widely studied, it has also been realized that the results of an exercise test must be interpreted with reference to Bayes' theorem. The prevalence of coronary artery disease in the population under study is very important. The predictive accuracy of a positive test increases with increasing prevalence of the disease in the population (Table 16.4). For a definition of terms, see Table 16.5.

Table 16.4 Predictive accuracy of the treadmill test

Patient	Pre-test likelihood of coronary disease (%)	Predictive accuracy of positive test (%)
Asymptomatic man	5	14–36
Man with angina pectoris	90	97

Assume exercise test with 80% sensitivity and 75% specificity.

Use in Asymptomatic Patients

It can be seen that exercise testing is of little value in screening asymptomatic individuals. The ST-segment response to exercise in this group has a poor predictive accuracy. In this group with a low pre-test likelihood of coronary disease, a positive test is often a false-positive test.

Use in Symptomatic Patients

In the high-risk group (e.g. men with angina) a positive test confirms a clinical diagnosis. A negative test may well be a false-negative test and has a low correlation with the absence of coronary disease. Thus exercise testing in

Table 16.5 Definition of terms

Term	Explanation	How calculated
Sensitivity	Percentage of all patients with coronary artery disease who have an abnormal exercise test	$\dfrac{TP}{TP+FN} \times 100$
Specificity	Percentage of negative exercise tests in normal patients without coronary artery disease	$\dfrac{TN}{TN+FP} \times 100$
Predictive accuracy	Percentage of positive exercise tests that are true positives	$\dfrac{TP}{TP+FP} \times 100$
False-positive response	Percentage of total positive exercise tests that are false positives (occurring in normal patients)	$\dfrac{FP}{TP+FP} \times 100$ (or 100% − predictive accuracy)
False-negative response	Percentage of total negative exercise tests that are false negatives (occurring in patients with coronary artery disease)	$\dfrac{FN}{TN+FN} \times 100$ (or 100% − predictive accuracy)
Risk ratio	Predictive accuracy related to false-negative response (predictive error)	$\dfrac{TP}{TP+FP} \Big/ \dfrac{FN}{TN+FN}$

FN, total false negatives; FP, total false positives; TN, total negatives; TP, total positives.

patients with cardiac symptoms has major limitations from the diagnosis point of view (coronary disease vs normal coronaries). Nevertheless it has great value in the assessment of cardiac function, the evaluation of symptoms, and total exercise time is of great pregnostic value.

Uses of Exercise Testing
- Confirmation of a diagnosis of coronary disease in a group with a high pre-test likelihood of the disease
- Evaluation of cardiac function and exercise capacity
- Prognosis after an MI
- Serial testing in evaluation of medical or surgical treatment
- Detection of exercise-induced arrhythmias
- Useful in rehabilitation and patient motivation.

Patient Safety
The patient should have avoided cigarettes or a recent meal before the test. A physician should be present at all exercise tests or in the immediate vicinity. The procedure is extremely safe, provided that strict criteria for stopping the exercise test are followed. Reported mortality rates are <1 in 10000 tests.

A defibrillator must be instantly available. A complete trolley of cardiac resuscitation equipment should be on hand, including intubation equipment and full range of cardiac drugs. Although cardiac resuscitation is very rarely necessary during or after exercise testing, occasional patients may develop refractory ventricular tachycardia requiring cardioversion.

Contraindications to Exercise Testing
Exercise testing should be avoided in the following cases:
- Severe aortic stenosis
- Acute myocarditis or pericarditis
- Any pyrexial or flu-like illness
- Severe left main-stem stenosis or its equivalent
- LV failure or congestive cardiac failure
- Adults with complete heart block
- Unstable or crescendo angina
- Frequent fast atrial or ventricular arrhythmias
- Renal failure
- Orthopaedic or neurological impairment
- Dissecting aneurysm
- Uncontrolled hypertension
- Thyrotoxicosis
- In any frail, elderly or sick patient
- Acute MI.

In patients who are fully mobile and capable of climbing one flight of stairs, exercise testing may be performed under careful supervision at about 7 days post-infarction, i.e. the day before hospital discharge.

Which Exercise Test?

It is now known that graduated treadmill exercise testing is superior to bicycle ergometry or step testing. Greater limits of exercise are achieved and maximal oxygen uptake is higher with treadmill testing than with other methods. Some patients are unable to pedal a bicycle efficiently, and many stop with 'tired legs' before reaching desired target heart rates.

There are numerous treadmill protocols (Table 16.6) with variations in increasing speed and gradient. Many centres start the test with a preliminary 'warm-up' period of 3 min (1.0 miles/h at 5% elevation).

There is no particular advantage of one protocol over another. Many centres use the Bruce protocol because its higher stages (6 and 7) are much more demanding than some other protocols. (More gradual protocols are available for less fit patients, e.g. those used in cardiac rehabilitation.) Most tests are now performed continuously. The blood pressure is recorded at every stage.

ECG Leads and Lead Systems

Many exercise tests are spoiled through inadequate skin preparation. The shaved skin should be cleaned with alcohol- or acetone-soaked gauze. The cleaned skin is gently abraded with dry gauze, sandpaper, a sterile needle or a dental burr. Silver/silver chloride pre-gelled electrodes are then applied (e.g. Cambmac Medicotest or Sentry medical products). The electrodes and leads are secured by Micropore tape. Electrically screened leads should be used.

The sensitivity for recording significant ST depression increases as more leads are used. Cardiac centres have now moved to 12-lead ECG recording.

Oxygen Consumption (Table 16.7)

The relationship between heart rate and oxygen consumption is linear for most patients during exercise. The slope of the relation is less for fitter and more athletic patients (i.e. greater oxygen consumption for less increment in heart rate). Maximum oxygen consumption is a good measure of maximum cardiac performance and is usually measured in millilitres O_2/kg per min or metabolic equivalents (METS). Resting O_2 consumption is approximately 3.5 ml O_2/kg per min, which is 1 METS.

In a male athlete Vo_{2max} is approximately 70–80 ml O_2/kg per min, and 60 ml O_2/kg for min for a female athlete.

Thus at stage 5 of the Bruce protocol (stage 7 of Sheffield protocol) the oxygen requirement is 56 ml O_2/kg per min or 16 METS.

End-points and When to Terminate the Exercise Test

First the test should be stopped when the target heart rate has been achieved. This may be maximum heart rate for age or submaximal (commonly 85% of maximum predicted heart rate) (Table 16.8).

Table 16.6 Table of standard treadmill protocols showing speed and elevation

Stage	Bruce (miles/h)	(%)	Sheffield (miles/h)	(%)	Naughton (miles/h)	(%)	Ellestad (miles/h)	(%)	Balke 3.0 (miles/h)	(%)	IMC 3.4 (miles/h)	(%)	Rehabilitation (miles/h)	(%)
1	1.7	10.0	1.7	0.0	1.0	0.0	1.7	10.0	3.0	6.0	3.4	0.0	2.0	0.0
2	2.5	12.0	1.7	5.0	2.0	0.0	3.0	10.0	3.0	8.0	3.4	4.0	2.5	0.0
3	3.4	14.0	1.7	10.0	2.0	0.0	4.0	10.0	3.0	10.0	3.4	8.0	2.5	3.0
4	4.2	16.0	2.5	12.0	2.0	3.5	5.0	10.0	3.0	12.0	3.4	12.0	2.5	6.0
5	5.0	18.0	3.4	14.0	2.0	7.0	5.0	15.0	3.0	14.0	3.4	16.0	2.5	9.0
6	5.5	20.0	4.2	16.0	2.0	10.5	6.0	15.0	3.0	16.0	3.4	20.0	2.5	12.0
7	6.0	22.0	5.0	18.0	2.0	14.0			3.0	18.0				

Stage 3 of the Sheffield protocol onwards is the same as stage 1 onwards of the Bruce protocol.

Table 16.7 Oxygen consumption at stages of exercise in various protocols

Stage	O₂ consumption (ml O₂/kg per min)		Balke 3.0
	Bruce	Sheffield	
1	17.5	8	18.0
2	24.5	12	21.0
3	34	17.5	24.0
4	46	24.5	28.0
5	56	34	32.0

A useful mental guide for heart rate (maximum) is 220 minus the age for men and 210 minus the age for women.

Second, the test should be stopped before maximum or submaximal heart rate if any of the following symptoms or signs occur:
• Progressive angina pectoris
• Undue dyspnoea
• Vasoconstriction with a clammy, sweaty skin
• Fatigue
• Musculoskeletal pain
• Feeling of faintness
• Atrial fibrillation or atrial tachycardia
• Premature ventricular contractions with increasing frequency
• Ventricular tachycardia
• Progressive ST-segment depression ⎫ with or without chest pain
• Progressive ST-segment elevation ⎭
• Failure of heart rate or blood pressure to rise with effort; this is very important and applies even in patients on β-blocking agents
• Excessive rise in peak systolic pressure (>230 mmHg)
• Electrical alternans

Table 16.8 Age-adjusted target heart rates

Age (years)	Submaximal heart rate (85% max.)	Maximal heart rate
30	165	194
35	160	188
40	155	182
45	150	176
50	145	171
55	140	165
60	135	159
65	130	153

- Development of LBBB
- Development of AV block.

Sometimes the greatest ECG abnormalities occur during the recovery period when the patient is lying down. Young unfit patients may develop a profound vagal bradycardia post-exercise requiring atropine. A period of 10–15 min is usually long enough for recovery. All haemodynamic criteria (heart rate and blood pressure) and the ECG should have returned to the pre-exercise state before the patient is moved.

Exercise Testing and Drugs

Digoxin frequently causes a false-positive exercise test and ST-segment changes at rest are common. If possible the drug should be stopped at least 1 week before exercise. Digoxin is not thought to cause false-negative responses.

β-*Blocking agents* do not need to be withdrawn before exercise and sudden withdrawal may be dangerous. The maximum heart rate response and maximum workload achieved will be reduced from normal. However, there is evidence that β blockade may help in converting false-positive results to negative ones, and allow true positive results to remain positive.

A single dose of a β-blocking agent may be taken 1.5–2 hours before the test if the patient is not on β blockade already and thought to have a false positive test. β Blockade will increase the specificity and predictive accuracy of the exercise test but reduce its sensitivity.

Exercise Testing after a Myocardial Infarction

In the absence of the contraindications listed, exercise testing may be safely performed after an MI and before hospital discharge (at about 7 days post-infarction), although exercise testing is sometimes delayed until about 1 month post-infarction. A limited treadmill test is useful in predicting recurrent angina or sudden death in the first year post-infarction. It helps to identify patients who need coronary angiography. Poor prognostic factors are shown in Section 5.7.

What Represents a Positive Test?

ST-segment Depression (Figure 16.16)

There must be ≥1.0 mm ST-segment depression 80 ms after the J point, using the PQ segment as the baseline in six consecutive cycles. If the J point is not clearly visible, the nadir of the S wave may be used instead. It does not matter if the ST segment is downsloping, horizontal or upsloping at the 80-ms point. Sometimes all three may occur in the same patient in different leads, and the ST segment changes should preferably be in more than one lead anyway. Some centres prefer to use 1.5-mm ST depression 80 ms after the J point if the ST segment is upsloping. If 1.5- or 2.0-mm ST depression is taken as the necessary hallmark of a positive test, the sensitivity of the test will fall, but the predictive accuracy will increase. T-wave inversion alone is of no value.

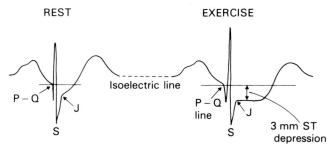

Figure 16.17 ECG at rest (left) and on exercise (right): the PQ function line is below the isoelectric line and is taken as the baseline for ST-segment analysis. The complex on the right shows 3 mm ST-segment depression 80 ms after the J point. If the J point is not clearly seen, the nadir of the S wave may be used.

The PQ junction is taken as the baseline because this junction is normally depressed on exercise below the classic isoelectric line. The Ta wave (P-wave repolarization) on exercise may extend through the QRS and influence the ST segment even in normal patients – hence the need for the 80-ms delay after the J point for test interpretation.

Although the degree of ST-segment depression is the diagnostic hallmark of a positive exercise test it is also important to note:
• How many and in which lead they occur
• The heart rate at which it first appears
• Its persistence in the recovery period.

Some equipment now integrates the area of ST-segment depression (in microvolt-seconds). It is also possible to run exercise tests using signal averaging of the QRS complex. This produces clear recordings with no electrical or myographic interference. However, the equipment is expensive, and meticulous attention to satisfactory electrode placement is all that is really necessary. Typically positive exercise tests are shown in Figure 16.17.

ST-segment Elevation (Figure 16.18)

This may occur during exercise in leads with Q waves and has the same significance as ST depression in other leads. It is a result of systolic outward wall movement over the infarct area.

Chest Pain

Taken in association with ST depression, chest pain increases the sensitivity of the exercise test to approximately 85% in a cohort of symptomatic patients. The nature of the pain is important. Unilateral chest pain is unlikely to be angina. Patients who experience 'walk through' or 'second wind' angina do not normally do so on an exercise test because the workload is progressive and not steady.

Other criteria (below) are not as useful as the ST segment in predicting coronary disease. However, they are important correlates of a positive test

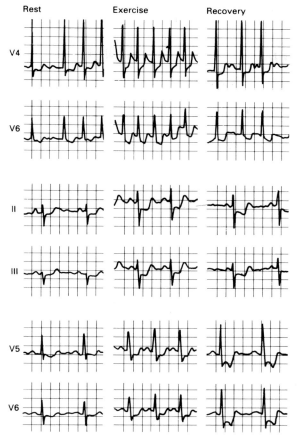

Figure 16.18 Changes in ST segments: this shows three examples of positive ST-segment depression. The top panel shows upsloping and downsloping ST-segment depression in different leads. The second panel shows a positive test persisting after β blockade. The bottom panel shows ST-segment depression getting progressive worse into the recovery stage. R-wave voltage increases (see below).

and increase the sensitivity of the test still further when combined with ST-segment analysis.

Increase in R-wave Voltage (see Figure 16.17, bottom panel)
In the normal patient, R-wave voltage decreases during exercise. Immediately after exercise R-wave voltage is at its smallest and then gradually returns to normal during the recovery period. The reduction in R-wave voltage is thought to be a result of the reduction of LVEDV with increasing exercise in the normal patient. The relationship of QRS voltage to LV blood volume is the Brody effect. LV volume also decreases on standing up from the supine position.

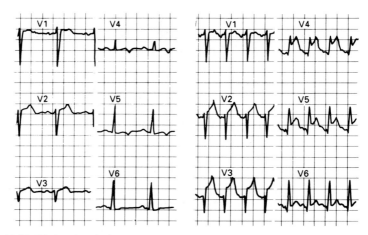

Figure 16.19 ST elevation during exercise test.

In patients with coronary disease, R-wave voltage usually remains unchanged or increases, especially in those with poor LV function. R-wave changes may be useful in patients with LBBB where ST changes lack sensitivity or specificity.

Unfortunately the R wave is related not only to LVEDV but also to other factors (e.g. respiration) see Section 16.1. R-wave voltage is best averaged for several cycles and leads rather than taking a mean of a single lead (e.g. V_5).

Inverted U Waves

Leads in which U waves are well seen may show U-wave inversion in patients with coronary disease. The changes may be transient and occur at peak exercise only. They are characterized by a concave depression in the T-P segment. The U wave is usually overlooked in exercise testing.

Abnormal Systolic Blood Pressure Response

Failure of the systolic blood pressure to rise during exercise is an important indicator of an abnormal LV and is an indication to stop the test. A decrease in systolic blood pressure during exercise is even more specific for severe coronary artery disease – assuming that there are no valve lesions and the patient is not on vasodilators.

Development of Ventricular Arrhythmias (see Figure 16.4)

The development of ventricular arrhythmias is not specific for coronary artery disease. Ventricular ectopics (>10/min), multifocal ectopics, ventricular tachycardia, etc., associated with ST-segment depression and chest pain, are more specific.

Auscultating Changes

Auscultation should be performed immediately in the recovery period. New mitral regurgitation or a fourth heart sound (S4) are highly significant.

Summary of Variables Developing During an Exercise Test Suggestive of Multiple Vessel Coronary Disease and a Poorer Prognosis

• ST depression: at low heart rate (<130/min off β blockade), >2mm in several leads, downsloping, persisting >5min into recovery period
• Blood pressure response: failure to rise or falling >10mmHg
• Ventricular arrhythmias developing at low exercise load
• Poor exercise tolerance: inability to complete Bruce protocol stage II or equivalent and a positive test with inappropriate tachycardia.

Patients with these results are generally referred for coronary angiography.

False-positive Results

An enormous number of conditions may be associated with false-positive exercise tests. They are particularly common in patients with a low pre-test likelihood of coronary artery disease (e.g. asymptomatic young women). Known associations of false-positive results in patients with normal coronaries are:
• hyperventilation
• prolapsing mitral valve
• hypertrophic cardiomyopathy
• dilated cardiomyopathy
• hypertension with LV hypertrophy
• LBBB
• aortic stenosis
• young women with chest pain
• Wolff–Parkinson–White syndrome
• drugs, e.g. digoxin, antidepressants
• anaemia
• coronary artery spasm
• hypokalaemia
• hypersensitivity to catecholamines
• observer variability.

Hyperventilation as a cause of a false-positive test can be excluded by asking the standing patient to hyperventilate for 30s before the exercise test. Patients with sympathetic overactivity, emotional lability and resting tachycardia are very likely to have a false-positive test. This functional condition has been called the hyperkinetic heart syndrome. β Blockade may abolish resting T-wave abnormalities on the ECG in these patients and will increase the specificity of the test by preventing the false-positive result.

16.3 Cardiac Catheterization

The advent of two-dimensional and Doppler echocardiography has reduced the need for cardiac catheterization in both congenital and adult heart disease. Newer forms of angiography, such as digital subtraction angiography and radionuclide angiography, together with magnetic resonance imaging, are reducing the need still further. However, it still plays a vital role in cardiac diagnosis. There has been a rapid increase in the use of intervention techniques that avoid the need for cardiac surgical treatment, as shown by the following.

Congenital Heart Disease
• Rashkind balloon septostomy in TGA. Balloon dilatation of coarctation, mustard baffle, pulmonary venous obstruction, Blalock anastomosis, valve stenosis, etc.

Percutaneous Coronary Intervention
• Native coronary vessels, vein grafts, internal mammary grafts
• Streptokinase infusion into main pulmonary artery in massive acute pulmonary embolism or rarely into the coronary artery in acute MI or during PCI.

Valvuloplasty
• Balloon dilatation of all four valves is now a recognized procedure.
Cardiac catheterization is usually merely a diagnostic procedure with well-defined mortality and morbidity risks. Since coronary arteriography was introduced by Mason Sones in 1962, great advances in techniques and equipment have occurred.

Percutaneous valve replacement
• Aortic and pulmonary valves are being replaced percutaneously.

Mortality and Morbidity
Mortality in most centres is now approximately 0.1% in patients having coronary arteriography. The deaths occur in patients with the most severe coronary disease. In addition there is a very small risk of an embolic CVA and a catheter-induced MI.

There is a definite morbidity relating to arterial entry site complications. The American Collaborative Study on Coronary Artery Surgery (CASS), published in 1979, suggested that the femoral entry site was safer. The brachial approach was safe only if the operator performed 80% or more of the procedures from the arm. Most cardiologists are able to catheterize from either route with no morbidity.

There is increasing use of the radial artery as an entry site using the percutaneous Seldinger technique. This route can be used in patients with peripheral vascular disease without the need for a cut-down. It is ideal for outpatient/day-case work because patients can sit up in a chair immediately after the procedure. Many units have started day-case angioplasty for simple cases using the radial approach.

What to Tell the Patient

The patient is told why the test is necessary and an explanation of what is involved and why local anaesthetic is preferred. The reasons that general anaesthesia is usually unnecessary are as follows: it interferes with haemodynamics and oxygen saturations; patients cannot indicate if they develop angina or other symptoms; patients are usually required to perform respiratory manoeuvres, coughing, etc.; and patients are very occasionally required to perform exercise during the test.

The procedure should be painless, although the patient should be warned of the hot flush associated with angiography, and the very small risks should be explained.

Which Route?

This is a matter of operator preference. Usually, however, the right brachial route (or brachial) is often used for the following:
• Patients on anticoagulants (unless a sealing device is used in the femoral artery)
• Coarctation of the aorta (or axillary cut-down in babies)
• Patients with intermittent claudication or those who have had aortoiliac surgery
• Occasionally aortic valve stenosis as a dominant lesion
• Hypertensive patients with high peak systolic pressures, because femoral haemostasis may be difficult.

The femoral route is usually preferred for patients with:
• atrial septal defects
• most types of congenital heart disease
• atypical chest pain in young women who may have small brachial arteries and a tendency to arterial spasm
• Raynaud's phenomenon
• several (two or more) previous brachial catheterizations
• presence of a right subclavian bruit.
• failed Allen's test
• LIMA graft to LAD

Premedication

Some form of premedication is important, because anxious patients may become vagal on arrival in the catheter laboratory or after withdrawal of the catheters. Anxiety may provoke angina before the procedure even starts in patients with ischaemic heart disease. The following is a suggested regimen.

Adults

Diazepam 10–20 mg orally 1–2 hours pre-catheter. A further dose (Diazemuls) may be given intravenously just before the catheter if the patient is still anxious. Fentanyl 25–50 mg i.v. is a useful additional analgesic given just before the catheter.

Children
<5 kg: Atropine only. 20 mcg/kg (or 40 mcg/kg orally)
5–10 kg: Triclofos orally 50 mg/kg. Elixir is 100 mg/ml
10–20 kg: Midazolam syrup orally 0.5 mg/kg
>20 kg: Temazepam orally. 0.5–1.0 mg/kg. Maximum 20 mg

Adults do not usually require general anaesthesia if these doses are used, but children usually have a general anaesthetic. Patients should be starved for >4 h pre-catheter. Their cardiac medication should not be discontinued, except for diuretics, which are best avoided on the morning of catheterization.

Polycythaemic patients with cyanotic congenital heart disease are at risk (if the haemoglobin level is > 18 g/100 ml) of both arterial and venous thromboses. A few days before cardiac catheter the patients should be admitted for venesection, with concurrent plasma exchange if the haemoglobin exceeds this level (see Section 2.10).

Renal Failure
This may occur after cardiac catheterization as a result of:
• pre-existing renal impairment
• dehydration
• contrast medium nephropathy
• prolonged hypotension.

It is essential to know the patient's serum creatinine before the procedure (in all but acute emergencies), and with simple measures the condition is largely preventable. Patients particularly at risk are those with diabetes, hypertension, congestive cardiac failure or known renal failure. The following routine is used in any patient with a serum creatinine >135 μmol/l:

• Administer 1 litre 0.9% saline over 12 h before the cardiac catheter. Give further volume during the procedure if necessary.
• Stop metformin, non-steroidal anti-inflammatory drugs and diuretics where possible 48 h pre-catheter and re-start them 48 h post-catheter if renal function satisfactory.
• Use as limited amount of contrast as possible during the procedure (aim for <3 ml/kg body weight)
• Use only a non-ionic, low osmolality contrast medium
• N-Acetylcysteine (NAC): the evidence that this is beneficial is not strong and largely based on meta-analysis of heterogeneous studies. It is a vasodilator and an antioxidant rapidly absorbed and converted in the liver to cysteine. The dose is 600 mg twice daily orally the day before and the day of the catheter. Some units continue 600 mg twice daily for 2 days after the procedure. One study using NAC in primary angioplasty found 1200 mg twice daily better than 600 mg twice daily in prevention of contrast nephropathy. An

intravenous preparation is also available: NAC ampoule is 2 g diluted to 10 ml with 50 ml 5% dextrose or 0.9% saline given over 15–30 min (intravenous dose is 600 mg = 3.0 ml of this solution).

The most important item here is pre-hydration. Try to arrange to do diabetic patients first on the catheter list. A renal film is also useful at the end of the procedure taken on the catheter table to check for renal size, function and any possible obstruction.

Cockcroft–Gault Equation for Estimation of Creatinine Clearance (1976)

An estimate of the creatinine clearance (in ml/min) can be made from the serum creatinine using the Cockcroft–Gault equation avoiding the need for a 24 h urine collection:

$$\frac{(140 - age) \times weight(kg) \times 1.23 \times (0.85 \text{ if female})}{\text{serum creatinine } (\mu mol/l)}$$

Severe renal dysfunction (creatinine clearance <30 ml/min) is known to be independently associated with an increased mortality and other adverse events after both PCI and CABG.

Coping with Catheter Complications Occurring on the Ward

Haemorrhage

Leg

This is controlled by firm pressure. A Johns Hopkins bandage is not effective and just obscures the puncture site. Firm pressure above the puncture site will help control the development of a haematoma. If the bleeding is not controlled after 30 min:

• Check the clotting screen. If the patient is on warfarin, fresh frozen plasma may help. Vitamin K is not recommended because it makes subsequent anti-coagulation very difficult. If the patient has just had heparin then check the APTT, because protamine reversal may help (dose=protamine 10 mg/1000 units heparin administered).
• Is the patient hypertensive? High peak systolic pressure will exacerbate bleeding.
• Call for help. Very rarely, femoral artery repair may be necessary for a false aneurysm. A hard, tender, pulsatile lump over the puncture site developing after cardiac catheterization suggests a false aneurysm/pseudoaneurysm (Figure 16.20). The diagnosis can be confirmed by ultrasonography.

A pseudoaneurysm is more likely with:
• low puncture site (more difficult to compress)
• obesity
• diabetes

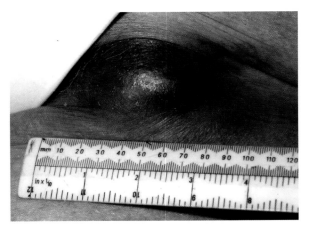

Figure 16.20 Right femoral artery pseudoaneurysm.

- women >70 years
- systemic hypertension.

Firm pressure with an ultrasound probe on the neck of the aneurysm for about 20–30 min can result in the false aneurysm thrombosing, avoiding the need for surgical repair in most cases. A femostop device can be used on the ward as an alternative. Most femoral false aneurysms can be dealt with in this way if the neck of the false aneurysm is small. It is painful and the patient will need sedation and analgesia. Occasionally, a false aneurysm thromboses spontaneously. The risk is greater with the larger sheaths used for PCI (especially atherectomy or rotablation). However, the use of devices to occlude the femoral artery puncture site (e.g. Angioseal, Perclose, Starclose) is of great value in these cases. Their use reduces haemorrhagic complications and allows for early mobilization.

Arm

The same principles apply, but in this case the artery has been repaired by direct suture. Bleeding is often venous oozing only. Firm brachial pressure should not occlude the radial pulse. Protamine is not usually given after brachial artery catheterization. Any haematoma development will require exploring and re-suturing of the brachial artery.

Radial Artery

This is a puncture site only and bleeding is dealt with by localized pressure. Generally complications after radial artery puncture are less than with femoral artery puncture (0.3% vs 2.8%), and a false aneurysm is rare (Figure 16.21) with current compression equipment.

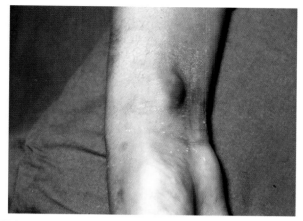

Figure 16.21 Right radial artery pseudoaneurysm.

Infection

Post-catheter pyrexia is usually the result of a dye reaction and settles within 24 h. Persistent pyrexia should be investigated and treated along the usual lines with blood cultures, urine cultures, etc. before antibiotics.

A tender pink area around the brachial cut-down should be treated with complete rest (arm resting on a pillow), and oral amoxicillin 500 mg three times daily and flucloxacillin 500 mg four times daily for 5 days.

Dye Reaction

This is commonly mild, causing: skin reaction, erythema, urticaria or even bullous eruption, nausea and vomiting, headache, hypotension, pyrexia, rigors. Very rarely, it causes more severe reactions: fits, transient cortical disturbance, e.g. cortical blindness, anaphylactic shock.

- Urticaria and skin reaction are usually helped by intravenous antihistamines (e.g. chlorpheniramine 10 mg i.v.) and more severe cases by additional intravenous hydrocortisone 100 mg.
- Nausea and/or vomiting: intravenous metoclopramide 10 mg.
- Hypotension: intravenous fluids may be necessary, especially in patients who have been excessively diuresed or who have had a lot of dye (e.g. >3 ml/kg).
- Pyrexia and rigors are usually transient. Rest and sedation are all that is necessary.
- Anaphylactic shock: occurs in the catheter laboratory rather than the ward, and should be treated by urgent volume replacement with intravenous plasma substitute or 0.9% saline, hydrocortisone 200 mg i.v., epinephrine 1 : 1000, 1 ml slowly subcutaneously.

• Cortical disturbances are rare and again usually transient. They are not necessarily embolic, and may result in part from vascular spasm or an osmotic effect of the dye. Fits are controlled as in grand mal epilepsy with intravenous diazepam.

Cyanotic Attacks
These typically occur in the small child with Fallot's tetralogy and severe infundibular stenosis. The combination of metabolic acidosis, hypoxia and hypovolaemia predisposes to infundibular shutdown or spasm. Catecholamine release secondary to pain and/or fear will also exacerbate this. Treatment depends on reversing these factors:
• Propranolol 0.025–0.1 mg/kg i.v.
• Morphine sulphate 0.1–0.2 mg/kg i.v. in severe cases
• Check the arterial acid–base balance; if the base deficit is or exceeds –5 give intravenous 8.4% $NaHCO_3$ as:

[Body weight (kg)/6] × Base deficit

then repeat the blood gases
• Exclude hypoglycaemia on above sample
• Oxygen via a facemask
• Placing the child in a knee–chest position acts, in the same way as 'squatting', by cutting off acidotic venous return from the legs; as an initial manoeuvre it may help while drugs are being prepared.

The Lost Radial Pulse after Brachial Artery Catheterization
This should be dealt with in the catheter laboratory at the time. If the patient is hypotensive, volume replacement with intravenous heparinization may help. Nitrates are of little benefit. Fifty per cent of patients who do not regain the radial pulse will not develop claudication symptoms. A few patients will regain the radial pulse once they warm up and brachial spasm regresses. Overall a lost radial pulse occurs in <1% of brachial catheterization cases.

A numb hand may occur in the presence of a good radial pulse. This is usually the effect of lidocaine on the median nerve at the catheter site and the sensation returns within 12 h. Residual median nerve damage is rare and probably a result of unnecessary manipulation of the nerve during the catheter procedure.

A loss of the foot pulses after femoral artery catheterization is also rare, but may be transient (24 h) in children. In adults, however, loss of the foot pulses is usually irreversible and requires femoral thrombectomy.

Angina
This may occur during or after coronary angiography, or as a result of paroxysmal tachycardia in the ischaemic patient. It usually responds to sublingual nitroglycerin and sedation. The ECG should be checked and if the angina

recurs the patient should be monitored. Occasionally diamorphine 2.5–5 mg i.m. or i.v. is required.

In severe cases with recurrent pain, intravenous nitrates should be started (see Section 5.4).

If ST-segment elevation occurs, the patient has probably occluded a major coronary artery as a result of thrombus or dissection after intubation or instrumentation of the coronary artery. Very occasionally it may be the result of coronary spasm. In either case treatment with intravenous nitrates is started. The next stage depends on the findings at cardiac catheterization. The patient may be suitable for an immediate angioplasty, or emergency CABG surgery may be necessary. If immediate surgery or PCI is not possible then intra-aortic balloon pumping is considered, which will help maintain coronary flow and reduce infarct size until a more definitive treatment is available. In elderly people, or those who have had a difficult salvage angioplasty, it may be felt that supportive medical treatment is appropriate (see Section 5.7).

Arrhythmias

These are usually transient and dealt with during catheterization. They may occasionally recur on the ward, e.g. paroxysmal AF or SVT, or more rarely paroxysmal VT. Each arrhythmia must be treated on its merits along the lines discussed in Sections 8.3–8.4.

Pericardial Tamponade

This should be considered in any patient who becomes hypotensive and anuric after catheterization. It is a very rare complication of routine cardiac catheterization but is a recognized complication of the transseptal puncture procedure or RV biopsy. Diagnosis is confirmed by M-mode and two-dimensional echocardiography. Pericardial aspiration may be required.

Valve Area Calculation (Table 16.9)

Calculation of aortic or mitral valve area from cardiac catheter data is possible if the cardiac output is measured together with simultaneous pressures from either side of the aortic or mitral valve. Calculations of tricuspid and pulmonary valve areas are perfectly possible but rarely needed.

Table 16.9 The range of aortic and mitral valve areas in adults

	Aortic (cm²)	Mitral (cm²)
Normal	2.5–3.5	4–6
Mild stenosis	1.0–1.5	1.5–2.0
Moderate stenosis	0.5–1.0	1.0–1.5
Severe stenosis	<0.5	<1

The calculation of valve area thus depends on:
- the mean valve gradient
- the forward flow across the valve
- a constant.

The constant used derives from the calculations of Gorlin and Gorlin (1951), which has been established by comparing calculated valve area and actual valve area measured at postmortem examination or surgery. As the calculation depends on 'forward flow' the method is invalidated in the presence of regurgitation unless an angiographic output is used.

Table 16.9 relates to native valves. The method can also be used for prosthetic valves. The Gorlin formula tends to overestimate the true valve area at high cardiac outputs and underestimate valve area at low cardiac outputs.

Aortic Valve Area (same formula for pulmonary valve) (Figure 16.21)

$$\text{Aortic valve area} = \frac{\text{Aortic valve flow (ml/sec)}}{44.5\sqrt{\text{Mean aortic gradient (mmHg)}}}$$

$$\text{Aortic valve flow} = \frac{\text{Cardiac output (ml/min)}}{\text{Systolic ejection period (sec/min)}}$$

The Gorlin constant for aortic (or pulmonary) valves is 44.5.

Mean aortic gradient is calculated by planimetry (five cycles in SR, ten in AF) of the area shown shaded in Figure 16.22.

Mitral Valve Area (same formula for tricuspid valve) (Figure 16.23)

$$\text{Mitral valve area} = \frac{\text{Mitral valve flow (ml/sec)}}{31\sqrt{\text{Mean mitral gradient (mmHg)}}}$$

$$\text{Mitral valve flow} = \frac{\text{Cardiac output (ml/min)}}{\text{Diastolic filling period (sec/min)}}$$

Mean mitral gradient is calculated by planimetry of the area shown in Figures 16.23, and 16.3 is the Gorlin constant for mitral (or tricuspid) valves (0.7×44.5) in the original calculation where LV mean diastolic pressure was assumed to be 5 mmHg.

With simultaneous measurement of LV and LA (or PAW) pressures the constants 38 or 40 are frequently used.

Angiographic Estimation of LV Volume (Figure 16.24 and Table 16.10)

In spite of the fact that gross assumptions are made about the shape of the LV cavity, magnification errors may arise and a single-plane cine is usually used, the angiographic assessment of LV volume correlates very closely with ventricular cast measurements or echocardiographic estimations of LV volume.

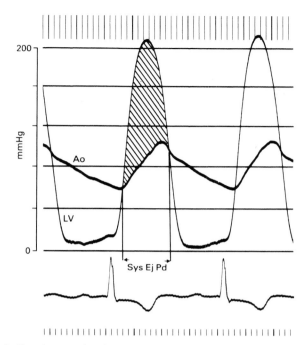

Figure 16.22 Aortic valve area: hatched area is planimetred for calculation of mean aortic gradient. Sys Ej Pd, systolic ejection period (s/min). Computerized catheter laboratory systems are programmed to calculate valve area automatically.

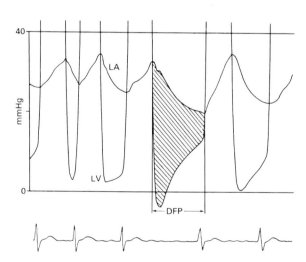

Figure 16.23 Mitral valve area: hatched area is planimetred for calculation of mitral valve area. Ten consecutive cycles should be measured for patients in AF. DFP, diastolic filling period (s/min).

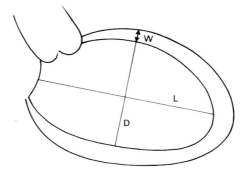

Figure 16.24 Estimation of LV volume by single-plane 30° RAO projection. L, major axis (cm); D, minor axis in two planes (cm); V, ventricular volume (ml); W, wall thickness (cm, see LV mass estimation).

Although formulae for biplane cineangiography have been produced, most centres use a single-plane 30° RAO projection for the LV cine. Most formulae assume that the left ventricular cavity is an ellipsoid of revolution, thus assuming that the minor axes in two planes are identical:

$$V = \frac{4\pi}{3} \times \frac{D}{2} \times \frac{D}{2} \times \frac{L}{2} = \frac{\pi}{2} \times D^2 \times L$$

(uncorrected for magnification).

The magnification factor (f) is calculated from filming a marked catheter or grid/ruler of known length (at central chest level). The corrected volume equation becomes:

$$V = \frac{\pi}{6} D^2.L.f^3 = 0.524.D^2.L.f^3 \text{ (Greene formula)}$$

The formula can be modified by calculation of the area (A in cm²) and length (L in cm) only. The area is measured by planimetry or more usually by a programmed computer system. Using this area–length method, the minor axis need not be measured as:

$$\frac{D}{2} = \frac{2A}{\pi L}$$

where A = area of LV in cm².

Table 16.10 Normal values for LV angiographic volumes (Kennedy)

LVEDVI	70 ± 20 (mean + SD) ml/m²
LVESVI	24 ± 10 ml/m²
Ejection fraction	0.67 ± 0.08
LV mass	92 ± 16 g
Wall thickness	10.9 ± 2.0 mm

Substituting this in the original volume equation we can simplify the equation to:

$$V = \frac{0.849 \times A^2 \times f^3}{L} \text{ (Dodge formula)}$$

Programming this formula into a computer, rapid sequential LV volume analysis is possible.

Formulae for the calculation of RV volume have been derived but each makes assumptions about RV cavity shape that are even more unfounded than the assumption of LV cavity shape.

Angiographic Assessment of LV Mass

The volume of the LV cavity is subtracted from the cavity and LV wall volume. Uniform wall thickness is assumed.

If W is the wall thickness at mid-point of intersection of the minor axis, and the specific gravity of heart muscle is 1.05 then:

$$\text{LV mass} = 1.05 \times \left[\frac{4}{3} \pi f^3 \left(\frac{D}{2} + W \right)^2 \left(\frac{L}{2} + W \right) \right] - \left[\frac{\pi}{6} f^3 . D^2 . L \right]$$

$$\underbrace{\qquad\qquad\qquad\qquad}_{\substack{\text{LV wall + cavity} \\ \text{volume}}} \qquad \underbrace{\qquad\qquad}_{\substack{\text{Cavity} \\ \text{volume}}}$$

In spite of the obvious invalidity of the assumptions involved in the calculation, this estimate of LV mass has been shown to correlate well with postmortem measurements.

Cardiac Output Calculations

Direct Fick Method

The main difficulty with this method is an accurate measurement of oxygen consumption:

$$\text{Cardiac output (CO)} = \frac{\text{Oxygen consumption}}{\text{Arteriovenous oxygen content difference}}$$

or

$$\text{CO (L/min)} = \frac{O_2 \text{ consumption (ml/min)}}{(A_o - PA) \, O_2 \text{ content (ml/dl)} \times 10}$$

Oxygen Content Calculation

The haemoglobin and oxygen saturation must be known.

O_2 content = (Hb × 1.34 × % saturation) + Plasma O_2 content

where Hb is haemoglobin; 1.34 is derived from the fact that 1 g Hb when 100% saturated combines with 1.34 ml O_2.

Plasma O_2 content in 100 ml plasma $= [100 \times 0.0258 \times Po_2]/760$.

Thus with Hb of 15 g/100 ml and 97% saturation, the arterial oxygen content is $(15 \times 1.34 \times 0.97) + 0.3 = 19.65$ ml/100 ml, where 0.3 is the plasma correction factor (Table 16.11).

It does not matter from which systemic artery the O_2 content is calculated. Only the pulmonary artery should be used for mixed venous oxygen content calculation.

Oxygen content can also be measured by specific equipment containing a galvanic fuel cell, which releases electrons on absorbing oxygen (Lexington instruments) or by a manometric method (Van Slyke).

Oxygen Consumption Calculation
Expired air is collected for 3–10 min of steady-state respiration. The method is only really possible or accurate in the basal state. Three methods are available:

1 Closed circuit spirometer: contains 100% oxygen and expired CO_2 is absorbed by soda-lime canister
2 Open circuit: with expired air collected in a Douglas bag
3 Fuel cell technique: with a sample of expired air measured for O_2 concentration using purpose-built equipment.

$$V_{O2} = V_E \, STP \, (Fio_2 - Feo_2) \times 10 \, \text{ml/min}$$

where V_{O2} = oxygen consumption in ml/min, $V_E STP$ = expired volume of air corrected for standard temperature and pressure, Fio_2 = concentration of inspired oxygen – in room air this is 20.93% and need not be measured – and Feo_2 = concentration of expired oxygen.

The correction of V_E for standard temperature and pressure is:

Table 16.11 Plasma correction factors

Saturation (%)	Correction
97	0.30
96	0.27
94	0.24
92	0.21
90	0.19
85	0.17
80	0.14
75	0.12
70	0.11
60	0.10
50	0.08
40	0.07
30	0.05
20	0.04

Table 16.12 Table of water vapour pressure (W) at various room temperatures (T)

Temp (°C)	W (mmHg)	Temp (°C)	W (mmHg)	Temp (°C)	W (mmHg)
15	12.79	21	18.65	27	26.74
16	13.63	22	19.83	28	28.35
17	14.53	23	21.07	29	30.04
18	15.48	24	22.38	30	31.82
19	16.48	25	23.76	31	33.70
20	17.54	26	25.21	32	35.60

$$V_{ESTP} = V_{EATP} \times \frac{273}{273+T} \times \frac{P-W}{P} \times \frac{P}{760}$$

where V_{EATP} = measured expired volume at atmospheric temperature and pressure, T = room temperature in °C, P = barometric pressure in the room (mmHg), and W = water vapour pressure (mmHg) (Table 16.12).

Indirect Fick Method

Using Table 16.13 for estimated oxygen consumption, the direct Fick measurement or an indicator dilution method can be checked. Table 16.13 is a guide and cannot be comprehensive for all ages at any heart rate.

Table 16.13 Mean oxygen consumption in the basal state per body surface area

Age (years)	Male (ml/min per m²)	Female (ml/min per m²)	Age (years)	Male (ml/min per m²)	Female (ml/ min per m²)
3	185	178	23	129	118
4	180	173	24	129	117
5	177	170	25	127	117
6	174	167	27	127	117
7	169	163	28	127	117
8	166	155	30	125	117
9	162	151	32	125	116
10	158	146	33	124	115
11	153	143	35	124	114
12	150	137	36	123	113
13	147	133	38	123	112
14	143	127	40	122	112
15	140	124	42	119	112
16	137	122	45	118	111
17	135	121	50	117	110
18	134	120	55	115	109
19	132	119	60	114	108
20	131	118	65	113	107
21	130	118	70	112	106
22	130	118	75	110	105

See body surface area nomogram, Appendix 1. Basal state: adults approximately 70 beats/min, children approximately 120 beats/min.

Cardiac Output by Indicator Dilution

Indocyanine green (peak absorption at 800 nm) is injected into the right heart or main PA. Downstream sampling is from the aorta, or brachial or femoral artery, through a densitometer. The Gilford densitometer is often used. It is insensitive to changes in O_2 saturation. Background dye causes a baseline shift.

The disadvantage of the technique is that two catheters are involved and that recirculation occurs. In addition a calibration factor (K) must be calculated from known concentrations of green dye in fresh heparinized blood from non-smokers. Then

$$K = \frac{\text{Indicator concentration in mg/l}}{\text{Deflection through densitometer (mm)}}$$

Several concentrations of dye in blood must first be prepared (e.g. 1–10 mg/l). From the Hamilton equation:

$$CO = \frac{I \times 60}{C \times t}$$

where I = amount of green dye injected (mg), C = mean concentration of dye (mg/l), t = duration of curve (s).

The product ($C \times t$) is the area under the curve excluding the recirculation component, the primary curve. There are two chief methods for calculation of the area. The most accurate is to reconstruct the primary curve by plotting the time–concentration curve on semi-logarithmic paper with the indicator concentration on the semi-log axis. The straight line on the descending limb is extrapolated and the primary curve reconstructed from the semi-log plot: it is assumed that the decay of the primary curve is exponential (Figure 16.25).

The second type of calculation employs short-cuts that ignore the recirculation component and do not involve reconstruction of the primary curve.

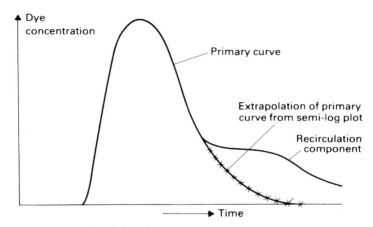

Figure 16.25 Reconstruction of the primary curve.

Reconstruction of the Primary Curve (Figure 16.24)

Once the primary curve has been constructed there are several methods for calculation of the area some of which are discussed below:

• By planimetry (Figure 16.26)
• Summation of 1-s interval concentration values (ordinates). This is easier if the curve is traced on to graph paper.

Thermodilution Method

This is usually performed using a Swan–Ganz catheter in the right heart. Doses of 5 or 10 ml 5% dextrose (at either room temperature or 4°C) are injected into the right atrium, and the thermistor at the catheter tip in the pulmonary artery senses the transient fall in temperature as a rise in resistance.

Advantages over green dye measurements are:

• the recirculation curve can be ignored
• only one catheter is needed
• the method can be repeated rapidly after drug intervention and the catheter may be left in the right heart for further assessment of the sick patient.

Various cardiac output computers are available that integrate electronically the area under the curve. Several methods are used, all of which assume that the downslope of the curve is exponential.

Shunt Quantitation by Oximetry

Oximetry is used to detect shunts rather than quantitate them accurately. Errors in quantitation arise from streaming and sampling in the wrong place. An estimation of shunt size can be made from saturation measurements during catheterization.

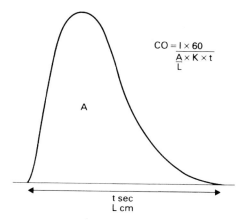

$$CO = \frac{I \times 60}{\frac{A}{L} \times K \times t}$$

t sec
L cm

Figure 16.26 Calculation of the basic area by planimetry. *A*, planimetred area of curve (cm²); *L*, length of baseline (cm); *K*, calibration factor; *t*, time of curve (s); *I*, quantity of dye injected (mg).

From the Fick equation:

$$\text{Pulmonary flow} = \frac{O_2 \text{ consumption}}{(PV - PA\ O_2 \text{ content})}$$

Pulmonary vein sampling is not possible unless there is an ASD or trans-septal catheterization is performed. PV saturation is assumed to be 98%.

The equation becomes:

$$\text{Pulmonary flow} = \frac{O_2 \text{ consumption}}{\dfrac{(98 - PA \text{ saturation})}{100} \times Hb \times 1.34 \times 10} \text{L/min} \qquad (1)$$

Similarly:

Systemic flow

$$= \frac{O_2 \text{ consumption}}{\dfrac{(Ao \text{ saturation} - \text{mixed venous saturation})}{100} \times Hb \times 1.34 \times 10} \text{L/min} \qquad (2)$$

Mixed venous saturation is calculated as:

$$\frac{(3 \times SVC \text{ saturation}) + (1 \times IVC \text{ saturation})}{4}$$

SVC saturation is usually lower than IVC saturation. Rather than measure O_2 consumption the ratio of pulmonary to systemic flow can be estimated by dividing Eqn (1) by Eqn (2), i.e.

$$\frac{\text{Pulmonary}}{\text{Systemic flow}} = \frac{Ao \text{ saturation} - \text{mixed venous saturation}}{98 - PA \text{ saturation}}$$

True PV saturation is substituted for 98% if it is obtained. Small left-to-right shunts may be missed by oximetry and green dye or ascorbate techniques are more sensitive. Oximetry will not usually detect a PDA or small VSD. A primum ASD may be mistaken on oximetry as a VSD with the oxygenated stream being missed in low right atrial sampling.

Nevertheless it provides a useful check during catheterization and an estimate of shunt size. A routine saturation run during catheterization usually involves sampling from:

High SVC: RV inflow
Low SVC: RV body
RA/SVC junction: RV outflow
High RA: main PA (RPA + LPA)
Mid-RA: LA and PV if possible
Low RA: LV
IVC: Ao.

Sampling through the right atrium is performed down the lateral RA wall to detect anomalous venous drainage. Bidirectional shunting can be detected but not accurately quantitated using oximetry.

Assessment of LV Function

The importance of the assessment of LV function to the cardiologist is in the prognosis after cardiac surgery. The importance lies, to the clinical pharmacologist, in the measurement of the effects of drugs and, to the physiologist, in the understanding of the heart as a pump.

The problem remains that there is no single index of LV function that can be used to diagnose early myocardial damage.

Compensatory mechanisms for volume or pressure overload result in many of the indices mentioned below remaining normal even in the presence of some myocardial damage or disease.

Myocardial mechanics is a complex subject, which cannot be covered here. The indices discussed briefly below are those that are most commonly used. None of the contractility indices is entirely independent of preload or afterload.

Compensatory Autoregulation Mechanisms

1 Frank–Starling effect (heterometric autoregulation): increasing fibre length results in increased velocity of contraction. Thus an increase in EDV results in an increased stroke volume. The descending limb of the curve does not exist in humans.
2 Anrep effect (homeometric autoregulation): increasing afterload resulting in increased contractility. This is possibly a result of norepinephrine release from the myocardium.
3 Bowditch effect (inochronic autoregulation): increasing heart rate resulting in increased contractility. Mediated via calcium flux.
These three mechanisms are independent of the sympathetic or parasympathetic system influences on the heart. During exercise the increase in cardiac output is primarily caused by an increase in heart rate (and not stroke volume) mediated via the sympathetic nervous system.

Parameters of Ventricular Function (see also Table 16.14)

1 *Angiographic*
LVEDV: LV mass
LVESV: LV ejection rate
Ejection fraction.

2 *Radionuclide*
Ejection fraction.

3 *Haemodynamic*
Cardiac index: minute work index
LVEDP: LV power
Stroke work index: myocardial O_2 consumption and efficiency.

Table 16.14 Common indices of cardiac function

Index	How derived	Normal range
Cardiac index	Cardiac output (CO)/body surface area	2.5–4.0 l/min per m^2
Stroke volume index (SVI)	Stroke volume/body surface area	40–70 ml/m^2
LV stroke work index (LVSWI)	Stroke volume index × 0.0136 × mean arterial − mean wedge pressure	40–80 g·m/m^2
LV minute work index (LVMWI)	Stroke work index × heart rate (HR)/1000	4.5–5.5 kg·m/m^2 per min
Systemic vascular resistance (SVR)	(a) $\dfrac{80(\overline{Ao}-\overline{RA})}{CO}$ or (b) $\dfrac{(\overline{Ao}-\overline{RA})}{CO}$	(a) 770–1500 dyn·s/cm^5, (b) 10–20 units
Pulmonary vascular resistance (PVR)	(a) $\dfrac{80(\overline{PA}-\overline{PAW})}{CO}$ or (b) $\dfrac{(\overline{PA}-\overline{PAW})}{CO}$	(a) <200 dyn·s/cm^5, (b) < 2.5 units
Tension time index (TTI)	LV pressure during ejection × HR × systolic ejection period (mmHg·s/min)	DPT:TTI ratio >0.7
Diastolic pressure time index (DPTI)	LV pressure during diastole × HR × diastolic filling period (mmHg·s/min)	
LV dP/dt max.	Differentiated LV pressure from micromanometer	Approximately 1000–2400 mmHg/s
V_{max}	See Figure 16.29	Developed pressure V_{max} approximately 2.0–3.3/s

4 *Pre-ejection/Isovolumic Phase Indices*
Systolic time intervals (see Figure 16.30)
Max. dP/dt, min. dP/dt
Derivatives of max. dP/dt correcting for preload, e.g.

max. dP/dt/LVEDP

V_{pm} = maximum measured rate of contractile element shortening from force–velocity loop, V_{max} = maximum rate of contractile element shortening at zero developed pressure (extrapolated from force–velocity loop) see Figure 16.29.

5 *Ejection Phase Indices*
Derived from echocardiogram or left ventricular angiogram, e.g. peak VCF.

6 *Diastolic Indices*
dP/dV (diastolic stiffness) or dV/dP (compliance).

Left Ventricular Work

Left Ventricular Stroke Work Index
Left ventricular work is commonly calculated as the LV stroke work index (LVSWI):

LVSWI = LV × SVI × 0.0136 g·m/m²

where LV = mean LV pressure (mmHg) during ejection (as in calculation of TTI, see Figure 16.27), SVI = stroke volume index (ml/m² per beat) (calculated from angiogram or thermodilution CO).

As planimetering the LV pressure during ejection to derive mean LV pressure is time-consuming, provided that there is no aortic valve gradient mean aortic pressure may be used. This calculates systolic work.

Net LV work is calculated as:

LVSWI = (LV − LVEDP) × SVI × 0.0136

or

(Ao − PAW) × SVI × 0.0136

where Ao = mean aortic pressure, PAW = mean pulmonary artery wedge pressure and LVEDP = LV end-diastolic pressure.

LV Minute Work Index
LVMWI is calculated as:

$$LVSWI \times \frac{HR}{1000} \ (kg·m/m²/min).$$

This allows consideration of heart rate in work calculations because the HR tends to have an inverse relationship with SVI.

Pressure–Volume Loops (Figure 16.27)
LV work may be calculated by measuring the area within a pressure–volume loop. Intraventricular pressure is measured during an LV angiogram. By recording ECG timing on cine film, instantaneous LV pressure can be calculated at any LV volume (Figure 16.27).

The pressure–volume loop is used to study LV compliance (dV/dP) and stiffness (dP/dV). There are major problems in the study of LV compliance as there are in contractility. The slope of the diastolic pressure–volume plot at any instant of volume is a measure of diastolic stiffness. Assumptions from the excised dog's heart that the diastolic pressure–volume relationship is exponential are not necessarily valid in humans.

Diastolic Pressure Time Index/Tension Time Index (Figure 16.28)
The diastolic pressure time index (DPTI)/tension time index (TTI) ratio is established as a measure of subendocardial ischaemia. The DPTI gives a measurement of myocardial oxygen supply and the TTI a measure of myocardial oxygen consumption. It is thus a supply/demand ratio (Buckberg and Hoffman):

DPTI = Mean LV pressure during diastole × Diastolic filling period × HR

TTI = Mean LV pressure during ejection x Systolic ejection period × HR.

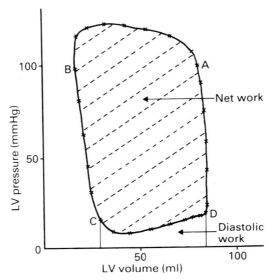

Figure 16.27 Pressure–volume loop to show calculation of net left ventricular work. A, aortic valve opening; B, aortic valve closure; C, mitral valve opening; D, mitral valve closure.

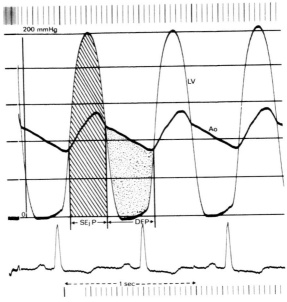

Figure 16.28 Calculation of tension time index and diastolic pressure time index in aortic stenosis. SEjP, systolic ejection period (s/min); DFP, diastolic filling period (s/min).

Figure 16.28 shows simultaneous pressure recordings of LV and aorta in a patient with aortic stenosis. The stippled area represents the area planimetred to calculate mean LV pressure in diastole and hence DPTI. The hatched area represents the area planimetred to calculate mean LV pressure in systole and hence TTI. Normal ratio = >0.7, typical range in aortic stenosis = 0.3–0.5.

Inotropes will reduce the ratio by increasing TTI and decreasing DPTI (by shortening diastole with the inevitable chronotropic effect). β Blockade will increase the ratio by reducing TTI and increasing DPTI (longer diastole).

Indices of Ventricular Contractility

The ideal index of contractility should be easily measurable in the human heart, reproducible and independent of changes in preload or afterload. No ideal index exists. Only two pre-ejection phase indices will be briefly discussed.

Max. dP/dt

The maximum rate of rise of LV pressure during the isovolumic phase is recorded via a catheter-tip micromanometer in the left ventricle with the pressure differentiated. It is known that max. dP/dt depends not only on the inotropic state of the muscle, but also on the preload, afterload and LV volume (end-diastolic fibre length). It is thus not a particularly useful index of contractility.

Attempts to avoid preload dependence by deriving other indices from max. dP/dt (e.g. max. $dP/dt \div$ LVEDP) do not solve the problem. Min. dP/dt (peak negative dP/dt) depends on the inotropic state of the muscle and on end-systolic volume.

V_{max} (Figure 16.29)

This index is defined as the maximum velocity of contractile element (VCE) shortening at zero load. As with max. dP/dt, it is derived from high-fidelity catheter-tip manometer recordings of LV pressure. The LV pressure is differentiated and divided by the instantaneous LV pressure. This is plotted on the vertical axis with LV pressure on the horizontal axis. Using numerous assumptions about the left ventricle it can be shown that:

$$VCE = \frac{dP/dt}{KP}$$

The force–velocity loop appears as shown in Figure 16.29.

Conversion of the vertical axis to a log scale allows for a straight-line extrapolation. The extrapolation distance is shorter if 'developed pressure' is used (i.e. LVEDP).

Some workers prefer to express results as KV_{max} because K, the coefficient of series elasticity, has not been calculated in humans. Many of the assumptions used to generate V_{max} are generally agreed to be invalid. It probably depends on preload.

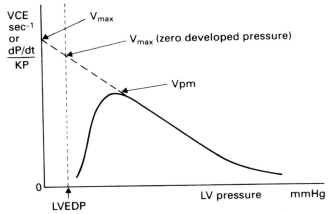

Figure 16.29 Force–velocity loop to show extrapolation of curve to zero developed pressure (LVEDP) to calculate V_{max}. VCE = velocity of contractile element shortening (s^{-1}), dP/dt = rate of rise of LV pressure (mmHg/s), K = coefficient of series elasticity (calculated in dogs as 28, but unknown in humans), P = instantaneous LV pressure — LVEDP, i.e. this is developed LV pressure.

Systolic Time Intervals (Table 16.15)

This non-invasive assessment of LV function is mainly used in the study of drugs on LV performance and in the follow-up of cardiac disease in a single patient. However, it should not really be used in interpatient comparisons. Intervals measured are shown in Figure 16.30.

Q–S_2

Onset of Q wave to onset of aortic valve closure. This is total electromechanical systole.

LVET

This is the LV ejection time, and is the onset of carotid upstroke to dicrotic notch. This interval has been shown to equal ejection time measured from the same interval in the aortic root.

Table 16.15 Predicted normal systolic time intervals (in ms)

	Male	Female
Q–S_2	$546 - 2.1 \times HR$	$549 - 2.0 \times HR$
LVET	$413 - 1.7 \times HR$	$418 - 1.6 \times HR$
PEP	$131 - 0.4 \times HR$	$133 - 0.4 \times HR$
PEP/LVET	0.35 ± 0.04 (1 SD)	

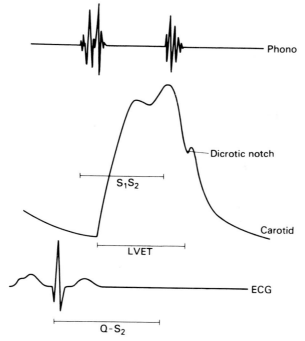

Figure 16.30 Systolic time intervals. Q–S$_2$, electromechanical systole. LVET, left ventricular ejection time.

PEP

This is the pre-ejection period, and is taken from the onset of the Q wave to aortic valve opening. However, unless taken at cardiac catheterization with LV and Ao pressures recorded the non-invasive measurement is:

PEP = Q–S$_2$ – LVET.

There are two components to the PEP:

1 The electromechanical interval (Q wave to onset of systolic rise of LV pressure)

2 The isovolumic contraction time (IVCT): onset of rise of LV pressure to aortic valve opening. IVCT = S$_1$–S$_2$ interval – LVET. The exact definition of the onset of mitral valve closure from the beginning of S$_1$ may be difficult. It is not usually measured non-invasively. The indices Q–S$_2$, PEP and LVET are dependent on HR. The ratio PEP/LVET has been widely used to avoid this dependence (Tables 16.15 and 16.16).

The ratio increases with a combination of prolonged PEP and shortened LVET. The ratio may also be increased by:

• LBBB (lengthens PEP)
• β blockade
• reduction in LV volume, diuretics, haemorrhage.

Table 16.16 Range of abnormality of PEP/LVET in LV dysfunction

Mild	Moderate	Severe
0.44–0.52	0.53–0.6	>0.6

The ratio decreases (shortening of PEP) if inotropes are given (digoxin or catecholamines). Moderate aortic valve disease also reduces the ratio by lengthening the LVET. As LV function in aortic valve disease deteriorates, the ratio returns towards normal. It is thus not a useful index in aortic valve disease. It has been found useful, however, in assessing prognosis after an MI.

Coronary Artery Nomenclature

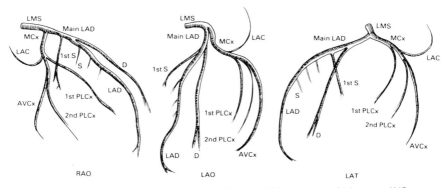

Figure 16.31 Left coronary artery. Key: A, atrial branch; AM, acute marginal artery; AVCx, atrioventricular groove branch of circumflex; AVN, atrioventricular node artery; CB, conus branch; D, diagonal branch of LAD; LAC, left atrial circumflex; LAD, left anterior descending; LAO, 30° left anterior oblique projection; LAT, left lateral projection; LMS, left main stem; LV, left ventricular branches; MCx, main circumflex; PD, posterior descending; PLCx, posterolateral circumflex branch (obtuse marginal); RA, right atrial branch; RAO, 30° right anterior oblique projection; RV, right ventricular branch; 1st S, first septal perforator; S, septal perforating arteries; SN, sinus node artery.

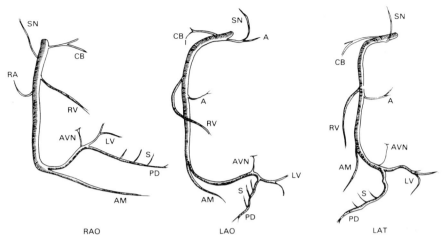

Figure 16.32 Right coronary artery. Key: A, atrial branch; AM, acute marginal artery; AVCx, atrioventricular groove branch of circumflex; AVN, atrioventricular node artery; CB, conus branch; D, diagonal branch of LAD; LAC, left atrial circumflex; LAD, left anterior descending; LAO, 30° left anterior oblique projection; LAT, left lateral projection; LMS, left main stem; LV, left ventricular branches; MCx, main circumflex; PD, posterior descending; PLCx, posterolateral circumflex branch (obtuse marginal); RA, right atrial branch; RAO, 30° right anterior oblique projection; RV, right ventricular branch; 1st S, first septal perforator; S, septal perforating arteries; SN, sinus node artery.

17 Echocardiography

Echocardiography is now a standard non-invasive cardiac investigation following the early pioneering work of Edler and Hertz in 1953.

Pulsed ultrasound of high frequency is generated by a piezo-electric crystal, which acts as both transmitter and receiver. Transmitted pulses of sound are produced by the transducer; reflected sound is converted back to an electrical signal and recorded.

The higher the frequency of the ultrasound used the greater the resolution of the image (with the shorter wavelength), but tissue attenuation (absorption of ultrasound) is greater.

17.1 Types of Scan (Figure 17.1)

A-mode (Amplitude Modulation)

The returned ultrasound signals are displayed on the oscilloscope as a series of vertical lines. The amplitude/height of each line represents the strength of the returning signals. The base is represented as distance (centimetres) from the transducer.

B-mode (Brightness Modulation)

The peaks of the A-mode scan are represented as a series of linear dots with the brightness representing the echo intensity.

M-mode (Motion Mode)

The B-mode scan is displayed on light-sensitive paper moving at constant speed to produce the conventional permanent record – a single dimension/time image.

Two-Dimensional ('Real Time')

A two-dimensional image of a segment of the heart is produced on the screen: a tine image or moving tomographic cut that can be stored. Frozen images

Swanton's Cardiology, sixth edition. By R. H. Swanton and S. Banerjee. Published 2008 Blackwell Publishing. ISBN 978-1-4051-7819-8.

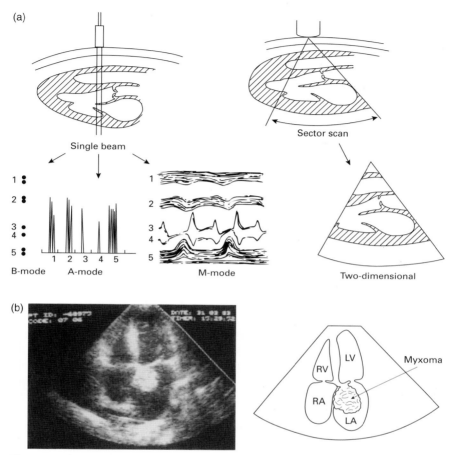

Figure 17.1 (a) Diagrammatic representation of types of echocardiogram. The numbers refer to the same structure in each type of scan: 1, anterior RV wall; 2, interventricular septum; 3, anterior mitral leaflet; 4, posterior mitral leaflet; 5, posterior LV wall. (b) An example of a two-dimensional scan in the four-chamber view, showing a left atrial myxoma.

can be hard copied. The two-dimensional image is produced either by rotating the scanning head rapidly through 80–90° (single crystal) or by a phased array (multicrystal) scanning head. In the phased array system the ultrasound crystals are excited in sequence or phase to produce a fan-shaped wave front.

The original multicrystal head in linear format (as used in abdominal ultra-sonography) is unsuitable for cardiac imaging because the ribs interfere with the ultrasound beams. An example of an LA myxoma seen on a two-dimensional scan is shown in Figure 17.1b (see also Stress Echocardiography and Three-dimensional Echocardiography, Figures 17.64 and 17.65).

17.2 The Normal Two-dimensional Echocardiographic Study

The normal sequence of views taken when recording an echocardiographic study are the parasternal long axis, parasternal short axis, apical four chamber, apical two chamber, subcostal and suprasternal views. Depending on the complexity of the case and the operator's experience, sometimes additional views are used.

For the purposes of this chapter we describe the areas best visualized by each of these standard views. After this introduction to basic echocardiography, we look at commonly found valvular and pericardial abnormalities and discuss the techniques required to demonstrate the abnormalities.

Parasternal Long Axis

The first view of the echocardiographic study is obtained by positioning the transducer just to the left of the sternum with the marker on the probe towards the left shoulder, usually in the second interspace. This view (Figure 17.2) clearly demonstrates the left atrium, mitral valve leaflets and subvalvar apparatus, left ventricle and part of the right ventricle.

The M-mode recording taken across the mitral valve shows the movement of the leaflets and is shown in Figures 17.3 and 17.4 (parts 1–3).

1 At point D the anterior and posterior mitral leaflets separate. The anterior leaflet has the greater excursion, which can be measured (D–E distance). The E point is the point of maximal opening and the anterior leaflet virtually touches the septum in the normal ventricle. In LV failure there is separation of the septum to E point and the greater the E point to septal distance the worse the LV function.

The mitral valve immediately starts to close again to the F point. The E–F slope is a measure of the rate of mitral valve closure. Normal E–F slope is 70–150 cm/s. It is reduced in mitral stenosis. The mitral valve reopens at end-diastole with the A wave. The leaflets meet at point C at the onset of systole. The movement of the posterior leaflet mirrors the anterior leaflet, but its excursion is less. It is more difficult to record on the M-mode echo.

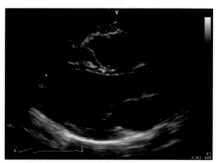
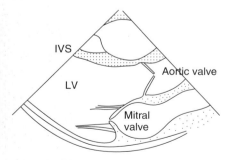
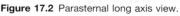

Figure 17.2 Parasternal long axis view.

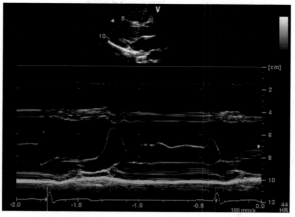

Figure 17.3 M-mode across mitral valve.

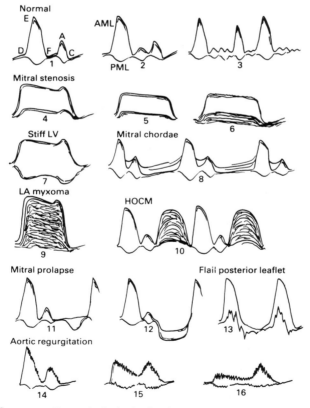

Figure 17.4 Common patterns of mitral valve involvement on M-mode echocardiogram.

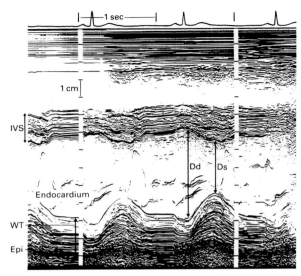

Figure 17.5 M-mode across LV in parasternal long axis.

2 The normal mitral valve with a slower heart rate in sinus rhythm. The movements are as in (1), but an extra excursion is seen in mid-diastole after the F point. This is normal and just represents mid-diastolic flow into LV.

3 The normal mitral valve in AF. Here the A wave disappears and the excursion of the E point varies depending on the R–R interval. Little fibrillation waves may be seen between the main mitral excursions.

The M-mode across the left ventricle (Figure 17.5) is helpful for measuring the LV dimensions. Diastolic dimensions are taken from leading edge to leading edge, in late diastole, as demonstrated by the Q wave on the ECG. Systolic dimensions are taken at the point of shortest distance between the septum and posterior wall.

Aortic valve opening on the M-mode rarely demonstrates the movement of the left coronary cusp (LCC), and usually shows right coronary cusp (RCC) and non-coronary cusp (NCC) movement. Aortic valve opening and closing is therefore a two-part movement seen as a box-like or parallelogram figure (Figure 17.6, parts 1–2):

1 The aortic cusps in diastole form a central closure line (CL). With LV ejection the cusps separate to the edge of the aortic wall: the RCC anteriorly and the posterior NCC (PCC) posteriorly. The LV ejection time can be measured from the point of cusp opening to cusp closure if good echoes are obtained.

2 In Figure 17.6 (parts 1–3) the LCC, which is rarely seen, is included. Systolic fluttering of the aortic cusps is not necessarily abnormal and may occur with high- or low-output states or causes of turbulence (e.g. subvalve stenosis).

Parasternal Short Axis

By rotating the transducer through 90° the next view in the sequence is obtained. Three short axis views or cuts (mitral valve, left ventricle and aortic

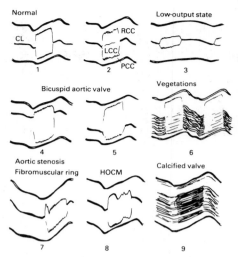

Figure 17.6 Common patterns of aortic valve movement on M-mode echocardiogram. CL, closure line; LCC, left coronary cusp; PCC, posterior non-coronary cusp; RCC, right coronary cusp.

valve) may be obtained by tilting the transducer along the imaginary line between the left hip and right shoulder.

The Mitral Valve

The mitral valve in this view is classically described as resembling a fish-mouth, as shown in Figure 17.7. This is a helpful view for looking at calcification of the leaflet tips and commissures and also for assessing the mitral valve area.

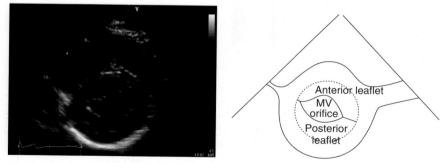

Figure 17.7 Parasternal short axis of mitral valve.

The Left Ventricle

Tilting the transducer down towards the apex from the mitral valve position opens up the left ventricular cavity, particularly at the level of the papillary muscles (Figure 17.8).

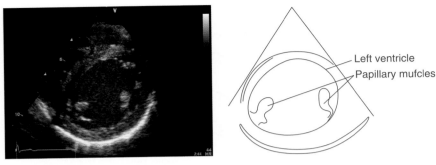

Figure 17.8 LV parasternal short axis.

The Aortic Valve

Tilting the probe in the opposite direction towards the right shoulder will open up a short axis view of the (usually) tricuspid aortic valve. This is classically described as resembling the Mercedes Benz sign and is shown in Figure 17.9.

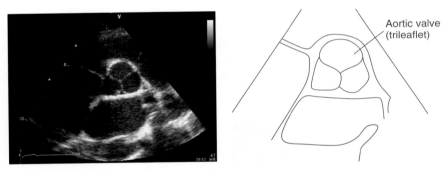

Figure 17.9 Aortic valve parasternal short axis.

The right heart wraps around the aortic valve in this position, and views of both atria, the right ventricle and pulmonary artery are possible.

Apical Four Chamber

In this view at the apex, the heart is visualized upside down (Figure 17.10). All four chambers are seen and this view is especially helpful for viewing the apex, the free wall and the complete right ventricle. A five-chamber view can be achieved by tilting the probe upwards (Figure 17.11). This opens up the

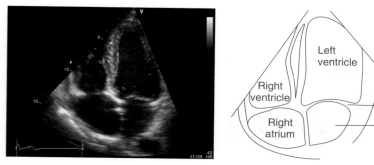

Figure 17.10 Four-chamber view.

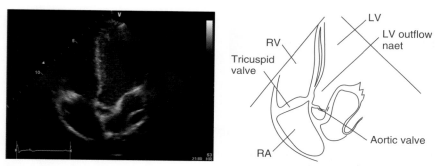

Figure 17.11 Five-chamber view.

LV outflow tract, and is useful for demonstrating aortic valve regurgitation with colour flow mapping.

Apical Two Chamber

Rotating the probe through 90° gives greater definition of the left ventricle (Figure 17.12), and is especially helpful for assessing LV function.

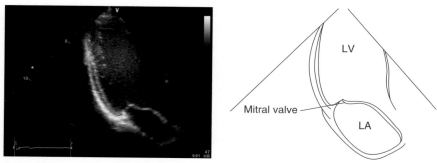

Figure 17.12 Apical two-chamber view.

Subcostal

This view is not always possible to obtain and is dependent on the patient's body habitus and general condition. It is useful for visualizing the pericardium and interatrial septum (Figure 17.13).

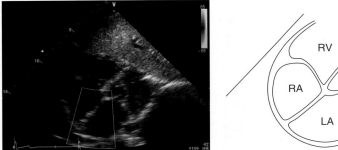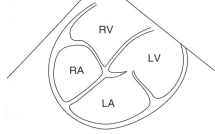

Figure 17.13 Subcostal view.

17.3 Doppler Ultrasonography

Doppler echocardiographic equipment compares the frequency of transmitted ultrasound with the received ultrasound frequency reflected off moving blood cells. Cells moving directly towards the transducer will result in a higher-frequency ultrasound, and cells moving away from the transducer a lower frequency.

This Doppler shift frequency is used to estimate the velocity of blood, i.e.

$$f_D = [2f(V \cos \theta)]/c$$

where f_D = Doppler shift frequency, V = velocity of blood, θ = angle between transmitted and reflected sound, f = transmitted frequency and c = velocity of sound.

Doppler ultrasonography has revolutionized cardiac diagnosis, particularly in paediatric cardiology, and has obviated the need for cardiac catheterization in many cases. It has proved very useful for estimating the severity of many cardiac lesions, e.g.

- aortic, mitral and pulmonary valve gradients and areas
- PA pressure (e.g. in children with VSDs)
- VSD closure (rising peak velocity of jet)
- PDA
- coarctation
- subaortic stenosis, infundibular stenosis
- PA branch stenosis
- severity of valve regurgitation.

Modes of Doppler Ultrasonography Used in Cardiology

Pulsed Wave (PW)

The pulsed wave Doppler signal of the normal mitral valve consists of an E wave caused by early diastolic flow, followed by an A wave, the result of atrial systole. It is a useful tool for identifying the exact site of stenosis, leak, etc. It is not useful, however, for quantitative measurements. Pulsed Doppler cannot detect high-frequency Doppler shifts because the pulse repetition frequency is limited. This results in 'aliasing' in which the signal may wrap around and appear on the other side of the baseline. This may introduce confusion as to the true direction of flow. PW Doppler across the normal MV is shown in Figure 17.14. Figure 17.15 shows how the PW measurements across the mitral

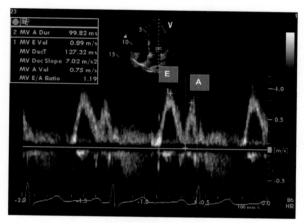

Figure 17.14 PW Doppler across the normal mitral valve. Arrows at E and A indicate PE and PA, respectively.

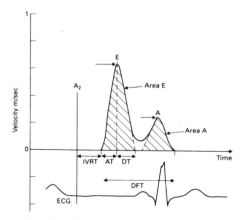

Figure 17.15 Calculation of diastolic indices from diagrammatic transmitral flow pattern. Arrows at E and A indicate PE and PA, respectively. A_2, aortic valve closure; IVRT, isovolumic relaxation time; AT, acceleration time; DT, deceleration time; DFT, diastolic filling time.

Table 17.1 Variables derived from transmitral diastolic Doppler flow recording (see Figure 17.15)

Variable	How derived	Normal range
PE	Peak early filling velocity (cm/s)	78 ± 15
PA	Peak late filling velocity (cm/s)	48 ± 12
E/A ratio	1.6 ± 0.2	
E area or integral	Rapid early (passive) filling velocity-time integral (area under the E portion of the Doppler profile) (cm^2)	0.1 ± 0.03
A area or integral	Late (active) filling velocity-time integral (area under the A portion of the Doppler profile) (cm^2)	0.06 ± 0.01
Total filling integral	E area + A area (cm^2)	0.16 ± 0.04
E area/A area		1.7 ± 0.4
E area/total area	Rapid early filling contribution to total filling, or early filling fraction	0.62 ± 0.05
A area/total area	Late filling contribution to total filling, atrial filling fraction	0.37 ± 0.07
IVRT	Isovolumic relaxation time (ms). Time between A_2 and onset of Doppler filling	48–65
Acceleration time	AT. Time from onset of diastolic flow to E point (ms)	70–90
Deceleration time	DT. Time from E point to point where the E–F slope hits the baseline (ms)	105–180
DFT	Total diastolic filling time (ms)	300–520

valve are used to calculate the diastolic indices from the transmitral flow pattern (Table 17.1).

Continuous Wave (CW)

This is needed to quantitate valve stenoses, etc. Aliasing does not occur. Blood flowing away from the transducer is represented as a spectral display below the baseline, and blood flowing towards it as a display above the baseline (Figure 17.16).

Colour Doppler

This colour codes for the direction of ultrasound shift, e.g. red indicating blood moving towards the transducer, blue indicating blood moving away from the transducer (Figure 17.17).

This enables the echocardiography technician to localize much more quickly the site and direction of abnormal blood flow (e.g. prosthetic valve regurgitation see Figure 9.10). It is not so useful in quantitating the severity of lesions.

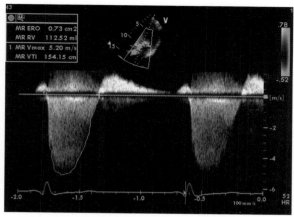

Figure 17.16 CW Doppler in mitral regurgitation.

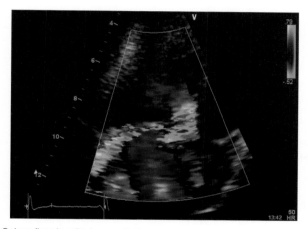

Figure 17.17 Colour flow in mitral regurgitation.

The Normal Doppler Examination

Normal blood velocity in adults (and children) is (in metres per second):

- tricuspid valve 0.3–0.7 m/s
- pulmonary valve 0.5–1.0 m/s
- mitral valve 0.6–1.3 m/s
- aortic valve 0.9–1.7 m/s.

Children with innocent murmurs have higher velocities in the ascending aorta. Low velocity in the ascending aorta is the result of a low cardiac output or a wide aorta (e.g. Marfan syndrome). Higher velocities occur in higher flow situations (e.g. post-exercise, anxiety) or in the right heart with left-to-right shunts.

Normal Valve Doppler Traces

Doppler examination has established that a very mild degree of regurgitation occurs through normal pulmonary and tricuspid valves. This regurgitation has a low peak velocity (e.g. < 1m/s through the pulmonary valve). Tricuspid and pulmonary regurgitation are more common in cases with pulmonary hypertension, older children or RBBB.

Laminar vs Turbulent Flow

With laminar flow all the velocities of the blood cells are similar and a thin waveform with minimal spectral broadening is produced. With turbulent flow, multiple different velocities are recorded and the Doppler signal is filled in with marked spectral broadening (Figures 17.18 and 17.19).

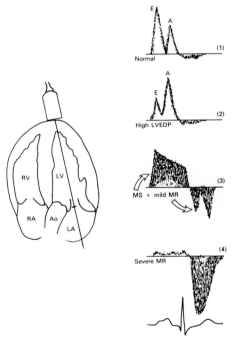

Figure 17.18 Apical CW Doppler echocardiography with sample volume in mitral valve orifice. (1) Normal laminar flow with minimal spectral broadening, A = contribution of atrial systole. (2) Normal laminar mitral flow but with high LVEDP. Early flow velocity *E* is reduced, but late velocity is increased with the A wave. (3) Mixed mitral valve disease. Turbulent flow in both directions produces multiple velocities and spectral broadening. The signal above the baseline is towards the transducer (stenotic jet), and the signal below is the regurgitation jet away from the transducer. (4) Severe mitral regurgitation. Complete envelope of turbulent flow. Early peak velocity of severe regurgitation.

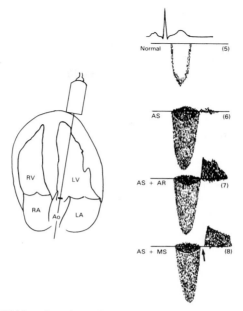

Figure 17.19 Apical CW Doppler echocardiography with sample volume in aortic valve orifice. (5) Normal velocity profile with laminar flow. (6) Aortic stenosis. Increased peak velocity with turbulent flow through the aortic valve. (7) Mixed aortic valve disease. Turbulent flow in both directions, the stenotic component being away from the transducer with its signal below the baseline, and the regurgitant component above. Forward and reversed flow are continuous. (8) Aortic and mural stenosis with no aortic regurgitation. The two jet signals are not continuous with a small gap between (arrowed). This helps to distinguish the signals of mitral stenosis from aortic regurgitation.

Doppler Mitral Valve Studies and Diastolic Function

(Figures 17.18 and 17.19)

Flow patterns through a normal mitral valve depend on LV stiffness, atrial systolic function and rhythm, the phases of respiration and heart rate. Using the apical four-chamber view with the sample volume in the mitral valve orifice (as in Figure 17.18), numerous variables are derived. Approximate normal ranges are shown in Table 17.2.

Recently it has been found that none of these indices is as sensitive to early increases in diastolic stiffness (caused by LV hypertrophy) as measurements made from acoustic quantification.

Acoustic Quantification (AQ)

The endocardial border of the left ventricle can be continuously outlined on a four-chamber view. This automatic border detection produces an LV area or volume/time curve (similar to the volume/time curve of LV angiography). Abnormalities can be demonstrated on area/volume curve filling rates by acoustic quantification even when the mitral flow Doppler pattern is still normal. It appears to be a very sensitive technique for early diastolic dysfunction.

It is important in calculations of LV function from echocardiograms to obtain good endocardial echoes from both the septum and the posterior LV wall (Table 17.3). The epicardium is a denser band of echoes visible at the back of the posterior LV wall (PLVW). The ratio of interventricular septal

---

Table 17.2 Normal echocardiographic values in an adult (see Figure 17.5)

Ventricular and atrial dimensions (ID, internal dimension)
LVIDd (end-diastole): 3.5–5.6 cm
LVIDs (end systole): 1.9–4.0 cm
Posterior LV wall thickness: 0.7–1.1 cm (at end diastole)
RVID (end diastole): 0.7–2.6 cm
Posterior LV wall excursion (amplitude): 0.8–1.2 cm
Interventricular septal thickness: 0.7–1.2 cm
LAID (end systole): 1.9.0 cm
Ratio of septum to posterior wall thickness = 1.3 : 1
Aorta and aortic valve
Aortic root internal diameter: 2.0–3.7 cm
Aortic valve opening: 1.6–2.6 cm
Mitral valve
E–F slope (closure rate): 70–150 cm/s
E point to septal distance: 0–5 mm
D–E distance: 20–30 mm
Ventricular function
Ejection fraction: 0.62–0.85
Velocity of circumferential fibre shortening of LV (Vcf) = 1.1–1.8 circ/s

---

Table 17.3 Formulae used in echocardiographic calculations of LV function (see Figure 17.5)

$LVEDV = (LVIDd)^3 = (Dd)^3$ ml (for normal ventricles)
$LVESV = (LVIDs)^3 = (Ds)^3$ ml
Stroke volume = $Dd^3 - Ds^3$ ml

$$\text{Ejection fraction} = \frac{Dd^3 - Ds^3}{Dd^3} 100\%$$

$$VCF = \frac{Dd - Ds}{Ds \times LVET} \text{circ/s}$$

LVET is measured from carotid pulse (see systolic time intervals).
Example from Figure 16.2:
$Dd = 5.0 \text{cm}$ $Dd^3 = 125$
$Ds = 2.9 \text{cm}$ $Ds^3 = 24.4$
Dd is taken as the maximum diastolic diameter at the point of augmentation caused by the A wave – at the timing of the R wave of the ECG

$$\text{Ejection fraction} = \frac{125 - 24.4}{125} \times 100 = 80\%$$

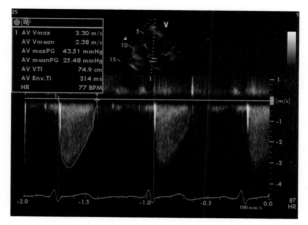

Figure 17.20 CW Doppler in aortic stenosis to assess peak gradient.

thickness (IVS) to posterior wall thickness (endocardium to epicardium at end-diastole) may be calculated and should be less than 1.3:1.

Valvular Defects

Valve Gradients

With good apical views using continuous wave, Doppler aortic and mitral valve gradients can be estimated. A suprasternal view of the aortic valve is needed in children (not possible in adults). Even using CW Doppler, it is possible to underestimate the aortic valve gradient if the cardiac output is low, the maximum jet is not recorded or the angle between the ultrasound beam and the blood jet $>20°$.

- Aortic valve: peak gradient (Figure 17.20). Peak systolic gradient = $4V_{max}^2$ where V_{max} is the measured peak velocity in m/s.
- Mitral valve: peak gradient = $4V_{max}^2$. Use CW from the apex.
- Mitral valve area: measurement of pressure half-time is needed to calculate mitral valve area (Figure 17.21).

$V_1 = 0.7 \times V_{max}$ and occurs at the time (t) when the pressure gradient has fallen to half its maximum value; t = pressure half time.

Mitral valve area = $220/t$

= $759/BT$, where BT is the base time of the slope extrapolated to zero ($t = 0.29 \times BT$).

These formulae cannot be used for the tricuspid valve.

Mitral Valve

Mitral Regurgitation (see also Section 3.3)

A number of different techniques in combination are used to assess the severity of mitral regurgitation including the CW trace (see Figure 17.16) the colour

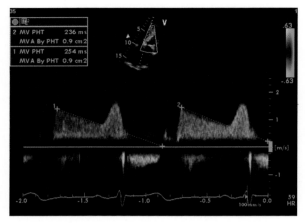

Figure 17.21 Mitral valve area by PHT.

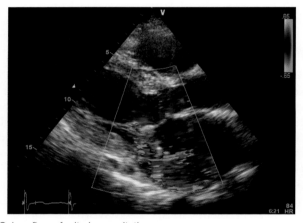

Figure 17.22 Colour flow of mitral regurgitation.

flow map (Figure 17.22), the LV effects, pulmonary venous flow and PA pressure assessment (Figure 17.23).

Estimation of PA pressure

First, a good recording of tricuspid regurgitation is obtained using CW Doppler (Figure 17.23). Peak velocity of the tricuspid regurgitation is measured (say 2 m/s). Then peak RV pressure = $4V^2$ of peak tricuspid regurgitation velocity (= 16). Add an extra 5 for estimated RA pressure, then peak RV pressure = 21 mmHg = peak PA pressure assuming no pulmonary stenosis.

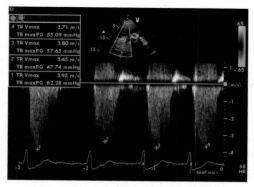

Figure 17.23 CW Doppler in tricuspid regurgitation to assess PA pressure.

Mitral Valve Prolapse (see also Section 3.3)

This is a common echocardiographic finding in an asymptomatic patient. Figures 17.24 and 17.25 show two-dimensional images of a prolapsing posterior leaflet in the parasternal long axis and four-chamber views. Figure 17.4, part 11 shows the late systolic prolapse of the mitral valve on M-mode. The point of separation of the anterior and posterior leaflets in mid-systole will coincide with the mid-systolic click if present. The late systolic murmur follows.

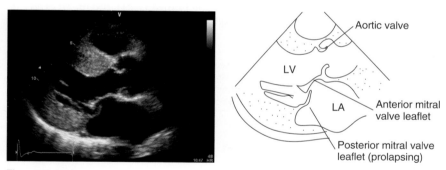

Figure 17.24 Mitral valve prolapse two-dimensional parasternal long axis.

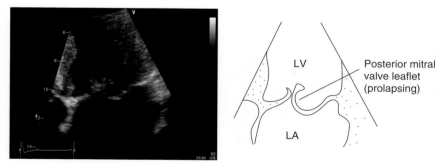

Figure 17.25 Mitral valve prolapse in two-dimensional four chamber.

Mitral Stenosis (Table 17.4) (see also Section 3.2)

The rheumatic mitral valve is best demonstrated in the two-dimensional, parasternal short axis view (Figure 17.26), which is useful for displaying the fused commissures and extensive calcification of the leaflets, and the long axis view (Figure 17.27) for demonstrating the thickening and contraction of the chordae resulting in restricted, staccato movement of the leaflets. This is often described as a dog's leg appearance (especially in rheumatic mitral valve disease).

The M-mode across the stenosed mitral valve (see Figure 17.4, part 4) shows that the mitral anterior leaflet excursion is reduced. The slope of mitral valve closure (E–F slope) is greatly reduced and in severe cases may be horizontal, giving a castellated appearance to the mitral valve. In mobile mitral stenosis still in SR a small A wave may be seen. The posterior leaflet moves anteriorly and may also exhibit an A wave.

In the next M-mode (Figure 17.4, part 5), mitral stenosis in AF, the A wave has disappeared and excursion is reduced. The final M-mode trace (Figure 17.4, part 6) shows calcific mitral stenosis with multiple hard horizontal bars on the posterior leaflet suggesting calcification.

The severity of mitral stenosis is again a multicomponent assessment, using the planimetered orifice area from the parasternal short axis view (Figure 17.28), in square centimetres, the pressure half-time (the rate of fall of the velocity signal – Figures 17.29, 17.30 and see Figure 17.21), the mean gradient across the valve and the assessment of resultant tricuspid regurgitation (see Figure 17.23).

Table 17.4 Assessment of severity of mitral stenosis

	Mild	Moderate	Severe
Planimetered orifice area (cm^2)	>1.5	1.0–1.5	<1.0
Pressure half-time	<150	150–200	>200
Mean gradient (mmHg)	<5	5–10	>10
TR V$_{max}$	<2.7	Variable	>3.0

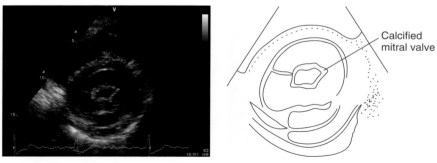

Calcified mitral valve

Figure 17.26 Mitral stenosis in parasternal short axis.

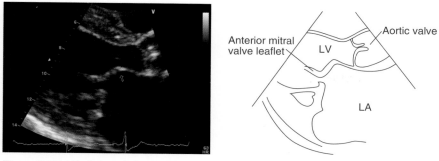

Figure 17.27 Mitral stenosis in parasternal long axis.

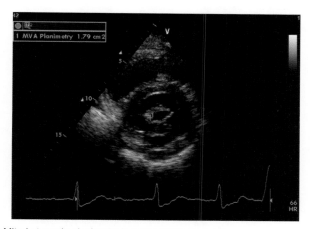

Figure 17.28 Mitral stenosis planimetry in parasternal short axis.

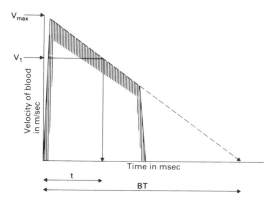

Figure 17.29 Calculation of mitral valve gradient and valve area from a diagrammatic apical continuous-wave Doppler signal.

Sinus rhythm.
Mild mitral stenosis. Peak velocity 1.07 m/s. Pressure half time 114 ms.
Valve area 1.92 cm². Prominent A waves

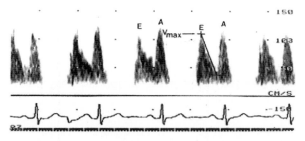

Severe mitral stenosis. Peak velocity 2.0 m/s. Pressure half time 211 ms.
Valve area 1.04 cm²

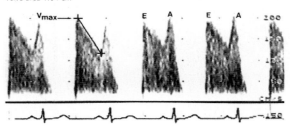

Atrial fibrillation.
Severe mitral stenosis. Peak velocity 2.0m/s. Pressure half time 180 ms.
Valve area 1.22 cm². Note loss of A wave

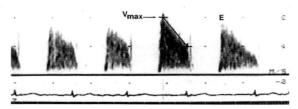

Figure 17.30 CW Doppler in mitral stenosis.

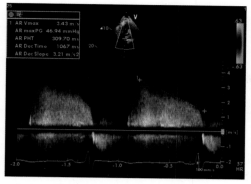

Figure 17.31 CW Doppler in aortic regurgitation.

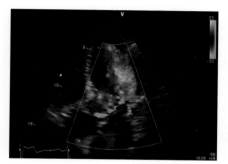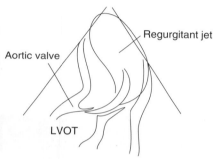

Figure 17.32 Colour flow aortic regurgitation.

Aortic Valve

Aortic Regurgitation (see also Section 3.5)

The assessment of the severity of AR is based on a number of individual assessments of the aortic valve. The CW Doppler trace assessment of pressure half-time (Figure 17.31) is reviewed with the colour Doppler looking at jet height as a percentage of outflow diameter. Diastolic flow reversal in the aorta also helps to quantify the severity of valve incompetence.

The severity of AR is dependent on the width of the regurgitant jet seen on colour flow (Figure 17.32). If the height of the jet is over 60% of the outflow diameter, the regurgitation is severe.

The effect of AR on the mitral valve M-mode is seen in Figure 17.4 (parts 14–16). Mild AR causes diastolic fluttering of the anterior leaflet only, with normal mitral valve excursion. As regurgitation becomes more severe, mitral valve excursion is reduced (premature mitral valve closure) and both anterior and posterior leaflets flutter. In very severe cases the mitral valve hardly opens until the A wave.

Aortic Stenosis (Table 17.5) (see also Section 3.4)

The assessment of the aortic valve may be fraught with inaccuracy because it is partially dependent on LV function, which can vary greatly and cause compounded error.

Table 17.5 Assessment of severity of aortic stenosis

	Mild	Moderate to severe	Severe
Aortic peak velocity (m/s)	<3	3–4.5	>4.5
Peak gradient (mmHg)	<30	30–80	>80
Mean gradient (mmHg)	<15	1 5–50	>50
Continuity equation area (cm^2)	>1.0	0.6–1.0	<0.6

The most basic assessment of leaflet mobility and calcification can be obtained from the two-dimensional parasternal short and long axis views (Figures 17.33 and 17.34), and excursion on the M-mode recordings (Figure 17.6, part 9).

Figure 17.6 (part 9) shows the M-mode in calcific aortic stenosis. Dense linear echoes, usually continuous through systole and diastole, are produced by one or more cusps. In more severe cases the entire aorta may be filled with these echoes and no discrete cusp movement is visible. However, the most accurate method is CW Doppler (Figure 17.35).

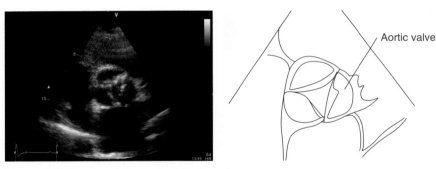

Figure 17.33 Parasternal short axis aortic stenosis.

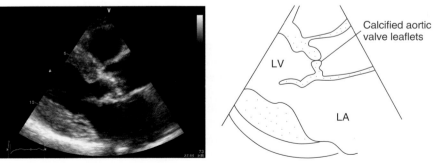

Figure 17.34 Parasternal long axis aortic stenosis.

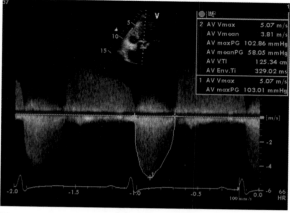

Figure 17.35 CW in aortic stenosis to assess peak gradient.

The velocity of blood flow across the aortic valve is directly related to the degree of stenosis. The simplified Bernouilli equation:

Pressure difference = $4 \times$ velocity^2

is a numerical summary of the statement that, within the heart at any point, the total potential and kinetic energy must be identical. As a result, the pressure drop or gradient (decreased potential energy) across a stenotic valve will be associated with an increase in the velocity (or kinetic energy) across the valve to maintain the constant.

Another assessment of severity of aortic stenosis is AV area. The continuity equation is based on the principle that as outflow area decreases, velocity must increase:

Valve area = [Subaortic cross-sectional area $\times$ Subaortic peak velocity]/
   Aortic peak velocity.

The Pulmonary Valve (see also Section 3.6)

This is the most difficult valve to visualize with the echo. Usually the posterior leaflet only is seen, and during pulmonary valve opening the echo often disappears to reappear as the valve closes.

Diagrammatic examples of pulmonary valve movement are shown in Figure 17.36:

1 Normal: atrial systole is transmitted to the pulmonary valve and causes a small posterior movement or A wave. Systolic opening occurs next (B–C). The valve drifts slightly anteriorly to point D later in systole and then closes rapidly (D–E). In diastole the valve drifts slowly posteriorly (E–F slope) in the presence of a low PA pressure before the next A wave.

2 Pulmonary hypertension: the A wave disappears and so does the normal posterior drift of the E–F slope. The E–F line is horizontal or may even be

Posterior leaflet

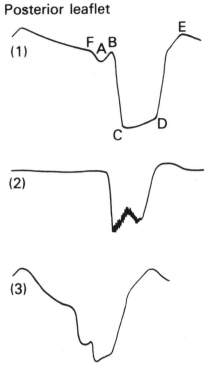

Figure 17.36 Normal pulmonary valve appearances on M-mode echocardiogram.

reversed. There is frequently coarse systolic fluttering of the pulmonary valve and mid-systolic closure.

3 Pulmonary stenosis (and see Figures 17.37 and 17.38): the A wave becomes increasingly prominent as the pulmonary stenosis becomes more severe. Unfortunately the size of the A wave is not a completely reliable guide to the severity of the pulmonary stenosis. Infundibular pulmonary stenosis produces diastolic and systolic fluttering of the pulmonary valve from turbu-

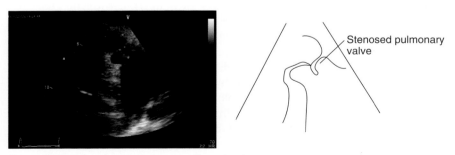

Figure 17.37 Pulmonary stenosis – two dimensional.

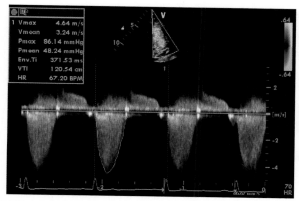

Figure 17.38 CW Doppler in pulmonary stenosis.

lence. The A wave disappears as the subpulmonary obstruction prevents its transmission to the valve.

The Tricuspid Valve

This is best visualized with two-dimensional imaging in the short axis or on the four-chamber view. Doppler studies may show tricuspid regurgitation. For calculation of PA pressure using the tricuspid regurgitant jet, see Figure 17.23. On M-mode imaging mitral and tricuspid valve movements are very similar with tricuspid closure occurring up to 40 ms after mitral closure. With wide RBBB, closure may be delayed up to 65 ms. In Ebstein's anomaly, in which tricuspid and mitral echoes are often seen well at the same time, tricuspid closure is delayed still further.

Many features of mitral valve disease echocardiographically also apply to the tricuspid valve (e.g. visualization of vegetations, posterior tricuspid leaflet prolapse).

In primum ASD with AV canal defect there may be a free-floating leaflet across the VSD component. Either the mitral or the tricuspid component of the valve may be seen to cross into the septum.

Septal Movement (see also Section 10.2)

The septum normally acts as part of the left ventricle with posterior movement in systole (see example under LV function). Some conditions result in paradoxical septal motion in which the septal's posterior movement is delayed; it moves anteriorly in systole acting as part of the RV. The main causes are the following:

- RV volume overload: ASD, tricuspid regurgitation, pulmonary regurgitation, partial or total anomalous pulmonary veins, Ebstein's anomaly
- Delayed or abnormal activation: LBBB, WPW syndrome, ventricular ectopics
- Septal abnormalities: ischaemic heart disease, dilated cardiomyopathy

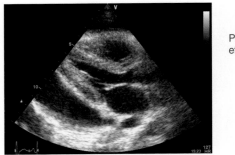
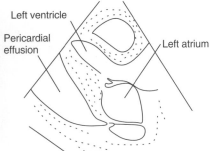

Figure 17.39 Large pericardial effusion 1.

- Pericardial disease: pericardial effusion, constrictive pericarditis, congenital absence of pericardium
- Open heart surgery: even in the absence of a conduction defect.

Pericardial Effusion (see also Section 10.2: see also Chapter 9)
The echocardiogram is very useful for detection of pericardial effusion. Pericardial fluid accumulates anterior to both ventricles and anterior and lateral to the right atrium. The pericardial reflection behind the left atrium limits the extension of effusion behind the left atrium and the pericardium tends to be adherent posteriorly. Pericardial fluid tends to be limited on the left side at the AV groove.

Thus an echo taken at ventricular level may show fluid in front of the RV wall and behind the posterior LV wall (Figure 17.39). Smaller effusions may be visualized only posteriorly. Usually an echocardiogram at the level of the aortic valve shows fluid anteriorly, but none behind the left atrium for the reasons given above.

The effect of the swinging heart inside the bag of fluid may produce paradoxical septal motion, pseudomitral prolapse and electrical alternans on the ECG (see Section 10.2).

Two-dimensional echocardiography shows the effusion clearly and the size of the effusion is the best predictor of tamponade. Diastolic collapse of the right ventricle and/or the right atrium may occur and the presence of diastolic collapse is an indication for pericardial aspiration. Fibrinous strands and exudates may be seen in chronic inflammatory effusions (Figure 17.40). A loculated pleural effusion may be mistaken for pericardial fluid.

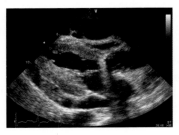
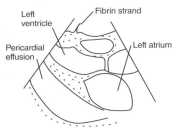

Figure 17.40 Fibrinous pericardial effusion.

17.4 Echo Library

This is a collection of fascinating two-dimensional and M-mode images of a variety of cardiac conditions.

Hypertrophic Cardiomyopathy (Figures 17.41–17.43 and Figure 17.4, part 10)

In HCM the mitral valve may be normal in diastole. In systole the entire mitral apparatus moves anteriorly producing the characteristic bulge illustrated.

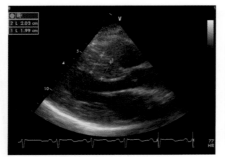

Figure 17.41 The interventricular septum in HCM.

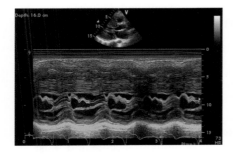

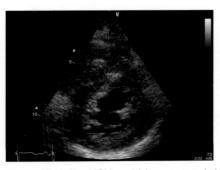

Figure 17.42 M-mode across HCM ventricle showing SAM.

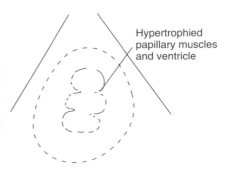

Figure 17.43 The HCM ventricle parasternal short axis.

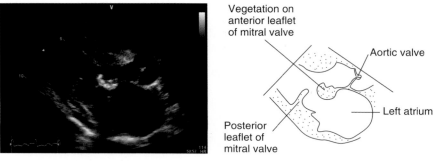

Vegetation on anterior leaflet of mitral valve

Aortic valve

Left atrium

Posterior leaflet of mitral valve

Figure 17.44 Vegetation anterior mitral valve leaflet.

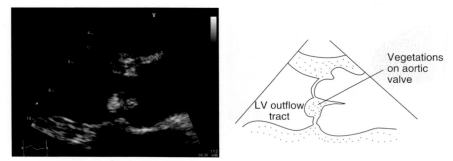

Vegetations on aortic valve

LV outflow tract

Figure 17.45 Aortic valve endocarditis.

This abuts the septum producing LVOTO. It is called the SAM (systolic anterior motion).

Endocarditis (Figures 17.44 and 17.45; see also Chapter 9)

Aortic valve vegetations will be visualized on M-mode only if they are >2 mm (see Figure 17.6, part 6). Small granular vegetations will be missed. Large aortic valve vegetations will be seen in both systole and diastole as dense horizontal lines. They may be confused with aortic valve calcification. Usually aortic valve vegetations are not continuous in systole and diastole, and are often seen only in diastole. Aortic valve calcification usually produces denser, more continuous, linear echoes. Unfortunately, there is no absolute guide to distinguishing them.

Bicuspid Aortic Valve (Figure 17.46 and see Figure 17.6, parts 4 and 5)

M-mode of bicuspid aortic valve: although the cusps separate normally the closure line is eccentric and may be either anterior (see Figure 17.6, part 4) or posterior (see Figure 17.6, part 5). Approximately 15% of bicuspid valves have a central closure line, and this sign cannot be relied on diagnostically. In addition, a tricuspid aortic valve with a subaortic VSD and prolapsing RCC may produce an eccentric closure line. Once a bicuspid valve is heavily calcified it cannot be distinguished from a tricuspid calcified valve by echocardiography.

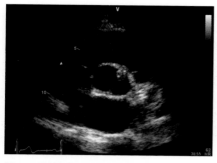
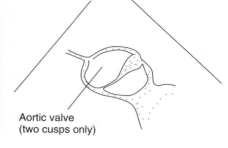

Aortic valve
(two cusps only)

Figure 17.46 Bicuspid aortic valve.

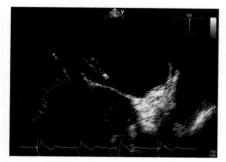
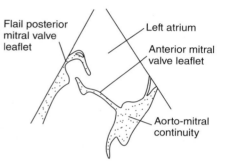

Flail posterior
mitral valve
leaflet

Left atrium

Anterior mitral
valve leaflet

Aorto-mitral
continuity

Figure 17.47 Flail posterior mitral valve leaflet.

Flail Posterior Mitral Valve Leaflet (Figure 17.47 and see Figure 17.4, parts 13)

M-mode of flail posterior MV leaflet: ruptured chordae can result in chaotic movement of the posterior leaflet (see Figure 17.4, part 13). The important diagnostic point is anterior movement and fluttering of the posterior leaflet in diastole.

LA Myxoma

M-mode of LA myxoma (see Figure 11.2 and Figure 17.4, part 9): a very characteristic appearance. Multiple echoes fill in the space behind and below the anterior leaflet. There may be an initial clear space before the echoes appear, i.e. the valve opens first, and then the tumour pops down into the mitral orifice. Differential diagnosis includes mitral valve vegetations, MV aneurysm and LA thrombus.

17.5 Transoesophageal Echocardiography (TOE) (Table 17.6)

This technique has proved of enormous diagnostic value in many aspects of both paediatric and adult cardiology. It has become an essential part in the management of prosthetic valve endocarditis, the search for the source of

Table 17.6 Cardiac structures best imaged by transoesophageal echocardiography

Structure	Possible abnormality
Right atrium	Thrombus, myxoma, pacing wire, central line
Left atrium	Thrombus, myxoma, spontaneous contrast
Left atrial appendage	Thrombus
Pulmonary veins	Anatomy, flow direction
Atrial septum	PFO, ASD, atrial septum aneurysm, shunts
Mitral valve	Anatomy, vegetations, strands, regurgitant jets, chordal rupture
Mitral valve prosthesis	Possible dehiscence, thrombosis, vegetations regurgitant jets, xenograft tears
Aortic valve prosthesis	Posterior ring abscess, valve dysfunction as in mitral
Ascending and descending aorta	Aortic dimensions, dissection, atheroma, patent duct
Coarctation	Site severity, gradient, possible post-dilatation aneurysms

systemic emboli, the diagnosis of aortic dissection or in the assessment of mitral valve repair and all valve replacements intraoperatively.

Standard transthoracic echocardiography (TTE) has been limited by poor tissue penetration of high-frequency transducers (5 MHz), although good definition (resolution) is better with these. Adequate transthoracic images can be very difficult to obtain even with the lower-frequency 2.25–2.5 MHz transducer in obese patients, or those with emphysema or chest deformities. Structures at the back of the heart may be missed altogether.

The Normal TOE Examination

TOE examinations may be performed without sedation, under light reversible sedation or under general anaesthetic. As a result patient tolerance of this procedure may be variable. For this reason, the purpose of the study should be ascertained before the study, so that this area is focused upon initially. If the patient fails to tolerate the procedure, the procedure will not be in vain if the critical information is gained from the outset.

The standard views for each structure are outlined in the following images, with the probe position and angulation.

Aortic Valve

TOE is especially useful for demonstrating aortic regurgitation, and for looking at prosthetic valve function, because excessive shatter (caused by the reflection of echo from the metallic prosthesis) can make visualization of the prosthetic valve difficult on TTE. The transgastric view is the most useful view for patients with aortic stenosis.

The short axis view (Figures 17.48 and 17.49) demonstrates the valve leaflet excursion and calcification. Colour Doppler can be used to demonstrate the regurgitant jet. The aortic valve area can be traced.

The LV outflow tract view can demonstrate the length and base of the regurgitant jet (Figure 17.50).

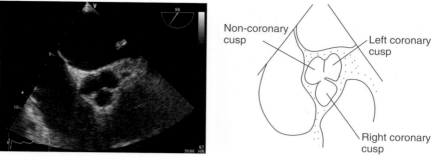

Figure 17.48 TOE short axis view of aortic valve.

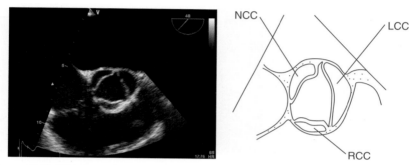

Figure 17.49 TOE short axis aortic valve open.

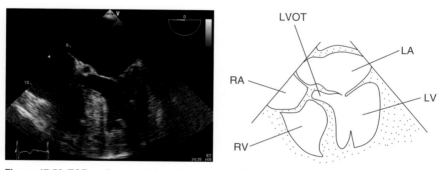

Figure 17.50 TOE outflow tract, five chamber of aortic valve.

The long axis view (Figure 17.51) is useful for the colour Doppler traces and for looking at the ascending aorta and potential entry points of aortic dissections. TOE is useful in possible aortic dissection (see Section 14.2) because it avoids the risks of aortography. The site and extent of the dissection are seen because both ascending aorta and descending thoracic aorta are imaged. Sometimes the tear or entry site can be seen with Doppler, which will show flow in the false lumen. It is important that the procedure be performed with careful BP monitoring and adequate sedation. Acute rises in systolic BP must be avoided.

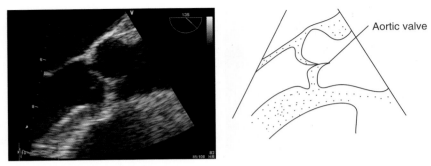

Figure 17.51 TOE LA aortic valve.

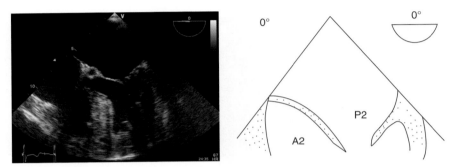

Figure 17.52 TOE of mitral valve, four chamber: 0°.

The transgastric view is the only view in which an outflow tract gradient can be measured. Stroke volume, cardiac output and aortic valve area (using the continuity equation) can be assessed, in addition to the pressure half-time for quantifying aortic regurgitation.

Mitral valve

The mitral valve sits just behind the oesophagus. With significant mitral stenosis and LA enlargement, symptoms of dysphagia can occur. Hence, the mitral valve is very clearly visualized from the oesophagus.

The transoesophageal study of the mitral valve can be very helpful to the surgeon for assessment of the valve before replacement or repair. The four-chamber view (Figure 17.52) can clearly show the mitral valve leaflets, chordae and papillary muscles. The diameter of the annulus and orifice area can be calculated.

The individual scallops of both leaflets of the mitral valve can be seen in particular views, by varying the cuts through the mitral valve orifice (Figures 17.52–17.55).

Left Ventricle

The transgastric view allows an assessment of regional wall motion across the short and long axes of the left ventricle. M-mode can be useful for quantifying LV function.

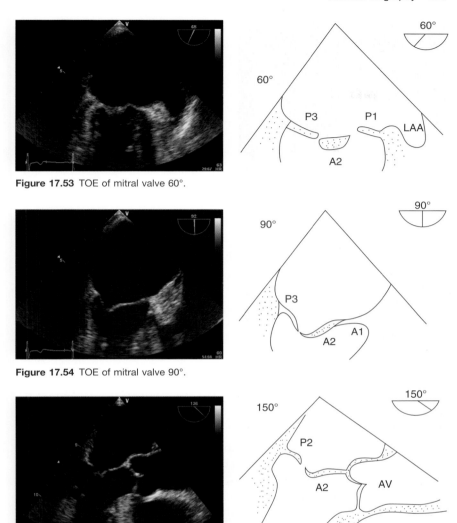

Figure 17.53 TOE of mitral valve 60°.

Figure 17.54 TOE of mitral valve 90°.

Figure 17.55 TOE of mitral valve 150°.

Interventricular Septum

The mobility of the septum is best seen in the four-chamber view (Figure 17.56), but also in the transgastric short axis view of the left ventricle. Colour Doppler enables the detection of defects in septal integrity.

Right Ventricle

In the midoesphagus, the four-chamber view allows assessment of RV function and size. The short axis transgastric view provides information for the right as for the left ventricle.

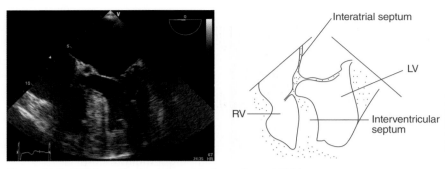

Figure 17.56 TOE four-chamber interventricular septum – LV/RV.

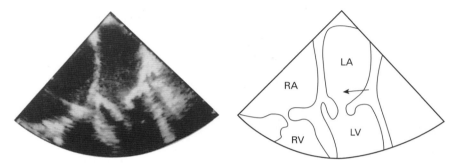

Figure 17.57 TOE in a woman with mitral and tricuspid stenosis showing spontaneous echo contrast in the left atrium (arrowed). RA = right atrium; RV = right ventricle; LA = left atrium; LV = left ventricle.

Pulmonary Valve

The views of the RV inflow and outflow tract are useful for visualizing the pulmonary valve. Colour Doppler can be used for demonstrating pulmonary regurgitation.

Tricuspid Valve

The four-chamber view and the view of the RV inflow and outflow tract are useful for visualizing the tricuspid valve. TR can be assessed by colour Doppler and assists in estimating RV systolic pressure (CVP = peak TR gradient).

The Atria

TOE allows clear visualization of both atria to exclude the presence of thrombus. This is especially useful before electrophysiological procedures where thrombus may be dislodged by catheters or provoked arrhythmias. TOE is essential before mitral valvuloplasty (see Section 3.2) and before DC cardioversion for AF if there is any doubt about the possibility of thrombus in the atrial appendage, or in those patients who have not received prior anticoagulation (see Section 8.3). Patients with spontaneous echo contrast (Figure 17.57) should also be anticoagulated first.

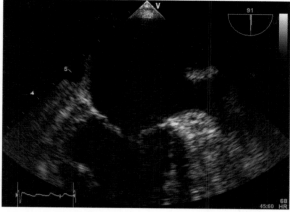

Figure 17.58 Left atrial appendage: view.

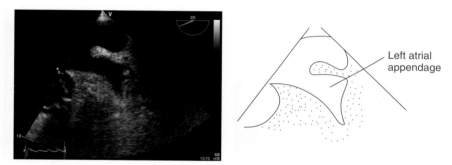

Left atrial
appendage

Figure 17.59 Close-up of left atrial appendage.

The right atrium is best seen in the four-chamber, RV inflow tract and bicaval views (90°). The left atrium is best assessed in a magnified four-chamber view for a closer look at the left atrial appendage especially the risk of thrombus, use pulse wave doppler to look at average velocities in the LAA (Figures 17.58, 17.59 and 17.60).

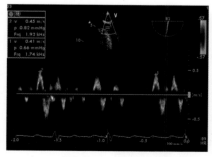

Figure 17.60 Left atrial appendage – PW Doppler.

Interatrial Septum (see also Section 2.2)
The four-chamber (Figure 17.61) and bicaval view (Figure 17.62) allow clear visualization of the interatrial septum. Contrast studies should be performed in studies checking the integrity of the septum. If there is any doubt, the study should be performed in both views.

If an ASD is detected, the pulmonary veins should be identified.

Great Vessels (Figure 17.63)
On withdrawing the probe, the probe should be rotated through 90° to assess the aorta and great vessels. The probe should be slowly withdrawn and the aorta scanned for atheroma.

Prosthetic Valve Endocarditis (see also Section 3.8 and Chapter 9)
TOE is able to detect small vegetations missed on TTE because it has a higher resolution image. All mechanical valves have a tiny puff of regurgitation through the centre of the valve as the ball or disc or discs close. Any regurgitant jet on the side of the valve is pathological and can easily be seen with TOE. Valve dehiscence, thrombosis or paravalve abscess are well seen. Acous-

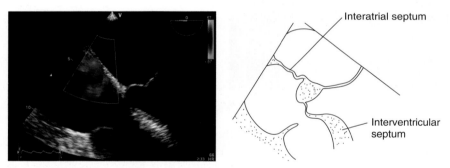

Figure 17.61 TOE four chamber of interatrial septum.

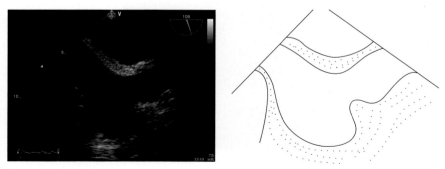

Figure 17.62 Bicaval view.

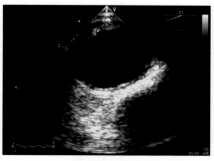 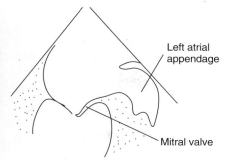

Left atrial appendage

Mitral valve

Figure 17.63 TOE of the aorta.

tic echoes from the mechanical valve struts prevent good visualization of the posterior aortic root in patients with an aortic valve replacement, and the back of the mitral valve and left atrium in patients with a mitral prosthesis. A negative TOE does not exclude infective endocarditis. Patients with infective endocarditis must have a TTE at least weekly and a TOE if their condition deteriorates. The two techniques are complementary not mutually exclusive.

TOE in ITU

TOE in ventilated patients is safe and useful in patients in ITU, e.g. in patients with low cardiac outputs, suspicious murmurs, or sepsis from an unknown source.

17.6 Stress Echocardiography (Table 17.7 and Figure 17.64)

Stress echocardiography is a technique that provides a functional, non-invasive assessment for the detection of myocardial ischaemia and

Table 17.7 Indications and contraindications for stress echocardiography

Indications

Prediction of coronary artery disease in patients unsuitable for exercise testing
To assess functional significance of coronary artery stenosis
Risk stratification in patients with known coronary artery disease
To assess completeness of revascularization
To assess myocardial viability after MI
Valve disease assessments

Contraindications

During admission with an acute coronary syndrome
Severe aortic stenosis
Hypertrophic cardiomyopathy
Significant dysrhythmia
Intercurrent illness including electrolyte imbalance, uncontrolled hypertension, DVT, pulmonary embolism.
Asthma (adenosine/dipyridamole stress)

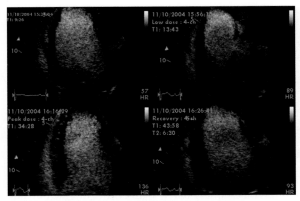

Figure 17.64 Stress echocardiography with contrast cavity opacification.

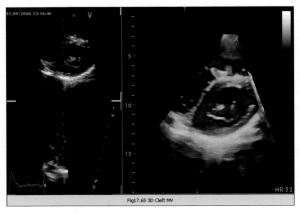

Figure 17.65 Three-dimensional echocardiogram of cleft MV.

hibernating myocardium. It has a high level of diagnostic accuracy. Reduced systolic wall thickening is the classic sign of myocardial ischaemia, during stress or exercise.

The stress part of the procedure can be provided by exercise, dobutamine or dipyridamole. Rest and stress images are assessed for LV size, shape and function.

17.7 Three-dimensional Echocardiography (Figure 17.65)

Over the last decade, significant developments in three-dimensional echocardiography have been made. Three-dimensional echocardiography has greatly improved the visualization of intracardiac structures and allows the measurement of specific cardiac structures such as valve areas, VSDs and ASDs. The potential applications of three-dimensional echocardiography may include assistance in the decision-making and planning of cardiac surgery, and in the diagnosis of complex cardiac lesions.

Appendices

APPENDIX 1

<table>
<tr><td>1</td><td colspan="2"><h1>Nomogram for Body Size</h1></td></tr>
</table>

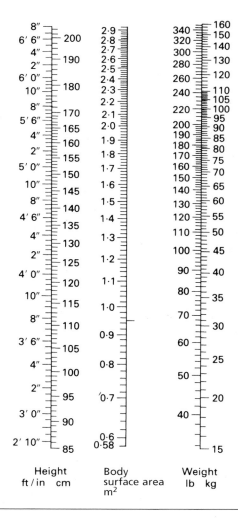

Height ft / in cm	Body surface area m²	Weight lb kg

Swanton's Cardiology, sixth edition. By R. H. Swanton and S. Banerjee. Published 2008 Blackwell Publishing. ISBN 978-1-4051-7819-8.

2 Rate Conversion Chart

Heart rate (beats/min)	R–R interval (ms)	Heart rate (beats/min)	R–R interval (ms)
30	2000	84	714
35	1714	86	698
40	1500	88	682
45	1333	90	667
50	1200	92	652
52	1154	94	638
54	1111	96	625
56	1071	98	612
58	1034	100	600
60	1000	110	545
62	968	120	500
64	938	130	462
66	909	140	429
68	882	150	400
70	857	160	375
72	833	170	353
74	811	180	330
76	789	190	315
78	769	200	300
80	750	210	286
82	732	220	273

Swanton's Cardiology, sixth edition. By R. H. Swanton and S. Banerjee. Published 2008
Blackwell Publishing. ISBN 978-1-4051-7819-8.

APPENDIX 3

3 | Further Reading

Bennett DH. *Cardiac Arrhythmias*, 7th edn. London: Hodder Arnold, 2006.

Braunwald E. Heart Disease. *A Text-Book of Cardiovascular Medicine*, 7th edn. Philadelphia: WB Saunders, 2006.

Camm AJ, Luscher TF, Serruys PW. *The European Society of Cardiology Textbook of Cardiovascular Medicine*. Oxford: Blackwell Science, 2006.

Carter SA, Bajec DF, Yannicelli, E, Wood EM. Estimation of left-to-right shunt from arterial dilution curves. *J Lab Clin* 1960;**55**:77.

Chambers JB. *Clinical Echocardiography*. London: BMJ Publishing Group, 1995.

Chugh SN. *Textbook of Electrocardiography*, 2nd edn. Tunbridge Wells: Anshan Ltd, 2006.

El Sherif N, Samet P. *Cardiac Pacing and Electrophysiology*. Philadelphia: WB Saunders, 1991.

Ellenbogen KA, Wood MA. *Cardiac Pacing and ICDs,* 4th edn. Cambridge, MA: Blackwell Science, 2005.

Feigenbaum H. *Echocardiography*. Philadelphia: Lea & Febiger, 1994.

Fogoros RN. *Electrophysiologic Testing*. Oxford: Blackwell Science, 1994.

Fuster VA, Alexander RW, O'Rourke RA (eds). *Hurst's The Heart*, 11th edn. New York: McGraw Hill, 2004.

Grossman W, Baim DS. *Cardiac Catheterization Angiography and Intervention*, 6th edn. Philadelphia: Lea & Febiger, 2001.

Hall RJC, Julian DC. *Diseases of the Cardiac Valves*. London: Churchill Livingstone, 1989.

Houston AB, Simpson I. *Cardiac Doppler Ultrasound. A clinical perspective*. London: Butterworth Scientific, 1988.

Jefferson K, Rees S. *Clinical Cardiac Radiology*. London: Butterworth, 1980.

Julian DG, Camm AJ, Fox KM, Hall RJC, Poole-Wilson PA. *Diseases of the Heart*. London: Baillière Tindall, 1996.

Kern MJ. *The Cardiac Catheterisation Handbook*. St Louis, MO: Mosby, 2003.

Little BB. *Drugs and Pregnancy – A handbook*. London: Hodder Education, 2006.

Lown B, Calvert AF, Armington R, Ryan M. Monitoring for serious arrhythmias and high risk of sudden death. *Circulation* 1975;**52**:189–98.

McMurray JJV, Pfeffer MA. *Heart Failure*. London: Taylor & Francis, 2003.

Miller G. *Invasive Investigation of the Heart*. Oxford: Blackwell Scientific Publications, 1989.

Swanton's Cardiology, sixth edition. By R. H. Swanton and S. Banerjee. Published 2008
Blackwell Publishing. ISBN 978-1-4051-7819-8.

Nanda NC, Domanski MJ. *Atlas of Transesophageal Echocardiography.* Baltimore, MA: Lippincott Williams & Wilkins, 2007.

Oakley CM, Warnes CA. *Heart Disease in Pregnancy.* London: BMJ Publishing, 2006.

Opie LH. *The Heart. Physiology from cell to circulation.* New York: Raven Press, 1997.

Opie LH. *Drugs for the Heart.* Philadelphia: WB Saunders, 2001.

Perloff JK, Child JS. *Congenital Heart Disease in Adults.* Philadelphia: WB Saunders, 1998.

Reaven GM. Role of insulin resistance in human disease. *Diabetes* 1988;**37**:1595–607.

Redington A, Shore D, Oldershaw P. *Congenital Heart Disease in Adults.* Philadelphia: WB Saunders, 1994.

Ross D, English T, McKay R. *Principles of Cardiac Diagnosis and Treatment – A Surgeons' Guide.* London: Springer-Verlag, 1992.

Schamroth L. *The 12 Lead Electrocardiogram.* Oxford: Blackwell Scientific Publications, 1989.

Sokolow M, Mdllroy MB, Cheitlin MD. *Clinical Cardiology.* Los Altos, CA: Lange Medical Publications, 1993.

Topol EJ. *Acute Coronary Syndromes.* New York: Marcel Dekker, 2005.

Uretsky BF. *Cardiac Catheterization: Concepts, techniques and applications.* Maiden , MA: Blackwell Science, 1997.

Ward DE, Camm AJ. *Clinical Electrophysiology of the Heart.* London: Edward Arnold, 1987.

Yang SS, Bentivoglio LG, Maranhao V, Goldberg H. *From Cardiac Catheterisation Data to Haemodynamic Parameters.* Philadelphia: FA Davis, 1978.

Yusuf S, Cairns JA, Camm AJ, Fallen E, Gersh BJ. *Evidence Based Cardiology*, 2nd edn. London: BMJ Books, 2003.

Zipes DM, Jalife J. *Cardiac Electrophysiology. From cell to bedside,* 4th edn. Philadelphia: WB Saunders, 2004.

4 References of Important Trials or Papers Quoted in the Text

Hyperlipidaemia

4S Study. Randomized trial of cholesterol lowering in 4444 patients with coronary heart disease: the Scandinavian Simvastatin Survival Study (4S): Scandinavian Simvastatin Survival Study Group. Secondary prevention teal of simvastatin in patients with hyper-cholesterolaemia followed for a median of 5.4 years. *Lancet* 1994;**344**:1383.

ASTEROID trial: Nissen SE, Nicholls SJ, Sipahi I *et al.* Effect of very high-intensity statin therapy on regression of coronary atherosclerosis. *JAMA* 2006;**295**:1556.

CARE study. Efficacy of pravastatin on coronary events after myocardial infarction in patients with average cholesterol levels: Sacks FM, Pfeffer MA, Moye LA *et al.* Five-year follow up of patients with starting cholesterol < 6.2 mmol/l treated with pravastatin. *N Engl J Med* 1996;**335**:1001.

CHAOS trial. Cambridge Heart Antioxidant Study. Randomised controlled trial of vitamin E in patients with coronary disease: Stephens NG, Parsons A, Schofield PM, Kelly F, Cheesman K, Mitchinson MI, Brown M. Reduction in non-fatal MI (but not cardiovascular death) in patients receiving vitamin E. *Lancet* 1996;**347**:781.

FATS study. Familial atherosclerosis treatment study: Brown GB, Albers JJ, Fisher LB *et al.* Regression of coronary artery disease as a result of intensive lipid lowering therapy in men with high levels of apolipoprotein B. *N Engl J Med* 1990;**323**:1289.

HPS. Heart protection study collaborative group. Collins R, Peto R, Armitage J; The MRC/BHF Heart Protection Study: preliminary results. *Int J Clin Pract* 2002;**56**:53. Nissen SE, Tsunoda T, Tuzcu EM, *et al;* The MRC/BHF Heart Protection Study of cholesterol lowering with simvastatin in 20,536 high-risk individuals: a randomised placebo-controlled trial: Reduction of major vascular events by one third after 5 years treatment with simvastatin 40 mg. *Lancet* 2002;**360**:7. Effect of recombinant Apo-A1 Milano on coronary atherosclerosis in patients with acute coronary syndromes: a randomised controlled trial. *JAMA* 2003;**290**:2292.

ILLUSTRATE trial: Nissen SE, Tardif JC, Nicholls SJ *et al.* Effect of torcetrapib on the progression of coronary atherosclerosis. *N Engl J Med* 2007;**356**:1304.

INTERHEART study: Yusuf S, Hawken S, Ounpuu S *et al.* Effect of potentially modifiable risk factors associated with myocardial infarction in 52 countries (the INTERHEART study): case–control study. *Lancet* 2004;**364**:912.

Swanton's Cardiology, sixth edition. By R. H. Swanton and S. Banerjee. Published 2008 Blackwell Publishing. ISBN 978-1-4051-7819-8.

POSCH study. Program on the surgical control of the hyperlipidaemias: Buchwald H, Varco RL, Matts PJ et al. Effect of partial ileal by-pass surgery on the mortality and morbidity from coronary heart disease in patients with hypercholesterolaemia. Report of the program on the surgical control of hyperlipidaemias. *N Engl J Med* 1990;**323**:946.

VA-HIT. Rubins HB, Robins SJ, Collins D et al; Veterans Affairs high-density lipoprotein-cholesterol intervention trial study group: Gemfibrozil therapy over 5 years significantly reduced coronary death and non-fatal myocardial infarction. *N Engl J Med* 1999;**341**:410.

WOSCOPS study. Prevention of coronary heart disease with pravastatin in men with hyper-cholesterolaemia: Shepherd J, Cobbe SM, Ford I et al. West of Scotland primary prevention trial in men followed for 4.9 years treated with pravastatin. *N Engl J Med* 1995;**333**:1301.

Catheter Ablation

Gallagher JJ, Svenson RH, Kasell JH et al. Catheter technique for closed-chest ablation of the atrio-ventricular conduction system. *N Engl J Med* 1982;**306**:194.

Jackman WM, Wang X, Friday K et al. Catheter ablation of accessory atrio-ventricular pathways (Wolff–Parkinson–White syndrome) by radiofrequency current. *N Engl J Med* 1991;**324**:1605.

Li-Fern Hsu, Jais P, Sanders P et al. Catheter ablation for atrial fibrillation in congestive cardiac failure. *N Engl J Med* **351** 2373. (2004)

Arrhythmias

ALIVE trial. Dorian P, Cass D, Schwartz B, et al; Amiodarone compared with lidocaine for shock-resistant ventricular fibrillation: In out of hospital arrests amiodarone improved survival to hospital compared to lidocaine (22.8% vs 12.0%). *N Engl J Med* 2002;**346**:884.

AVID trial. Causes of death in the Antiarrhythmic Versus Implantable Defibrillators (AVID) trial: ICDs significantly better at reducing arrhythmic deaths in patients who had survived VF or sustained VT. *J Am Coll Cardiol* 1999;**34**:1552.

CAMIAT trial. Randomised trial of outcome after myocardial infarction in patients with frequent or repetitive ventricular premature depolarisations: The Canadian amiodarone myocardial infarction arrhythmia trial investigators. Amiodarone reduced arrhythmic death. *Lancet* 1997;**349**:675.

CASH trial: Cardiac Arrest Study Hamburg: Kuck KH, Cappato R, Siebels J, et al. A non significant reduction in mortality in survivors of a cardiac arrest treated with an ICD compared to amiodarone. *Circulation* 2000;**102**:748.

CAST study: Echt DS, Liebson PR, Mitchell B et al. The cardiac arrhythmia suppression trial: Mortality and morbidity in patients receiving encainide, flecainide or placebo. *N Engl J Med* 1991;**324**:781.

CIDS trial: Canadian Implantable Defibrillator Study: Connolly SJ, Gent M, Roberts RS, et al; A non significant reduction in all cause mortality in patients resuscitated from ventricular arrhythmia treated with an ICD compared to amiodarone. *Circulation* 2000;**101**:1297.

COMPANION trial. Comparison of Medical therapy, Pacing, and Defibrillation in Heart failure trial: Bristow MR, Saxon LA, Boehmer J, et al; Cardiac resynchronisation therapy with or without an implantable defibrillator in advanced chronic heart failure. *N Engl J Med* 2004;**350**:2140.

DEFINITE TRIAL: Kadish A, Dyer A, Daubert JP, et al; Defibrillators in Non-Ischemic Cardiomyopathy Treatment Evaluation (DEFINITE) Investigators. Prophylactic defibrillator implantation in patients with nonischemic dilated cardiomyopathy. *N Engl J Med* 2004;**350**:2151.

EMIAT trial. Randomised trial of effect of amiodarone on mortality in patients with left ventricular dysfunction after recent myocardial infarction: Julian DG *et al*. for the European myocardial infarct amiodarone trial investigators. Amiodarone reduced arrhythmic deaths but not overall mortality. *Lancet* 1997;**349**:667.

ESVEM trial. Electrophysiologic study versus electrocardiographic monitoring: Mason JM for the ESVEM investigators. A comparison of electrophysiologic testing with Holter monitoring to predict anti-arrhythmic drug efficacy for ventricular tachyarrhythmias. *N Engl J Med* 1993;**329**:445.

MADIT trial. Moss AJ, Hall WJ, Cannom DS *et al*. Improved survival with an implanted defilbrillator in patients with coronary disease at high risk for ventricular tachycardia: The ICD reduced mortality over a 5-year period, but drug therapy did not influence mortality. *N Engl J Med* 1996;**335**:1933.

MADIT II trial: Moss AJ, Zareba W, Hall WJ *et al*. Multicenter Automatic Defibrillator Implantation trial II. Prophylactic implantation of a defibrillator in patients with myocardial infarction and reduced ejection fraction. Reduction in sudden death in asymptomatic patients not documented to have ventricular arrhythmias. *N Engl J Med* 2002;**346**:877.

MUSTT trial. Multicenter Unsustained Tachycardia Trial. A randomised study of the prevention of sudden death in patients with coronary artery disease: Buxton AE, Lee KL, Fisher JD *et al*. Reduction of sudden cardiac death in patients with ischaemic LV dysfunction using electrophysiologically guided ICD therapy. *N Engl J Med* 1999;**341**:1882

OPTIC trial: Optimal pharmacology therapy in cardioverter defibrillator patients. Connolly SJ, Dorian P, Roberts RS *et al*; Comparison of beta-blockers, amiodarone plus beta-blockers, or sotalol for prevention of shocks from implantable cardioverter defibrillators. Amiodarone plus beta-blocker reduced shocks by 73% in a group of secondary prevention patients. *JAMA* 2006;**295**:165.

PROMISE trial. Prospective randomised milrinone survival evaluation: Packer M, Carver JR, Rodeheffer RJ *et al*. Effect of oral milrinone on mortality in severe chronic heart failure. *N Engl J Med* 1991;**325**:1468.

Coronary Angioplasty and Unstable Angina

ACME study. Angioplasty compared to medicine: Parisi AF, Folland ED, Hartigan P *et al*. A comparison of angioplasty with medical therapy in the treatment of single vessel coronary disease. *N Engl J Med* 1992;**326**:10.

ADMIRAL study. Abciximab before direct angioplasty and stenting in myocardial infarction: Montalescot G, Barragon P, Wittenberg O *et al*. Platelet glycoprotein IIb/IIIa inhibition with coronary stenting for acute myocardial infarction. Abciximab lowered the 30 day composite endpoint in patients being stented for acute MI. *N Engl J Med* 2001;**344**:1895.

ARTS trial. Arterial Revascularisation Therapies Study Group: Serruys PW, Unger F, Sousa JE *et al*. Comparison of coronary artery by-pass surgery and stenting for the treatment of multivessel disease. *N Engl J Med* 2001;**344**:1117.

Bavry AA *et al*. Benefit of early invasive therapy in acute coronary syndromes: A meta-analysis of contemporary randomized clinical trials. *J Am Coll Cardiol* 2006;**48**:1319.

BENESTENT study. A comparison of balloon expandable stent implantation with balloon angioplasty in patients with coronary artery disease: Serruys PW, de Jaegere P, Kiemeneij F *et al*. Stent implantation compared with balloon dilatation alone reduced restenosis rate in arteries of 3.0 mm or more from 32% to 20% at 7 months. *N Engl J Med* 1994;**331**:489.

CAVEAT study. Coronary angioplasty versus excisional atherectomy: Topol EJ, Leya F, Pinkerton CA *et al.* A comparison of directional atherectomy with coronary angioplasty in patients with coronary artery disease. *N Engl J Med* 1993;**329**:221.

CCAT study. Canadian coronary atherectomy trial: Adelman AG, Cohen EA, Kimball BP *et al.* A comparison of directional atherectomy with balloon angioplasty for lesions of the left anterior descending coronary artery. *N Engl J Med* 1993;329:**228**.

COURAGE trial: Boden WE, O'Rourke RA, Teo KT *et al.* Optimal medical therapy with or without PCI for stable coronary disease. *N Engl J Med* 2007;**356**:1503.

CURE trial. Clopidogrel in Unstable angina to prevent Recurrent Events: Effects of clopidogrel in addition to aspirin in patients with acute coronary syndromes without ST-segment elevation. The CURE investigators. *N Engl J Med* 2001;**345**:494.

EPIC trial. Randomised trial of coronary intervention with antibody against platelet IIb/IIIa intergrin for reduction of clinical restenosis: result at 6 months: Topol EJ, Califf RM, Weisman HF *et al.* Evaluation of c7E3 for the prevention of ischaemic complications. c7E3 reduced acute events following PCI and also the need for revascularization at 6 months. *Lancet* 1994;**343**:881.

EPISTENT trial. Evaluation of platelet IIb/IIIa inhibitor for stenting: Randomised placebo controlled and balloon angioplasty controlled trial to assess safety of coronary stenting with use of glycoprotein IIb/IIIa blockade. *Lancet* 1998;**352**:87.

FRISC II trial. Fragmin and fast revascularization during instability in coronary artery disease: Invasive compared with non-invasive treatment in unstable coronary artery disease: FRISC II prospective randomised multicentre study. *Lancet* 1999;**354**:708. Lindahl B, Toss H, Siegbahn *et al.* for the FRISC study group. Markers of myocardial damage and inflammation in relation to long term mortality in unstable coronary artery disease. *N Engl J Med* 2000;**343**:1139.

Furberg CD, Psaty BM, Meyer JV Nifedipine. Dose related increase in mortality in patients with coronary heart disease. *Circulation* 1995;**92:**1326.

ISAR-REACT 2 trial: Abciximab in patients with acute coronary syndromes undergoing percutaneous coronary intervention after clopidogrel treatment. *JAMA* 2006;**295**:13.

Keeley EC, Boura JA, Grines CL. Primary angioplasty versus intravenous thrombolytic therapy for acute myocardial infarction: a quantitative review of 23 randomised trials. *Lancet* 2003;**361**:13–20.

OAT investigators. Occluded Artery Trial: Hochman JS, Lamas GA, Buller CE *et al.* Coronary intervention for persistent occlusion after myocardial infarction. There was no benefit in late PCI (3–28 days after an MI) over a 4 year period. *N Engl J Med* 2006;**355**:2395.

OPTICUS trial: Mudra H, diMario C, de Jaegere P *et al.* Optimisation with intracoronary ultrasound to reduce stent restenosis. IVUS guided stent deployment did not reduce the need for repeat PCI. *Circulation* 2001;**104**:1343.

PRAIS-UK trial. Prospective Registry of Acute Ischaemic syndromes in the UK: Collinson J, Flather MD, Fox KAA *et al.* Clinical outcomes, risk stratification and practice patterns of unstable angina and myocardial infarction without ST elevation. *Eur Heart J* 2000;**21**:1450.

PRAMI trial. Primary angioplasty in myocardial infarction study group: Grines CL, Browne KF, Marco J *et al.* A comparison of immediate angioplasty with thrombolytic therapy for acute myocardial infarction. *N Engl J Med* 1993;**328**:673.

RITA trial. Randomised intervention treatment of angina: RITA trial participants. Coronary angioplasty versus coronary artery by-pass surgery. *Lancet* 1993;**341**:573.

SHOCK trial. Should we urgently revascularize occluded coronaries for cardiogenic shock?: Early revascularisation in acute MI complicated by cardiogenic shock. Hochman JS, Sleeper LA, Webb JG *et al. N Engl J Med* 1999;**341**:625.

Sigwart U., Puel J., Mirkovitch V *et al.* Intravascular stents to prevent occlusion and restenosis after transluminal angioplasty. *New Eng J Med* 1987;**316**:701.

STENT-PAMI trial: Grines C, Cox DA, Stone GW *et al.* Coronary angioplasty with or without stent implantation for acute myocardial infarction. Stents superior to balloons alone at reducing 6 month target vessel revascularisation and major adverse cardiac events. *N Engl J Med* 1999;**341**:1949.

STRESS trial. Stent restenosis study: Fischman DL, Leon MB, Baim DS *et al.* A randomised comparison of coronary stent placement and balloon angioplasty in the treatment of coronary artery disease. *N Engl J Med* 1994;**331**:496.

TACTICS-TIMI 18 trial: Cannon CP, Weintraub WS, Demopoulos LA, *et al.* Comparison of early invasive and conservative strategies in patients with unstable coronary syndromes treated with the glycoprotein IIb/IIIa inhibitor tirofiban. *N Engl J Med* 2001;**344**:1879.

TARGET trial: Comparison of two glycoprotein IIb/IIIa inhibitors, tirofiban and abciximab, for the prevention of ischaemic events with percutaneous coronary revascularization. Topol EJ, Moliterno DJ, Herrmann HC *et al. N Engl J Med* 2001;**344**:1888.

TYPHOON trial: Spaulding C, Henry P, Teiger E *et al.* Sirolimus eluting stents in acute myocardial infarction reduced the rate of target vessel revascularisation at 1 year compared with bare metal stents. *N Engl J Med* 2006;**355**:1093.

VANQWISH trial. Veteran Affairs non-Q wave Infarction Strategies in Hospital: Outcomes in patients with acute non-Q wave MI randomly assigned to an invasive as compared with a conservative strategy. Boden WE, O'Rourke RA, Crawford MH *et al. N Engl J Med* 1998;**338**:1785.

Myocardial Infarction and Thrombolysis

AIMS trial. APSAC intervention mortality study: Long-term effects of intravenous anistreplase in acute myocardial infarction: final report of the AIMS study. *Lancet* 1990;**335**:427.

ASSET study. Anglo-Scandinavian study of early thrombolysis: Wilcox RG, von der Lippe G, Olsson CG *et al.* Trial of tissue plasminogen activator for mortality reduction in acute myocardial infarction. *Lancet* 1988;**ii**:525.

DAVITT II trial. Danish study group on verapamil in myocardial infarction: Effect of verapamil on mortality and major events after an acute myocardial infarction. *Am J Cardiol* 1990;**66**:779.

GISSI 1 trial. Gruppo Italiano per to studio delta streptochinasi nell'infarto miocardico: Effectiveness of intravenous thrombolytic treatment in acute myocardial infarction. *Lancet* 1986;**i**;397.

GISSI 2 trial: A factorial randomised trial of alteplase versus streptokinase and heparin versus no heparin among 12,490 patients with acute myocardial infarction. *Lancet*, 1990;**336**:65.

GUSTO trial. Global utilisation of streptokinase and tissue plasminogen activator for occluded coronary arteries: An international randomised trial comparing four thrombolytic strategies far acute myocardial infarction. The GUSTO Investigators. *N Engl J Med* 1993;**329**:673.

GUSTO V trial: Reperfusion therapy for acute myocardial infarction with fibrinolytic therapy or combination reduced fibrinolytic therapy and platelet glycoprotein IIb/IIIa inhibition. Topol EJ. *Lancet* 2001;**357**:1905.

ISIS 2 trial. Second international study of infarct survival: Collaborative group. Randomised trial of intravenous streptokinase, oral aspirin, both or neither among 17 187 cases of suspected acute myocardial infarction. *Lancet* 1988;**ii**:349.

ISIS 3. Third international study of infarct survival: A randomised comparison of streptokinase vs. tissue plasminogen activator vs. anistreplase and of aspirin plus heparin vs. aspirin alone among 41,299 cases of suspected acute myocardial infarction. *Lancet* 1992;**339**;753.

LIMIT 2 trial. Leicester intravenous magnesium intervention: Intravenous magnesium sulphate in suspected acute myocardial infarction: results of the second Leicester intravenous magnesium intervention LIMIT 2 trial. Woods KL, Fletcher S, Roffe C *et al. Lancet* 1992;**339**:1553.

REACT trial: Gershlick A *et al.* Rescue angioplasty versus conservative treatment or repeat thrombolysis. *N Engl J Med* 2005;**353**:2758.

SWIFT trial. Should we intervene following thrombolysis?: SWIFT trial of delayed elective intervention vs. conservative treatment after thrombolysis with anistreplase in acute myocardial infarction. *BMJ* 1991;**302**:555.

TIMI II. Thrombolysis in myocardial infarction. Phase II trial: Comparison of invasive and conservative strategies after treatment with intravenous tissue plasminogen activator in acute myocardial infarction. *N Engl J Med* 1989;**320**:618.

TIMI IIIB. Thrombolysis in myocardial infarction. Effects of tissue plasminogen activator and a comparison of early invasive and conservative strategies in unstable angina and non-Q-wave MI. *Circulation* 1994;**89**:1545.

Heart Failure

A-HeFT trial. African–American Heart Failure trial: A combination of isosorbide dinitrate and hydralazine reduced all cause mortality in black patients with grade III or IV heart failure by 43% when compared to standard therapy over a 10 month mean follow up. *N Engl J Med* 2004;**351**:2049.

CAPRICORN trial. Carvedilol Post-Infarct Survival Control in LV dysfunction: Effect of carvedilol on outcome after myocardial infarction in patients with left ventricular dysfunction. The CAPRICORN randomised controlled trial. *Lancet* 2001;**357**:1385.

CIBIS II trial. The cardiac insufficiency Bisoprolol Study II: A randomised trial. *Lancet* 1999;**353**:9.

CONSENSUS I. The cooperative North Scandinavian enalapril survival study: The CONSENSUS trial study group. Effects of enalapril on mortality in severe congestive heart failure: results of the North Scandinavian enalapril survival study. *N Engl J Med* 1987;**316**:1429.

CONSENSUS II. The cooperative new Scandinavian enalapril survival study: Swedberg K, Held P, Kjekshus J *et al.* Effects of the early administration of enalapril on mortality in patients with acute myocardial infarction. *N Engl J Med* 1992;**327**:678.

COPERNICUS trial. Carvedilol Prospective/Randomised Cumulative Survival Study: Packer M, Coats A, Fowler M *et al.* Effect of carvedilol on survival in severe heart failure. *N Engl J Med* 2001;**344**:1651.

DIG trial. The effect of digoxin on mortality and morbidity in patients with heart failure: The Digitalis Investigation Group. Digoxin did not reduce mortality in chronic CCF but did reduce hospital admissions for heart failure. *N Engl J Med* 1997;**336**:525.

ELITE trial. Randomised trial of losartan versus captopril in patients over 65 with heart failure. (Evaluation of losartan in the elderly study, ELITE): Pitt B, Segal R, Martinez FA *et al.* Lower mortality in patients treated with losartan compared to captopril. *Lancet* 1997;**349**:747.

ELITE II trial. Losartan Heart failure survival study: Effect of losartan compared with captopril on mortality in patients with symptomatic heart failure. *Lancet* 2000;**355**: 1582.

EPHESUS trial: Pitt B, Remme W, Zannad F *et al.* Eplerenone, a selective aldosterone blocker, in patients with left ventricular dysfunction after myocardial infarction. *N Engl J Med* 2003;**348**:1309.

HOPE trial. Heart Outcomes Prevention Evaluation study: Yusuf S, Sleight P *et al.* Effects of an angiotensin-converting-enzyme-inhibitor, ramipril, on cardiovascular events in high risk patients. *N Engl J Med* 2000;**342**:145.

LIDO trial. Levosimendan infusion vs Dobutamine study: Follath F, Cleland JGF, Just H *et al.* Efficacy and safety of intravenous levosimendan compared with dobutamine in severe low output heart failure. A randomised double blind trial. *Lancet* 2002;**360**:196.

MERIT HF trial. Effect of metoprolol CR/XL in chronic heart failure: Metoprolol CR/XL randomised intervention trial in congestive cardiac failure: Beneficial effects of metoprolol in CCF. *Lancet* 1999;**353**:2001.

MUSTIC trial. Multisite Stimulation in Cardiomyopathies: Cazeau S, Petrie MC *et al.* Effects of multisite biventricular pacing in patients with heart failure and intraventricular conduction delay. *N Engl J Med* 2001;**344**:215.

OVERTURE trial: Packer M, Califf RM, Konstam MA *et al.* Comparison of omapatrilat and enalapril in patients with chronic heart failure: the Omaptrilat Versus Enalapril Randomised Trial of Utility in Reducing Events (OVERTURE). *Circulation* 2002;**106**:920.

PRAISE trial. The effect of amlodipine on morbidity and mortality in severe chronic heart failure: Packer M, O'Connor C.M, Ghali JK *et al.* Amlodipine did not increase mortality in severe chronic CCF and possibly reduced it in dilated cardiomyopathy. *N Engl J Med* 1996;**335**:1107.

RADIANCE trial. Randomised Assessment of effect of Digoxin on Inhibitors of ACE study: Packer M, Gheorghiade M, Young JB *et al*; Withdrawal of digoxin from patients with chronic heart failure treated with ACE inhibitor. *N Engl J Med* 1993;**329**:1.

RALES study group. Randomised aldactone evaluation study: Effectiveness of spironolactone added to an angiotensin-converting enzyme inhibitor and a loop diuretic for severe chronic congestive cardiac failure. *Am J Cardiol* 1996;**78**:902.

SAVE trial: Pfeffer M, Braunwald E, Moye L *et al.* Survival and ventricular enlargement trial Effect of captopril on mortality and morbidity in patients with left ventricular dysfunction after myocardial infarction. *N Engl J Med* 1992;**327**:669.

SCD-HeFT trial. Sudden Cardiac Death in Heart Failure Trial: Bardy GH, Lee KL, Mark DB *et al*; Amiodarone or an Implantable Cardioverter-Defibrillator for congestive cardiac failure. *N Engl J Med* 2005;**352**;225.

SOLVD study: The SOLVD investigators. Studies of left ventricular dysfunction: Effects of enalapril on mortality and the development of heart failure in asymptomatic patients with reduced left ventricular ejection fractions. *N Engl J Med* 1992;**327**:685.

Low-molecular-weight Heparins

ESSENCE trial: ESSENCE study group. A comparison of low-molecular-weight heparin with unfractionated heparin for unstable coronary artery disease: Enoxaparin was more effective than unfractionated heparin (both with aspirin) at reducing ischaemic events in unstable angina. *N Engl J Med* 1997;**337**:447.

FRISC trial: Fragmin during instability in coronary artery disease (FRISC) study group. Low molecular weight heparin during instability in coronary artery disease: Fragmin reduced myocardial infarcts and deaths in patients on aspirin in unstable angina. *Lancet* 1996;**347**:561.

Hypertension

ASCOT-BPLA. Anglo-Scandinavian Cardiac Outcomes Trial. Poulter NR, Wedel H, Dahlöf B *et al*; Blood pressure lowering arm: An amlodipine based regimen (with additional perindopril if necessary) was better at preventing cardiovascular events than an atenolol based regime (with additional thiazide). *Lancet* 2005;**366**:907.
LIFE. Losartan Intervention For Endpoint reduction in hypertension study: Dahlof B, Devereux RB, Kjeldsen SE *et al*. Losartan was superior to atenolol at stroke prevention in spite of similar blood pressure reduction. *Lancet* 2002;**359**:995.

Pregnancy

Brach Prever S, Sheppard MN, Somerville J. Fatal outcomes in pregnancy in Eisenmenger's syndrome. *Cardiol Young* 1997;**7**:238.
Chan WS, Anand S, Ginsberg JS. Anticogulation of pregnant women with mechanical heart valves: a systematic review of the literature. *Arch Intern Med* 2000;**160**(2):191–6.
Elkayam U, Tummala PP, Rao K *et al*. Maternal and fetal outcomes of subsequent pregnancies in women with peripartum cardiomyopathy. *N Engl J Med* 2001;**344**:1567.
Fett JD, Christie LG, Carraway RD, Murphy JG. Five-year prospective study of the incidence and prognosis of peripartum cardiomyopathy at a single institution. *Mayo Clin Proc* 2005;**80**(12):1602-1606.
Gleicher N, Midwall J, Hochberger D, Jqffin H. Eisenmenger's syndrome and pregnancy. *Obstet Gynecol Surv* 1979;**34**:721.
Head CEG, Thorne SA. Congenital heart disease in pregnancy. *Postgrad Med J* 2005;**81**: 292.
James AH, Biswas MS, Swamy GK. Acute myocardial infarction in pregnancy. A United States Population-Based Study. *Circulation* 2006;**113**:1564.
Khairy P, Ouyang DW, Fernandes SM, Lee-Parritz A, Economy KE, Landzberg MJ. Pregnancy outcomes in women with congenital heart disease. *Circulation* 2006;**113**:517.
Magee LA, Ornstein MP, von Dadelzen P. Management of hypertension in pregnancy. *BMJ* 1999;**318**:1332.
Nakagawa M, Katou S, Ichinose M *et al*. Characteristics of new-onset ventricular arrhythmias in pregnancy. *J Electrocard* 2004;**37**:47–53.
Natale A, Davidson T, Geiger MJ, Newley K. Implantable cardioverter-defibrillators and pregnancy: A safe combination? *Circulation* 1997;**96**;808.
Nelson-Piercy C. *Handbook of Obstetric Medicine*. Informa, 2006.
Ostrezega E, Mehra A, Widerhorn J. Evidence for increased incidence of arrhythmias during pregnancy: a study of 104 pregnant women with symptoms of palpitations, dizziness or syncope. *J Am Coll Cardiol* 1992;**19**:125.
Pearson GD, Veille JC, Rahimtoola S *et al*. Peripartum cardiomyopathy: National Heart Lung and Blood Institute and Office of Rare Diseases (National Institutes of Health) workshop recommendations and review. *JAMA* 2000;**283**(9):1183-1188.
Prasad AK, Ventura HO. Valvular heart disease and pregnancy. *Postgrad Med* 2001;**110**: | 69.

Rashba EJ, Zareba W, Moss AJ *et al.* Influence of pregnancy on the risk of cardiac events in patients with hereditary long QT syndrome. *Circulation* 1998;**97**:451.

Reinold SC, Rutherford JD. Valvular heart disease in pregnancy. *N Engl J Med* 2003;**349**:52.

Royal College of Obstetricians and Gynaecologists: *Confidential Enquiry into Maternal Death 2000–2002.*

Sliwa K, Fett J, Elkayam U. Peripartum cardiomyopathy. *Lancet* 2006;**368**:687.

Stout K. Pregnancy in women with congenital heart disease: the importance of evaluation and counselling. *Heart* 2005;**91**:713.

Tawan M, Levine J, Mendelson M *et al.* Effect of pregnancy on paroxysmal supraventricular tachycardia. *Am J Cardiol* 1993;**72**:838.

Thaman R, Varnava A, Hamid MS *et al.* Pregnancy related complications in women with hypertrophic cardiomyopathy. *Heart* 2003;**89**:752.

Thorne SA. Pregnancy in heart disease. *Heart* 2004;**90**:450.

Uebing A, Steer PJ, Yentis SM, Gatzoulis MA. Pregnancy and congenital heart disease. *BMJ* 2006;**332**:401.

Webber MD, Halligan RE, Schumacher JA. Acute infarction, intracoronary thrombolysis and primary PCI in pregnancy. *Catheter Cardiovascular Diagnosis* 1997;**42**:28–43.

Echocardiography

Binder TM, Rosenhek R, Porenta G, Maurer G, Baumgartner H. Improved assessment of mitral valve stenosis by volumetric real-time three-dimensional echocardiography. *J Am Coll Cardiol* 2000;**36**:1355–1361.

Edler I, Hertz CH. The early work of ultrasound in medicine at the University of Lund. *J Clin Ultrasound* 1977;**5**:352–6.

Maron BJ, Pelliccia A, Spirito P. Cardiac disease in young trained athletes: Insights into methods for distinguishing athlete's heart from structural heart disease with particular emphasis on hypertrophic cardiomyopathy. *Circulation* 1995;**91**:1596–1601.

Senior R, Chambers JB. Stress echocardiography – current status. *Br J Cardiol* 2007;**14**:90–97.

Siu SC, Levine RA, Rivera JM *et al.* Three-dimensional echocardiography improves non-invasive assessment of left ventricular volume and performance. *Am Heart J* 1995;**130**:812–822.

Miscellaneous

Durack DT, Lukes AS, Bright DK. New criteria for diagnosis of infective endocarditis: utilization of specific echocardiographic findings. Duke Endocarditis Service. *Am J Med* 1994;**96**:200–9.

Gorlin R, Gorlin SG. Hydraulic formula for calculation of the area of the stenotic mitral valve, other cardiac valves, and central circulatory shunts. *I Am Heart J* 1951 Jan;**41**:1–29.

Kennedy JW, Trenholme SE, Kasser IS. Left ventricular volume and mass from single-plane cineangiocardiogram. A comparison of anteroposterior and right anterior oblique methods. *Am Heart J* 1970;**80**:343.

Swanton RH, Brooksby IA, Davies MJ *et al.* Systolic and diastolic ventricular function in cardiac amyloidosis. Studies in six cases diagnosed with endomyocardial biopsy. *Am J Cardiol* 1977;**39**:658–64.

Wheat MW, Palmer RF, Bartley TD *et al.* Treatment of dissecting aneurysms of the aorta without surgery. *J Thorac Cardiovasc Surg.* 1965;**50**:364.

5   Useful Addresses and Hyperlinks

American College of Cardiology, Heart House, 9111 Old Georgetown Road, Bethesda, MD 20814, USA www.acc.org

American Heart Association or Circulation, 7320 Greenville Avenue, Dallas, TX 75231 www.amhrt.org

American Heart Journal, CV Mosby Co, 11830 Westline Industrial Drive, St Louis, MO 63141, USA

American Society of Echocardiography www.asecho.org

American Society of Hypertension www.ash-us.org

American Society of Nuclear Cardiology www.asnc.org

American Journal of Cardiology, 875 Third Avenue, New York, NY 10022, USA

British Cardiovascular Society, 9 Fitzroy Square, London W1P 5AH. Tel: 020 7383 3887 www.bcs.com

British Cardiovascular Intervention Society (BCIS) www.bcis.org.uk

Heart Rhythm UK (HRUK) www.bcs.com/affiliates/hruk.html

British Society of Echocardiography (BSE) www.bsecho.org

British Nuclear Cardiology Society (BNCS) www.bncs.org.uk

Society for Cardiological Science and Technology (SCST) www.bcs.com/affiliates/scst.html

British Congenital Cardiac Association (BCCA) www.bcs.com/affiliates/bcca.html

British Association for Cardiac Rehabilitation (BACR) www.bcs.com/affiliates/bacr.html

British Association for Cardiovascular Research (BSCR) www.bcs.com/affiliates/bscr.html

British Association for Nursing in Cardiac Care (BANCC) www.www.bcs.com/affiliates/bancc.html

British Medical Association, Tavistock Square, London WC1 www.bma.org.uk

} Addresses as for British Cardiovascular Society

Swanton's Cardiology, sixth edition. By R. H. Swanton and S. Banerjee. Published 2008 Blackwell Publishing. ISBN 978-1-4051-7819-8.

British Heart Foundation, 14 Fitzhardinge Street, London W1H
4DH. Tel: 020 7935 0185 www.bhf.org.uk

British Atherosclerosis Society (BAS) www.britathsoc.ac.uk

British Junior Cardiologists Association (BJCA) www.bcs.com/
affiliates/bjca.html

British Society for Heart Failure (BSH) www.bcs.com/affiliates/
bsh.html

Primary Care Cardiovascular Society (PCCS) www.pccs.org.uk

} Addresses as for British Cardiovascular Society

Canadian Cardiovascular Society www.ccs.ca

Cardiovascular Research, Elsevier Science, PO Box 211, 1000 AE Amsterdam, The
Netherlands www.elsevier.com/locate/cardiores

Central Cardiac Audit Database (CCAD) ccad3.biomed.gla.ac.uk/ccad

Driving and Vehicle Licensing Authority: DVLA www.dvla.gov.uk

European Heart Journal (Journal of the European Society of Cardiology), Oxford University
Press: Editorial Office: Gasthuisberg University Hospital, Department of Cardiology Her-
estraat 49, B-3000 Leuven, Belgium www.euroheartj.org

European Society of Cardiology: European Heart House, 2035 Route des Colles, Les Templi-
ers, BP 179, 06903 Sophia Antipolis Cedex, France www.escardio.org

General Medical Council www.gmc-uk.org

Heart (formerly British Heart Journal) www.heart.bmjjournals.com/ifora (for authors and
reviewers)

Heart Care Partnership UK (HCPUK) www.bcs.com

International Society and Federation of Cardiology www.isfc.org

Journal of the American College of Cardiology, Elsevier Science Publishing Co Inc, 52 Van-
derbilt Avenue, New York, NY 10017, USA

NASPE, North American Society of Pacing and Electrophysiology, 13 Eaton Court, Wellesley
Hills, MA 02181, USA. Tel: 00 1 617 237 1866

National Institute for Health and Clinical Excellence (NICE) www.nice.org.uk

Resuscitation Council UK www.nda.ox.ac.uk/rc-uk

Society of Cardiothoracic Surgeons of Great Britain and Ireland, c/o The Royal College of
Surgeons, 35/43 Lincoln's Inn Fields, London WC2A 3PN www.scts.org

Scottish Intercollegiate Guidelines Network (SIGN) www.show.scot.nhs.uk/sign/home.
html

6   Driving and Cardiovascular Disease in the UK

Introduction

Detailed guidance may be obtained from the publication *At a Glance Guide to the Current Medical Standards of Fitness to Drive* and the website www.dvla.gov. uk. This is updated twice a year and is available in pdf format for personal use. Hard copies can be obtained from: DVLA, Longview Road, Morriston, Swansea SA99 1TU (01792 7761337) at a cost of £4.50. The DVLA does not always require notification of a condition.

Temporary cessation of driving will be necessary for disabling events such as giddiness, syncope, paroxysmal dysrhythmia or systemic embolism until the cause has been established and successfully treated.

In the event of a debarring condition it is the doctor's responsibility to advise a patient that he or she should not drive, and then the patient's legal obligation to contact the DVLA. If a patient continues to drive in spite of this advice, the doctor is strongly advised to inform the DVLA of the situation following GMC guidelines, and to inform the patient of this. After discussion the DVLA may then contact the patient to open a medical enquiry or to revoke the licence. In general patients with cardiovascular disorders should see a cardiologist before (re-)licensing.

The medical standards refer to two groups of driving licence:

1 Group 1 licences: ordinary driving licences for motor cars and motor cycles. Licence valid age 17–70, then renewable every 3 years with a medical self-declaration form.

2 Group 2 licences: occupational driving licences (includes LGV/PCV licences). Large lorries and buses. A group 2 licence is now required for all drivers of lorries >3.5 metric tonnes, or passenger vehicles carrying more than eight passengers (excluding the driver). A group 2 licence is normally valid from age 21 to age 45, renewable every 5 years till age 65, and then annually.

Swanton's Cardiology, sixth edition. By R. H. Swanton and S. Banerjee. Published 2008 Blackwell Publishing. ISBN 978-1-4051-7819-8.

Medical restrictions are more stringent for group 2 drivers than for group 1 drivers. Those with known cardiovascular disease must have a regular medical review. Those with coronary artery disease will need an exercise test every 3 years.

Taxi licences: these are not regulated by the DVLA. Standards and medical requirements are determined by the Public Carriage Office in the London Metropolitan area, and the local authority in other areas.

DVLA Medical Advice

If a doctor has any doubts about a particular condition, DVLA medical advisers are available in office hours to discuss the problem:

England, Scotland and Wales
The Medical Adviser
Drivers Medical Group
DVLA
Longview Road
Morriston
Swansea
Tel: 01792 761119 (Medical practitioners
    only)

Northern Ireland
Driver and Vehicle Licensing
Northern Ireland
Castlerock Road
Coleraine
BT51 3TB

Tel: 028 70341369

Summary of Cardiovascular Disorders and Driving 1

Condition	Group 1 entitlement	Group 2 entitlement
1. Angina	Driving must cease if angina occurs at rest or at the wheel. Driving may restart once the angina is controlled. DVLA need not be notified	Disqualifies from driving for at least 6 weeks. Relicensing may be permitted after this time provided that the treadmill exercise test requirements can be met and there is no other disqualifying condition. See Appendix 6 for test details
2. Coronary/Angioplasty	No driving for 1 week. As above. Restart provided there is no other disqualifying condition. DVLA need not be notified	As above
3. Acute coronary syndromes including acute MI	No driving for at least 4 weeks. Driving may restart provided that there is no other disqualifying condition. DVLA need not be notified	As above
4. CABG, valve or any open heart surgery	As in (3) above	As above
5. New pacemaker implant or box change	No driving for 1 week	No driving for 6 weeks. May be relicensed subject to specialist evaluation
6. Successful catheter ablation	No driving for 1 week. DVLA need not be notified	Driving may be permitted if the arrhythmia has been controlled for 3 months, and the LVEF is >0.4, and there is no other disqualifying condition
7. Arrhythmia, e.g. sinoatrial disease, AF, atrial flutter second- and third-degree AV block, atrial or ventricular tachycardias	Driving must cease if the arrhythmia distracts the driver's attention or is likely to cause incapacity. Driving may be permitted if the cause has been identified and controlled for at least 4 weeks DVLA should be notified only if the symptoms are disabling	As above
8. Implantable cardioverter defibrillator (ICD)	Driving may restart if: the first device has been implanted for >6 months. There has been no shock therapy. There has been no antitachycardia pacing in the last 6 months. No syncope with previous therapy	Permanently disbarred

Summary of Cardiovascular Disorders and Driving 2

Condition	Group 1 entitlement	Group 2 entitlement
9. Hypertension	Driving may continue unless treatment causes unacceptable side effects. DVLA need not be notified	Disqualified if BP consistently >180/100. Relicensing may be permitted once BP is controlled and if therapy does not cause symptoms affecting driving capability
10. Heart failure, DCM, heart or heart–lung transplantation	Driving may continue provided that there are no symptoms that might distract the driver's attention. DVLA need not be notified	Disqualified if symptomatic. Relicensing may be considered provided that the exercise test requirements can be met (see above) and the LVEF is >0.4 and there is no other disqualifying condition
11. HCM	Driving may continue provided that there is no other disqualifying condition	Disqualified if symptomatic. Relicensing may be possible after specialist evaluation
12. Heart valve disease	Driving may continue provided that there is no other disqualifying condition	Disqualified if symptomatic, and for 1 year after cerebral embolism. Specialist evaluation required
13. Ascending, descending or abdominal aortic aneurysm	DVLA should be notified if the aneurysm reaches 6 cm in spite of treatment. Licensing will then be permitted subject to annual review. BP control or surgical repair must be satisfactory. An aneurysm ≥6.5 cm disqualifies from driving	Disqualified if the aortic diameter >5.5 cm. Relicensing may be possible after satisfactory medical or surgical treatment. For abdominal aortic aneurysm the exercise test requirement (see above) must be met
14. Chronic aortic dissection	Driving may continue after satisfactory BP control or surgery. DVLA need not be notified	Relicensing may be considered if: (1) BP is well controlled. (2) False lumen is completely thrombosed. (3) Maximum aortic diameter (including false lumen) is <5.5 cm
15. Marfan syndrome	DVLA need not be notified unless there is an aortic aneurysm	Relicensing permitted if: the requirements for aneurysm are met (see above). Satisfactory medical treatment. Annual review to include aortic root measurement. Aortic root replacement debars

Special Conditions Relating to Group 2 Licence Applicants

1 A LVEF < 0.4 is considered a bar to group 2 entitlement.

2 The treadmill exercise test is a requirement for group 2 drivers with several conditions including 1, 2, 3, 4, 10 and 11 above.

Drivers must be instructed to discontinue all antianginal medication 48 h before the exercise test. They may, however, continue taking antihypertensive medication where appropriate. ACE inhibitors are allowed. They must be able to complete three stages of the standard Bruce protocol (9-min exercise) with no abnormal ECG changes, i.e. usually >2 mm horizontal or downsloping ST-segment depression. There should be no symptoms to suggest cardiovascular dysfunction such as angina, syncope, VT or hypotension. Limitation as a result of peripheral vascular disease will usually require another functional procedure such as a stress myocardial perfusion scan or a stress echocardiogram. Patients with LBBB or RBBB who require a group 2 licence will require a functional test other than treadmill testing.

3 Coronary angiography is not usually required by the DVLA because it is not a functional test. If the exercise test is equivocal or uninterpretable (e.g. in the presence of LBBB), myocardial perfusion scanning or stress echocardiography may be requested. Antianginal medication should be discontinued as in (2) above before the test. With either of these tests there should be no more than 10% of the myocardium showing reversible ischaemia.

7 List of Abbreviations

ACE	angiotensin-converting enzyme
ACS	acute coronary syndrome
AF	atrial fibrillation
AML	anterior mural leaflet
ANF	antinuclear factor
AP	aortopulmonary
APD	action potential duration
APSAC	anisoylated plasminogen streptokinase activator complex
APTT	activated partial thromboplastin time
APVD	anomalous pulmonary venous drainage
AR	aortic regurgitation
AIIRA	angiotensin II receptor antagonist
ARB	angiotensin receptor blocker
AS	aortic stenosis
ASD	atrial septal defect
ASO	anti-streptolysin-O titre
AV	atrioventricular
AVID	aortic valve disease
AVR	aortic valve replacement
BCR	British corrected ratio
CABG	coronary artery bypass grafting
CAD	coronary artery disease
CCF	congestive cardiac failure
CFT	complement fixation test
CPB	cardiopulmonary bypass
CPK-MB	creative phosphokinase isoenzyme of cardiac muscle
CPR	cardiopulmonary resuscitation
CRP	C-reactive protein

Swanton's Cardiology, sixth edition. By R. H. Swanton and S. Banerjee. Published 2008 Blackwell Publishing. ISBN 978-1-4051-7819-8.

CVA	cerebrovascular accident
CVP	central venous pressure
CVS	cardiovascular system
CW	continuous wave
DC	direct current
DCM	dilated cardiomyopathy
Dd	diastolic dimension
DFP	diastolic filling period
DOLV	double-outlet left ventricle
DORV	double-outlet right ventricle
DPTI	diastolic pressure time index
DTPA	diethylenetriamine penta-acetic acid
DXT	deep X-ray therapy
EDM	early diastolic murmur
EFE	endocardial fibroelastosis
EP	electrophysiological
ERP	effective refractory period
ESR	erythrocyte sedimentation rate
FBC	full blood count
FDPs	fibrin degradation products
FEV,	forced expiratory volume in 1 second
FFA	free fatty acids
GTN	glyceryl trinitrate
GUCH	grown-up congenital heart disease
HBD	hydroxybutyrate dehydrogenase
HCM	hypertrophic cardiomyopathy
HFABP	heart fatty acid-binding protein
HMG	hydroxymethylglutaryl
HR	heart rate
HRAE	high right atrial electrogram
H-V	His-ventricular
IABP	intra-aortic balloon pumping
ICD	implantable cardioverter defibrillator
INR	international normalized ratio
ISA	intrinsic sympathomimetic activity
ITU	intensive therapy unit
IUGR	intrauterine growth retardation
IVC	inferior vena cava
IVS	interventricular septum
IVU	intravenous urogram
NIP	jugular venous pulse
LA	left atrium
LAD	left axis deviation; left anterior descending
LAHB	left anterior hemiblock
LAID	left atrial internal dimension

LAO	left anterior oblique
LAT	lateral
LBBB	left bundle-branch block
LDH	lactic dehydrogenase
LFT	liver function test
LIMA	left internal mammary artery
LPHB	left posterior hemiblock
LSE	left sternal edge
LV	left ventricular/left ventricle
LVEDP	left ventricular end-diastolic pressure
LVEDV	left ventricular end-diastolic volume
LVEF	left ventricular ejection fraction
LVESV	left ventricular end-systolic volume
LVET	left ventricular ejection time
LVF	left ventricular failure
LVFP	left ventricular filling pressure
LVIDd	left ventricular internal dimension at end-diastole
LVIDs	left ventricular internal dimension at end-systole
LVMWI	left ventricular minute work index
LVOTO	left ventricular outflow tract obstruction
LVSWI	left ventricular stroke work index
MAOIs	monoamine oxidase inhibitors
METS	metabolic equivalents
MIC	minimum inhibitory concentration
MR	mitral regurgitation
MS	mitral stenosis
MUGA	multiple gated acquisition
MV	mitral valve
MVR	mitral valve replacement
NICE	National Institute for Health and Clinical Excellence
NSTEMI	Non ST elevation myocardial infarction
NYHA	New York Heart Association
PA	pulmonary artery
PAEDP	pulmonary artery end-diastolic pressure
PATB	paroxysmal atrial tachycardia with varying block
PAW	pulmonary artery wedge
PDA	patent ductus arteriosus
PDE	phosphodiesterase
PE	pulmonary embolism
PEA	pulseless electrical activity
PEEP	positive end-expiratory pressure
PEP	pre-ejection period
PFO	patent foramen ovate
PGE_2	prostaglandin E_2
PGI_2	prostaglandin I_2 (prostacyclin)

PHT	pulmonary hypertension
PLVW	posterior left ventricular wall
PND	paroxysmal nocturnal dyspnoea
PR	pulmonary regurgitation
PS	pulmonary stenosis
PCI	percutaneous transluminal coronary angioplasty
PV	pulmonary vein
PVC	premature ventricular contraction
PVR	pulmonary vascular resistance
PW	pulsed wave
PXE	pseudoxanthoma elasticum
RA	right atrial/right atrium
RAID	right axis deviation
RAO	right anterior oblique
RBBB	right bundle-branch block
REM	rapid eye movement
RF	radiofrequency
rtPA	recombinant tissue plasminogen activator
RV	right ventricle
RVEDP	right ventricular end-diastolic pressure
RVF	right ventricular failure
RVID	right ventricular internal dimension
RVOT	right ventricular outflow tract
SACT	sinoatrial conduction time
SAM	systolic anterior movement of the mitral valve
SBE	subacute bacterial endocarditis
SEjP	systolic ejection period
SLE	systemic lupus erythematosus
SNRT	sinus node recovery time
SR	sinus rhythm
SSS	sick sinus syndrome
STEMI	ST elevation myocardial infarction
SV	stroke volume
SVC	superior vena cava
$S\bar{v}o_2$	mixed venous oxygen saturation
SVR	systemic vascular resistance
SVT	supraventricular tachycardia
TAPVD	total anomalous pulmonary venous drainage
TGA	transposition of the great arteries
TGF	transforming growth factor
TNF	tumour necrosis factor
TOE	transoesophageal echocardiography
tPA	tissue plasminogen activator
TPHA	*Treponema pallidum* haemagglutination
TR	tricuspid regurgitation

TS	tricuspid stenosis
TSH	thyroid stimulating hormone
TTE	transthoracic echocardiography
TTI	tension time index
TV	tricuspid valve
TxA_2	thromboxane A_2
U&Es	urea and electrolytes
VCE	velocity of contractile element shortening
VCF	velocity of circumferential fibre shortening
VDRL	Venereal Disease Reference Laboratory
VF	ventricular fibrillation
VPB	ventricular premature beats
VSD	ventricular septal defect
VT	ventricular tachycardia
WPW	Wolff–Parkinson–White
WT	wall thickness

Index

Page numbers in *italics* refer to figures, those in **bold** refer to tables.